Current Research in Adrenal Cortex Disorders

Current Research in Adrenal Cortex Disorders

Editor: Leroy Finch

AMERICAN
MEDICAL PUBLISHERS
www.americanmedicalpublishers.com

AMERICAN
MEDICAL PUBLISHERS
www.americanmedicalpublishers.com

Cataloging-in-Publication Data

Current research in adrenal cortex disorders / edited by Leroy Finch.
p. cm.
Includes bibliographical references and index.
ISBN 979-8-88740-038-9
1. Adrenal cortex--Diseases. 2. Adrenal glands--Diseases. 3. Adrenal cortex--Diseases--Research.
4. Adrenal glands--Diseases--Research. 5. Adrenal cortex--Diseases--Diagnosis.
6. Adrenal cortex--Diseases--Treatment. I. Finch, Leroy.
RC659 .C87 2023
61645--dc23

American Medical Publishers,
41 Flatbush Avenue,
1st Floor, New York,
NY 11217, USA

ISBN 979-8-88740-038-9 (Hardback)

Contents

Preface

The adrenal cortex is the outer region of the adrenal gland. It is also the largest part of an adrenal gland. The specific zones of adrenal cortex synthesize different hormones that control sex (androgens, estrogens), salt balance in the blood (aldosterone) and sugar balance (cortisol). The excess or deficient secretion of each type of adrenal hormone causes severe disorders that include hypercortisolism, adrenal insufficiency, hyperaldosteronism, hypoaldosteronism, and androgen excess. Hypocortisolism, also known as Addison's disease, is a disorder marked by inadequate production of the steroid hormones cortisol and aldosterone that causes adrenal inefficiency. The signs and symptoms of this disease are abdominal pain and gastrointestinal abnormalities, weakness, weight loss, and darkening of skin in certain areas. Cushing syndrome is caused due to excessive release of cortisol hormone in the body. This syndrome leads to weight gain and fatty tissue deposits, slow healing of cuts, insect bites and infections, acne, etc. This book explores all the important aspects of adrenal cortex disorders in the present day scenario. The readers would gain knowledge that would broaden their perspective about these disorders.

This book has been the outcome of endless efforts put in by authors and researchers on various issues and topics within the field. The book is a comprehensive collection of significant researches that are addressed in a variety of chapters. It will surely enhance the knowledge of the field among readers across the globe.

It gives us an immense pleasure to thank our researchers and authors for their efforts to submit their piece of writing before the deadlines. Finally in the end, I would like to thank my family and colleagues who have been a great source of inspiration and support.

Editor

1

Circadian Clocks, Stress, and Immunity

Rebecca Dumbell*[†]*, Olga Matveeva*[†] *and Henrik Oster**

Chronophysiology Group, Medical Department I, University of Lübeck, Lübeck, Germany

****Correspondence:***
Henrik Oster
henrik.oster@uni-luebeck.de

[†]Rebecca Dumbell and Olga Matveeva contributed equally.

In mammals, molecular circadian clocks are present in most cells of the body, and this circadian network plays an important role in synchronizing physiological processes and behaviors to the appropriate time of day. The hypothalamic–pituitary–adrenal endocrine axis regulates the response to acute and chronic stress, acting through its final effectors – glucocorticoids – released from the adrenal cortex. Glucocorticoid secretion, characterized by its circadian rhythm, has an important role in synchronizing peripheral clocks and rhythms downstream of the master circadian pacemaker in the suprachiasmatic nucleus. Finally, glucocorticoids are powerfully anti-inflammatory, and recent work has implicated the circadian clock in various aspects and cells of the immune system, suggesting a tight interplay of stress and circadian systems in the regulation of immunity. This mini-review summarizes our current understanding of the role of the circadian clock network in both the HPA axis and the immune system, and discusses their interactions.

Keywords: circadian clock, HPA axis, immune system, glucocorticoids, stress

INTRODUCTION

Life on Earth has evolved in the context of a rhythmic environment, characterized largely by the regular succession of night and day. This has led to the evolution of intrinsic circadian (from Latin *circa diem* - about the day) clock systems, in order to optimally time physiological and behavioral processes. Disruption of circadian timing, such as with inter-time zone travel, shift work, and mistimed eating, can have consequences for cardiovascular, metabolic, and mental health and, crucially, immune function. The hypothalamic–pituitary–adrenal (HPA) axis and the immune system show extensive crosstalk, in particular with regard to the strong anti-inflammatory effects of glucocorticoids (cortisol in humans and corticosterone in rodents). However, less well studied is the interaction of the HPA axis and immune system with regard to the circadian clock. This mini-review will summarize current knowledge regarding the role of the circadian clock in each of these systems, and the interactions that can occur in the context of disrupted circadian rhythmicity.

THE CIRCADIAN CLOCK

Circadian rhythms are synchronized to external time by cues known as zeitgebers (German for time givers), such as light and food. In mammals, the clock system is organized in a hierarchical manner, with a master pacemaker residing in the hypothalamic suprachiasmatic nuclei (SCN), acting to synchronize peripheral clocks in all other tissues *via* endocrine and autonomic signals (1). At the cellular level, circadian clocks coordinate gene expression programs to control physiological processes over the course of the day. The primary zeitgeber for the SCN is light. From the eye, signals are relayed *via* the retinohypothalamic tract to the SCN, which in turn coordinates peripheral tissue clocks. Other zeitgebers can influence circadian rhythms, with mistimed feeding in particular being able to reset peripheral clocks independent from the SCN (2, 3).

The molecular circadian clock consists of interlocked transcriptional–translational feedback loops [TTLs; discussed in detail elsewhere (4, 5)]. Briefly, during the day, the transcription factors CLOCK (circadian locomotor output cycles kaput) or NPAS2 (neuronal PAS domain-containing protein 2) in complex with BMAL1 (brain and muscle aryl hydrocarbon receptor nuclear translocator-like 1) bind to *E-box* (enhancer box) promoter elements to drive expression of *Period* (*Per1-3*) and *Cryptochrome* (*Cry1/2*), along with other clock controlled genes (inset in **Figure 1**). PER/CRY protein complexes accumulate in the cytoplasm over the day and later relocate into the nucleus where they inhibit the activity of the CLOCK–BMAL1 (or NPAS2–BMAL1) complex. This shuts down *Per*/*Cry* transcription during the night. After degradation of nuclear PER/CRY complexes toward the next morning, the inhibition of CLOCK–BMAL1 is released and a new cycle begins.

CIRCADIAN AND STRESS REGULATION OF THE HPA AXIS

The HPA axis is a key in the regulation of stress responses, with glucocorticoids mediating intermediate and chronic adaptation to stressful stimuli, complementing the rapid response of catecholamines, both secreted from the adrenal gland. The rhythmic regulation of catecholamines and other adrenal hormones is discussed elsewhere (6). Rhythmic regulation of glucocorticoid release (**Figure 1**) allows for anticipation of daily timing of energy-demanding situations. In addition, glucocorticoid rhythms play a key role in the systemic coordination of circadian rhythms by resetting cellular clocks downstream of the SCN.

During stress, the brainstem and limbic forebrain stimulate corticotrophin-releasing hormone (CRH) and arginine vasopressin (AVP) secretion from neurosecretory neurons of the paraventricular nucleus of the hypothalamus (PVN) (7). *Via* the hypophyseal portal system, these reach anterior pituitary corticotrophs, which secrete adrenocorticotrophic hormone (ACTH).

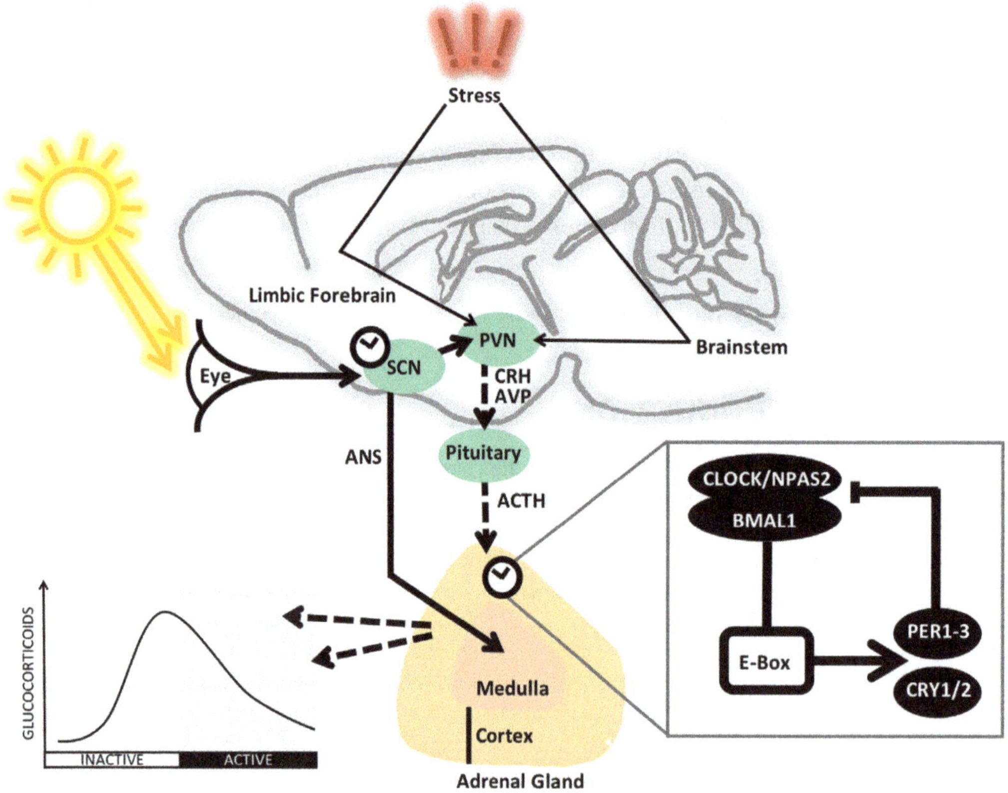

FIGURE 1 | The rhythmic control of the HPA axis is regulated at several levels. The master clock residing in the suprachiasmatic nucleus (SCN) is synchronized by light information received *via* the retinohypothalamic tract from the eye in order to exert autonomic (ANS) and hormonal influence on the clocks and rhythms of downstream tissues of the body. In addition to the direct innervation of the adrenal, the SCN influences the paraventricular nucleus (PVN) to secrete corticotropin-releasing hormone (CRH) and arginine vasopressin (AVP), which reach the pituitary *via* the blood portal system to stimulate secretion of adrenocorticotropic hormone (ACTH), which activates production and release of glucocorticoids. In addition, local adrenal clocks are thought to regulate responsiveness to ACTH in a circadian fashion. The baseline circadian rhythm of circulating glucocorticoids peaks just before the beginning of the active phase (day in humans and night in rodents). Stress-induced stimulation of the HPA axis acts *via* afferent signals from the limbic forebrain and brainstem to the PVN. Inset: the core transcriptional–translational feedback loop (TTL) that makes up the molecular circadian clockwork. In the positive arm of the clock, CLOCK or NPAS2 form a complex with BMAL1 and bind to *E-Box* elements in the gene promotors of PERs and CRYs, which make up the negative arm and act to inhibit the activity of CLOCK–BMAL1 or NPAS2–BMAL1, with a cycle of roughly 24 h. For further detail, see the main text.

ACTH then acts at melanocortin type-2 receptors (MC2R) in the adrenal cortex to stimulate production and release of glucocorticoids. Negative feedback from glucocorticoids acts at the level of CRH in the hypothalamus and ACTH in the pituitary (8, 9). In addition, PVN CRH expression is indirectly controlled by the SCN (8–11).

Glucocorticoids bind to glucocorticoid (GR) and mineralocorticoid receptors (MR) in target tissues. Unlike the MR, which is almost constantly activated by glucocorticoids, GR – widely expressed in the brain and periphery, but not in the SCN (12) – activation occurs only during glucocorticoid peak levels (13). This means that GR activation may occur during the peak of the circadian rhythm even during the ultradian trough, but ultradian peaks during the circadian nadir may not be sufficient for activation (14, 15). GR binds to glucocorticoid response elements (*GRE* or *nGRE*) to regulate transcription of target genes (16). *GRE* are present in the promoter region of the clock genes *Per1, Per2, Npas2,* and various clock controlled genes involved in the synchronization of peripheral circadian rhythms (17).

Glucocorticoid circadian rhythms peak slightly before the onset of the active phase, which is during the night for most rodent species and during the day for humans (18). This rhythm overlays a more dynamic ultradian pattern for both ACTH and glucocorticoid secretion (19) driven by feedback between glucocorticoids and ACTH release at the pituitary (20) and intra-adrenal feedback of glucocorticoids (21). The presence of GR in the adrenal cortex (22, 23) and the demonstrated inhibitory effects of exogenous corticosterone on the ACTH-stimulated corticosteroid synthesis could potentially play a role in local regulation of glucocorticoid secretion in the adrenal gland. Circadian glucocorticoid rhythms can persist independent of the SCN (24–26). Given the influence that circadian rhythmicity of glucocorticoids may have on peripheral clock function, it is perhaps not surprising that the HPA axis, which is acutely activated in stressful situations, is unlikely to be the main driver of the circadian rhythm of these hormones. Indeed, there are several components of the HPA axis which, although they express circadian rhythmicity, do not synchronize well enough to explain downstream endocrine rhythms (3, 10, 27). The circadian influence of the SCN on the HPA axis also occurs through autonomic innervation of the adrenal gland (28, 29), with SCN-dependent rapid induction of *Per1* expression being stimulated in the adrenal gland following a light pulse (30). In line with this, splanchnic nerve transection results in dampened circadian glucocorticoid rhythm in rats (31, 32).

LOCAL REGULATION OF GLUCOCORTICOID RHYTHMS

A circadian rhythm of steroid release was first demonstrated in isolated Syrian hamster adrenals [*Mesocricetus auratus*, See Ref. (33)], and rhythmic glucocorticoid concentrations persist under constant peripheral CRH infusion in *CRH* knockout mice (34), or in hamsters with natural loss of ACTH rhythm (35). Adrenal circadian rhythms can however be altered by ACTH, which stimulates *PER1* and *BMAL1* expression *ex vivo* in human tissue (36) and shifts clock rhythms in isolated adrenals of *Per2:LUC* reporter mice (37).

Circadian clocks within the adrenal gland also play a role in the rhythmic regulation of the HPA axis, both in glucocorticoid production and in sensitivity to ACTH. Robust clock gene expression rhythms have been demonstrated in the adrenal cortex of rodents and primates (38–43), and several steroidogenic genes show circadian expression (31, 40, 44). Work in transgenic mice has shown that those lacking genes of the positive arm of the TTL produce lower levels of corticosterone (45, 46), while those with mutations in the negative arm are chronical hypersecreters (47, 48). Evidence for the importance of adrenocortical clocks in regulating ACTH sensitivity comes from isolated adrenal tissue responses to ACTH, which differs across the day and is very low in mice deficient for *Per2* and *Cry1* (41) or *Bmal1* (46). This is further supported by evidence from primate adrenal explant studies, where knockdown of *Cry2* and subsequent downregulation of *Bmal1* lead to attenuated ACTH responses (49). Together, these studies suggest that the local adrenal clock is important for regulating the circadian glucocorticoid rhythm independent of systemic influences such as during stress, and may explain the high amplitude of glucocorticoid rhythm in the face of comparably low variations in ACTH concentrations.

HPA AXIS INTERACTION WITH THE IMMUNE SYSTEM

A bidirectional communication exists between the HPA axis and the immune system (**Figure 2**). It is well understood that immune cells can activate the HPA axis *via* cytokines such as tumor necrosis factor-alpha (TNF-α), interleukins (IL-1, IL-6), and the type-I interferons (IFNs) (50–53). Interestingly, some cytokines can activate the HPA axis *via* different mechanisms. Although primarily acting on the PVN to stimulate CRH release (54–56), they also have direct action at the level of the pituitary and adrenal (57, 58).

At the same time, glucocorticoids can affect viability and function of many immune cell types, including T cells, B cells, monocytes, macrophages, and granulocytes (59, 60). Glucocorticoids suppress the synthesis and release of cytokines, thereby protecting the host organism from the detrimental consequences of a long-term hyperactivity of the immune system [reviewed in Ref. (61)]. Pioneering work by Hench, Kendall, and Reichstein demonstrated the immunosuppressive actions of glucocorticoids almost 70 years ago (62). Nevertheless, glucocorticoids are still the most widely used and most effective treatment to control allergic, autoimmune, inflammatory, and hematological disorders (63). GR are found in almost all types of immune cells, and upon activation tether and trans-represses pro-inflammatory regulators such as nuclear factor kappa-light-chain-enhancer of activated B-cells (NF-κB) and activator protein 1 (AP-1) (61, 64) by activating anti-inflammatory molecules such as glucocorticoid-induced-leucine zipper [GILZ (65)], MAPK phosphatase-1 [MKP-1 (66)], annexin-1 (67), mitogen-inducible gene-6 [Mig-6 (68)], and SRC-like adaptor protein 1 [SLAP (69)].

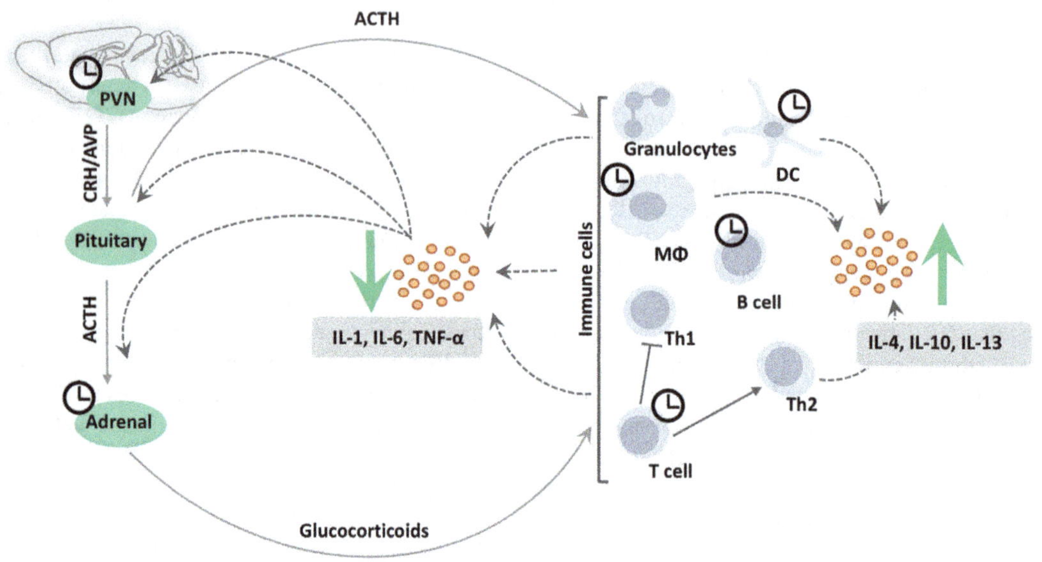

FIGURE 2 | Circadian clocks in HPA axis-immune system crosstalk. Immune cells can activate the HPA axis *via* cytokines such as tumor necrosis factor-alpha (TNF-α) and interleukins (IL-1/6) at the level of the paraventricular nucleus (PVN) of the hypothalamus as well as at the pituitary and adrenal, stimulating the production of glucocorticoids. Glucocorticoids in turn act on the receptors on the surface or in the cytoplasm of immune cells to suppress the induction of pro-inflammatory responses, and to promote a shift from T helper cell type 1 (Th1) toward T helper cell type 2 (Th2)-mediated humoral immunity. This inhibits the production of pro-inflammatory cytokines, while promoting the production of anti-inflammatory cytokines, such as interleukin-4, interleukin-10, and interleukin-13 (IL-4/10/13) by various immune cells. In addition, ACTH exerts direct anti-inflammatory and immune-modulating effects *via* the melanocortin system. CRH, corticotropin-releasing hormone; AVP, arginine vasopressin; DC, dendritic cell; MΦ, macrophage.

In contrast to the well-described immunosuppressive effects recent studies indicate that glucocorticoids can also have permissive or even stimulatory effects on immune processes [reviewed in Ref. (70–72)]. It is thought that acute stress enhances, while chronic stress suppresses the peripheral immune response (70), but the mechanism of this dual role is not well understood. Several studies report that glucocorticoids induce expression of innate immune-related genes, including members of the toll-like receptor (TLR) family, such as TLR2 and TLR4 (73–75). Glucocorticoids also rapidly induce a central component of the inflammasome, NLRP3, in macrophages, which stimulates secretion of pro-inflammatory cytokines (76).

In addition, glucocorticoids regulate adaptive immune responses by influencing cell trafficking to the sites of inflammation and by suppressing T helper cell type 1 (Th1) and enhancing T helper cell type 2 (Th2) cytokine-driven responses (77, 78). Consequently, in contrast to the traditional view of glucocorticoids as generally immunosuppressive hormones, glucocorticoids are now more accurately regarded as immune modulators.

As an alternative to the glucocorticoid treatment of chronic inflammatory diseases such as multiple sclerosis, the use of ACTH has recently been re-employed, appearing to act not only indirectly by stimulating glucocorticoid production but also by a direct anti-inflammatory effect *via* the melanocortin system [reviewed in Ref. (79–81)]. Melanocortin receptors (MCRs) are found on lymphocytes and macrophages (82–84). Anti-inflammatory effects of ACTH are mediated primarily by MC1R and MC3R, while immune-regulatory effects rely on MC5R (80). Such glucocorticoid-independent effects of ACTH have been demonstrated after lipo-polysaccharide (LPS)-stimulated production of IL-1ß and TNF-α in human blood samples (85), in a rat gout model (86), and in TNF-α-induced acute kidney disease in rats (87). Furthermore, ACTH can reduce neutrophil infiltration *via* MC3R (88).

CIRCADIAN INTERACTION OF THE HPA AXIS WITH IMMUNE FUNCTION

In mammals, the circadian clock is an important regulator of the immune system, allowing the organism to anticipate daily changes in activity and the associated risk of antigen encounter. Circadian rhythms are found in multiple aspects of immune function, such as recruitment of immune cells to tissues, antigen presentation, lymphocyte proliferation, TLR function, and cytokine gene expression (89, 90). Furthermore, several inflammatory diseases, such as bronchial asthma and rheumatoid arthritis vary in severity over the course of the day, implicating a circadian regulation of vulnerability (91, 92). Animal studies have revealed that circadian rhythm disruption by shift work or chronic jet lag leads to a dysregulation of the immune system and a higher risk for several pathologies (93, 94).

Molecular clocks have been characterized in various immune cells, including macrophages, dendritic cells, and T and B lymphocytes (95–97). In humans, under constant routine conditions, administration of exogenous glucocorticoids 10 h after awakening can entrain circadian rhythms in peripheral blood mononuclear cells (PBMCs) without changing plasma melatonin and cortisol rhythms, thus linking HPA axis regulation to immune cell function. In line with this, oral administration of synthetic hydrocortisone shifts the expression of *BMAL1* and *PER2/3* in PBMCs by 9.5–11.5 h (98).

Stress-induced alterations of HPA axis rhythmicity can lead to wide-spread alterations in innate and adaptive immune responses and contribute to the development and progression of some types of cancer in animals (99, 100). In humans, data are less clear, with a positive association between stress and breast cancer observed in some (101), but not in other studies (102). In another context, stress-induced inflammatory priming of microglia was influenced by time of day in rats. Animals exposed to stress during the rest phase showed enhanced neuroinflammatory responses to an LPS challenge compared with animals experiencing stress during the active phase (103). Whether these effects involve circadian alterations remains to be shown. Of interest in this context, pulmonary antibacterial responses in mice appear to be gated by circadian clocks residing in the epithelial club cells lining the pulmonary airways, entrained by glucocorticoids (104).

Not only does the circadian clock regulate the immune system but immune status also feeds back on circadian rhythms. For example, administration of LPS resets activity rhythms in mice (105), and transiently suppresses *Per2* and *Dbp* expression in the SCN and liver of rats (106). LPS treatment increases AVP release from SCN explants (107), and TNF-α treatment downregulates SCN *Dbp* expression and causes prolonged rest periods during the active phase in rodents (108).

Recent studies reveal blunted circadian cortisol rhythms and attenuated stress responses in patients with allergic diseases, such as bronchial asthma, allergic rhinitis, atopic dermatitis, and extensive nasal polyposis (109–112). In patients with sepsis hypercortisolism persists despite low ACTH levels, suggesting that non-ACTH-mediated mechanisms are involved in the maintenance of high glucocorticoid levels. Interestingly, circadian rhythm of both ACTH and cortisol secretion were shown to be blunted in these patients (113). Furthermore, neonatal endotoxin exposure reprograms HPA axis development in rats, leading to ACTH and corticosterone hyper-responsiveness later in life (114).

CONCLUSION

Cellular circadian clocks in central and peripheral tissues interact to regulate the activity of the main endocrine axes. Our improved understanding about the systemic regulation of HPA axis circadian rhythms and the interplay of clock and stress functions in this context may help to optimize current treatment strategies for many immunological disorders. For example, in chronic diseases such as rheumatoid arthritis, timed administration of exogenous glucocorticoids at specific times of day may improve therapeutic effectiveness and reduce negative side effects, since lower doses are required (115). At the same time, the importance of glucocorticoids in the coordination of the circadian timing system itself has so far been largely neglected in clinical settings. Stabilizing circadian HPA axis regulation may protect against adverse external influences such as stress and infection, thus protecting the body against some of the most frequent threats of the 24/7 globalized society.

AUTHOR CONTRIBUTIONS

RD, OM, and HO discussed the concept, compiled the literature, and wrote the paper.

ACKNOWLEDGMENTS

This work was supported by grants from the Volkswagen Foundation (Lichtenberg Fellowship to HO) and the German Research Association (DFG; SFB-654 and a single project grant to HO).

REFERENCES

1. Dibner C, Schibler U, Albrecht U. The mammalian circadian timing system: organization and coordination of central and peripheral clocks. *Annu Rev Physiol* (2010) **72**:517–49. doi:10.1146/annurev-physiol-021909-135821
2. Damiola F, Le Minh N, Preitner N, Kornmann B, Fleury-Olela F, Schibler U. Restricted feeding uncouples circadian oscillators in peripheral tissues from the central pacemaker in the suprachiasmatic nucleus. *Genes Dev* (2000) **14**(23):2950–61. doi:10.1101/gad.183500
3. Girotti M, Weinberg MS, Spencer RL. Diurnal expression of functional and clock-related genes throughout the rat HPA axis: system-wide shifts in response to a restricted feeding schedule. *Am J Physiol Endocrinol Metab* (2009) **296**(4):E888–97. doi:10.1152/ajpendo.90946.2008
4. Zhang EE, Kay SA. Clocks not winding down: unravelling circadian networks. *Nat Rev Mol Cell Biol* (2010) **11**(11):764–76. doi:10.1038/nrm2995
5. Brown SA, Kowalska E, Dallmann R. (Re)inventing the circadian feedback loop. *Dev Cell* (2012) **22**(3):477–87. doi:10.1016/j.devcel.2012.02.007
6. Leliavski A, Dumbell R, Ott V, Oster H. Adrenal clocks and the role of adrenal hormones in the regulation of circadian physiology. *J Biol Rhythms* (2015) **30**(1):20–34. doi:10.1177/0748730414553971
7. Ulrich-Lai YM, Herman JP. Neural regulation of endocrine and autonomic stress responses. *Nat Rev Neurosci* (2009) **10**(6):397–409. doi:10.1038/nrn2647
8. Watts AG. Glucocorticoid regulation of peptide genes in neuroendocrine CRH neurons: a complexity beyond negative feedback. *Front Neuroendocrinol* (2005) **26**(3–4):109–30. doi:10.1016/j.yfrne.2005.09.001
9. Dallman MF, Akana SF, Cascio CS, Darlington DN, Jacobson L, Levin N. Regulation of ACTH secretion: variations on a theme of B. *Recent Prog Horm Res* (1987) **43**:113–73.
10. Watts AG, Tanimura S, Sanchez-Watts G. Corticotropin-releasing hormone and arginine vasopressin gene transcription in the hypothalamic paraventricular nucleus of unstressed rats: daily rhythms and their interactions with corticosterone. *Endocrinology* (2004) **145**(2):529–40. doi:10.1210/en.2003-0394
11. Girotti M, Weinberg MS, Spencer RL. Differential responses of hypothalamus-pituitary-adrenal axis immediate early genes to corticosterone and circadian drive. *Endocrinology* (2007) **148**(5):2542–52. doi:10.1210/en.2006-1304
12. Balsalobre A, Brown SA, Marcacci L, Tronche F, Kellendonk C, Reichardt HM, et al. Resetting of circadian time in peripheral tissues by glucocorticoid signaling. *Science* (2000) **289**(5488):2344–7. doi:10.1126/science.289.5488.2344
13. de Kloet ER, Joels M, Holsboer F. Stress and the brain: from adaptation to disease. *Nat Rev Neurosci* (2005) **6**(6):463–75. doi:10.1038/nrn1683
14. Reul JM, de Kloet ER. Two receptor systems for corticosterone in rat brain: microdistribution and differential occupation. *Endocrinology* (1985) **117**(6):2505–11. doi:10.1210/endo-117-6-2505
15. Spencer RL, Miller AH, Moday H, Stein M, McEwen BS. Diurnal differences in basal and acute stress levels of type I and type II adrenal steroid

receptor activation in neural and immune tissues. *Endocrinology* (1993) **133**(5):1941–50. doi:10.1210/en.133.5.1941

16. Surjit M, Ganti KP, Mukherji A, Ye T, Hua G, Metzger D, et al. Widespread negative response elements mediate direct repression by agonist-liganded glucocorticoid receptor. *Cell* (2011) **145**(2):224–41. doi:10.1016/j.cell.2011.03.027
17. So AY, Bernal TU, Pillsbury ML, Yamamoto KR, Feldman BJ. Glucocorticoid regulation of the circadian clock modulates glucose homeostasis. *Proc Natl Acad Sci U S A* (2009) **106**(41):17582–7. doi:10.1073/pnas.0909733106
18. Lightman SL, Conway-Campbell BL. The crucial role of pulsatile activity of the HPA axis for continuous dynamic equilibration. *Nat Rev Neurosci* (2010) **11**(10):710–8. doi:10.1038/nrn2914
19. Dickmeis T, Weger BD, Weger M. The circadian clock and glucocorticoids – interactions across many time scales. *Mol Cell Endocrinol* (2013) **380**(1–2):2–15. doi:10.1016/j.mce.2013.05.012
20. Walker JJ, Spiga F, Waite E, Zhao Z, Kershaw Y, Terry JR, et al. The origin of glucocorticoid hormone oscillations. *PLoS Biol* (2012) **10**(6):e1001341. doi:10.1371/journal.pbio.1001341
21. Walker JJ, Spiga F, Gupta R, Zhao Z, Lightman SL, Terry JR. Rapid intra-adrenal feedback regulation of glucocorticoid synthesis. *J R Soc Interface* (2015) **12**(102):20140875. doi:10.1098/rsif.2014.0875
22. Paust HJ, Loeper S, Else T, Bamberger AM, Papadopoulos G, Pankoke D, et al. Expression of the glucocorticoid receptor in the human adrenal cortex. *Exp Clin Endocrinol Diabetes* (2006) **114**(1):6–10. doi:10.1055/s-2005-873007
23. Loose DS, Do YS, Chen TL, Feldman D. Demonstration of glucocorticoid receptors in the adrenal cortex: evidence for a direct dexamethasone suppressive effect on the rat adrenal gland. *Endocrinology* (1980) **107**(1):137–46. doi:10.1210/endo-107-1-137
24. Moore RY, Eichler VB. Loss of a circadian adrenal corticosterone rhythm following suprachiasmatic lesions in the rat. *Brain Res* (1972) **42**(1):201–6. doi:10.1016/0006-8993(72)90054-6
25. Stephan FK, Zucker I. Circadian rhythms in drinking behavior and locomotor activity of rats are eliminated by hypothalamic lesions. *Proc Natl Acad Sci U S A* (1972) **69**(6):1583–6. doi:10.1073/pnas.69.6.1583
26. Husse J, Leliavski A, Tsang AH, Oster H, Eichele G. The light-dark cycle controls peripheral rhythmicity in mice with a genetically ablated suprachiasmatic nucleus clock. *FASEB J* (2014) **28**(11):4950–60. doi:10.1096/fj.14-256594
27. Henley DE, Russell GM, Douthwaite JA, Wood SA, Buchanan F, Gibson R, et al. Hypothalamic-pituitary-adrenal axis activation in obstructive sleep apnea: the effect of continuous positive airway pressure therapy. *J Clin Endocrinol Metab* (2009) **94**(11):4234–42. doi:10.1210/jc.2009-1174
28. Buijs RM, Wortel J, Van Heerikhuize JJ, Feenstra MG, Ter Horst GJ, Romijn HJ, et al. Anatomical and functional demonstration of a multisynaptic suprachiasmatic nucleus adrenal (cortex) pathway. *Eur J Neurosci* (1999) **11**(5):1535–44. doi:10.1046/j.1460-9568.1999.00575.x
29. Engeland WC. Sensitization of endocrine organs to anterior pituitary hormones by the autonomic nervous system. *Handb Clin Neurol* (2013) **117**:37–44. doi:10.1016/B978-0-444-53491-0.00004-3
30. Ishida A, Mutoh T, Ueyama T, Bando H, Masubuchi S, Nakahara D, et al. Light activates the adrenal gland: timing of gene expression and glucocorticoid release. *Cell Metab* (2005) **2**(5):297–307. doi:10.1016/j.cmet.2005.09.009
31. Ulrich-Lai YM, Arnhold MM, Engeland WC. Adrenal splanchnic innervation contributes to the diurnal rhythm of plasma corticosterone in rats by modulating adrenal sensitivity to ACTH. *Am J Physiol Regul Integr Comp Physiol* (2006) **290**(4):R1128–35. doi:10.1152/ajpregu.00042.2003
32. Wotus C, Lilley TR, Neal AS, Suleiman NL, Schmuck SC, Smarr BL, et al. Forced desynchrony reveals independent contributions of suprachiasmatic oscillators to the daily plasma corticosterone rhythm in male rats. *PLoS One* (2013) **8**(7):e68793. doi:10.1371/journal.pone.0068793
33. Andrews RV, Folk GE Jr. Circadian metabolic patterns in cultured hamster adrenal glands. *Comp Biochem Physiol* (1964) **11**:393–409. doi:10.1016/0010-406X(64)90006-4
34. Muglia LJ, Jacobson L, Weninger SC, Luedke CE, Bae DS, Jeong KH, et al. Impaired diurnal adrenal rhythmicity restored by constant infusion of corticotropin-releasing hormone in corticotropin-releasing hormone-deficient mice. *J Clin Invest* (1997) **99**(12):2923–9. doi:10.1172/JCI119487
35. Lilley TR, Wotus C, Taylor D, Lee JM, de la Iglesia HO. Circadian regulation of cortisol release in behaviorally split golden hamsters. *Endocrinology* (2012) **153**(2):732–8. doi:10.1210/en.2011-1624
36. Campino C, Valenzuela FJ, Torres-Farfan C, Reynolds HE, Abarzua-Catalan L, Arteaga E, et al. Melatonin exerts direct inhibitory actions on ACTH responses in the human adrenal gland. *Horm Metab Res* (2011) **43**(5):337–42. doi:10.1055/s-0031-1271693
37. Yoder JM, Brandeland M, Engeland WC. Phase-dependent resetting of the adrenal clock by ACTH in vitro. *Am J Physiol Regul Integr Comp Physiol* (2014) **306**(6):R387–93. doi:10.1152/ajpregu.00519.2013
38. Bittman EL, Doherty L, Huang L, Paroskie A. Period gene expression in mouse endocrine tissues. *Am J Physiol Regul Integr Comp Physiol* (2003) **285**(3):R561–9. doi:10.1152/ajpregu.00783.2002
39. Lemos DR, Downs JL, Urbanski HF. Twenty-four-hour rhythmic gene expression in the rhesus macaque adrenal gland. *Mol Endocrinol* (2006) **20**(5):1164–76. doi:10.1210/me.2005-0361
40. Oster H, Damerow S, Hut RA, Eichele G. Transcriptional profiling in the adrenal gland reveals circadian regulation of hormone biosynthesis genes and nucleosome assembly genes. *J Biol Rhythms* (2006) **21**(5):350–61. doi:10.1177/0748730406293053
41. Oster H, Damerow S, Kiessling S, Jakubcakova V, Abraham D, Tian J, et al. The circadian rhythm of glucocorticoids is regulated by a gating mechanism residing in the adrenal cortical clock. *Cell Metab* (2006) **4**(2):163–73. doi:10.1016/j.cmet.2006.07.002
42. Fahrenkrug J, Hannibal J, Georg B. Diurnal rhythmicity of the canonical clock genes Per1, Per2 and Bmal1 in the rat adrenal gland is unaltered after hypophysectomy. *J Neuroendocrinol* (2008) **20**(3):323–9. doi:10.1111/j.1365-2826.2008.01651.x
43. Valenzuela FJ, Torres-Farfan C, Richter HG, Mendez N, Campino C, Torrealba F, et al. Clock gene expression in adult primate suprachiasmatic nuclei and adrenal: is the adrenal a peripheral clock responsive to melatonin? *Endocrinology* (2008) **149**(4):1454–61. doi:10.1210/en.2007-1518
44. Son GH, Chung S, Choe HK, Kim HD, Baik SM, Lee H, et al. Adrenal peripheral clock controls the autonomous circadian rhythm of glucocorticoid by causing rhythmic steroid production. *Proc Natl Acad Sci U S A* (2008) **105**(52):20970–5. doi:10.1073/pnas.0806962106
45. Turek FW, Joshu C, Kohsaka A, Lin E, Ivanova G, McDearmon E, et al. Obesity and metabolic syndrome in circadian clock mutant mice. *Science* (2005) **308**(5724):1043–5. doi:10.1126/science.1108750
46. Leliavski A, Shostak A, Husse J, Oster H. Impaired glucocorticoid production and response to stress in Arntl-deficient male mice. *Endocrinology* (2014) **155**(1):133–42. doi:10.1210/en.2013-1531
47. Lamia KA, Papp SJ, Yu RT, Barish GD, Uhlenhaut NH, Jonker JW, et al. Cryptochromes mediate rhythmic repression of the glucocorticoid receptor. *Nature* (2011) **480**(7378):552–6. doi:10.1038/nature10700
48. Barclay JL, Shostak A, Leliavski A, Tsang AH, Johren O, Muller-Fielitz H, et al. High fat diet-induced hyperinsulinemia and tissue-specific insulin resistance in Cry deficient mice. *Am J Physiol Endocrinol Metab* (2013) **304**(10):E1053–63. doi:10.1152/ajpendo.00512.2012
49. Torres-Farfan C, Abarzua-Catalan L, Valenzuela FJ, Mendez N, Richter HG, Valenzuela GJ, et al. Cryptochrome 2 expression level is critical for adrenocorticotropin stimulation of cortisol production in the capuchin monkey adrenal. *Endocrinology* (2009) **150**(6):2717–22. doi:10.1210/en.2008-1683
50. Besedovsky H, del Rey A, Sorkin E, Dinarello CA. Immunoregulatory feedback between interleukin-1 and glucocorticoid hormones. *Science* (1986) **233**(4764):652–4. doi:10.1126/science.3014662
51. van der Meer MJ, Sweep CG, Rijnkels CE, Pesman GJ, Tilders FJ, Kloppenborg PW, et al. Acute stimulation of the hypothalamic-pituitary-adrenal axis by IL-1 beta, TNF alpha and IL-6: a dose response study. *J Endocrinol Invest* (1996) **19**(3):175–82. doi:10.1007/BF03349862
52. Turnbull AV, Rivier CL. Regulation of the hypothalamic-pituitary-adrenal axis by cytokines: actions and mechanisms of action. *Physiol Rev* (1999) **79**(1):1–71.
53. Saphier D. Neuroendocrine effects of interferon-alpha in the rat. *Adv Exp Med Biol* (1995) **373**:209–18. doi:10.1007/978-1-4615-1951-5_29
54. Berkenbosch F, van Oers J, del Rey A, Tilders F, Besedovsky H. Corticotropin-releasing factor-producing neurons in the rat activated by interleukin-1. *Science* (1987) **238**(4826):524–6. doi:10.1126/science.2443979

55. Sapolsky R, Rivier C, Yamamoto G, Plotsky P, Vale W. Interleukin-1 stimulates the secretion of hypothalamic corticotropin-releasing factor. *Science* (1987) **238**(4826):522–4. doi:10.1126/science.2821621
56. Kovacs KJ, Elenkov IJ. Differential dependence of ACTH secretion induced by various cytokines on the integrity of the paraventricular nucleus. *J Neuroendocrinol* (1995) **7**(1):15–23. doi:10.1111/j.1365-2826.1995.tb00662.x
57. Harbuz MS, Stephanou A, Sarlis N, Lightman SL. The effects of recombinant human interleukin (IL)-1 alpha, IL-1 beta or IL-6 on hypothalamo-pituitary-adrenal axis activation. *J Endocrinol* (1992) **133**(3):349–55. doi:10.1677/joe.0.1330349
58. Ehrhart-Bornstein M, Hinson JP, Bornstein SR, Scherbaum WA, Vinson GP. Intraadrenal interactions in the regulation of adrenocortical steroidogenesis. *Endocr Rev* (1998) **19**(2):101–43. doi:10.1210/edrv.19.2.0326
59. Ashwell JD, Lu FW, Vacchio MS. Glucocorticoids in T cell development and function*. *Annu Rev Immunol* (2000) **18**:309–45. doi:10.1146/annurev.immunol.18.1.309
60. Caramori G, Adcock I. Anti-inflammatory mechanisms of glucocorticoids targeting granulocytes. *Curr Drug Targets Inflamm Allergy* (2005) **4**(4):455–63. doi:10.2174/1568010054526331
61. Vandevyver S, Dejager L, Tuckermann J, Libert C. New insights into the anti-inflammatory mechanisms of glucocorticoids: an emerging role for glucocorticoid-receptor-mediated transactivation. *Endocrinology* (2013) **154**(3):993–1007. doi:10.1210/en.2012-2045
62. Hench PS, Kendall EC, Slocumb CH, Polley HF. The effect of a hormone of the adrenal cortex (17-hydroxy-11-dehydrocorticosterone; compound E) and of pituitary adrenocorticotropic hormone on rheumatoid arthritis. *Proc Staff Meet Mayo Clin* (1949) **24**(8):181–97.
63. Rhen T, Cidlowski JA. Antiinflammatory action of glucocorticoids – new mechanisms for old drugs. *N Engl J Med* (2005) **353**(16):1711–23. doi:10.1056/NEJMra050541
64. De Bosscher K, Vanden Berghe W, Haegeman G. Cross-talk between nuclear receptors and nuclear factor kappaB. *Oncogene* (2006) **25**(51):6868–86. doi:10.1038/sj.onc.1209935
65. D'Adamio F, Zollo O, Moraca R, Ayroldi E, Bruscoli S, Bartoli A, et al. A new dexamethasone-induced gene of the leucine zipper family protects T lymphocytes from TCR/CD3-activated cell death. *Immunity* (1997) **7**(6):803–12. doi:10.1016/S1074-7613(00)80398-2
66. Lasa M, Abraham SM, Boucheron C, Saklatvala J, Clark AR. Dexamethasone causes sustained expression of mitogen-activated protein kinase (MAPK) phosphatase 1 and phosphatase-mediated inhibition of MAPK p38. *Mol Cell Biol* (2002) **22**(22):7802–11. doi:10.1128/MCB.22.22.7802-7811.2002
67. Perretti M, D'Acquisto F. Annexin A1 and glucocorticoids as effectors of the resolution of inflammation. *Nat Rev Immunol* (2009) **9**(1):62–70. doi:10.1038/nri2470
68. Xu D, Makkinje A, Kyriakis JM. Gene 33 is an endogenous inhibitor of epidermal growth factor (EGF) receptor signaling and mediates dexamethasone-induced suppression of EGF function. *J Biol Chem* (2005) **280**(4):2924–33. doi:10.1074/jbc.M408907200
69. Park SK, Beaven MA. Mechanism of upregulation of the inhibitory regulator, src-like adaptor protein (SLAP), by glucocorticoids in mast cells. *Mol Immunol* (2009) **46**(3):492–7. doi:10.1016/j.molimm.2008.10.011
70. Dhabhar FS. Stress-induced augmentation of immune function – the role of stress hormones, leukocyte trafficking, and cytokines. *Brain Behav Immun* (2002) **16**(6):785–98. doi:10.1016/S0889-1591(02)00036-3
71. Cruz-Topete D, Cidlowski JA. One hormone, two actions: anti- and pro-inflammatory effects of glucocorticoids. *Neuroimmunomodulation* (2015) **22**(1–2):20–32. doi:10.1159/000362724
72. Dhabhar FS. Enhancing versus suppressive effects of stress on immune function: implications for immunoprotection and immunopathology. *Neuroimmunomodulation* (2009) **16**(5):300–17. doi:10.1159/000216188
73. Galon J, Franchimont D, Hiroi N, Frey G, Boettner A, Ehrhart-Bornstein M, et al. Gene profiling reveals unknown enhancing and suppressive actions of glucocorticoids on immune cells. *FASEB J* (2002) **16**(1):61–71. doi:10.1096/fj.01-0245com
74. Homma T, Kato A, Hashimoto N, Batchelor J, Yoshikawa M, Imai S, et al. Corticosteroid and cytokines synergistically enhance toll-like receptor 2 expression in respiratory epithelial cells. *Am J Respir Cell Mol Biol* (2004) **31**(4):463–9. doi:10.1165/rcmb.2004-0161OC
75. Chinenov Y, Rogatsky I. Glucocorticoids and the innate immune system: crosstalk with the toll-like receptor signaling network. *Mol Cell Endocrinol* (2007) **275**(1–2):30–42. doi:10.1016/j.mce.2007.04.014
76. Busillo JM, Azzam KM, Cidlowski JA. Glucocorticoids sensitize the innate immune system through regulation of the NLRP3 inflammasome. *J Biol Chem* (2011) **286**(44):38703–13. doi:10.1074/jbc.M111.275370
77. Daynes RA, Araneo BA. Contrasting effects of glucocorticoids on the capacity of T cells to produce the growth factors interleukin 2 and interleukin 4. *Eur J Immunol* (1989) **19**(12):2319–25. doi:10.1002/eji.1830191221
78. Agarwal SK, Marshall GD Jr. Dexamethasone promotes type 2 cytokine production primarily through inhibition of type 1 cytokines. *J Interferon Cytokine Res* (2001) **21**(3):147–55. doi:10.1089/107999001750133159
79. Catania A, Gatti S, Colombo G, Lipton JM. Targeting melanocortin receptors as a novel strategy to control inflammation. *Pharmacol Rev* (2004) **56**(1):1–29. doi:10.1124/pr.56.1.1
80. Ross AP, Ben-Zacharia A, Harris C, Smrtka J. Multiple sclerosis, relapses, and the mechanism of action of adrenocorticotropic hormone. *Front Neurol* (2013) **4**:21. doi:10.3389/fneur.2013.00021
81. Montero-Melendez T. ACTH: the forgotten therapy. *Semin Immunol* (2015) **27**(3):216–26. doi:10.1016/j.smim.2015.02.003
82. Johnson EW, Hughes TK Jr, Smith EM. ACTH receptor distribution and modulation among murine mononuclear leukocyte populations. *J Biol Regul Homeost Agents* (2001) **15**(2):156–62.
83. Andersen GN, Hagglund M, Nagaeva O, Frangsmyr L, Petrovska R, Mincheva-Nilsson L, et al. Quantitative measurement of the levels of melanocortin receptor subtype 1, 2, 3 and 5 and pro-opio-melanocortin peptide gene expression in subsets of human peripheral blood leucocytes. *Scand J Immunol* (2005) **61**(3):279–84. doi:10.1111/j.1365-3083.2005.01565.x
84. Cooper A, Robinson SJ, Pickard C, Jackson CL, Friedmann PS, Healy E. Alpha-melanocyte-stimulating hormone suppresses antigen-induced lymphocyte proliferation in humans independently of melanocortin 1 receptor gene status. *J Immunol* (2005) **175**(7):4806–13. doi:10.4049/jimmunol.175.7.4806
85. Catania A, Garofalo L, Cutuli M, Gringeri A, Santagostino E, Lipton JM. Melanocortin peptides inhibit production of proinflammatory cytokines in blood of HIV-infected patients. *Peptides* (1998) **19**(6):1099–104. doi:10.1016/S0196-9781(98)00055-2
86. Getting SJ, Christian HC, Flower RJ, Perretti M. Activation of melanocortin type 3 receptor as a molecular mechanism for adrenocorticotropic hormone efficacy in gouty arthritis. *Arthritis Rheum* (2002) **46**(10):2765–75. doi:10.1002/art.10526
87. Si J, Ge Y, Zhuang S, Wang LJ, Chen S, Gong R. Adrenocorticotropic hormone ameliorates acute kidney injury by steroidogenic-dependent and -independent mechanisms. *Kidney Int* (2013) **83**(4):635–46. doi:10.1038/ki.2012.447
88. Getting SJ, Gibbs L, Clark AJ, Flower RJ, Perretti M. POMC gene-derived peptides activate melanocortin type 3 receptor on murine macrophages, suppress cytokine release, and inhibit neutrophil migration in acute experimental inflammation. *J Immunol* (1999) **162**(12):7446–53.
89. Scheiermann C, Kunisaki Y, Frenette PS. Circadian control of the immune system. *Nat Rev Immunol* (2013) **13**(3):190–8. doi:10.1038/nri3386
90. Geiger SS, Fagundes CT, Siegel RM. Chrono-immunology: progress and challenges in understanding links between the circadian and immune systems. *Immunology* (2015) **146**(3):349–58. doi:10.1111/imm.12525
91. Gibbs JE, Ray DW. The role of the circadian clock in rheumatoid arthritis. *Arthritis Res Ther* (2013) **15**(1):205. doi:10.1186/ar4146
92. Durrington HJ, Farrow SN, Loudon AS, Ray DW. The circadian clock and asthma. *Thorax* (2014) **69**(1):90–2. doi:10.1136/thoraxjnl-2013-203482
93. Castanon-Cervantes O, Wu M, Ehlen JC, Paul K, Gamble KL, Johnson RL, et al. Dysregulation of inflammatory responses by chronic circadian disruption. *J Immunol* (2010) **185**(10):5796–805. doi:10.4049/jimmunol.1001026
94. Knutsson A. Health disorders of shift workers. *Occup Med (Lond)* (2003) **53**(2):103–8. doi:10.1093/occmed/kqg048
95. Silver AC, Arjona A, Hughes ME, Nitabach MN, Fikrig E. Circadian expression of clock genes in mouse macrophages, dendritic cells, and B cells. *Brain Behav Immun* (2012) **26**(3):407–13. doi:10.1016/j.bbi.2011.10.001

96. Keller M, Mazuch J, Abraham U, Eom GD, Herzog ED, Volk HD, et al. A circadian clock in macrophages controls inflammatory immune responses. *Proc Natl Acad Sci U S A* (2009) **106**(50):21407–12. doi:10.1073/pnas.0906361106
97. Bollinger T, Leutz A, Leliavski A, Skrum L, Kovac J, Bonacina L, et al. Circadian clocks in mouse and human CD4+ T cells. *PLoS One* (2011) **6**(12):e29801. doi:10.1371/journal.pone.0029801
98. Cuesta M, Cermakian N, Boivin DB. Glucocorticoids entrain molecular clock components in human peripheral cells. *FASEB J* (2015) **29**(4):1360–70. doi:10.1096/fj.14-265686
99. Reiche EM, Nunes SO, Morimoto HK. Stress, depression, the immune system, and cancer. *Lancet Oncol* (2004) **5**(10):617–25. doi:10.1016/S1470-2045(04)01597-9
100. Ben-Eliyahu S, Page GG, Yirmiya R, Shakhar G. Evidence that stress and surgical interventions promote tumor development by suppressing natural killer cell activity. *Int J Cancer* (1999) **80**(6):880–8. doi:10.1002/(SICI)1097-0215(19990315)80:6<880::AID-IJC14>3.0.CO;2-Y
101. Nielsen NR, Zhang ZF, Kristensen TS, Netterstrom B, Schnohr P, Gronbaek M. Self reported stress and risk of breast cancer: prospective cohort study. *BMJ* (2005) **331**(7516):548. doi:10.1136/bmj.38547.638183.06
102. Protheroe D, Turvey K, Horgan K, Benson E, Bowers D, House A. Stressful life events and difficulties and onset of breast cancer: case-control study. *BMJ* (1999) **319**(7216):1027–30. doi:10.1136/bmj.319.7216.1027
103. Fonken LK, Weber MD, Daut RA, Kitt MM, Frank MG, Watkins LR, et al. Stress-induced neuroinflammatory priming is time of day dependent. *Psychoneuroendocrinology* (2016) **66**:82–90. doi:10.1016/j.psyneuen.2016.01.006
104. Gibbs J, Ince L, Matthews L, Mei J, Bell T, Yang N, et al. An epithelial circadian clock controls pulmonary inflammation and glucocorticoid action. *Nat Med* (2014) **20**(8):919–26. doi:10.1038/nm.3599
105. Marpegan L, Bekinschtein TA, Costas MA, Golombek DA. Circadian responses to endotoxin treatment in mice. *J Neuroimmunol* (2005) **160**(1–2):102–9. doi:10.1016/j.jneuroim.2004.11.003
106. Okada K, Yano M, Doki Y, Azama T, Iwanaga H, Miki H, et al. Injection of LPS causes transient suppression of biological clock genes in rats. *J Surg Res* (2008) **145**(1):5–12. doi:10.1016/j.jss.2007.01.010
107. Nava F, Carta G, Haynes LW. Lipopolysaccharide increases arginine-vasopressin release from rat suprachiasmatic nucleus slice cultures. *Neurosci Lett* (2000) **288**(3):228–30. doi:10.1016/S0304-3940(00)01199-X
108. Cavadini G, Petrzilka S, Kohler P, Jud C, Tobler I, Birchler T, et al. TNF-alpha suppresses the expression of clock genes by interfering with E-box-mediated transcription. *Proc Natl Acad Sci U S A* (2007) **104**(31):12843–8. doi:10.1073/pnas.0701466104
109. Buske-Kirschbaum A, von Auer K, Krieger S, Weis S, Rauh W, Hellhammer D. Blunted cortisol responses to psychosocial stress in asthmatic children: a general feature of atopic disease? *Psychosom Med* (2003) **65**(5):806–10. doi:10.1097/01.PSY.0000095916.25975.4F
110. Wamboldt MZ, Laudenslager M, Wamboldt FS, Kelsay K, Hewitt J. Adolescents with atopic disorders have an attenuated cortisol response to laboratory stress. *J Allergy Clin Immunol* (2003) **111**(3):509–14. doi:10.1067/mai.2003.140
111. Fei GH, Liu RY, Zhang ZH, Zhou JN. Alterations in circadian rhythms of melatonin and cortisol in patients with bronchial asthma. *Acta Pharmacol Sin* (2004) **25**(5):651–6.
112. Fidan V, Alp HH, Kalkandelen S, Cingi C. Melatonin and cortisol rhythm in patients with extensive nasal polyposis. *Am J Otolaryngol* (2013) **34**(1):61–4. doi:10.1016/j.amjoto.2012.09.001
113. Michalaki M, Margeli T, Tsekouras A, Gogos CH, Vagenakis AG, Kyriazopoulou V. Hypothalamic-pituitary-adrenal axis response to the severity of illness in non-critically ill patients: does relative corticosteroid insufficiency exist? *Eur J Endocrinol* (2010) **162**(2):341–7. doi:10.1530/EJE-09-0883
114. Shanks N, Larocque S, Meaney MJ. Neonatal endotoxin exposure alters the development of the hypothalamic-pituitary-adrenal axis: early illness and later responsivity to stress. *J Neurosci* (1995) **15**(1 Pt 1):376–84.
115. Buttgereit F, Doering G, Schaeffler A, Witte S, Sierakowski S, Gromnica-Ihle E, et al. Efficacy of modified-release versus standard prednisone to reduce duration of morning stiffness of the joints in rheumatoid arthritis (CAPRA-1): a double-blind, randomised controlled trial. *Lancet* (2008) **371**(9608):205–14. doi:10.1016/S0140-6736(08)60132-4

2

Stress-Related and Circadian Secretion and Target Tissue Actions of Glucocorticoids: Impact on Health

Nicolas C. Nicolaides[1,2], Evangelia Charmandari[1,2], Tomoshige Kino[3] and George P. Chrousos[1,2]*

[1] Division of Endocrinology, Metabolism and Diabetes, First Department of Pediatrics, National and Kapodistrian University of Athens Medical School, 'Aghia Sophia' Children's Hospital, Athens, Greece, [2] Division of Endocrinology and Metabolism, Center of Clinical, Experimental Surgery and Translational Research, Biomedical Research Foundation of the Academy of Athens, Athens, Greece, [3] Division of Experimental Genetics, Sidra Medical and Research Center, Doha, Qatar

***Correspondence:**
Nicolas C. Nicolaides
nnicolaides@bioacademy.gr

Living organisms are highly complex systems that must maintain a dynamic equilibrium or homeostasis that requires energy to be sustained. Stress is a state in which several extrinsic or intrinsic disturbing stimuli, the stressors, threaten, or are perceived as threatening, homeostasis. To achieve homeostasis against the stressors, organisms have developed a highly sophisticated system, the stress system, which provides neuroendocrine adaptive responses, to restore homeostasis. These responses must be appropriate in terms of size and/or duration; otherwise, they may sustain life but be associated with detrimental effects on numerous physiologic functions of the organism, leading to a state of disease-causing disturbed homeostasis or cacostasis. In addition to facing a broad spectrum of external and/or internal stressors, organisms are subject to recurring environmental changes associated with the rotation of the planet around itself and its revolution around the sun. To adjust their homeostasis and to synchronize their activities to day/night cycles, organisms have developed an evolutionarily conserved biologic system, the "clock" system, which influences several physiologic functions in a circadian fashion. Accumulating evidence suggests that the stress system is intimately related to the circadian clock system, with dysfunction of the former resulting in dysregulation of the latter and *vice versa*. In this review, we describe the functional components of the two systems, we discuss their multilevel interactions, and we present how excessive or prolonged activity of the stress system affects the circadian rhythm of glucocorticoid secretion and target tissue effects.

Keywords: stress, stress system, hypothalamic–pituitary–adrenal axis, glucocorticoids, glucocorticoid receptor, circadian endocrine rhythms, clock system

THE STRESS SYSTEM

The stress system consists of the locus caeruleus/norepinephrine autonomic nervous systems and the hypothalamic–pituitary–adrenal (HPA) axis. These two components interact with each other, as well as with other brain subsystems, such as the mesocortical and the mesolimbic dopaminergic system, which is involved in reward and motivation, the central nucleus of the amygdalae, which generate fear and/or anger, and the arcuate nucleus of the hypothalamus participating in stress system control (1–4). The activity of the stress system is influenced by several neurochemical modulators (e.g., serotonin, acetylcholine, γ-aminobutyric acid, glutamate and endogenous cannabinoids, and benzodiazepines) (1–4). When homeostasis is threatened or perceived by the individual as threatened by stressors, the locus caeruleus/norepinephrine/autonomic nervous systems release norepinephrine in the brain and the systemic circulation, while epinephrine is secreted by the adrenal medulla. On the other hand, the HPA axis is associated with the production and secretion of glucocorticoids by the *zona fasciculata* of the adrenal cortex (1–4). Glucocorticoids play a fundamental role in the maintenance of basal and stress-related homeostasis, regulating many physiologic functions through genomic actions mediated by their cognate intracellular receptor, the glucocorticoid receptor (GR); the latter belongs to the steroid receptor family of the nuclear receptor superfamily of transcription factors (4–8).

The human glucocorticoid receptor (hGR) is encoded by the *NR3C1* gene, which is located in the long arm of chromosome 5 and is composed of 10 exons. The alternative splicing of exon 9 generates the two main protein isoforms of the receptor, the hGRα and the hGRβ. Expressed in every tissue except the suprachiasmatic nucleus (SCN) of the hypothalamus, the hGRα is activated following binding of natural or synthetic glucocorticoids to its ligand-binding domain and binds to the regulatory regions of glucocorticoid-responsive genes through its DNA-binding domain and/or interacts with other transcription factors altering their transcriptional activities (*vide infra*) (6–10). On the other hand, the hGRβ isoform is an enigma in endocrine physiology. Exclusively localized in the nucleus of certain cell types, such as endothelial cells, the hGRβ acts as a dominant-negative inhibitor of hGRα-induced transcriptional activity through well-delineated molecular mechanisms (11–13). Interestingly, this receptor isoform can influence the transcription rate of several genes independently of hGRα (14, 15). Recent studies have demonstrated that hGRβ may be involved in insulin signaling and implicated in gluconeogenesis and inflammation in mouse liver (16, 17). New evidence suggests a pivotal role of the GRβ isoform in the molecular cascades of glioma formation and bladder cancer cells migration (18–20). Further to the alternative splicing of exon 9, Lu and Cidlowski showed that the initiation of the hGRα mRNA translation might occur through eight different sites giving rise to receptor isoforms with variable N-terminal domains: hGRα-A (classic GRα), hGRα-B, hGRα-C1, hGRα-C2, hGRα-C3, hGRα-D1, hGRα-D2, and hGRα-D3, which have distinct properties in terms of intracellular localization and transcriptional activity (10, 21). We assume similar translation processing of the GRβ isoform.

At the cellular level, the glucocorticoid signaling pathway is initiated by ligand-induced activation of the primarily cytoplasmic hGRα, which dissociates from chaperon heat shock proteins and immunophillins, and translocates into the nucleus, where it binds, as homo- or heterodimer, to specific DNA sequences, the glucocorticoid response elements, within the regulatory regions of target genes, thereby influencing their transcription in a positive or negative fashion (4, 6–8, 10). In addition to direct hGRα binding to glucocorticoid-responsive genes, glucocorticoids can influence the transcription of several other genes independently of DNA binding. Indeed, the activated hGRα isoform can interact, possibly as a monomer, with other transcription factors, such as the nuclear factor-κB, the activator protein-1, and the signal transducers and activators of transcription, suppressing or inducing their transcriptional activity (4, 6–8, 10). In addition to the well-described genomic actions, glucocorticoids can induce some cellular effects in a very short-time frame. These effects are referred to as "non-genomic glucocorticoid actions" and are likely to be mediated by membrane-bound GRs, which may trigger the activation of kinase signaling pathways (22–24).

THE CIRCADIAN CLOCK SYSTEM

To adjust their daily activities to light/dark changes, organisms have developed a highly conserved timekeeping system, the circadian clock system (from the Latin "circa diem" meaning "approximately a day"), which creates internal rhythmicity under the influence of day/night cycles. This regulatory system is composed of a central "master" clock located in the SCN of hypothalamus, and peripheral "slave" clocks, which are ubiquitously expressed in all tissues (25–27). Importantly, peripheral clocks are tightly synchronized to the central clock through as yet unknown possibly neural or neuroendocrine mechanisms. The central clock influences virtually all physiologic functions, such as sleep/wakefulness, feeding, thermoregulation, energy expenditure, glucose homeostasis, and the activity of the HPA axis. Similarly, peripheral clocks regulate several functions of their residing tissues, ultimately contributing to the homeostasis of living organisms (25–28).

At the cellular level, the circadian clock system is composed of transcriptional/translational loops, which create an intrinsic, self-oscillating circadian rhythm in both the central and peripheral clocks (**Figure 1**). At the molecular level, these feedback loops are mediated by the circadian locomotor output cycle kaput/brain–muscle–arnt-like protein 1 (CLOCK/BMAL1) heterodimer and other negative transcription factors, such as the Periods (PER1, PER2, and PER3) and Cryptochromes (CRY1 and CRY2). In the principal or core transcription loop, the activated CLOCK/BMAL1 heterodimer binds to the E-box response elements and induces the expression of *Pers* and *Crys*. These proteins associate with casein kinase (Csnk) 1ε and δ and undergo phosphorylation (29–31). The phosphorylated isoforms then translocate to the nucleus and suppress the transcriptional activity of the CLOCK/BMAL1 heterodimer. In addition, several other clock-related genes, such as retinoic acid receptor-related orphan receptor α (RORα) and reverse viral erythroblastosis oncogene product (REV-ERBα), are upregulated by the CLOCK/BMAL1 heterodimer, forming an auxiliary loop, which stabilizes the transcriptional activity of the core loop. The transcription factors of both principal and auxiliary loops can modulate the expression of many clock-responsive genes in various tissues (27, 29–31).

In addition to light/dark signals, the circadian clock system is strongly influenced by several metabolic inputs, particularly those associated with ingestion of food (**Figure 1**) (33–39). Indeed, the

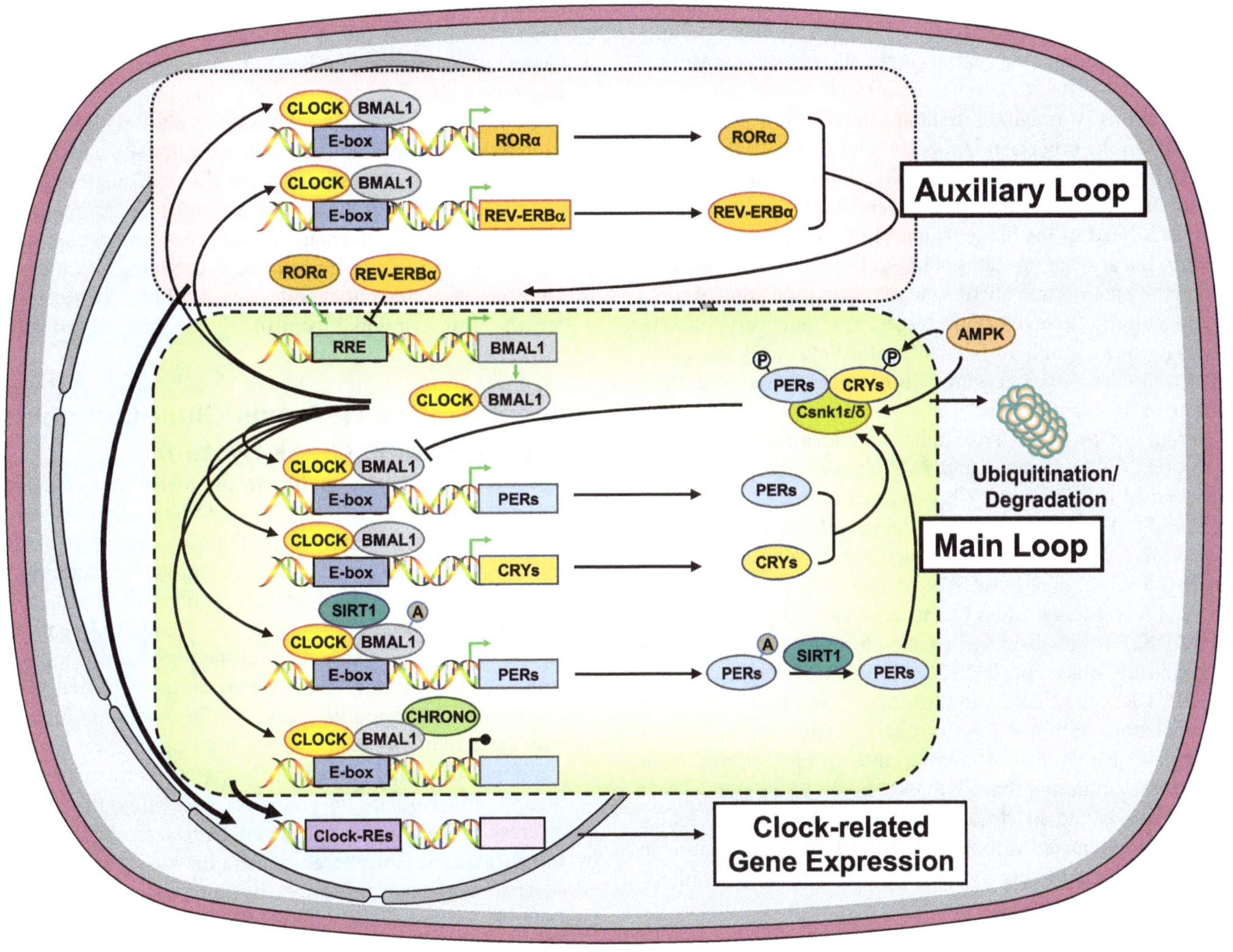

FIGURE 1 | Molecular components of the main and auxiliary transcriptional/translational loops of the circadian clock system. In the main transcription loop, the heterodimer CLOCK/BMAL1 causes upregulation of *Pers* and *Crys*. PERs and CRYs undergo phosphorylation by the Csnk1ε/δ and translocate to the nucleus suppressing the transcriptional activity of the CLOCK/BMAL1. Moreover, CLOCK/BMAL1 influences the transcription rate of several other clock-related genes, such as RORα and REV-ERBα, giving rise to an auxiliary transcription loop. AMPK participates in the main transcription loop by phosphorylating CRYs, PERs, and Csnk1ε. SIRT1 functions as a counter-regulatory mechanism for the acetyltransferase activity of the CLOCK by deacetylating BMAL1, PER2, and histone 3. CHRONO, a recently identified BMAL target was found to interact with BMAL1, repressing the main transcription loop *via* recruitment of histone deacetylase 1. A, acetyl residue on the acetylated molecules; AMPK, adenosine monophosphate-activated protein kinase; BMAL1, brain–muscle–arnt-like protein 1; CHRONO, ChIP-derived repressor of network oscillator; CLOCK, circadian locomotor output cycle kaput; CRYs, cryptochromes; Csnk1ε/δ, casein kinase 1ε/δ; P, phosphate residue on the phosphorylated molecules; PERs, periods; RORα, retinoic acid receptor-related orphan nuclear receptor α; SIRT1, sirtuin 1. Modified from Ref. (32).

adenosine monophosphate-activated protein kinase (AMPK), a tissue sensor and master regulator of energy balance, seems to influence the activity of the clock system through energy-dependent signals. AMPK does so by phosphorylating CRYs and PERs leading to their degradation. AMPK can also cause destabilization of PERs indirectly by increasing the activity of Csnk1ε through phosphorylation, resulting in Csnk1ε-mediated degradation of PERs (**Figure 1**) (33–36). In addition to AMPK, the longevity and metabolism-associated sirtuin 1 (SIRT1) was demonstrated to deacetylate BMAL1, PER2, and histone 3 depending on the NAD+ cellular levels, possibly functioning as a counter-regulatory mechanism for the histone acetyltransferase activity of the CLOCK (**Figure 1**) (35–39).

MOLECULAR INTERRELATIONS BETWEEN THE HPA AXIS AND THE CIRCADIAN CLOCK SYSTEM: THE PIVOTAL ROLE OF GLUCOCORTICOIDS

Influence of the Circadian Clock System on the HPA Axis

A growing body of evidence suggests that the stress-responsive HPA axis and the circadian clock system interact with each other at multiple levels (27, 32, 40–45). Indeed, the central clock in the SCN projects neurons in the paraventricular nucleus (PVN) of the hypothalamus providing the basis for the diurnal oscillation of circulating glucocorticoid concentrations, which are higher during the day for diurnal species and at night for nocturnal species (28). In addition, the central clock influences the sensitivity of the adrenal cortex to adrenocorticotropic hormone (ACTH) concentrations through a multisynaptic neuronal pathway (46, 47). On the other hand, in peripheral tissues, the CLOCK/BMAL1 heterodimer represses the hGRα-induced transcriptional activity through CLOCK-mediated acetylation of multiple lysine residues located in the hinge region of the receptor (48–51). In humans, the acetylation status of hGRα is higher in the morning than in the evening, and mirrors the circadian oscillation of cortisol concentrations; therefore, the target tissue glucocorticoid sensitivity reaches a zenith during the evening hours (52). Moreover, CRY1 and CRY2 interact with hGRα leading to reduced DNA binding of the receptor (53).

Recent *in vitro* and *in vivo* studies have identified a novel circadian CLOCK component and BMAL target gene, the *Gm129*, later termed as "*Chrono*" ("ChIP-derived repressor of network oscillator") (**Figure 1**) (54, 55). *Chrono* mRNA was found to oscillate in a circadian fashion, which was antiphasic to that of *Bmal1* mRNA, in the mouse SCN, as well as in many peripheral tissues. *Chrono* was showed to encode a 45-kDa protein, called "CHRONO," which displayed robust circadian oscillation with the opposite phase of BMAL1. CHRONO interacted with BMAL1, CRY2, and DEC2 and functioned as a repressor of the principal transcriptional loop through recruitment of histone deacetylase 1 (55, 56). Moreover, interesting findings from these studies indicated that CHRONO might be a potential link between the circadian clock system and the HPA axis, since this protein interacted with the GR, and *Chrono* knockout mice had increased circulating serum corticosterone concentrations, compared to wild-type mice (56, 57).

Influence of the Circadian Clock System on Glucocorticoid Secretion

Glucocorticoids, the end products of the HPA axis, play a pivotal role in mediating the stress response and contribute to the tight synchronization of peripheral clocks. These steroid hormones are secreted into the systemic circulation in an ultradian, circadian, and stress-related fashion (58). The ultradian or pulsatile pattern of glucocorticoid release is characterized by a time period of 80–110 min in humans, and its activity is independent of SCN input (59). The circadian release of glucocorticoids is influenced by three factors: (i) the SCN-activated HPA axis, (ii) the SCN-derived autonomic innervation of the adrenal glands through the splanchnic nerve, and (iii) local adrenal clocks (60). As mentioned earlier, SCN neurons send projections into the area of PVN of hypothalamus, thereby creating the diurnal fluctuation of corticotropin-releasing hormone (CRH), arginine vasopressin (AVP), ACTH, and glucocorticoids (28). Furthermore, SCN neurons transmit light information to the adrenal glands *via* splanchnic nerve innervation and increase glucocorticoid release in an HPA-independent fashion (46, 47). The transmission of the light signal to the adrenal cortex is likely to be mediated by catecholamines and/or neuropeptides produced by the adrenal medulla (61). In addition to the photic transmission, the SCN-guided autonomic innervation also alters the sensitivity of the adrenal cortex to ACTH concentrations (46, 47). As already known in the 1960s and as recently confirmed, isolated adrenal gland tissues and cells display robust circadian secretion of steroids, suggesting that the SCN input is not the only prerequisite for diurnal oscillation of the adrenal transcriptome (62). Indeed, adrenal glands harbor their own circadian clocks influencing the rhythmic expression of approximately 10% of the adrenal genome (63). Among genes regulated by adrenal circadian clocks, the steroidogenic acute regulatory protein, a rate-limiting gene encoding a cholesterol transporter into the mitochondria, is rhythmically expressed under the transcriptional control of the adrenal circadian BMAL1 (64).

Influence of the HPA Axis/Glucocorticoids on the Circadian Clock System

Glucocorticoids, through binding to the hGRα, can effectively reset the activity of peripheral clocks, adding another level of interaction between the HPA axis and the circadian clock system (65). Glucocorticoids alter circadian oscillations of several clock-related genes, including *Pers*, by phase shifting their expression in peripheral organs (66). Therefore, *Per1* and *Per2* genes are upregulated, causing a phase delay of the peripheral clocks, but not the SCN master clock (67). Moreover, the activated hGRα transrepresses the *Rev-ERBα* and *RORα* genes, influencing directly the activity of the auxiliary transcriptional/translational loop and indirectly that of the main loop (68). At the tissue level, glucocorticoids regulate several local oscillators in different brain areas, as well as in peripheral tissues, as demonstrated by rodent studies. Chronic administration of prednisolone or adrenalectomy strongly influences the expression of clock-related genes [reviewed in Ref. (69)]. In the PVN, adrenalectomy causes a reduction in the amplitude of the expression of *Per1*, whereas acute stress results in the increased expression of the same gene (70, 71). In several limbic areas, many clock genes are suppressed by adrenalectomy, such as the *Per2*. The expression of the latter was shown to be restored when adrenalectomized rats were given corticosterone placed in their drinking water (72). In the hippocampus, the expression of *Per1* was influenced by glucocorticoids (73). In peripheral tissues, glucocorticoids modulate local clocks (74–78). In kidney, adrenalectomy causes phase delay in *Per1* oscillations (74). In white adipose tissue, dexamethasone increases the amplitude of oscillations of clock genes in preadipocytes and attenuates them in differentiated adipocytes (75). In bronchial epithelial cells of the lung, the administration of dexamethasone resulted in upregulation of the *Per1* (76). In cardiac muscle tissue, dexamethasone phase shifts the expression of local clock genes (77). In cornea, adrenalectomy causes a phase delay in *Per1* (74). Finally, the bone local clock can be reset by dexamethasone (78).

Interplay between Stress and Circadian Clock Systems on the HPA Axis/Glucocorticoids

In the absence of stressors, the central clock regulates the HPA axis activity and influences the sensitivity of the adrenal cortex to

ACTH (28, 46, 47). These two mechanisms are responsible for the diurnal fluctuation of circulating glucocorticoid concentrations (28, 46, 47). The peripheral clocks are synchronized to the activity of the central clock through as yet unknown, perhaps neural or endocrine mechanisms (79, 80). In addition, the peripheral clocks suppress the hGRα-induced transcriptional activity through acetylation of the receptor by the CLOCK/BMAL1 heterodimer, possibly functioning as a counter-regulatory mechanism against the circulating glucocorticoid concentrations (48) (**Figure 2**).

Under stressful conditions, acute stressors induce HPA axis activity, thereby increasing the synthesis and secretion of glucocorticoids by the adrenal cortex. Upon binding to the GRα, secreted glucocorticoids phase shift the expression of several clock-related genes, such as *Per1* and *Per2*, and reset peripheral clocks but not the central clock, granted that GRα is not expressed in SCN neurons (65, 66, 68, 81, 82) (**Figure 2**). Therefore, the circadian rhythm in peripheral clocks phase shifts from that of central clock under the regulation of the HPA axis, leading to transient uncoupling of the central and peripheral clocks (48). Following termination of the acute stress, the central clock can reset peripheral clocks to their initial phase within a few days (65, 83). hGRα-induced transcriptional activity may be influenced by

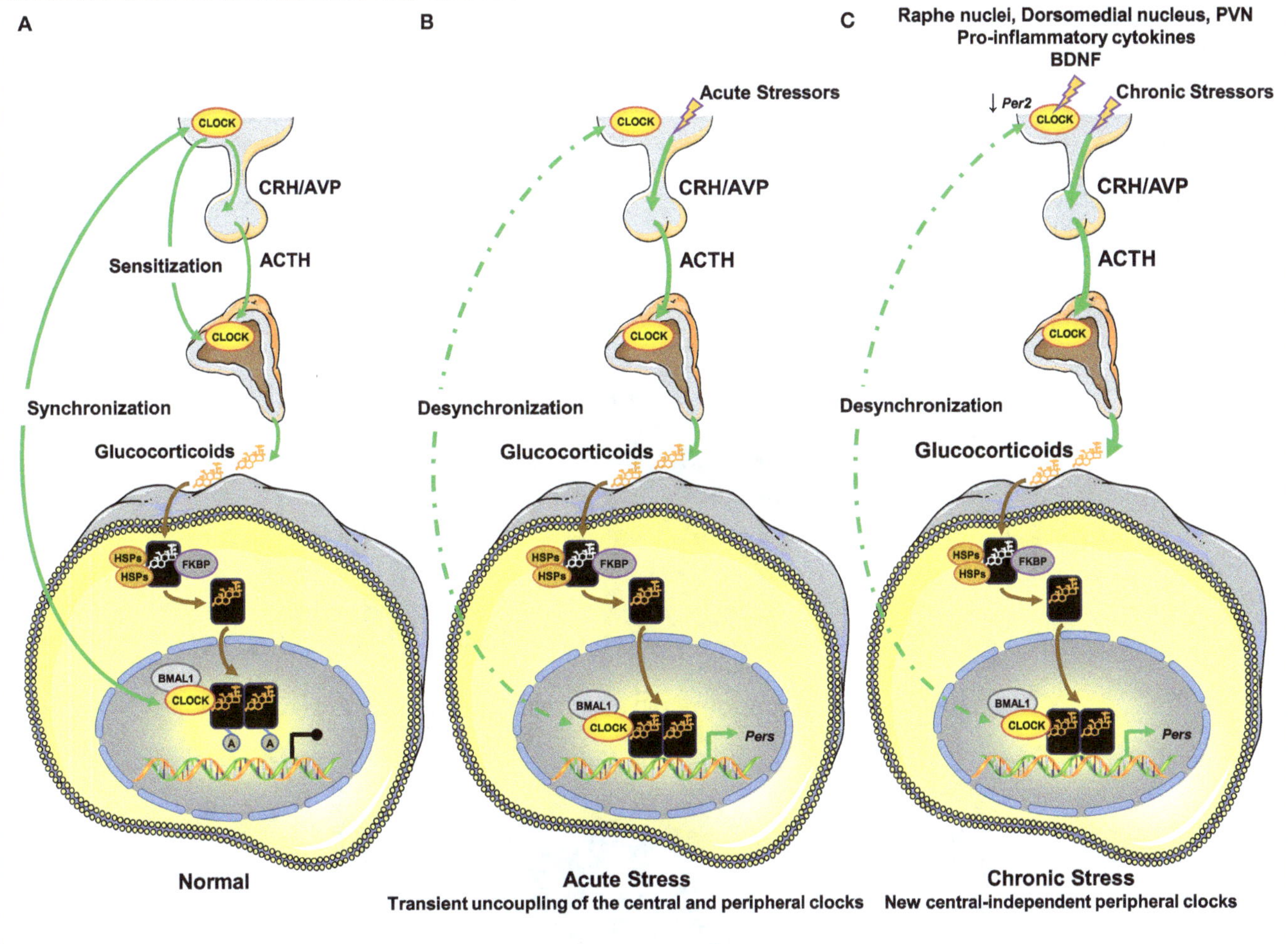

FIGURE 2 | Molecular interactions between the hypothalamic–pituitary–adrenal (HPA) axis and the circadian clock system. (A) In the absence of stressors, **(B)** under acute stressors, and **(C)** under chronic stressors. **(A)** In normal conditions, the central suprachiasmatic nucleus (SCN) clock creates the diurnal fluctuation of glucocorticoid concentrations by regulating the activity of the HPA axis through neuronal projections and by influencing the adrenal cortex sensitivity to ACTH through the splanchnic nerves. The peripheral clocks are synchronized to the circadian activity of the central clock through unknown mechanisms and suppress the transcriptional activity of the hGRα by CLOCK-mediated acetylation of the receptor. **(B)** Under stressful conditions, acute stressors activate the HPA axis leading to increased glucocorticoid concentrations independently of the central clock-mediated circadian regulation of the HPA axis. In peripheral tissues, glucocorticoids phase shift and reset peripheral clocks leading to uncoupling of the latter from the central clock, granted that the GRα protein is not expressed in the SCN. In addition, the transcriptional activity of the hGRα may be influenced by the phase-shifted peripheral clocks by unknown mechanisms. Following termination of the acute stress, the central clock can reset peripheral clocks to their initial phase. **(C)** In the presence of chronic stressors, the SCN receives indirect glucocorticoid feedback from raphe nuclei, the hypothalamic dorsomedial nucleus, and the paraventricular nucleus. Its activity is also influenced by pro-inflammatory cytokines and BDNF. Chronic stressors trigger the release of glucocorticoids by the adrenal cortex independently of the central clock-mediated diurnal regulation of the HPA axis. This stress-induced glucocorticoid secretion phase shifts and resets peripheral clocks leading to uncoupling of the latter from the central clock. A, acetyl residue on the acetylated molecules; ACTH, adrenocorticotropic hormone; AVP, arginine vasopressin; BDNF, brain-derived neurotrophic factor; BMAL1, brain–muscle–arnt-like protein 1; CLOCK, circadian locomotor output cycle kaput; CRH, corticotropin-releasing hormone; FKBP, FK506-binding protein; GR, glucocorticoid receptor; HSPs, heat shock proteins; PERs, periods.

phase-shifted peripheral clocks in local tissues, but the specific mechanisms remain to be elucidated (**Figure 2**).

In the presence of chronic or repeated stressors, accumulating evidence suggests that the non-expressing GRα SCN receives indirect glucocorticoid feedback from peripheral tissues expressing GRα, such as the raphe nuclei, the hypothalamic dorsomedial nucleus, and the PVN (84, 85) (**Figure 2**). Indeed, chronic stressors reduce the expression of *Per2* in the SCN, suggesting an impact of chronic stress on SCN function (86, 87). In addition to glucocorticoids, several other molecules in the periphery (e.g., pro-inflammatory cytokines, brain-derived neurotrophic factor, etc.) provide feedback to the central SCN clock during chronic stress (88, 89) (**Figure 2**). As chronic or repeated stressors trigger the secretion of glucocorticoids into the systemic circulation independently of the central clock-mediated diurnal regulation of the HPA axis, stress-related glucocorticoid secretion phase shifts and resets peripheral clocks leading to uncoupling of the latter and the central clock (48) (**Figure 2**). We speculate that a prolonged and/or excessive or deficient adaptive response may not allow the proper rhythmicity of peripheral clocks under the control of the central clock, ultimately leading to several pathologic conditions.

CLINICAL IMPLICATIONS

Alterations in circadian release of glucocorticoids have been found in several pathologic conditions, such as mood, metabolic and inflammatory disorders, as well as in cancers (60). On the other hand, chronically stressed (CS) humans, rotating shift workers and subjects frequently exposed to jet lag because of trans-timezone traveling have been demonstrated to be at increased risk for cardiometabolic disorders and their sequelae myocardial infarction and stroke (69). Compared to normal subjects, CS individuals might display an uncoupling between the circadian clock and the HPA axis, a decreased variance between evening nadir and morning zenith cortisol concentrations, as well as an inadequate response to a low-dose dexamethasone suppression test as a result of chronic hyperactivation of PVN CRH and vasopressin secretion (90) (**Figure 3**). We hypothesize that shift workers or trans-timezone travelers might show a phase-altered curve of cortisol concentrations (**Figure 3**). Individuals with alterations in circadian secretion of glucocorticoids might develop psychiatric diseases (e.g., anxiety and depression) and autoimmune/inflammatory conditions, with

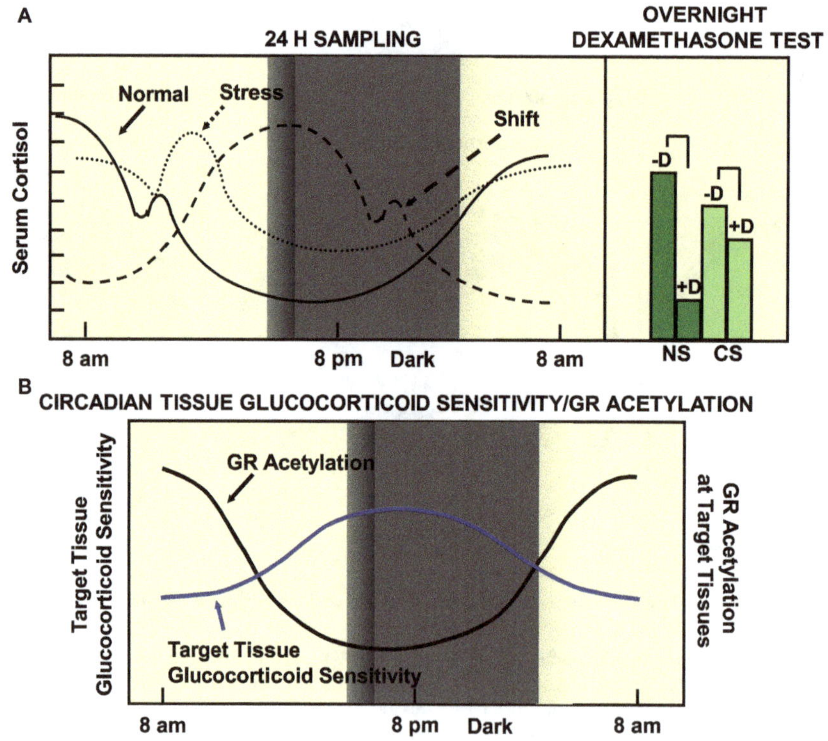

FIGURE 3 | (A) Circadian pattern of cortisol secretion in normal humans, CS subjects and rotating shift workers (left panel), and the responses of normal and stressed subjects to overnight dexamethasone suppression test. **(B)** The target tissue sensitivity is lower in the morning and higher at night, mirroring the status of GR acetylation. **(A)** A population of 284 51-year-old men were examined by obtaining a detailed medical history, by performing anthropometry, and by measuring a series of diurnal salivary cortisol concentrations. Participants were asked to fill in a questionnaire about self-perceived stress and underwent a low-dose overnight dexamethasone suppression test. Normal participants were characterized by increased variance, distant zeniths in the morning and nadirs in the evening, and an appropriate suppression in the morning salivary cortisol concentrations following a low-dose dexamethasone suppression test. On the other hand, CS participants showed a decreased variance, evening nadir elevations and morning zenith decreases of cortisol concentrations, as well as an inadequate response to a low-dose dexamethasone suppression test. We speculate that rotating shift workers might be characterized by a phase-delayed curve of salivary cortisol concentrations, compared to that of normal participants. CS, chronically stressed individuals; D, midnight dexamethasone administration; NS, non-stressed individuals. Modified from Ref. (35, 90).

rheumatoid arthritis and asthma as representative examples (91). Furthermore, chronic stress with loss of a proper cortisol circadian rhythm result in glucocorticoid excess-related increased appetite, splachnic obesity, and metabolic disturbances, such as hyperglycemia, insulin resistance, dyslipidemia, osteopenia/osteoporosis, and hypertension (27). All the above pieces of evidence strongly suggest that any dysfunction of the stress system may cause dysregulation of the circadian clock system and *vice versa*.

Several studies in animals and humans have shown that diurnal fluctuations of cortisol concentrations are flattened in obesity. Indeed, genetically obese rats, *db/db* mice, and obese adults display dampened glucocorticoid circadian rhythms (92, 93). In addition, childhood overweight and obesity are associated with a reduction in the amplitude of ultradian glucocorticoid secretion (94). Moreover, subjects carrying specific *Clock* polymorphisms are more susceptible to develop obesity and metabolic syndrome (95, 96). Not only in obesity but also in diabetes mellitus there is a flattened 24-h pattern of cortisol concentrations. In diabetic adults, salivary cortisol was low in the morning and high in the afternoon and evening (97). Finally, mice deficient in the *Cry* gene had a defective suppression of HPA axis, ultimately leading to glucose intolerance and metabolic syndrome (98).

Disruption of circadian rhythms, as often observed in shift workers, may cause mood disorders (99). Mice exposed to a short 7-h light/dark change have higher concentrations of corticosterone and exhibit depressive symptoms (100). On the other hand, subjects suffering from major depression have flattened diurnal glucocorticoid rhythms, probably due to altered secretion of CRH and AVP in the brain (101). They also display defective clock-related gene expression in the peripheral blood cells, as well as in brain tissues (102, 103). Indeed, the rhythmic expression of core clock transcription factor genes, such as *Bmal1*, *Per1-3*, *Dec1/2*, and *Rev-erbα* is attenuated in brain regions influencing mood, compared to healthy controls. In addition to depression, several other psychiatric conditions, including bipolar disorder, posttraumatic stress disorder, attention deficit hyperactivity disorder, schizophrenia, and chronic alcoholism, are examples in which the interconnection between the stress system and the circadian clock system is dysregulated (104).

Chronic inflammatory disorders, such as rheumatoid arthritis and asthma, are characterized by worsening symptoms in early morning hours (60). This phenomenon has been attributed to the circadian fluctuation of circulating cytokines, such as interleukin (IL)-1α, IL-6, and tumor necrosis factor-α, which strongly participate in the pathogenesis of these diseases (105, 106). These inflammatory cytokines reach their peak concentrations earlier than cortisol; however, the target tissue glucocorticoid sensitivity is low during that time because of CLOCK-mediated suppressed hGRα-transcriptional and transrepressive activities (48). Furthermore, night-shift workers have increased risk for common infections and multiple sclerosis, indicating that dysregulation of the circadian clock system contributes undoubtedly to the development of inflammatory diseases (107, 108).

Subjects with prolonged night-shift work are also more susceptible to develop several cancers (109). Previous studies have shown that SCN damage, chronic jet lag, as well as *Per2* deficiency contribute to cancer initiation and progression (110–112). On the other hand, patients with breast, ovarian, lung, and kidney cancers have flattened or antiphasic diurnal oscillations of cortisol, compared to normal subjects (60). Future studies are still needed to clarify the molecular mechanisms underlying the association between stress, circadian rhythms, and carcinogenesis.

In addition to metabolic, psychiatric, autoimmune/inflammatory, and malignant disorders, sleep disturbances and disorders have been associated with alterations in circadian secretion of glucocorticoids (69). Indeed, a prolonged or excessive activation of the HPA axis results in insufficient sleep, which, in turn, may cause an elevation of glucocorticoid concentrations and cytokines in the early evening, forming a vicious cycle (69). Moreover, sleep deprivation has been associated with an increase in HPA axis activity in the evening hours, thereby altering the ability of the latter to properly autoregulate itself (113–115). Idiopathic chronic insomnia has been associated with evening hypercortisolism and hypercytokinemia influencing substantially the transcription rate of numerous genes in the brain (116, 117). On the other hand, a dysfunctional HPA axis could promote insomnia (69) or be affected by obstructive sleep apnea (118, 119). Not only chronic insomnia but also chronic fatigue syndrome, fibromyalgia and posttraumatic stress disorder have been linked to consistent alterations in HPA axis activity (120, 121).

CONCLUDING REMARKS AND FUTURE DIRECTIONS: SYNTHETIC GLUCOCORTICOIDS IN THE ERA OF CHRONOTHERAPY

Synthetic glucocorticoids have been widely used in the treatment of several inflammatory disorders and hematologic malignancies (122). Since target tissue glucocorticoid sensitivity is lower in the morning and higher in the evening, glucocorticoid analogs should be administered in a time-of-day dependent fashion to achieve a beneficial therapeutic outcome and to avoid their detrimental side effects, such as osteoporosis, weight gain, glucose intolerance, and psychiatric symptoms. Therefore, patients with autoimmune disorders are treated with prednisolone or other synthetic glucocorticoids in the evening, given that the hGRα is less acetylated during that time (106). In addition to inflammatory disorders, chronic administration of glucocorticoids is frequently used as substitution treatment of hypocortisolemic disorders, such as adrenal insufficiency, regardless of its etiology. Approximately two-thirds of hydrocortisone dose is usually given in the morning, while the remainder one-third is administered in two doses (in the mid-day and in the early evening) (123). Recent advances in the therapeutic manipulation of adrenal insufficiency have shown that a dual-release hydrocortisone formulation, which resembles circadian cortisol secretion, results in improved quality of life, decreased body weight and blood pressure, and improved glucose tolerance (124, 125).

Although we have gained important insight in the molecular communication between the stress system and the circadian clock system, there are many physiologic and pathophysiologic aspects of their interrelation that still elude us. The molecular mechanisms underlying resetting of peripheral clocks by glucocorticoids are under intense investigation both in normal and pathologic conditions. Moreover, the tight synchronization of peripheral clocks with the central clock remains poorly understood. Furthermore, our understanding on the function and significance of local adrenal clocks is still increasing. Future *in vitro* and *in vivo* studies will shed light on the functional significance of the cross talk between the stress system and the circadian clock system of living organisms to increase survival chance. Importantly, in parallel with the tremendous progress of molecular, cellular, and structural biology, significant advances in the field of mathematical and computer biosciences will undoubtedly help us have a deeper understanding of system interrelations. Interestingly, accumulating evidence suggests that stress-related "static" signaling pathways can be effectively transformed into functionally predictive computerized kinetic models (126–129). Such efforts will be useful for accurate predictions of a system response to acute or chronic stress, as well as to pharmacotherapy with novel medications.

AUTHOR CONTRIBUTIONS

All authors contributed equally to the conception of the work, drafted the manuscript or revisited it critically for important intellectual content, finally approved the version to be published, and agreed to be accountable for all aspects of the work in ensuring that questions related to the accuracy or integrity of any part of the work are appropriately investigated and resolved.

REFERENCES

1. Chrousos GP, Gold PW. The concepts of stress and stress system disorders: overview of physical and behavioral homeostasis. *JAMA* (1992) 267:1244–52. doi:10.1001/jama.1992.03480090092034
2. Charmandari E, Tsigos C, Chrousos GP. Endocrinology of the stress response. *Annu Rev Physiol* (2005) 67:259–84. doi:10.1146/annurev.physiol.67.040403.120816
3. Chrousos GP. Stress and disorders of the stress system. *Nat Rev Endocrinol* (2009) 5(7):374–81. doi:10.1038/nrendo.2009.106
4. Nicolaides NC, Kyratzi E, Lamprokostopoulou A, Chrousos GP, Charmandari E. Stress, the stress system and the role of glucocorticoids. *Neuroimmunomodulation* (2015) 22(1–2):6–19. doi:10.1159/000362736
5. Chrousos GP, Charmandari E, Kino T. Glucocorticoid action networks – an introduction to systems biology. *J Clin Endocrinol Metab* (2004) 89:563–4. doi:10.1210/jc.2003-032026
6. Chrousos GP, Kino T. Intracellular glucocorticoid signaling: a formerly simple system turns stochastic. *Sci STKE* (2005):e48. doi:10.1126/stke.3042005pe48
7. Rhen T, Cidlowski JA. Anti-inflammatory action of glucocorticoids – new mechanisms for old drugs. *N Engl J Med* (2005) 353:1711–23. doi:10.1056/NEJMra050541
8. Nicolaides NC, Galata Z, Kino T, Chrousos GP, Charmandari E. The human glucocorticoid receptor: molecular basis of biologic function. *Steroids* (2010) 75(1):1–12. doi:10.1016/j.steroids.2009.09.002
9. Zhou J, Cidlowski JA. The human glucocorticoid receptor: one gene, multiple proteins and diverse responses. *Steroids* (2005) 70:407–17. doi:10.1016/j.steroids.2005.02.006
10. Oakley RH, Cidlowski JA. The biology of the glucocorticoid receptor: new signaling mechanisms in health and disease. *J Allergy Clin Immunol* (2013) 132(5):1033–44. doi:10.1016/j.jaci.2013.09.007
11. Bamberger CM, Bamberger AM, de Castro M, Chrousos GP. Glucocorticoid receptor β, a potential endogenous inhibitor of glucocorticoid action in humans. *J Clin Invest* (1995) 95:2435–41. doi:10.1172/JCI117943
12. Yudt MR, Jewell CM, Bienstock RJ, Cidlowski JA. Molecular origins for the dominant negative function of human glucocorticoid receptor β. *Mol Cell Biol* (2003) 23:4319–30. doi:10.1128/MCB.23.12.4319-4330.2003
13. Charmandari E, Chrousos GP, Ichijo T, Bhattacharyya N, Vottero A, Souvatzoglou E, et al. The human glucocorticoid receptor (hGR) β isoform suppresses the transcriptional activity of hGRα by interfering with formation of active coactivator complexes. *Mol Endocrinol* (2005) 19:52–64. doi:10.1210/me.2004-0112
14. Kino T, Manoli I, Kelkar S, Wang Y, Su YA, Chrousos GP. Glucocorticoid receptor (GR) beta has intrinsic, GRalpha-independent transcriptional activity. *Biochem Biophys Res Commun* (2009) 381(4):671–5. doi:10.1016/j.bbrc.2009.02.110
15. Kino T, Su YA, Chrousos GP. Human glucocorticoid receptor isoform beta: recent understanding of its potential implications in physiology and pathophysiology. *Cell Mol Life Sci* (2009) 66(21):3435–48. doi:10.1007/s00018-009-0098-z
16. Stechschulte LA, Wuescher L, Marino JS, Hill JW, Eng C, Hinds TD Jr. Glucocorticoid receptor β stimulates Akt1 growth pathway by attenuation of PTEN. *J Biol Chem* (2014) 289:17885–94. doi:10.1074/jbc.M113.544072
17. He B, Cruz-Topete D, Oakley RH, Xiao X, Cidlowski JA. Human glucocorticoid receptor β regulates gluconeogenesis and inflammation in mouse liver. *Mol Cell Biol* (2015) 36(5):714–30. doi:10.1128/MCB.00908-15
18. Yin Y, Zhang X, Li Z, Deng L, Jiao G, Zhang B, et al. Glucocorticoid receptor β regulates injury-mediated astrocyte activation and contributes to glioma pathogenesis via modulation of β-catenin/TCF transcriptional activity. *Neurobiol Dis* (2013) 59:165–76. doi:10.1016/j.nbd.2013.07.013
19. Wang Q, Lu PH, Shi ZF, Xu YJ, Xiang J, Wang YX, et al. Glucocorticoid receptor β acts as a co-activator of T-cell factor 4 and enhances glioma cell proliferation. *Mol Neurobiol* (2015) 52(3):1106–18. doi:10.1007/s12035-014-8900-9
20. McBeth L, Nwaneri AC, Grabnar M, Demeter J, Nestor-Kalinoski A, Hinds TD Jr. Glucocorticoid receptor beta increases migration of human bladder cancer cells. *Oncotarget* (2016) 7(19):27313–24. doi:10.18632/oncotarget.8430
21. Lu NZ, Cidlowski JA. Translational regulatory mechanisms generate N-terminal glucocorticoid receptor isoforms with unique transcriptional target genes. *Mol Cell* (2005) 18:331–42. doi:10.1016/j.molcel.2005.03.025
22. Ayroldi E, Cannarile L, Migliorati G, Nocentini G, Delfino DV, Riccardi C. Mechanisms of the anti-inflammatory effects of glucocorticoids: genomic and nongenomic interference with MAPK signaling pathways. *FASEB J* (2012) 26:4805–20. doi:10.1096/fj.12-216382
23. Song IH, Buttgereit F. Non-genomic glucocorticoid effects to provide the basis for new drug developments. *Mol Cell Endocrinol* (2006) 246:142–6. doi:10.1016/j.mce.2005.11.012
24. Lee SR, Kim HK, Youm JB, Dizon LA, Song IS, Jeong SH, et al. Non-genomic effect of glucocorticoids on cardiovascular system. *Pflugers Arch* (2012) 464:549–59. doi:10.1007/s00424-012-1155-2
25. Takahashi JS, Hong HK, Ko CH, McDearmon EL. The genetics of mammalian circadian order and disorder: implications for physiology and disease. *Nat Rev Genet* (2008) 9(10):764–75. doi:10.1038/nrg2430
26. Ko CH, Takahashi JS. Molecular components of the mammalian circadian clock. *Hum Mol Genet* (2006) 15:R271–7. doi:10.1093/hmg/ddl207
27. Nader N, Chrousos GP, Kino T. Interactions of the circadian CLOCK system and the HPA axis. *Trends Endocrinol Metab* (2010) 21:277–86. doi:10.1016/j.tem.2009.12.011
28. Kalsbeek A, Palm IF, La Fleur SE, Scheer FA, Perreau-Lenz S, Ruiter M, et al. SCN outputs and the hypothalamic balance of life. *J Biol Rhythms* (2006) 21(6):458–69. doi:10.1177/0748730406293854
29. Kondratov RV, Kondratova AA, Lee C, Gorbacheva VY, Chernov MV, Antoch MP. Post-translational regulation of circadian transcriptional CLOCK(NPAS2)/BMAL1 complex by CRYPTOCHROMES. *Cell Cycle* (2006) 5(8):890–5. doi:10.4161/cc.5.8.2684
30. Kiyohara YB, Tagao S, Tamanini F, Morita A, Sugisawa Y, Yasuda M, et al. The BMAL1 C terminus regulates the circadian transcription feedback loop. *Proc Natl Acad Sci U S A* (2006) 103(26):10074–9. doi:10.1073/pnas.0601416103

31. Padmanabhan K, Robles MS, Westerling T, Weitz CJ. Feedback regulation of transcriptional termination by the mammalian circadian clock PERIOD complex. *Science* (2012) 337(6094):599–602. doi:10.1126/science.1221592
32. Nicolaides NC, Charmandari E, Chrousos GP, Kino T. Circadian endocrine rhythms: the hypothalamic-pituitary-adrenal axis and its actions. *Ann N Y Acad Sci* (2014) 1318:71–80. doi:10.1111/nyas.12464
33. Lamia KA, Sachdeva UM, DiTacchio L, Williams EC, Alvarez JG, Egan DF, et al. AMPK regulates the circadian clock by cryptochrome phosphorylation and degradation. *Science* (2009) 326:437–40. doi:10.1126/science.1172156
34. Um JH, Yang S, Yamazaki S, Kang H, Viollet B, Foretz M, et al. Activation of 5'-AMP-activated kinase with diabetes drug metformin induces casein kinase I epsilon (CKIepsilon) dependent degradation of clock protein mPer2. *J Biol Chem* (2007) 282:20794–8. doi:10.1074/jbc.C700070200
35. Jordan SD, Lamia KA. AMPK at the crossroads of circadian clocks and metabolism. *Mol Cell Endocrinol* (2013) 366(2):163–9. doi:10.1016/j.mce.2012.06.017
36. Lee Y, Kim EK. AMP-activated protein kinase as a key molecular link between metabolism and clockwork. *Exp Mol Med* (2013) 45:e33. doi:10.1038/emm.2013.65
37. Asher G, Gatfield D, Stratmann M, Reinke H, Dibner C, Kreppel F, et al. SIRT1 regulates circadian clock gene expression through PER2 deacetylation. *Cell* (2008) 134:317–28. doi:10.1016/j.cell.2008.06.050
38. Nakahata Y, Kaluzova M, Grimaldi B, Sahar S, Hirayama J, Chen D, et al. The NAD+-dependent deacetylase SIRT1 modulates CLOCK-mediated chromatin remodeling and circadian control. *Cell* (2008) 134:329–40. doi:10.1016/j.cell.2008.07.002
39. Nakahata Y, Sahar S, Astarita G, Kaluzova M, Sassone-Corsi P. Circadian control of the NAD+ salvage pathway by CLOCK-SIRT1. *Science* (2009) 324:654–7. doi:10.1126/science.1170803
40. Dickmeis T. Glucocorticoids and the circadian clock. *J Endocrinol* (2009) 200(1):3–22. doi:10.1677/JOE-08-0415
41. Dickmeis T, Foulkes NS. Glucocorticoids and circadian clock control of cell proliferation: at the interface between three dynamic systems. *Mol Cell Endocrinol* (2011) 331(1):11–22. doi:10.1016/j.mce.2010.09.001
42. Son GH, Chung S, Kim K. The adrenal peripheral clock: glucocorticoid and the circadian timing system. *Front Neuroendocrinol* (2011) 32(4):451–65. doi:10.1016/j.yfrne.2011.07.003
43. Barclay JL, Tsang AH, Oster H. Interaction of central and peripheral clocks in physiological regulation. *Prog Brain Res* (2012) 199:163–81. doi:10.1016/B978-0-444-59427-3.00030-7
44. Kalsbeek A, van der Spek R, Lei J, Endert E, Buijs RM, Fliers E. Circadian rhythms in the hypothalamo-pituitary-adrenal (HPA) axis. *Mol Cell Endocrinol* (2012) 349(1):20–9. doi:10.1016/j.mce.2011.06.042
45. Ota T, Fustin JM, Yamada H, Doi M, Okamura H. Circadian clock signals in the adrenal cortex. *Mol Cell Endocrinol* (2012) 349(1):30–7. doi:10.1016/j.mce.2011.08.010
46. Ulrich-Lai YM, Arnhold MM, Engeland WC. Adrenal splanchnic innervations contributes to the diurnal rhythm of plasma corticosterone in rats by modulating adrenal sensitivity to ACTH. *Am J Physiol Regul Integr Comp Physiol* (2006) 290(4):R1128–35. doi:10.1152/ajpregu.00042.2003
47. Ishida A, Mutoh T, Ueyama T, Bando H, Masubuchi S, Nakahara D, et al. Light activates the adrenal gland: timing of gene expression and glucocorticoid release. *Cell Metab* (2005) 2(5):297–307. doi:10.1016/j.cmet.2005.09.009
48. Nader N, Chrousos GP, Kino T. Circadian rhythm transcription factor CLOCK regulates the transcriptional activity of the glucocorticoid receptor by acetylating its hinge region lysine cluster: potential physiological implications. *FASEB J* (2009) 23(5):1572–83. doi:10.1096/fj.08-117697
49. Han DH, Lee YJ, Kim K, Kim CJ, Cho S. Modulation of glucocorticoid receptor induction properties by core circadian clock proteins. *Mol Cell Endocrinol* (2014) 383(1–2):170–80. doi:10.1016/j.mce.2013.12.013
50. Kino T, Chrousos GP. Circadian CLOCK-mediated regulation of target-tissue sensitivity to glucocorticoids: implications for cardiometabolic diseases. *Endocr Dev* (2011) 20:116–26. doi:10.1159/000321232
51. Kino T, Chrousos GP. Acetylation-mediated epigenetic regulation of glucocorticoid receptor activity: circadian rhythm-associated alterations of glucocorticoid actions in target tissues. *Mol Cell Endocrinol* (2011) 336(1–2):23–30. doi:10.1016/j.mce.2010.12.001
52. Charmandari E, Chrousos GP, Lambrou GI, Pavlaki A, Koide H, Ng SS, et al. Peripheral CLOCK regulates target-tissue glucocorticoid receptor transcriptional activity in a circadian fashion in man. *PLoS One* (2011) 6(9):e25612. doi:10.1371/journal.pone.0025612
53. Lamia KA, Papp SJ, Yu RT, Barish GD, Uhlenhaut NH, Jonker JW, et al. Cryptochromes mediate rhythmic repression of the glucocorticoid receptor. *Nature* (2011) 480(7378):552–6. doi:10.1038/nature10700
54. Annayev Y, Adar S, Chiou YY, Lieb JD, Sancar A, Ye R. Gene model 129 (Gm129) encodes a novel transcriptional repressor that modulates circadian gene expression. *J Biol Chem* (2014) 289(8):5013–24. doi:10.1074/jbc.M113.534651
55. Anafi RC, Lee Y, Sato TK, Venkataraman A, Ramanathan C, Kavakli IH, et al. Machine learning helps identify CHRONO as a circadian clock component. *PLoS Biol* (2014) 12(4):e1001840. doi:10.1371/journal.pbio.1001840
56. Goriki A, Hatanaka F, Myung J, Kim JK, Yoritaka T, Tanoue S, et al. A novel protein, CHRONO, functions as a core component of the mammalian circadian clock. *PLoS Biol* (2014) 12(4):e1001839. doi:10.1371/journal.pbio.1001839
57. Robinson R. Chronos: stress makes the clock tick. *PLoS Biol* (2014) 12(4):e1001838. doi:10.1371/journal.pbio.1001838
58. Dickmeis T, Weger BD, Weger M. The circadian clock and glucocorticoids-interactions across many time scales. *Mol Cell Endocrinol* (2013) 380(1–2):2–15. doi:10.1016/j.mce.2013.05.012
59. Waite EJ, McKenna M, Kershaw Y, Walker JJ, Cho K, Piggins HD, et al. Ultradian corticosterone secretion is maintained in the absence of circadian cues. *Eur J Neurosci* (2012) 36(8):3142–50. doi:10.1111/j.1460-9568.2012.08213.x
60. Leliavski A, Dumbell R, Ott V, Oster H. Adrenal clocks and the role of adrenal hormones in the regulation of circadian physiology. *J Biol Rhythms* (2015) 30(1):20–34. doi:10.1177/0748730414553971
61. Engeland WC. Sensitization of endocrine organs to anterior pituitary hormones by the autonomic nervous system. *Handb Clin Neurol* (2013) 117:37–44. doi:10.1016/B978-0-444-53491-0.00004-3
62. Andrews RV, Folk GE Jr. Circadian metabolic patterns in cultured hamster adrenal glands. *Comp Biochem Physiol* (1964) 11:393–409. doi:10.1016/0010-406X(64)90006-4
63. Oster H, Damerow S, Hut RA, Eichele G. Transcriptional profiling in the adrenal gland reveals circadian regulation of hormone biosynthesis genes and nucleosome assembly genes. *J Biol Rhythms* (2006) 21:350–61. doi:10.1177/0748730406293053
64. Son GH, Chung S, Choe HK, Kim HD, Baik SM, Lee H, et al. Adrenal peripheral clock controls the autonomous circadian rhythm of glucocorticoid by causing rhythmic steroid production. *Proc Natl Acad Sci U S A* (2008) 105(52):20970–5. doi:10.1073/pnas.0806962106
65. Balsalobre A, Brown SA, Marcacci L, Tronche F, Kellendonk C, Reichardt HM, et al. Resetting of circadian time in peripheral tissues by glucocorticoid signaling. *Science* (2000) 289(5488):2344–7. doi:10.1126/science.289.5488.234
66. Yamamoto T, Nakahata Y, Tanaka M, Yoshida M, Soma H, Shinohara K, et al. Acute physical stress elevates mouse period1 mRNA expression in mouse peripheral tissues via a glucocorticoid-responsive element. *J Biol Chem* (2005) 280(51):42036–43. doi:10.1074/jbc.M509600200
67. So AY, Bernal TU, Pillsbury ML, Yamamoto KR, Feldman BJ. Glucocorticoid regulation of the circadian clock modulates glucose homeostasis. *Proc Natl Acad Sci U S A* (2009) 106(41):17582–7. doi:10.1073/pnas.0909733106
68. Torra IP, Tsibulsky V, Delaunay F, Saladin R, Laudet V, Fruchart JC, et al. Circadian and glucocorticoid regulation of Rev-erbalpha expression in liver. *Endocrinology* (2000) 141(10):3799–806. doi:10.1210/endo.141.10.7708
69. Oster H, Challet E, Ott V, Arvat E, de Kloet ER, Dijk DJ, et al. The functional and clinical significance of the 24-h rhythm of circulating glucocorticoids. *Endocr Rev* (2016) 17:er20151080. doi:10.1210/er.2015-1080
70. Su Y, van der Spek R, Foppen E, Kwakkel J, Fliers E, Kalsbeek A. Effects of adrenalectomy on daily gene expression rhythms in the rat suprachiasmatic and paraventricular hypothalamic nuclei and in white adipose tissue. *Chronobiol Int* (2015) 32:211–24. doi:10.3109/07420528.2014.963198
71. Takahashi S, Yokota S, Hara R, Kobayashi T, Akiyama M, Moriya T, et al. Physical and inflammatory stressors elevate circadian clock gene mPer1 mRNA levels in the paraventricular nucleus of the mouse. *Endocrinology* (2001) 142:4910–7. doi:10.1210/endo.142.11.8487
72. Segall LA, Perrin JS, Walker CD, Stewart J, Amir S. Glucocorticoid rhythms control the rhythm of expression of the clock protein, Period2, in oval nucleus of the bed nucleus of the stria terminalis and central nucleus of the amygdala in rats. *Neuroscience* (2006) 140:753–7. doi:10.1016/j.neuroscience.2006.03.037

73. Conway-Campbell BL, Sarabdjitsingh RA, McKenna MA, Pooley JR, Kershaw YM, Meijer OC, et al. Glucocorticoid ultradian rhythmicity directs cyclical gene pulsing of the clock gene period 1 in rat hippocampus. *J Neuroendocrinol* (2010) 22:1093–100. doi:10.1111/j.1365-2826.2010.02051.x
74. Pezuk P, Mohawk JA, Wang LA, Kalsbeek M. Glucocorticoids as entraining signals for peripheral circadian oscillators. *Endocrinology* (2012) 153:4775–83. doi:10.1210/en.2012-1486
75. Barnea M, Madar Z, Froy O. Dexamethasone induces high-amplitude rhythms in preadipocytes, but hinders circadian expression in differentiated adipocytes. *Chronobiol Int* (2013) 30:837–42. doi:10.3109/07420528.2013.767824
76. Burioka N, Takata M, Okano Y, Ohdo S, Fukuoka Y, Miyata M, et al. Dexamethasone influences human clock gene expression in bronchial epithelium and peripheral blood mononuclear cells in vitro. *Chronobiol Int* (2005) 22:585–90. doi:10.1081/CBI-200062416
77. van der Veen DR, Shao J, Xi Y, Li L, Duffield GE. Cardiac atrial circadian rhythms in PERIOD2:LUCIFERASE and per1:luc mice: amplitude and phase responses to glucocorticoid signaling and medium treatment. *PLoS One* (2012) 7:e47692. doi:10.1371/journal.pone.0047692
78. Fujihara Y, Kondo H, Noguchi T, Togari A. Glucocorticoids mediate circadian timing in peripheral osteoclasts resulting in the circadian expression rhythm of osteoclast related genes. *Bone* (2014) 61:1–9. doi:10.1016/j.bone.2013.12.026
79. Cermakian N, Sassone-Corsi P. Multilevel regulation of the circadian clock. *Nat Rev Mol Cell Biol* (2000) 1:59–67. doi:10.1038/35036078
80. Green CB, Menaker M. Circadian rhythms. Clocks on the brain. *Science* (2003) 301:319–20. doi:10.1126/science.1087824
81. Le Minh N, Damiola F, Tronche F, Schütz G, Schibler U. Glucocorticoid hormones inhibit food-induced phase-shifting of peripheral circadian oscillators. *EMBO J* (2001) 20:7128–36. doi:10.1093/emboj/20.24.7128
82. Cheon S, Park N, Cho S, Kim K. Glucocorticoid-mediated Period2 induction delays the phase of circadian rhythm. *Nucleic Acids Res* (2013) 41:6161–74. doi:10.1093/nar/gkt307
83. Bartlang MS, Savelyev SA, Johansson AS, Reber SO, Helfrich-Förster C, Lundkvist GB. Repeated psychosocial stress at night, but not day, affects the central molecular clock. *Chronobiol Int* (2014) 31:996–1007. doi:10.3109/07420528.2014.940085
84. Kiessling S, Eichele G, Oster H. Adrenal glucocorticoids have a key role in circadian resynchronization in a mouse model of jet lag. *J Clin Invest* (2010) 120:2600–9. doi:10.1172/JCI41192
85. Malek ZS, Sage D, Pevet P, Raison S. Daily rhythm of tryptophan hydroxylase-2 messenger ribonucleic acid within raphe neurons is induced by corticoid daily surge and modulated by enhanced locomotor activity. *Endocrinology* (2007) 148:5165–72. doi:10.1210/en.2007-0526
86. Jiang WG, Li SX, Zhou SJ, Jiang WG, Li SX, Zhou SJ. Chronic unpredictable stress induces a reversible change of PER2 rhythm in the suprachiasmatic nucleus. *Brain Res* (2011) 1399:25–32. doi:10.1016/j.brainres.2011.05.001
87. Kinoshita C, Miyazaki K, Ishida N. Chronic stress affects PERIOD2 expression through glycogen synthase kinase-3beta phosphorylation in the central clock. *Neuroreport* (2012) 23:98–102. doi:10.1097/WNR.0b013e32834e7ec2
88. Cermakian N, Lange T, Golombek D, Sarkar D, Nakao A, Shibata S, et al. Crosstalk between the circadian clock circuitry and the immune system. *Chronobiol Int* (2013) 30:870–88. doi:10.3109/07420528.2013.782315
89. Liang FQ, Sohrabji F, Miranda R, Earnest B, Earnest D. Expression of brain-derived neurotrophic factor and its cognate receptor, TrkB, in the rat suprachiasmatic nucleus. *Exp Neurol* (1998) 151:184–93. doi:10.1006/exnr.1998.6804
90. Rosmond R, Dallman MF, Björntorp P. Stress-related cortisol secretion in men: relationships with abdominal obesity and endocrine, metabolic and hemodynamic abnormalities. *J Clin Endocrinol Metab* (1998) 83:1853–9. doi:10.1210/jcem.83.6.4843
91. Chung S, Son GH, Kim K. Circadian rhythm of adrenal glucocorticoid: its regulation and clinical implications. *Biochim Biophys Acta* (2011) 1812(5):581–91. doi:10.1016/j.bbadis.2011.02.003
92. Walker CD, Scribner KA, Stern JS, Dallman MF. Obese Zucker (fa/fa) rats exhibit normal target sensitivity to corticosterone and increased drive to adrenocorticotropin during the diurnal trough. *Endocrinology* (1992) 131:2629–37. doi:10.1210/endo.131.6.1332842
93. Ahima RS, Prabakaran D, Flier JS. Postnatal leptin surge and regulation of circadian rhythm of leptin by feeding: implications for energy homeostasis and neuroendocrine function. *J Clin Invest* (1998) 101:1020–7. doi:10.1172/JCI1176
94. Kjölhede EA, Gustafsson PE, Gustafsson PA, Nelson N. Overweight and obese children have lower cortisol levels than normal weight children. *Acta Paediatr* (2014) 103(3):295–9. doi:10.1111/apa.12499
95. Sookoian S, Gemma C, Gianotti TF, Burgueño A, Castaño G, Pirola CJ. Genetic variants of Clock transcription factor are associated with individual susceptibility to obesity. *Am J Clin Nutr* (2008) 87(6):1606–15.
96. Scott EM, Carter AM, Grant PJ. Association between polymorphisms in the clock gene, obesity and the metabolic syndrome in man. *Int J Obes (Lond)* (2008) 32:658–62. doi:10.1038/sj.ijo.0803778
97. Lederbogen F, Hummel J, Fademrecht C, Krumm B, Kuhner C, Deuschle M, et al. Flattened circadian cortisol rhythm in type 2 diabetes. *Exp Clin Endocrinol Diabetes* (2011) 119(9):573–5. doi:10.1055/s-0031-1275288
98. Barclay JL, Shostak A, Leliavski A, Tsang AH, Johren O, Muller-Fielitz H, et al. High fat diet-induced hyperinsulinemia and tissue-specific insulin resistance in Cry deficient mice. *Am J Physiol Endocrinol Metab* (2013) 304(10):E1053–63. doi:10.1152/ajpendo.00512.2012
99. Albrecht U. Circadian clocks and mood-related behaviors. *Handb Exp Pharmacol* (2013) 217:227–39. doi:10.1007/978-3-642-25950-0_9
100. LeGates TA, Altimus CM, Wang H, Lee HK, Yang S, Zhao H, et al. Aberrant light directly impairs mood and learning through melanopsin-expressing neurons. *Nature* (2012) 491(7425):594–8. doi:10.1038/nature11673
101. Jarcho MR, Slavich GM, Tylova-Stein H, Wolkowitz OM, Burke HM. Dysregulated diurnal cortisol pattern is associated with glucocorticoid resistance in women with major depressive disorder. *Biol Psychol* (2013) 93(1):150–8. doi:10.1016/j.biopsycho.2013.01.018
102. Li JZ, Bunney BG, Meng F, Hagenauer MH, Walsh DM, Vawter MP, et al. Circadian patterns of gene expression in the human brain and disruption in major depressive disorder. *Proc Natl Acad Sci U S A* (2013) 110(24):9950–5. doi:10.1073/pnas.1305814110
103. Li SX, Liu LJ, Xu LZ, Gao L, Wang XF, Zhang JT, et al. Diurnal alterations in circadian genes and peptides in major depressive disorder before and after escitalopram treatment. *Psychoneuroendocrinology* (2013) 38(11):2789–99. doi:10.1016/j.psyneuen.2013.07.009
104. Landgraf D, McCarthy MJ, Welsh DK. Circadian clock and stress interactions in the molecular biology of psychiatric disorders. *Curr Psychiatry Rep* (2014) 16(10):483. doi:10.1007/s11920-014-0483-7
105. Straub RH, Cutolo M. Circadian rhythms in rheumatoid arthritis: implications for pathophysiology and therapeutic management. *Arthritis Rheum* (2007) 56(2):399–408. doi:10.1002/art.22368
106. Kino T, Charmandari E, Chrousos GP. Glucocorticoid receptor: implications for rheumatic diseases. *Clin Exp Rheumatol* (2011) 29(5 Suppl 68):S32–41.
107. Mohren DC, Jansen NW, Kant IJ, Galama J, van den Brandt PA, Swaen GM. Prevalence of common infections among employees in different work schedules. *J Occup Environ Med* (2002) 44(11):1003–11. doi:10.1097/00043764-200211000-00005
108. Hedström AK, Åkerstedt T, Hillert J, Olsson T, Alfredsson L. Shift work at young age is associated with increased risk for multiple sclerosis. *Ann Neurol* (2011) 70(5):733–41. doi:10.1002/ana.22597
109. Stevens RG, Hansen J, Costa G, Haus E, Kauppinen T, Aronson KJ, et al. Considerations of circadian impact for defining 'shift work' in cancer studies: IARC Working Group Report. *Occup Environ Med* (2011) 68(2):154–62. doi:10.1136/oem.2009.053512
110. Fu L, Pelicano H, Liu J, Huang P, Lee C. The circadian gene Period2 plays an important role in tumor suppression and DNA damage response in vivo. *Cell* (2002) 111(1):41–50. doi:10.1016/S0092-8674(02)01223-0
111. Filipski E, Li XM, Levi F. Disruption of circadian coordination and malignant growth. *Cancer Causes Control* (2006) 17(4):509–14. doi:10.1007/s10552-005-9007-4
112. Filipski E, Subramanian P, Carriere J, Guettier C, Barbason H, Levi F. Circadian disruption accelerates liver carcinogenesis in mice. *Mutat Res* (2009) 680(1–2):95–105. doi:10.1016/j.mrgentox.2009.10.002
113. Spiegel K, Leproult R, Van Cauter E. Impact of sleep debt on metabolic and endocrine function. *Lancet* (1999) 354(9188):1435–9. doi:10.1016/S0140-6736(99)01376-8

114. Spiegel K, Leproult R, L'Hermite-Baleriaux M, Copinschi G, Penev PD, Van Cauter E. Leptin levels are dependent on sleep duration: relationships with sympathovagal balance, carbohydrate regulation, cortisol, and thyrotropin. *J Clin Endocrinol Metab* (2004) 89(11):5762–71. doi:10.1210/jc.2004-1003
115. Leproult R, Copinschi G, Buxton O, Van Cauter E. Sleep loss results in an elevation of cortisol levels the next evening. *Sleep* (1997) 20(10):865–70.
116. Vgontzas AN, Bixler EO, Lin HM, Prolo P, Mastorakos G, Vela-Bueno A, et al. Chronic insomnia is associated with nyctohemeral activation of the hypothalamicpituitary-adrenal axis: clinical implications. *J Clin Endocrinol Metab* (2001) 86(8):3787–94. doi:10.1210/jcem.86.8.7778
117. Mongrain V, Hernandez SA, Pradervand S, Dorsaz S, Curie T, Hagiwara G, et al. Separating the contribution of glucocorticoids and wakefulness to the molecular and electrophysiological correlates of sleep homeostasis. *Sleep* (2010) 33(9):1147–57.
118. Buckley TM, Schatzberg AF. On the interactions of the hypothalamic-pituitary-adrenal (HPA) axis and sleep: normal HPA axis activity and circadian rhythm, exemplary sleep disorders. *J Clin Endocrinol Metab* (2005) 90(5):3106–14. doi:10.1210/jc.2004-1056
119. Balbo M, Leproult R, Van Cauter E. Impact of sleep and its disturbances on hypothalamo-pituitary-adrenal axis activity. *Int J Endocrinol* (2010) 2010:759234. doi:10.1155/2010/759234
120. Papadopoulos AS, Cleare AJ. Hypothalamic-pituitary-adrenal axis dysfunction in chronic fatigue syndrome. *Nat Rev Endocrinol* (2011) 8(1):22–32. doi:10.1038/nrendo.2011.153
121. Yehuda R, Seckl J. Minireview: stress-related psychiatric disorders with low cortisol levels: a metabolic hypothesis. *Endocrinology* (2011) 152(12): 4496–503. doi:10.1210/en.2011-1218
122. Busillo JM, Cidlowski JA. The five Rs of glucocorticoid action during inflammation: ready, reinforce, repress, resolve, and restore. *Trends Endocrinol Metab* (2013) 24(3):109–19. doi:10.1016/j.tem.2012.11.005
123. Husebye ES, Allolio B, Arlt W, Badenhoop K, Bensing S, Betterle C, et al. Consensus statement on the diagnosis, treatment and follow-up of patients with primary adrenal insufficiency. *J Intern Med* (2014) 275(2):104–15. doi:10.1111/joim.12162
124. Nilsson AG, Marelli C, Fitts D, Bergthorsdottir R, Burman P, Dahlqvist P, et al. Prospective evaluation of long-term safety of dual-release hydrocortisone replacement administered once daily in patients with adrenal insufficiency. *Eur J Endocrinol* (2014) 171(3):369–77. doi:10.1530/EJE-14-0327
125. Johannsson G, Nilsson AG, Bergthorsdottir R, Burman P, Dahlqvist P, Ekman B, et al. Improved cortisol exposure-time profile and outcome in patients with adrenal insufficiency: a prospective randomized trial of a novel hydrocortisone dual-release formulation. *J Clin Endocrinol Metab* (2012) 97(2):473–81. doi:10.1210/jc.2011-1926
126. Čupić Ž, Marković VM, Maćešić S, Stanojević A, Damjanović S, Vukojević V, et al. Dynamic transitions in a model of the hypothalamic-pituitary-adrenal axis. *Chaos* (2016) 26(3):033111. doi:10.1063/1.4944040
127. Marković VM, Čupić Ž, Vukojević V, Kolar-Anić L. Predictive modeling of the hypothalamic-pituitary-adrenal (HPA) axis response to acute and chronic stress. *Endocr J* (2011) 58(10):889–904. doi:10.1507/endocrj.EJ11-0037
128. Jelić S, Cupić Z, Kolar-Anić L. Mathematical modeling of the hypothalamic-pituitary-adrenal system activity. *Math Biosci* (2005) 197(2):173–87. doi:10.1016/j.mbs.2005.06.006
129. Walker JJ, Spiga F, Gupta R, Zhao Z, Lightman SL, Terry JR. Rapid intra-adrenal feedback regulation of glucocorticoid synthesis. *J R Soc Interface* (2015) 12(102):20140875. doi:10.1098/rsif.2014.0875

3

From Bioinactive ACTH to ACTH Antagonist: The Clinical Perspective

*Chiraz Ghaddhab[1], Jean-Marc Vuissoz[2] and Johnny Deladoëy[1]**

[1] Endocrinology Service and Research Center, Sainte-Justine University Hospital Center, Department of Pediatrics, Université de Montréal, Montreal, QC, Canada, [2] Division of Pediatric Endocrinology, University Children's Hospital Basel (UKBB), University of Basel, Basel, Switzerland

***Correspondence:**
Johnny Deladoëy
johnny.deladoey@umontreal.ca

The adrenocorticotropic hormone (ACTH) is a pituitary hormone derived from a larger peptide, the proopiomelanocortin (POMC), as are the MSHs (α-MSH, β-MSH, and γ-MSH) and the β-LPH-related polypeptides (**Figure 1A**). ACTH drives adrenal steroidogenesis and growth of the adrenal gland. ACTH is a 39 amino acid polypeptide that binds and activates its cognate receptor [melanocortin receptor 2 (MC2R)] through the two regions $H_6F_7R_8W_9$ and $K_{15}K_{16}R_{17}R_{18}P_{19}$. Most POMC-derived polypeptides contain the $H_6F_7R_8W_9$ sequence that is conserved through evolution. This explains the difficulties in developing selective agonists or antagonists to the MCRs. In this review, we will discuss the clinical aspects of the role of ACTH in physiology and disease, and potential clinical use of selective ACTH antagonists.

Keywords: stress, cortisol, adrenals, ACTH, antagonist

FROM THE CONCEPT OF "STRESS" TO THE DISCOVERY OF ADRENOCORTICOTROPIC HORMONE (ACTH)

Adrenocorticotropic hormone and cortisol are nowadays associated with the physiological response to stress. Historically, the concept of stress was first introduced in 1936 by Hans Selye (1). It was first called the "general adaptation syndrome" and later renamed by Selye as "stress response." Stress results from the balance between the stressor, an agent that produces stress at any time, and the body's adaptive response to it. His experiments on rats in 1936 have shown that a stressor often alters the adrenal cortex, the immune system, and the gut. Indeed, rats exposed to various nocuous chemical or physical stimuli had a hypertrophy of the adrenals, an involution of the lymphatic nodes and developed gastric erosions (2).

In the 1930s–1940s, Selye performed extensive structure–function studies, resulting in the first classification of steroid hormones, e.g., corticoids, testoids/androgens, and folliculoids/estrogens (3, 4). During those years, he recognized the respective anti- and pro-inflammatory actions of gluco- and mineralocorticoids (named by Selye) in animal models, several years before demonstration of anti-rheumatic actions of cortisone and ACTHs in patients. In 1935 and 21 years after having isolated thyroxine in crystalline form, Kendall isolated and identified the structure of cortisone, and in 1936, Reichstein identified the structure of cortisol. In 1948, Hench and Kendall demonstrated that cortisone and ACTH exert a profound anti-inflammatory effect in patients with rheumatoid arthritis. In 1950, Hench, Kendall, and Reichstein were awarded the Nobel Prize in Physiology and Medicine for these discoveries. In the same year, Harris established that ACTH

Abbreviations: ACTH, adrenocorticotropin; PBMAH, primary bilateral macronodular adrenal hyperplasia; AGRP, agouti-related protein; ASIP, agouti signaling protein; CAH, congenital adrenal hyperplasia; FGD, family glucocorticoid deficiency; MSH, melanocyte-stimulating hormone; MCR, melanocortin receptor; MRAP, melanocortin receptor-associated protein; POMC, proopiomelanocortin.

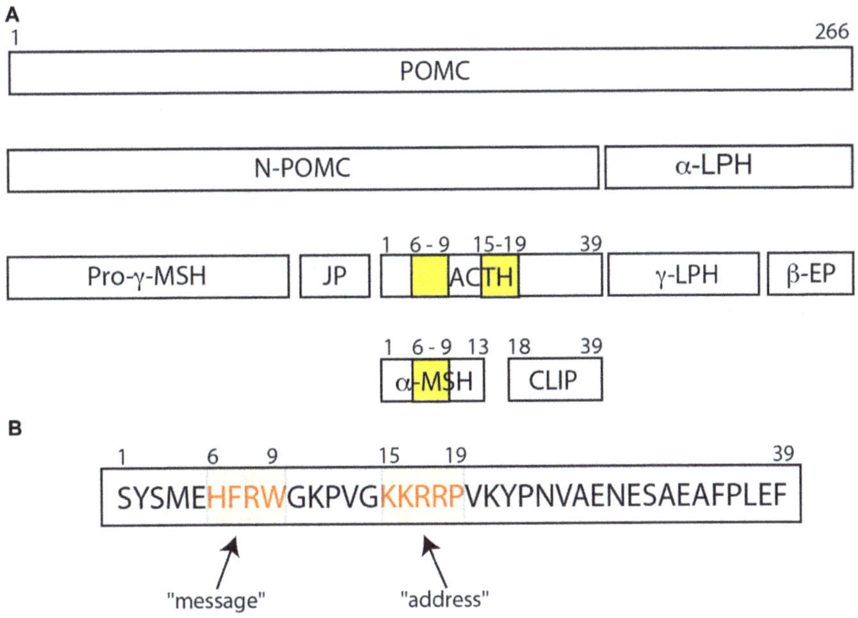

FIGURE 1 | (A) The POMC protein and its various peptide cleavage products: the yellow bands correspond to the amino acid sequences $His^6Phe^7Arg^8Trp^9$ and $Lys^{15}Lys^{16}Arg^{17}Arg^{18}Pro^{19}$. $His^6Phe^7Arg^8Trp^9$ is important for binding and signal transduction of α-MSH. **(B)** $His^6Phe^7Arg^8Trp^9$ sequence is important for adrenocorticotropic hormone (ACTH) signal transduction and for ACTH binding to melanocortin receptor 2 (MC2R) (26), and was called the "message" sequence (13). The amino acids $Lys^{15}Lys^{16}Arg^{17}Arg^{18}Pro^{19}$ was initially defined as the "address" sequence allowing specific ACTH binding to MC2R (27).

secretion involves "neuronal control *via* the hypothalamus and the hypophyseal portal vessels of the pituitary stalk" (5). ACTH was first isolated in 1943 and then synthesized in the 1960s and 1970s by different groups (6–9). Next, the amino acid sequences of ACTH from four mammalian species were elucidated between 1954 and 1961 by three groups of Bell, Li, and Lerner (6, 10, 11). In 1955, Guillemin (a former student of Selye's) and Rosenberg demonstrated in rats the existence of CRF, the hypothalamic factor that allows ACTH release (12).

ACTH STRUCTURE AND FUNCTION

Adrenocorticotropic hormone, adrenocorticotropin, corticotropin, or ACTH, transmits information from the anterior lobe of the pituitary to the adrenal cortex. ACTH is a linear non-atriacontapeptide with species differences in the COOH terminal two-third of the molecule (13). Initially, an analysis of the ACTH crystal structure was still lacking. In the early 1970s, different polypeptides were isolated from different lobes of the vertebrate pituitary (14). Lowry showed that ACTH and β-lipotropin (β-LPH) shared the same amino acid motif $H_6F_7R_8W_9$ even if they have different functions (14, 15) (**Figure 1**). α-MSH and β-MSH were found to be embedded within the primary sequences of ACTH and β-LPH, respectively, in the melanocorticotropic cells (in the intermediate pituitary) (16). A few years later, the prediction that ACTH, the MSHs, and the β-LPH-related polypeptides were derived from the same precursor (17) was confirmed by the cloning of the proopiomelanocortin gene (POMC) mRNA (18). Initially, Schwyzer and Sieber suggested that ACTH is a linear polypeptide (19). Later, Schiller showed that residues 10–21 have a flexible conformation (20). Squire and Bewley had already suggested that a small region close to N-terminus had a tendency to form a helical structure (21). Low et al. have confirmed that a helical structure is produced in a solvent, the trifluoroethanol (22). It was suggested that this conformational change could occur when ACTH binds its receptor, to ensure a kinetically and a thermodynamically optimal hormone–receptor contact (23, 24). Later, Hruby et al. showed that the N terminal region of ACTH, between residues 4 and 10, adopts a β-turn conformation (25). Molecular modeling supports this hypothesis, given the presence of an N-terminal helical structure in the wild-type ACTH model (**Figure 2A**). This helical secondary structure is disrupted by validated inactivating mutations, which suggests that it is essential for ACTH bioactivity (**Figure 2B**).

Due to different bioassay systems, several research teams screened the biological activity of C terminally truncated analogs of ACTH (1–39) (30). ACTH (1–24) was as potent as ACTH (1–39) to induce glucocorticoid production by adrenal cells in culture (31), while ACTH (1–16) was unable to do so. It was concluded that the critical portion of ACTH for activating adrenal cells resided between residues 17 and 24 (31). However, the analog ACTH (11–24) was unable to induce glucocorticoid production and was even an antagonist at high concentrations (31). Fauchère et al. showed that dimers of ACTH (11–24) and ACTH (7–24) were potent antagonists, whereas ACTH (1–24) dimers remained agonists but were 70 times less potent when compared to its monomeric ACTH (1–24) (32–34).

Altogether, Schwyzer concluded that residues 17–24 were important for recognition of ACTH by its adrenal receptor, and he coined the term "address sequence" to indicate that

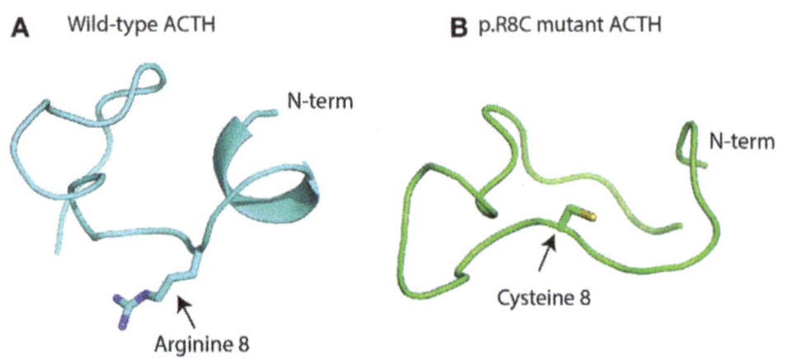

FIGURE 2 | Structure of wild-type (A) and mutant adrenocorticotropic hormone (ACTH) (B) after a 100-ns molecular dynamics simulation in implicit water (28, 29): (A) to retain full bioactivity, the N-terminal "message" sequence has to conserve its helical secondary structure as postulated by Schwyzer 40 years ago (13). (B) Naturally occurring bioinactive ACTH mutation (p.R8C) disrupts the helical conformation and hampers proper binding and activation of the melanocortin receptor 2 (26).

these residues allowed the ligand to find the cognate receptor (**Figure 1B**) (13, 27). As Costa et al. suggested, the position 20 should be included in the address site (35). To activate the adrenal receptor, a "message" region is needed. Several studies suggested that the $H_6F_7R_8W_9$ motif should be considered as the "message sequence" (13) (**Figure 1B**). Indeed, both address and message sequences are necessary to activate the adrenal receptor: the address sequence interacts with the adrenal receptor and then the message sequence enters in contact with the receptor to induce the conformation change in the receptor that activates the adrenal cell (27). This could explain why α-MSH could not activate adrenal cells, even if it has the $H_6F_7R_8W_9$ motif. On the other hand, Schwyzer considered also the effect of analogs of ACTH (1–39) on the activation of melanocytes. All analogs of ACTH (N-terminally as well as C terminally truncated forms) were able to activate melanocytes as long as the $H_6F_7R_8W_9$ motif was intact (13, 27), and the $H_6F_7R_8W_9$ motif is probably both the message and the address sequence in these cells.

In the 1990s, five melanocortin receptor (MCR) genes were identified in the genome of mammals, tetrapods, birds, bony fish, and cartilaginous fish (36–39). MC1R mediates pigmentation, MC2R activates glucocorticoid biosynthesis in the adrenal cortex, MC3R and MC4R influence metabolic homeostasis in the central nervous system and periphery (40), and MC5R regulates sebaceous gland secretions (41). The MCRs belong to the rhodopsin family of G protein-coupled receptors (GPCRs) (37, 42). They induce intracellular cyclic AMP production following activation by ligands (43, 44). ACTH (1–39) or α-MSH can activate MC1R, MC3R, MC4R, and MC5R (37), but MC2R can only be activated by ACTH and not by α-MSH or other analogs (45). The MCR genes have now been cloned and expressed in cell lines, allowing *in vitro* binding and activation assays of ACTH analogs against all MCRs. Recently, it has been shown that MC2R requires the presence of the melanocortin receptor-associated protein (MRAP) to be expressed and active at the cell surface (46–49).

Although ACTH and α-MSH both have the $H_6F_7R_8W_9$ motif, only ACTH can activate MC2R. This raises the question of differences between the $H_6F_7R_8W_9$-binding site in MC2R when compared to the other MCRs. Due to a crystal structure of the $H_6F_7R_8W_9$-binding site and site-directed mutagenesis analyses of human MC4R, we know that vertebrate MCRs have a common $H_6F_7R_8W_9$-binding site (50–53), which further confirms that the $H_6F_7R_8W_9$ motif is both the message sequence and the address sequence for the α-MSH. Dores hypothesized that, prior to stimulation, MC1, MC3, MC4, or MC5 receptors have a binding site that is in an open conformation for the ligand. When the ligand interacts with the receptor, it leads to a conformational change (a "docking event") that activates the receptor (27). Therefore, the activation of MC2R may be a multistep process that requires (i) a conformational change after docking of the $H_6F_7R_8W_9$ motif on its MC2R-binding site and, in the second step, (ii) docking of the $K_{15}K_{16}R_{17}R_{18}P_{19}$ motif of ACTH to activate the MC2R receptor (27, 54). This could explain the differential ligand selectivity of the MCRs. However, further analyses and experiments are necessary to confirm this hypothesis.

FAMILIAL GLUCOCORTICOID DEFICIENCY (FGD) AND POMC DEFICIENCY

Familial Glucocorticoid Deficiency

The glucocorticoid deficiency syndrome (FGD) is an autosomal recessive disorder characterized by insensitivity to ACTH action on the adrenal cortex (55), thereby resulting in glucocorticoid insufficiency with intact mineralocorticoid secretion. It may manifest during early neonatal life but can be diagnosed later during childhood. Clinical manifestations include recurrent hypoglycemia that may lead to seizures and coma, chronic fatigue, failure to thrive, recurrent infections, and skin hyperpigmentation. Typically, plasma cortisol levels are very low or undetectable without response to ACTH, while endogenous ACTH levels are very high, which clearly shows a specific resistance to the action of ACTH in these patients. The aldosterone and renin levels are usually normal and correctly match the activation of the renin–angiotensin axis. Even if congenital adrenal hyperplasia (CAH) (due to defects in the glucocorticoid synthesis pathway), congenital adrenal hypoplasia, and X-linked adrenoleukodystrophy are associated with high ACTH and low cortisol levels, they are distinct from FGD.

So far, mutations in five genes have been associated with isolated FGD and four with FGD associated with various syndromic features. In all these genetic disorders, low cortisol and a high ACTH suggest ACTH resistance. Causative genes of *isolated* FGD are the ACTH receptor (*MC2R*; also formerly defined as FGD 1) (56), the melanocortin receptor-associated protein (*MRAP*; also formerly defined as FGD 2) (46), the DAX1 transcription factor (*NR0B1*) (57), nicotinamide nucleotide transhydrogenase (*NNT*) (58–60), and mitochondrial thioredoxin reductase (*TXNRD2*) (61). Interestingly, NNT and thioredoxin reductase (TXNRD2) are crucial enzymes for the production of sufficient NADPH to maintain the redox potential in the steroid-producing cells. Four *syndromes* have been reported with FDG: (i) the AAA(A) syndrome (ACTH resistance, alacrimia, achalasia, and autonomous system dysfunction) due to *AAAS* mutations (62); (ii) the IMAGe syndrome (intrauterine growth restriction, metaphyseal dysplasia, adrenal hypoplasia congenita, and genital anomalies) due to *CDKN1C* mutations (63); (iii) a syndrome with short stature, recurrent infection due to natural killer cell deficiency, and chromosomal fragility associated with mutation of the DNA helicase, minichromosome maintenance 4 (*MCM4*) (64); and (iv) the MIRAGE syndrome (myelodysplasia, infection, restriction of growth, adrenal hypoplasia, genital phenotypes, and enteropathy) due to mutations in *SAMD9* (65).

POMC Deficiency

Proopiomelanocortin (POMC) deficiency causes severe monogenic obesity that begins at an early age, adrenal insufficiency, red hair, and pale skin. Affected infants have a normal weight at birth, but they develop early hyperphagia that leads to excessive weight gain starting in the first year of life. During the neonatal period, patients usually present with hypoglycemic seizures, hyperbilirubinemia, and cholestasis due to secondary hypocorticism (66). Subclinical hypothyroidism was also reported. The incidence is very low, about one in 1 million. Complete POMC deficiency is an autosomal recessive disorder and is caused by homozygous or compound heterozygous loss-of-function mutations in the POMC gene on chromosome 2p23.3.

POMC is regulated by leptin and is cleaved by prohormone convertases to produce ACTH and MSH α, β, and γ. In POMC deficiency, the serum concentrations of these cleavage products are low. The red hair pigmentation, adrenal insufficiency, and obesity are caused by inability to activate the MC1, MC2, and MC4 receptors, respectively (66). In addition to complete POMC deficiency, isolated deficiency of β-MSH has been described. This isolated deficiency of β-MSH leads to severe obesity without adrenal insufficiency or red hair (67, 68).

A few years ago, we reported glucocorticoid deficiency in two unrelated patients with apparent ACTH resistance due to an unusual mutation in POMC: the p.R8C mutation in the sequence encoding ACTH and α-MSH (26). The patients (a 4-year-old girl and a 4-month-old boy) presented with hypoglycemia, low cortisol, normal electrolytes, and high ACTH. Both patients had red hair, adrenal insufficiency, and developed early-onset obesity. They were initially treated with gluco- and mineralocorticoids, but after the identification of the mutation in POMC, mineralocorticoid treatment was discontinued in both patients. Whole exome sequencing revealed that the girl was compound heterozygous for POMC mutations: one previously described null allele and one novel p.R8C mutation in the sequence encoding ACTH and α-MSH. The boy was homozygous for the p.R8C mutation. We demonstrated that even if ACTH-R8C was immunoreactive, it failed to bind and activate cAMP production in melanocortin-2 receptor (MC2R)-expressing cells. We demonstrated also that α-MSH-R8C failed to bind and stimulate cAMP production in MC1R- and MC4R-expressing cells.

Discovery of this mutation indicates that in humans, unlike rodents, the amino acid sequence $H_6F_7R_8W_9$ is important not only for cAMP activation but also for ACTH binding to the MC2R. Furthermore, *in silico* modeling suggested that the pR8C mutation disrupts the secondary structure of ACTH, which implies that this secondary structure may have a crucial role for M2R activation (**Figure 2**).

Diagnosis of complete POMC deficiency may be suspected on the basis of clinical manifestations and can be confirmed by identification of mutations in the *POMC* gene. To treat POMC-deficient patients, only hydrocortisone substitution is currently available and is required. An intranasal administration of the ACTH 4–10 melanocortin fragment did not lead to a reduction in body weight. Administration of thyroid hormone had no effect on obesity (69). Recently, two extremely obese POMC patients have been substituted with a MC4R agonist (setmelanotide), and a significant reduction of their weight has been achieved (more than 10% after 10 weeks of treatment) (70). This paves the way for treatment of this condition with specific MC4R agonists and should also prompt research into developing agonists to other MCRs such as MC2R.

PERSPECTIVES: A ROLE FOR SPECIFIC ACTH ANTAGONISTS IN HUMAN DISEASE

Specific ACTH antagonists would be of great value especially to treat two conditions: CAH and primary bilateral macronodular adrenal hyperplasia (PBMAH). Moreover, MC2R antagonists could represent a valuable alternative to anticortisolic drugs in clinical management of ACTH-dependent hypercortisolism, essentially Cushing's disease, when removal of the source of ACTH excess is impossible or incomplete.

Congenital Adrenal Hyperplasia

Adrenocorticotropic hormone drives the synthesis and secretion of cortisol as well as androgens from the adrenal gland. In CAH due to 21 hydroxylase deficiency, excess of ACTH leads to overandrogenization. CAH is due to the enzymatic defect in the cortisol synthesis pathway, with subsequent hypocortisolism, ACTH overproduction, accumulation of androgen precursors, and adrenal gland hyperplasia. Treatment with glucocorticoids at physiological doses is life saving but is not sufficient to suppress the elevated ACTH levels and androgen overproduction. Failure to suppress excess androgens results in height acceleration, advanced skeletal maturation, and eventually leads to decreased final adult height. Other effects of androgen excess include clitoromegaly and hirsutism in females, isosexual pseudoprecocious puberty in males, and acne and deepening of the voice in both sexes. Only supraphysiological doses of glucocorticoids suppress ACTH in CAH but at the cost of hypercortisolemia with its adverse effects such as hyperglycemia, arterial hypertension, reduced growth, and osteoporosis. Since MC2R is expressed only in the adrenals, it could become a specific target. Therefore, an adjuvant drug able to specifically block the MC2R would obviate the need for supraphysiological dose of glucocorticoids in CAH and prevent the undesirable effects inherent to glucocorticoid overtreatment.

MC2R Expressing PBMAH

Primary bilateral macronodular adrenal hyperplasia (also known as ACTH-independent macronodular adrenal hyperplasia) is a rare, sporadic disease affecting men and women with an almost equal ratio. PBMAH has a bimodal age distribution: during the first year of life (minority) when it may be associated with the McCune–Albright syndrome (71) and during the fifth decade of life (majority) (72). Occurrence of familial cases of PBMAH and involvement of both adrenal glands (even in sporadic cases) strongly suggest involvement of germline genetic predisposition in PBMAH. Indeed, inactivating mutations of the armadillo repeat containing 5 (*ARMC5*) have been reported in 25–55% of patients with sporadic PBMAH (73–75).

The most frequent clinical manifestation of PBMAH is Cushing syndrome. In PBMAH, one previously believed that glucocorticoid secretion is ACTH independent given that, most of the time, plasma ACTH levels are undetectable, and high-dose dexamethasone administration fails to suppress cortisol secretion. This notion has been revised following the demonstration of local production of ACTH. Indeed, Cheitlin et al. studied the adrenal cells from a patient with PBMAH *in vitro*; the cells were cultured on an extracellular matrix and demonstrated rapid growth and a high rate of cortisol secretion in the absence of ACTH (76). Not only the MC2R was expressed in PBMAH tissue (77) but also ACTH was abnormally expressed, further stimulating the cortisol secretion through a paracrine effect (78). These findings represent a strong incentive to treat PBMAH-associated hypercortisolism with MC2R antagonists. This contrasts with primary pigmented nodular adrenocortical disease, sporadic large benign adenomas, and adrenocortical carcinomas, which are mostly ACTH unresponsive (79).

Even if these observations suggest that specific MC2R antagonist could help patients with PBMAH, the specific structure of the ACTH produced by PBMAH cells (78) and in ectopic Cushing's syndrome (80) might raise unexpected difficulties. Indeed, these bioactive ACTH are not detected by antibodies directed to the ACTH C terminal portion. This may result from extrapituitary sources of ACTH producing increased amounts of precursors (pre-ACTH and POMC) due to impaired POMC processing (81, 82). Reports on receptor affinity and steroidogenic potency of ACTH precursors are conflicting (81), which may complicate the design of MC2R antagonists that also block ACTH precursors.

A Specific MC2R Antagonist: An Elusive Target

In the last four decades, extensive studies that have been performed to determine the molecular basis of the interaction of ACTH with cognate MCRs have shown inconsistent results, mainly due to technical limitations. First, the expression at the cell membrane of human MC2R in cell lines was not possible until the discovery of the melanocortin receptor-associated protein (MRAP) (46), which is required to address MC2R at the cell membrane. Second, studies on putative ACTH antagonists failed to perform a systematic analysis of ACTH antagonists' activation and binding against all cognate MCRs to assess specificity (83, 84).

Melanocortin receptors belong to the GPCRs family that has natural agonists and antagonists. The melanocortin antagonists, agouti-related protein (AGRP) and agouti signaling protein (ASIP), are the only two endogenous antagonists of MCRs identified to date (85–87). The primary sequences of the endogenous agonists (MSHs) and antagonists (AGRP and ASIP) are different, and they interact differently with the MCRs to produce the active and inactive conformations of the ligand–receptor complex.

The design of a specific peptide remains a challenge that has not been resolved because of the difficulty of designing a peptide specific for one MCR (e.g., MC2R) (37). Indeed, all melanocortin ligands receptors shared the same $H_6F_7R_8W_9$ motif, which is important for MCR binding and stimulation (88) and which bind to all MCR receptors. Development of selective ligands for the melanocortin system is challenging due to the conserved amino acid sequences of the MCRs and of their structural similarity in the seven-transmembrane GPCR fold (89). The limited structural variations of the endogenous melanotropin ligands further reduce options in the design of MCR ligands for achieving selectivity. If they are not selective, these peptides could be the source of severe undesirable effects due to the numerous specific roles of the five MCRs. Of note, some ACTH fragments show variable specificity across species. For example, ACTH (7–38) fragment antagonizes the human MC2 receptor but stimulates aldosterone secretion from the rat adrenal cortex through a mechanism involving the angiotensin receptor (90). Variable specificity between species is therefore another challenge for the preclinical phase of the development of new ACTH receptor agonists. A table listing MC2R agonists and antagonists is available in Table S1 in Supplemental Material.

Designing molecules that possess both functional selectivity and human melanocortin receptor (hMCR) subtype selectivity from the melanotropin core sequence $H_6F_7R_8W_9$ has been difficult. Many peptides are conformationally flexible in aqueous solution, but upon interacting with their biologically relevant molecule, they assume a preferred conformation. The reduction of conformational freedom may eventually lead to the receptor bound conformation, which results in the selective interaction of a ligand with a receptor. A major step is to determine which peptide conformation is required for binding to the receptor and resulting in an agonist or antagonist effect. A critical approach is to understand if changes in ACTH three-dimensional (3D) conformation are associated with antagonist properties (**Figure 2**). X-ray crystal structures provide 3D conformation but may be misleading in terms of function. Incorporation of these X-ray coordinates into a computer-aided examination of function into 3D space is being pursued (91). This allows one to further explore the region/site or the surrounding 3D space occupied by the key amino acids of the protein (where the potent ligand has an affinity) so as to better understand biological actions. Nevertheless, the numerous physiological functions of the five known subtypes of hMCRs continue to be a stimulus for the production of selective melanocortin agonists and antagonists (92).

CONCLUSION

The ACTH is the pituitary hormone that allows growth and development of the adrenal cortex and glucocorticoid synthesis. Even if the structure of ACTH has been known for decades, the exact mechanism of activation of MC2R, the specific ACTH receptor on adrenal cells, is still unknown. Understanding this activation and the development of specific MC2R antagonists would allow the treatment of some difficult-to-treat diseases such as CAH or PBMAH.

AUTHOR CONTRIBUTIONS

CG wrote the review and revised the final version; J-MV performed bioinformatic analysis and revised the final version; and JD wrote the review and revised the final version.

FUNDING

This work has been supported by Clinical Fellowship Award of the CHU Ste-Justine—Université de Montréal and Academic Medical Interdisciplinary Research Association (AMIR) of the Université Libre de Bruxelles to CG and Clinician-Scientist scholarship of the Fonds de Recherche du Québec—Santé (FRQS) to JD.

REFERENCES

1. Selye H. A syndrome produced by diverse nocuous agents. 1936. *J Neuropsychiatry Clin Neurosci* (1998) 10:230–1. doi:10.1176/jnp.10.2.230a
2. Selye H, Collip JB. Fundamental factors in the interpretation of stimuli influencing endocrine glands. *Endocrinology* (1936) 20:667–72. doi:10.1210/endo-20-5-667
3. Selye H. *Encyclopedia of Endocrinology*. Montreal: A.W.T. Franks Publishing (1943).
4. Szabo S, Tache Y, Somogyi A. The legacy of Hans Selye and the origins of stress research: a retrospective 75 years after his landmark brief "letter" to the editor# of nature. *Stress* (2012) 15:472–8. doi:10.3109/10253890.2012.710919
5. Harris GW. The hypothalamus and endocrine glands. *Br Med Bull* (1950) 6:345–50.
6. Li CH, Geschwind II, Levy AL, Harris JI, Dixon JS, Pon NG, et al. Isolation and properties of alpha-corticotrophin from sheep pituitary glands. *Nature* (1954) 173:251–3. doi:10.1038/173251b0
7. Li CH, Simpson ME, Evans HM. Isolation of adrenocorticotropic hormone from sheep pituitaries. *Science* (1942) 96:450. doi:10.1126/science.96.2498.450
8. Ramachandran J, Chung D, Li CH. Synthesis of biologically active peptides related to ACTH. *Metabolism* (1964) 13(Suppl):1043–58. doi:10.1016/S0026-0495(64)80024-X
9. Nishimura O, Hatanaka C, Fujino M. Synthesis of peptides related to corticotropin (ACTH). IX. Application of N-hydroxy-5-norbornene-2,3-dicarboximide active ester procedure to the synthesis of human adrenocorticotropic hormone (alphah-ACTH). *Chem Pharm Bull (Tokyo)* (1975) 23:1212–20.
10. Clayton GW, Bell WR, Guillemin R. Stimulation of ACTH-release in humans by non-pressor fraction from commercial extracts of posterior pituitary. *Proc Soc Exp Biol Med* (1957) 96:777–9. doi:10.3181/00379727-96-23605
11. Lee TH, Lerner AB, Buettner-Janusch V. On the structure of human corticotropin (adrenocorticotropic hormone). *J Biol Chem* (1961) 236:2970–4.
12. Guillemin R, Rosenberg B. Humoral hypothalamic control of anterior pituitary: a study with combined tissue cultures. *Endocrinology* (1955) 57:599–607. doi:10.1210/endo-57-5-599
13. Schwyzer R. ACTH: a short introductory review. *Ann N Y Acad Sci* (1977) 297:3–26. doi:10.1111/j.1749-6632.1977.tb41843.x
14. Lowry PJ, Bennett HP, McMartin C. The isolation and amino acid sequence of an adrenocorticotrophin from the pars distalis and a corticotrophin-like intermediate-lobe peptide from the neurointermediate lobe of the pituitary of the dogfish *Squalus acanthias*. *Biochem J* (1974) 141:427–37. doi:10.1042/bj1410427
15. Lowry PJ, Chadwick A. Interrelations of some pituitary hormones. *Nature* (1970) 226:219–22. doi:10.1038/226219a0
16. Lowry PJ, Scott AP. The evolution of vertebrate corticotrophin and melanocyte stimulating hormone. *Gen Comp Endocrinol* (1975) 26:16–23. doi:10.1016/0016-6480(75)90211-7
17. Eipper BA, Mains RE. Structure and biosynthesis of pro-adrenocorticotropin/endorphin and related peptides. *Endocr Rev* (1980) 1:1–27. doi:10.1210/edrv-1-1-1
18. Nakanishi S, Inoue A, Kita T, Nakamura M, Chang AC, Cohen SN, et al. Nucleotide sequence of cloned cDNA for bovine corticotropin-beta-lipotropin precursor. *Nature* (1979) 278:423–7. doi:10.1038/278423a0
19. Schwyzer R, Sieber P. Total synthesis of adrenocorticotrophic hormone. *Nature* (1963) 199:172–4. doi:10.1038/199172b0
20. Schiller PW. Study of adrenocorticotropic hormone conformation by evaluation of intramolecular resonance energy transfer in N-dansyllysine 21-ACTH-(1-24)-tetrakosipeptide. *Proc Natl Acad Sci U S A* (1972) 69:975–9. doi:10.1073/pnas.69.4.975
21. Squire PG, Bewley T. Adrenocorticotropins. XXXV. The optical rotatory dispersion of sheep adrenocorticotropic hormone in acidic and basic solutions. *Biochim Biophys Acta* (1965) 109:234–40.
22. Low M, Kisfaludy L, Fermandjian S. Proposed preferred conformation of ACTH. *Acta Biochim Biophys Acad Sci Hung* (1975) 10:229–31.
23. Schwyzer R. Chemical structure and biological activity in the field of polypeptide hormones. *Pure Appl Chem* (1963) 6:265–95. doi:10.1351/pac196306030265
24. Schwyzer R. Organization and read-out of biological information in polypeptides. *Proc IV Int Congr Pharmacol* (1970) 5:196–209.
25. Hruby VJ, Sharma SD, Toth K, Jaw JY, al-Obeidi F, Sawyer TK, et al. Design, synthesis, and conformation of superpotent and prolonged acting melanotropins. *Ann N Y Acad Sci* (1993) 680:51–63. doi:10.1111/j.1749-6632.1993.tb19674.x
26. Samuels ME, Gallo-Payet N, Pinard S, Hasselmann C, Magne F, Patry L, et al. Bioinactive ACTH causing glucocorticoid deficiency. *J Clin Endocrinol Metab* (2013) 98:736–42. doi:10.1210/jc.2012-3199
27. Dores RM. Adrenocorticotropic hormone, melanocyte-stimulating hormone, and the melanocortin receptors: revisiting the work of Robert Schwyzer: a thirty-year retrospective. *Ann N Y Acad Sci* (2009) 1163:93–100. doi:10.1111/j.1749-6632.2009.04434.x
28. Hess B, Kutzner C, van der Spoel D, Lindahl E. GROMACS 4: algorithms for highly efficient, load-balanced, and scalable molecular simulation. *J Chem Theory Comput* (2008) 4:435–47. doi:10.1021/ct700301q
29. Inoue M, Tawata M, Yokomori N, Endo T, Onaya T. Expression of thyrotropin receptor on clonal osteoblast-like rat osteosarcoma cells. *Thyroid* (1998) 8:1059–64. doi:10.1089/thy.1998.8.1059
30. Schwyzer R, Schiller P, Seelig S, Sayers G. Isolated adrenal cells: log dose response curves for steroidogenesis induced by ACTH(1-24), ACTH(1-10), ACTH(4-10) and ACTH(5-10). *FEBS Lett* (1971) 19:229–31.
31. Seelig S, Lindley BD, Sayers G. A new approach to the structure-activity relationship for ACTH analogs using isolated adrenal cortex cells. *Methods Enzymol* (1975) 39:347–59. doi:10.1016/S0076-6879(75)39031-9
32. Fauchère JL, Rossier M, Capponi A, Vallotton MB. Potentiation of the antagonistic effect of ACTH11-24 on steroidogenesis by synthesis of covalent dimeric conjugates. *FEBS Lett* (1985) 183:283–6. doi:10.1016/0014-5793(85)80794-8
33. Feuilloley M, Stolz MB, Delarue C, Fauchère JL, Vaudry H. Structure-activity relationships of monomeric and dimeric synthetic ACTH fragments in perifused frog adrenal slices. *J Steroid Biochem* (1990) 35:583–92. doi:10.1016/0022-4731(90)90202-4
34. Fauchère JL, Pelican GM. [Specific covalent attachment of adrenocorticotropin and angiotensin II derivatives to polymeric matrices for use

in affinity chromatography (author's transl)]. *Helv Chim Acta* (1975) 58:1984–94. doi:10.1002/hlca.19750580713
35. Costa JL, Bui S, Reed P, Dores RM, Brennan MB, Hochgeschwender U. Mutational analysis of evolutionarily conserved ACTH residues. *Gen Comp Endocrinol* (2004) 136:12–6. doi:10.1016/j.ygcen.2003.11.005
36. Cone RD, Mountjoy KG, Robbins LS, Nadeau JH, Johnson KR, Roselli-Rehfuss L, et al. Cloning and functional characterization of a family of receptors for the melanotropic peptides. *Ann N Y Acad Sci* (1993) 680:342–63. doi:10.1111/j.1749-6632.1993.tb19694.x
37. Cone RD. Studies on the physiological functions of the melanocortin system. *Endocr Rev* (2006) 27:736–49. doi:10.1210/er.2006-0034
38. Ringholm A, Fredriksson R, Poliakova N, Yan YL, Postlethwait JH, Larhammar D, et al. One melanocortin 4 and two melanocortin 5 receptors from zebrafish show remarkable conservation in structure and pharmacology. *J Neurochem* (2002) 82:6–18. doi:10.1046/j.1471-4159.2002.00934.x
39. Ringholm A, Klovins J, Fredriksson R, Poliakova N, Larson ET, Kukkonen JP, et al. Presence of melanocortin (MC4) receptor in spiny dogfish suggests an ancient vertebrate origin of central melanocortin system. *Eur J Biochem* (2003) 270:213–21. doi:10.1046/j.1432-1033.2003.03371.x
40. Begriche K, Girardet C, McDonald P, Butler AA. Melanocortin-3 receptors and metabolic homeostasis. *Prog Mol Biol Transl Sci* (2013) 114:109–46. doi:10.1016/B978-0-12-386933-3.00004-2
41. Chen W, Kelly MA, Opitz-Araya X, Thomas RE, Low MJ, Cone RD. Exocrine gland dysfunction in MC5-R-deficient mice: evidence for coordinated regulation of exocrine gland function by melanocortin peptides. *Cell* (1997) 91:789–98. doi:10.1016/S0092-8674(00)80467-5
42. Fredriksson R, Schiöth HB. The repertoire of G-protein-coupled receptors in fully sequenced genomes. *Mol Pharmacol* (2005) 67:1414–25. doi:10.1124/mol.104.009001
43. Gallo-Payet N, Battista MC. Steroidogenesis-adrenal cell signal transduction. *Compr Physiol* (2014) 4:889–964. doi:10.1002/cphy.c130050
44. Gallo-Payet N. 60 years of POMC: adrenal and extra-adrenal functions of ACTH. *J Mol Endocrinol* (2016) 56:T135–56. doi:10.1530/JME-15-0257
45. Mountjoy KG, Robbins LS, Mortrud MT, Cone RD. The cloning of a family of genes that encode the melanocortin receptors. *Science* (1992) 257:1248–51. doi:10.1126/science.1325670
46. Metherell LA, Chapple JP, Cooray S, David A, Becker C, Rüschendorf F, et al. Mutations in MRAP, encoding a new interacting partner of the ACTH receptor, cause familial glucocorticoid deficiency type 2. *Nat Genet* (2005) 37:166–70. doi:10.1038/ng1501
47. Cooray SN, Clark AJ. Melanocortin receptors and their accessory proteins. *Mol Cell Endocrinol* (2011) 331:215–21. doi:10.1016/j.mce.2010.07.015
48. Hinkle PM, Sebag JA. Structure and function of the melanocortin2 receptor accessory protein (MRAP). *Mol Cell Endocrinol* (2009) 300:25–31. doi:10.1016/j.mce.2008.10.041
49. Hinkle PM, Serasinghe MN, Jakabowski A, Sebag JA, Wilson KR, Haskell-Luevano C. Use of chimeric melanocortin-2 and -4 receptors to identify regions responsible for ligand specificity and dependence on melanocortin 2 receptor accessory protein. *Eur J Pharmacol* (2011) 660:94–102. doi:10.1016/j.ejphar.2010.10.113
50. Chai BX, Pogozheva ID, Lai YM, Li JY, Neubig RR, Mosberg HI, et al. Receptor-antagonist interactions in the complexes of agouti and agouti-related protein with human melanocortin 1 and 4 receptors. *Biochemistry* (2005) 44:3418–31. doi:10.1021/bi0478704
51. Pogozheva ID, Chai BX, Lomize AL, Fong TM, Weinberg DH, Nargund RP, et al. Interactions of human melanocortin 4 receptor with nonpeptide and peptide agonists. *Biochemistry* (2005) 44:11329–41. doi:10.1021/bi0501840
52. Li J, Edwards PC, Burghammer M, Villa C, Schertler GF. Structure of bovine rhodopsin in a trigonal crystal form. *J Mol Biol* (2004) 343:1409–38. doi:10.1016/j.jmb.2004.08.090
53. Fowler CB, Pogozheva ID, LeVine H III, Mosberg HI. Refinement of a homology model of the mu-opioid receptor using distance constraints from intrinsic and engineered zinc-binding sites. *Biochemistry* (2004) 43:8700–10. doi:10.1021/bi036067r
54. Davis P, Franquemont S, Liang L, Angleson JK, Dores RM. Evolution of the melanocortin-2 receptor in tetrapods: studies on *Xenopus tropicalis* MC2R and *Anolis carolinensis* MC2R. *Gen Comp Endocrinol* (2013) 188:75–84. doi:10.1016/j.ygcen.2013.04.007
55. Meimaridou E, Hughes CR, Kowalczyk J, Guasti L, Chapple JP, King PJ, et al. Familial glucocorticoid deficiency: new genes and mechanisms. *Mol Cell Endocrinol* (2013) 371:195–200. doi:10.1016/j.mce.2012.12.010
56. Clark AJ, McLoughlin L, Grossman A. Familial glucocorticoid deficiency associated with point mutation in the adrenocorticotropin receptor. *Lancet* (1993) 341:461–2. doi:10.1016/0140-6736(93)90208-X
57. Muscatelli F, Strom TM, Walker AP, Zanaria E, Récan D, Meindl A, et al. Mutations in the DAX-1 gene give rise to both X-linked adrenal hypoplasia congenita and hypogonadotropic hypogonadism. *Nature* (1994) 372:672–6. doi:10.1038/372672a0
58. Meimaridou E, Kowalczyk J, Guasti L, Hughes CR, Wagner F, Frommolt P, et al. Mutations in NNT encoding nicotinamide nucleotide transhydrogenase cause familial glucocorticoid deficiency. *Nat Genet* (2012) 44:740–2. doi:10.1038/ng.2299
59. Hasselmann C, Deladoey J, Vuissoz J-M, Patry L, Alirezaie N, Schwartzentruber J, et al. Expanding the phenotypic spectrum of nicotinamide nucleotide transhydrogenase (NNT) mutations and using whole exome sequencing to discover potential disease modifiers. *J. Genomes Exomes* (2013) 2:19–30. doi:10.4137/JGE.S11378
60. Scott R, Van Vliet G, Deladoëy J. Association of adrenal insufficiency with insulin-dependent diabetes mellitus in a patient with inactivating mutations in nicotinamide nucleotide transhydrogenase: a phenocopy of the animal model. *Eur J Endocrinol* (2017) 176(3):C1–2. doi:10.1530/EJE-16-0970
61. Prasad R, Chan LF, Hughes CR, Kaski JP, Kowalczyk JC, Savage MO, et al. Thioredoxin Reductase 2 (TXNRD2) mutation associated with familial glucocorticoid deficiency (FGD). *J Clin Endocrinol Metab* (2014) 99:E1556–63. doi:10.1210/jc.2013-3844
62. Tullio-Pelet A, Salomon R, Hadj-Rabia S, Mugnier C, de Laet MH, Chaouachi B, et al. Mutant WD-repeat protein in triple-A syndrome. *Nat Genet* (2000) 26:332–5. doi:10.1038/81642
63. Arboleda VA, Lee H, Parnaik R, Fleming A, Banerjee A, Ferraz-de-Souza B, et al. Mutations in the PCNA-binding domain of CDKN1C cause IMAGe syndrome. *Nat Genet* (2012) 44:788–92. doi:10.1038/ng.2275
64. Hughes CR, Guasti L, Meimaridou E, Chuang CH, Schimenti JC, King PJ, et al. MCM4 mutation causes adrenal failure, short stature, and natural killer cell deficiency in humans. *J Clin Invest* (2012) 122:814–20. doi:10.1172/JCI60224
65. Narumi S, Amano N, Ishii T, Katsumata N, Muroya K, Adachi M, et al. SAMD9 mutations cause a novel multisystem disorder, MIRAGE syndrome, and are associated with loss of chromosome 7. *Nat Genet* (2016) 48:792–7. doi:10.1038/ng.3569
66. Krude H, Biebermann H, Luck W, Horn R, Brabant G, Grüters A. Severe early-onset obesity, adrenal insufficiency and red hair pigmentation caused by POMC mutations in humans. *Nat Genet* (1998) 19:155–7. doi:10.1038/509
67. Challis BG, Pritchard LE, Creemers JW, Delplanque J, Keogh JM, Luan J, et al. A missense mutation disrupting a dibasic prohormone processing site in pro-opiomelanocortin (POMC) increases susceptibility to early-onset obesity through a novel molecular mechanism. *Hum Mol Genet* (2002) 11:1997–2004. doi:10.1093/hmg/11.17.1997
68. Lee YS, Challis BG, Thompson DA, Yeo GS, Keogh JM, Madonna ME, et al. A POMC variant implicates beta-melanocyte-stimulating hormone in the control of human energy balance. *Cell Metab* (2006) 3:135–40. doi:10.1016/j.cmet.2006.01.006
69. Krude H, Biebermann H, Schnabel D, Tansek MZ, Theunissen P, Mullis PE, et al. Obesity due to proopiomelanocortin deficiency: three new cases and treatment trials with thyroid hormone and ACTH4-10. *J Clin Endocrinol Metab* (2003) 88:4633–40. doi:10.1210/jc.2003-030502
70. Kühnen P, Clément K, Wiegand S, Blankenstein O, Gottesdiener K, Martini LL, et al. Proopiomelanocortin deficiency treated with a melanocortin-4 receptor agonist. *N Engl J Med* (2016) 375:240–6. doi:10.1056/NEJMoa1512693
71. Kirk JM, Brain CE, Carson DJ, Hyde JC, Grant DB. Cushing's syndrome caused by nodular adrenal hyperplasia in children with McCune-Albright syndrome. *J Pediatr* (1999) 134:789–92. doi:10.1016/S0022-3476(99)70302-1
72. Lieberman SA, Eccleshall TR, Feldman D. ACTH-independent massive bilateral adrenal disease (AIMBAD): a subtype of Cushing's syndrome with major diagnostic and therapeutic implications. *Eur J Endocrinol* (1994) 131:67–73. doi:10.1530/eje.0.1310067

73. Assié G, Libé R, Espiard S, Rizk-Rabin M, Guimier A, Luscap W, et al. ARMC5 mutations in macronodular adrenal hyperplasia with Cushing's syndrome. *N Engl J Med* (2013) 369:2105–14. doi:10.1056/NEJMoa1304603
74. Espiard S, Drougat L, Libé R, Assié G, Perlemoine K, Guignat L, et al. ARMC5 mutations in a large cohort of primary macronodular adrenal hyperplasia: clinical and functional consequences. *J Clin Endocrinol Metab* (2015) 100:E926–35. doi:10.1210/jc.2014-4204
75. Fragoso MC, Alencar GA, Lerario AM, Bourdeau I, Almeida MQ, Mendonca BB, et al. Genetics of primary macronodular adrenal hyperplasia. *J Endocrinol* (2015) 224:R31–43. doi:10.1530/JOE-14-0568
76. Cheitlin RA, Westphal M, Cabrera CM, Fujii DK, Snyder J, Fitzgerald PA. Cushing's syndrome due to bilateral adrenal macronodular hyperplasia with undetectable ACTH: cell culture of adenoma cells on extracellular matrix. *Horm Res* (1988) 29:162–7. doi:10.1159/000180995
77. Bourdeau I, D'Amour P, Hamet P, Boutin JM, Lacroix A. Aberrant membrane hormone receptors in incidentally discovered bilateral macronodular adrenal hyperplasia with subclinical Cushing's syndrome. *J Clin Endocrinol Metab* (2001) 86:5534–40. doi:10.1210/jcem.86.11.8062
78. Louiset E, Duparc C, Young J, Renouf S, Tetsi Nomigni M, Boutelet I, et al. Intraadrenal corticotropin in bilateral macronodular adrenal hyperplasia. *N Engl J Med* (2013) 369:2115–25. doi:10.1056/NEJMoa1215245
79. Matsukura S, Kakita T, Sueoka S, Yoshimi H, Hirata Y, Yokota M, et al. Multiple hormone receptors in the adenylate cyclase of human adrenocortical tumors. *Cancer Res* (1980) 40:3768–71.
80. Smallridge RC, Bourne K, Pearson BW, Van Heerden JA, Carpenter PC, Young WF. Cushing's syndrome due to medullary thyroid carcinoma: diagnosis by proopiomelanocortin messenger ribonucleic acid in situ hybridization. *J Clin Endocrinol Metab* (2003) 88:4565–8. doi:10.1210/jc.2002-021796
81. Stewart PM, Gibson S, Crosby SR, Penn R, Holder R, Ferry D, et al. ACTH precursors characterize the ectopic ACTH syndrome. *Clin Endocrinol (Oxf)* (1994) 40:199–204. doi:10.1111/j.1365-2265.1994.tb02468.x
82. Gibson S, Ray DW, Crosby SR, Dornan TL, Jennings AM, Bevan JS, et al. Impaired processing of proopiomelanocortin in corticotroph macroadenomas. *J Clin Endocrinol Metab* (1996) 81:497–502. doi:10.1210/jcem.81.2.8636257
83. Kovalitskaya YA, Zolotarev YA, Kolobov AA, Sadovnikov VB, Yurovsky VV, Navolotskaya EV. Interaction of ACTH synthetic fragments with rat adrenal cortex membranes. *J Pept Sci* (2007) 13:513–8. doi:10.1002/psc.873
84. Kapas S, Cammas FM, Hinson JP, Clark AJ. Agonist and receptor binding properties of adrenocorticotropin peptides using the cloned mouse adrenocorticotropin receptor expressed in a stably transfected HeLa cell line. *Endocrinology* (1996) 137:3291–4. doi:10.1210/en.137.8.3291
85. Nijenhuis WA, Oosterom J, Adan RA. AgRP(83-132) acts as an inverse agonist on the human-melanocortin-4 receptor. *Mol Endocrinol* (2001) 15:164–71. doi:10.1210/mend.15.1.0578
86. Yang YK, Dickinson C, Lai YM, Li JY, Gantz I. Functional properties of an agouti signaling protein variant and characteristics of its cognate radioligand. *Am J Physiol Regul Integr Comp Physiol* (2001) 281:R1877–86.
87. McNulty JC, Jackson PJ, Thompson DA, Chai B, Gantz I, Barsh GS, et al. Structures of the agouti signaling protein. *J Mol Biol* (2005) 346:1059–70. doi:10.1016/j.jmb.2004.12.030
88. Hruby VJ, Wilkes BC, Hadley ME, Al-Obeidi F, Sawyer TK, Staples DJ, et al. Alpha-melanotropin: the minimal active sequence in the frog skin bioassay. *J Med Chem* (1987) 30:2126–30. doi:10.1021/jm00394a033
89. Barrett P, MacDonald A, Helliwell R, Davidson G, Morgan P. Cloning and expression of a new member of the melanocyte-stimulating hormone receptor family. *J Mol Endocrinol* (1994) 12:203–13. doi:10.1677/jme.0.0120203
90. Malendowicz LK, Rebuffat P, Nussdorfer GG, Nowak KW. Corticotropin-inhibiting peptide enhances aldosterone secretion by dispersed rat zona glomerulosa cells. *J Steroid Biochem Mol Biol* (1998) 67:149–52. doi:10.1016/S0960-0760(98)00081-8
91. Cai M, Hruby VJ. The melanocortin receptor system: a target for multiple degenerative diseases. *Curr Protein Pept Sci* (2016) 17(5):488–96. doi:10.2174/1389203717666160226145330
92. Bouw E, Huisman M, Neggers SJ, Themmen AP, van der Lely AJ, Delhanty PJ. Development of potent selective competitive-antagonists of the melanocortin type 2 receptor. *Mol Cell Endocrinol* (2014) 394:99–104. doi:10.1016/j.mce.2014.07.003

4

Dual Topology of the Melanocortin-2 Receptor Accessory Protein is Stable

*Zachary J. Maben, Sundeep Malik, Liyi H. Jiang and Patricia M. Hinkle**

Department of Pharmacology and Physiology, University of Rochester Medical Center, Rochester, NY, USA

***Correspondence:**
Patricia M. Hinkle
patricia_hinkle@urmc.rochester.edu

Melanocortin 2 receptor accessory protein (MRAP) facilitates trafficking of melanocortin 2 (MC2) receptors and is essential for ACTH binding and signaling. MRAP is a single transmembrane domain protein that forms antiparallel homodimers. These studies ask when MRAP first acquires this dual topology, whether MRAP architecture is static or stable, and whether the accessory protein undergoes rapid turnover. To answer these questions, we developed an approach that capitalizes on the specificity of bacterial biotin ligase, which adds biotin to lysine in a short acceptor peptide sequence; the distinct mobility of MRAP protomers of opposite orientations based on their *N*-linked glycosylation; and the ease of identifying biotin-labeled proteins. We inserted biotin ligase acceptor peptides at the *N*- or C-terminal ends of MRAP and expressed the modified proteins in mammalian cells together with either cytoplasmic or endoplasmic reticulum-targeted biotin ligase. MRAP assumed dual topology early in biosynthesis in both CHO and OS3 adrenal cells. Once established, MRAP orientation was stable. Despite its conformational stability, MRAP displayed a half-life of under 2 h in CHO cells. The amount of MRAP was increased by the proteasome inhibitor MG132 and MRAP underwent ubiquitylation on lysine and other amino acids. Nonetheless, when protein synthesis was blocked with cycloheximide, MRAP was rapidly degraded even when MG132 was included and all lysines were replaced by arginines, implicating non-proteasomal degradation pathways. The results show that although MRAP does not change orientations during trafficking, its synthesis and degradation are dynamically regulated.

Keywords: accessory protein, ACTH, biotin ligase, cAMP, MC2 receptor, MRAP, membrane protein topology, ubiquitin

INTRODUCTION

The hypothalamic/pituitary/adrenal axis comprises a classical endocrine loop in which hypothalamic corticotropin-releasing hormone stimulates synthesis and release of ACTH from corticotropes of the anterior pituitary gland, ACTH stimulates glucocorticoid production in the adrenal gland, and glucocorticoids exert feedback control centrally. ACTH stimulates multiple steps in the glucocorticoid biosynthetic pathway, acting via a receptor coupled to the heterotrimeric Gs protein to activate adenylyl cyclase and elevate intracellular cAMP. ACTH also exerts receptor-dependent but cAMP-independent effects (1).

Abbreviations: AP, acceptor peptide; BirAcyt, cytoplasmic biotin ligase; BirAER, ER-targeted biotin ligase-KDEL; Ccyt, cytoplasmic carboxyterminus; Cexo, extracellular carboxyterminus; CRE, cAMP response element; ER, endoplasmic reticulum; MC2R, melanocortin-2 receptor; MRAP, MC2 receptor accessory protein; Ncyt, intracellular aminoterminus; Nexo, extracellular aminoterminus.

The receptor for ACTH was identified almost 25 years ago by Mountjoy et al. (2). The melanocortin 2 (MC2) (ACTH) receptor is one of five structurally related G protein-coupled melanocortin receptors, MCl through MC5, all of which are activated by peptides derived from pro-opiomelanocortin, or POMC. The MC2 receptor was found to differ from the other four melanocortin receptors in two important ways. First, it could not be activated by α-, β-, or γ-MSH but only by the longer ACTH peptide. Second, it was not functional unless it was expressed in adrenal or melanoma cells. This led to speculation that the MC2 receptor required an additional protein present in a limited number of cell types.

The nature of the hypothetical accessory protein remained a mystery for more than a decade, when Metherell et al. (3) identified the gene encoding MC2 receptor accessory protein (MRAP) from individuals with familial glucocorticoid deficiency type 2, which is characterized by resistance to ACTH despite normal MC2 receptor genes. MRAP encodes a small protein with a single predicted transmembrane domain. Two splice variants of human MRAP (α and β) are identical in the aminoterminal and transmembrane regions. When MRAP was co-expressed with MC2 receptor, the receptor was able to traffic to the plasma membrane and respond to ACTH with an increase in cAMP in cells that were otherwise non-responsive. MRAP and MC2 receptors have been shown to interact closely by a variety of approaches including co-precipitation (4, 5), fluorescence microscopy (6, 7), bimolecular fluorescence complementation (8), and co-internalization in response to ACTH (9). Recent data establish that two MRAP dimers can interact with one MC2 receptor and that two MC2 receptors can interact with one MRAP, but it is unclear whether this happens normally (10). MRAP2, an MRAP paralog, co-precipitates with the MC2 receptor and all other members of the melanocortin receptor family (5) but does not support signaling by MC2 receptors (11).

Using an alanine-scanning mutagenesis approach and focusing on the highly conserved aminoterminus of MRAP, we discovered that MRAP lacking a critical tyrosine-rich region was able to promote MC2 receptor trafficking but not signaling (11). This established that MRAP has two distinct functions, one to enable MC2 receptor trafficking to the cell surface, perhaps because it assists protein folding, and a second to enable signal transduction. Importantly, when MC2 receptors were expressed with a mutated MRAP, receptors were localized on the plasma membrane but completely unable to bind ACTH. As a result, ACTH cannot be expected to exert any effect - cAMP-dependent or otherwise - in cells lacking MRAP.

It is well established that mRNA encoding MC2 receptor undergoes feed-forward regulation, increasing in response to stress or ACTH (12). MRAP mRNA levels also increase, and do so within minutes, in response to either an imposed stress or ACTH (13, 14). MC2 receptor and MRAP mRNAs rise dramatically when cultured adrenal cells are incubated with ACTH, establishing a direct action at the adrenal gland (15). It is not known whether MC2 receptor and MRAP protein levels also change on a rapid time scale. One of the goals of the experiments described here was to characterize MRAP turnover in an isolated cell system.

The architecture of MRAP is extremely unusual. MRAP appears to form antiparallel homodimers. This conclusion is based on the following: (1) immunological findings showing dual topology, where antibodies identify both the amino and carboxyterminal ends of MRAP facing outwards on the cell surface (4); (2) quantitative co-precipitation of differentially tagged MRAPs, pointing to a multimeric structure (4); (3) biochemical experiments showing that approximately half of MRAP undergoes glycosylation at the single predicted site for *N*-linked glycosylation, a process that takes place in the interior of the endoplasmic reticulum (ER) and Golgi apparatus (4); (4) bimolecular fluorescence complementation (8) and bioluminescence resonance energy transfer (16) in configurations consistent with an antiparallel dimeric structure; and (5) evidence that a concatenated protein made by fusing two MRAPs to the extracellular aminoterminus of the MC2 receptor is ACTH-responsive (10). The latter studies established that the tyrosine-rich domain of the MRAP aminoterminus is necessary on the outer surface of the cell, likely allowing ACTH to bind.

Taken together, these data provide strong evidence that MRAP forms antiparallel homodimers. MRAP and MRAP2 are the only single transmembrane domain proteins thought to exist in this configuration. It is not yet known when MRAP conformation is established, whether MRAP orientation changes during synthesis and trafficking, whether dual topology predominates in adrenal cells, and whether MRAP is stable. We designed the experiments reported here to address these unresolved issues and describe several approaches to probe the topology of the MRAP protein at different times after biosynthesis and estimate its half-life.

MATERIALS AND METHODS

Reagents

Melanocortin 2 receptor accessory protein plasmids that have not been described previously (4, 8, 11) were constructed using QuikChange from Stratagene with standard molecular biological techniques and verified by sequencing. MRAP-V5-3xFlag contained mMRAP followed by GKPIPNPLLGLDSTGRDY KDHDGDYKDHDIDYKDDDDK at the C-terminus. AP-MRAP contained the minimal AP sequence GLNDIFEAQKIEWHE immediately after the initiating Met followed by mMRAP or mMRAP-V5-3xFlag. MRAP-AP contained the same AP sequence at the C-terminus of mMRAP or mMRAP-V5-3xFlag followed by a stop codon. MRAPs containing the AP sequence but no epitope tags were constructed similarly. On figures, these constructs are shown as AP-MRAP or MRAP-AP and epitope tags are described in the legends. V5-MART1-AP and AP-MART1-V5 were constructed by adding V5 epitope (GKPIPNPLLGLDST) and AP sequence (GLNDIFEAQKIEWHE) to opposite ends of mMART1. (4K to R)MRAP refers to V5-mMRAP-3xFlag with the four Lys in native mMRAP mutated to Arg. 3xHA-hMC2 receptor, referred to as MC2 receptor, was from Missouri cDNA Resource Center and plasmid encoding eGFP from Clontech. BirA in pcDNA3 and $BirA_{ER}$ in pDisplay vectors were generously donated by Dr. Alice Ting (Massachusetts Institute of Technology) and CRE-luciferase by Dr. George Holz (SUNY Upstate Medical University). Plasmid encoding HA-ubiquitin (HA-Ub) has been described (17). Monoclonal antibodies were from the following: Sigma (M2 anti-Flag and immobilized M2 anti-Flag), Covance (HA-11 anti-HA), and AbDSerotec (anti-V5). Streptavidin–HRP and streptavidin–agarose were from Thermo Scientific, immobilized Protein A/G beads from Santa Cruz Biotechnology, and HRP-labeled antibody against mouse heavy and light chains from BioRad.

Cell Growth and Transfection

CHO cells were from American Type Culture Collection and OS3 adrenal cells (18) from Dr. Bernard Schimmer (University of Toronto). CHO and OS3 cells were maintained in DMEM/F12 medium containing 5% fetal bovine serum at 37°C in 5% CO_2-95% air and passaged with trypsin. Transfection was performed using FugeneHD or Lipofectamine 3000 according to manufacturers' instructions. Stable cell lines were generated by transfecting with plasmids encoding an MRAP, BirA, or $BirA_{ER}$ and selecting with 1 mg/ml G418. Pooled cells were used for experiments. Biotin-labeling experiments were performed by adding 2.5 μM biotin to complete medium at the time of transfection unless otherwise noted.

cAMP Responses

In brief, cells were grown in white 96-well plates and transfected with 40–50 ng total DNA/well, usually with equal parts of MC2 receptor, MRAP construct and CRE-luciferase, a reporter containing multiple cAMP response elements from the rat insulin promoter (19). After 24 h cells were challenged for 4–5 h with hACTH(1–24) or 20 μM forskolin in DMEM with 0.1% BSA. Medium was replaced with Firefly Reagent from Nanolight and luminescence read in a BioTek platereader. Unless noted, results are expressed as percent of the forskolin response measured in the same experiment.

Immunoprecipitation, SDS-PAGE, and Immunoblotting

Cells were washed with PBS and lysed on ice in Tris/Mg/EGTA buffer (150 mM NaCl, 50 mM Tris-Cl, 1 mM EDTA, and 1% Triton X-100, pH 8.0) containing protease inhibitors. Iodoacetamide (10 mM) was included in lysis buffers when ubiquitin labeling was being assessed. Samples were centrifuged at 10,000 × *g* for 20 min to remove nuclei and supernatants used for analysis. In some cases, HA- or Flag-labeled proteins were immunoprecipitated by incubating overnight at 4°C with 1:1000 dilutions of antibody and collected on Protein A/G beads. Biotin-labeled proteins were pelleted following overnight incubation with streptavidin–agarose beads. Samples were taken up in NuPage LDS sample buffer with a final concentration of 50 mM dithiothreitol. For analysis by SDS-PAGE samples were run on Lonza PagR or BioRad TGX gels. Proteins were transferred to nitrocellulose, blocked in TBST (Tris-buffered saline with 0.05% Tween 20) with 5% non-fat dry milk, and incubated overnight at 4°C in either monoclonal anti-V5, anti-HA, or anti-Flag antibody at 1:5000 in TBST/milk. After washing, antibody blots were incubated in 1:5000 HRP-anti-mouse heavy and light chain, washed and visualized using Western Lightning chemiluminescent reagent. To visualize biotin-labeled proteins, blots were incubated in 1:10,000 HRP–streptavidin in TBST with 0.5–1% BSA, because milk contains biotin, washed and developed. In some cases, blots were subsequently incubated in 0.1% sodium azide to inactivate HRP and blotted with antibody as described above.

Cell Surface ELISA

Expression of proteins on the plasma membrane was quantified as described previously (4, 11). Cells grown in 12- or 24-well plates were fixed with 2 or 3% paraformaldehyde for 10–20 min at room temperature, washed with PBS, and incubated for ~1 h with 1:5000 monoclonal anti-HA, anti-V5, or anti-Flag antibodies in PBS containing 5% non-fat dry milk. Cells were then washed extensively and incubated for ~1 h with 1:5000 HRP-labeled anti-mouse IgG, and washed prior to the addition of tetramethylbenzidine substrate (Sigma) and measurement of absorbance at 450 nm.

Fluorescence Microscopy

For microscopy, CHO cells stably expressing $BirA_{cyt}$ or $BirA_{ER}$ were grown on glass coverslips and transfected with AP-tagged MRAP constructs. After overnight incubation, live cells were incubated with anti-Flag antibody (1:250 in serum-containing medium) for 30 min at 37°C, washed, and then incubated with 1:500 Alexa488-labeled anti-mouse M2 and 1:500 Alexa555-labeled streptavidin and incubated for 30 min at room temperature. Cells were washed, fixed in paraformaldehyde, washed again and mounted in Prolong Gold (InVitrogen), and viewed in a Nikon epifluorescence microscope with a 40× oil objective. Images showing Flag and streptavidin were obtained using 500 and 2500 ms exposures, respectively. All Flag and all streptavidin micrographs were processed identically.

Miscellaneous

To deglycosylate proteins, cell lysates were denatured and incubated with PNGaseF from New England Biolabs following manufacturer's instructions; control lysates were incubated identically in reactions lacking enzyme. All experiments were repeated a minimum of two times. Error bars indicate mean and range or SE of duplicate or triplicate determinations in representative experiments. Significance of differences between two values was determined by Student's *t*-test.

RESULTS

When Is MRAP Topology Established?

The strategy used to determine whether MRAP is first synthesized in dual orientations is outlined schematically in **Figure 1A**. Biotin labeling of a protein modified to contain a decarboxylase biotin acceptor domain was used previously to characterize membrane insertion of bacterial lactose permease (20). The biotin-labeling approach described here uses a small acceptor sequence and exogenous BirAs to provide a new means to analyze MRAP architecture. The bacterial enzyme biotin ligase (BirA) attaches a biotin residue to the single Lys residue in a specific acceptor peptide sequence (AP). When expressed in mammalian cells, bacterial biotin ligase is localized in the cytoplasm; addition of a carboxyterminal KDEL sequence targets the enzyme to the ER (21, 22). Because there are relatively low concentrations of

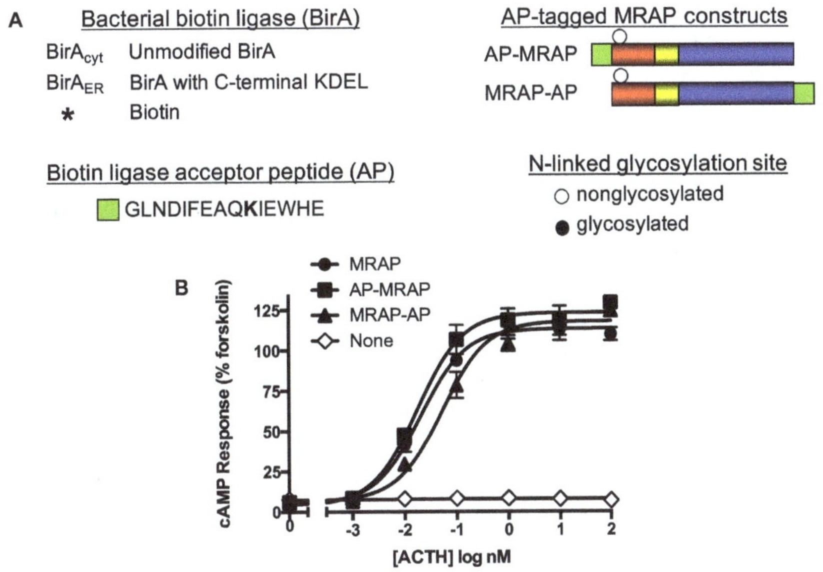

FIGURE 1 | Use of biotin tagging to discern MRAP orientation. (A) Schematic representation showing the sequence of the acceptor peptide (AP) for bacterial biotin ligase that catalyzes addition of biotin to Lys. Addition of C-terminal KDEL sequence to BirA targets it to the ER. Circles depict a potential *N*-linked glycosylation site (Asn-X-Ser/Thr) with or without glycosylation. An AP sequence was added immediately after the initiating Met in AP–MRAP or at the C-terminus in MRAP–AP as detailed in Section "Materials and Methods." **(B)** ACTH responses of CHO cells expressing a cAMP-responsive CRE-luciferase reporter, MC2 receptor, and MRAP constructs.

biotin in standard serum-supplemented tissue culture media, it is straightforward to initiate biotin labeling of a protein tagged with an AP sequence by adding exogenous biotin. Mouse MRAP contains a single *N*-linked glycosylation site at Asn3 of the aminoterminus and *N*-glycosylation occurs exclusively in the inside of the ER and Golgi apparatus, which is topologically equivalent to the exoplasmic face of the plasma membrane. Glycosylated MRAP, which migrates more slowly than non-glycosylated MRAP on SDS-PAGE, must, therefore, be in the N_{exo}/C_{cyt} orientation unless it has changed orientations during trafficking. We engineered MRAPs with an AP sequence at either the aminoterminal or carboxyterminal end of the protein; each of these MRAP constructs also contained a Flag epitope. As shown in **Figure 1B**, control MRAP, AP–MRAP (*N*-terminal AP sequence), and MRAP–AP (C-terminal AP sequence) all supported comparable ACTH-stimulated increases in a cAMP reporter.

MRAP, AP–MRAP, and MRAP–AP were expressed in CHO cells stably expressing either cytoplasmic BirA or ER-targeted $BirA_{ER}$. The upper left panel of **Figure 2** shows a Flag immunoblot identifying total MRAP. In every case, monomeric glycosylated and non-glycosylated MRAP species ran as a doublet at ~20 and 25 kDa. Enzymatic degradation with the glycosidase PNGaseF confirmed that the two major bands represented MRAP with and without *N*-linked glycosylation (4) and **Figure 11** below. Higher MW bands are likely MRAP multimers and their mobility shifts following PNGaseF treatment (not shown). The upper right panel of **Figure 2A** shows the same blot probed with streptavidin to detect only biotin-labeled proteins. Despite having identical molecular weights, AP–MRAP and MRAP–AP consistently displayed different mobilities on SDS-PAGE, as do AP–MART1 and MART1–AP (**Figure 3** below). It is possible that the proteins undergo different post-translational modifications but the behavior of membrane proteins on SDS-PAGE is not always predictable.

Endogenous biotinylated carboxylases are visible in all lanes at high molecular weight (75 kDa and above) in the blot on the upper right. These metabolically labeled proteins do not depend on transfected BirA. The three control lanes shown on the left of each blot in **Figure 2** demonstrate that MRAP lacking the biotin acceptor peptide was expressed well but not labeled with biotin. Cytoplasmic BirA catalyzed the addition of biotin to the faster-migrating, non-glycosylated form of AP–MRAP (situation *a* in **Figure 2B**), whereas ER-targeted $BirA_{ER}$ added biotin to the higher molecular weight glycosylated form of AP–MRAP (situation *b*). The reverse was found when cytoplasmic BirA and ER-targeted $BirA_{ER}$ were expressed with MRAP–AP. In this case, $BirA_{cyt}$ preferentially labeled glycosylated MRAP–AP and $BirA_{ER}$ preferentially labeled non-glycosylated MRAP–AP (situations *c* and *d*, respectively). These results support the conclusion that the great majority of MRAP molecules achieve an antiparallel orientation when first synthesized. The finding of some biotin-labeled but non-glycosylated AP–MRAP with $BirA_{ER}$ could result from (1) biotin labeling of AP–MRAP that is incompletely glycosylated, (2) incomplete import of overexpressed $BirA_{ER}$ into the ER leaving some active enzyme in the cytoplasm, or (3) a change in orientation of a small portion of MRAP after synthesis. The finding of a biotin-labeled and glycosylated MRAP–AP band with $BirA_{ER}$ is consistent with incomplete $BirA_{ER}$ import. After overnight incubation in biotin-supplemented media, essentially all AP-tagged MRAP could be collected on streptavidin–agarose beads, implying nearly quantitative biotinylation.

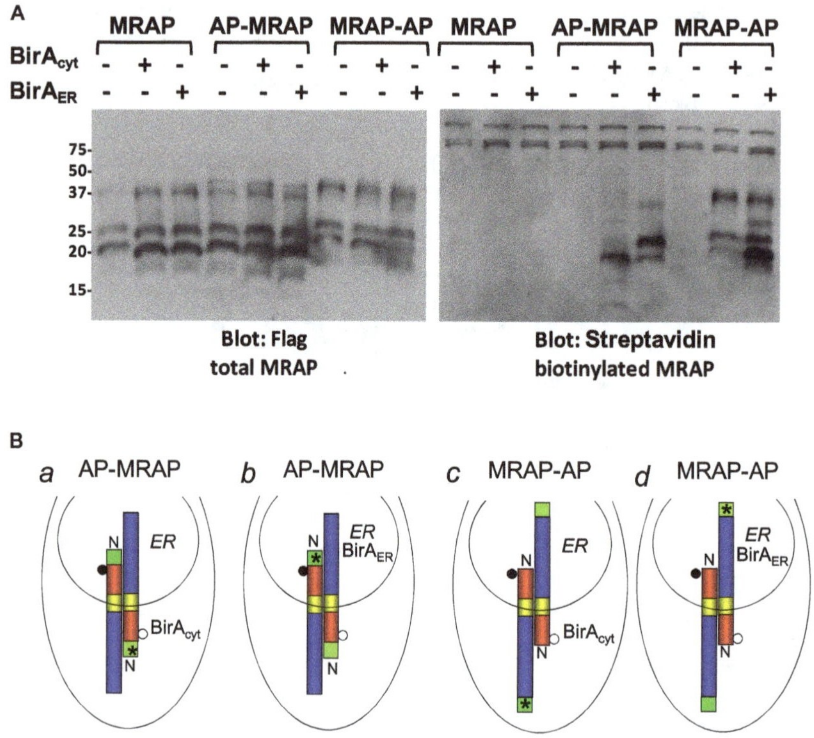

FIGURE 2 | Biotin labeling confirms dual topology of MRAP. (A) CHO cells stably expressing $BirA_{cyt}$ or $BirA_{ER}$ were transfected with MRAP, AP–MRAP, or MRAP–AP; these plasmids also contained a Flag epitope. Following detergent solubilization, proteins were resolved on SDS-PAGE and probed with monoclonal anti-Flag antibody and HRP-anti-mouse IgG or HRP–streptavidin. **(B)** Expected localization of BirA and predicted orientation of newly synthesized MRAPs. Filled and open circles depict glycosylated and non-glycosylated MRAP and red stars represent biotin.

As an additional control for this approach, we studied MART1 (also called Melan-A), a melanosome protein with a single transmembrane domain, strongly predicted N_{exo}/C_{cyt} orientation, and size close to that of mouse MRAP (18 vs. 14 kDa without epitopes or carbohydrate). We engineered plasmids encoding MART1 with AP tags at one end or the other and V5 tags at the opposite ends. We used a previously described fixed cell ELISA protocol (4) in which antibodies were added to intact cells to detect epitopes localized on the outside of the plasma membrane (**Figure 3A**). MART1 was found in the predicted N_{exo}/C_{cyt} orientation, whereas MRAPs with the AP sequence at either end were found in dual N_{exo}/C_{cyt} and N_{cyt}/C_{exo} orientations. MRAP but not MART1 increased surface expression of co-expressed MC2 receptor (**Figure 3B**). MART1 was then tested in an experiment identical to that shown in **Figure 2** for MRAP. AP–MART1 was expressed strongly but labeled only by ER-localized $BirA_{ER}$ and labeling was rather weak (**Figure 3C**). By contrast, MART1–AP was expressed weakly but labeled strongly by cytoplasmic BirA and slightly by $BirA_{ER}$. Labeling by $BirA_{ER}$ probably occurred because of incomplete import of $BirA_{ER}$ into the ER, which left some biotin ligase in the cytoplasm.

Does MRAP Change Orientation after Biosynthesis?

To isolate MRAP that had trafficked to the plasma membrane, we localized cell surface biotin-labeled MRAP by fluorescence microscopy. Cells stably expressing cytoplasmic or ER-targeted BirA were transiently transfected to express either AP–MRAP–Flag or MRAP–Flag–AP. After incubation with biotin, live cells were stained with monoclonal anti-Flag antibody or fluorescent streptavidin. Because MRAP forms an antiparallel structure, both AP–MRAP–Flag and MRAP–Flag–AP were detectable on the cell surface with anti-Flag antibody, as expected (**Figure 4A**). On the other hand, if AP–MRAP–Flag and MRAP–Flag–AP did not change orientations following biosynthesis, only ER-localized $BirA_{ER}$ would be able to label acceptor peptide in the ER lumen and, after trafficking, the extracellular side of the plasma membrane (**Figure 4B**). This result was obtained, with cell surface MRAP clearly labeled in all configurations but cell surface biotin-labeled MRAP visible only in cells expressing $BirA_{ER}$. The results of this experiment are not confounded by incomplete import of $BirA_{ER}$ into the ER.

A kinetic approach was also undertaken to determine whether MRAP changes orientation after biosynthesis (**Figure 5**). To avoid the ambiguity present in experiments using $BirA_{ER}$, cells were transfected with cytoplasmic BirA and either AP–MRAP or MRAP–AP and incubated overnight in the absence of added biotin. During this period MRAP synthesis took place with very little biotin labeling (zero time point). Cells were then treated with added biotin for times up to 24 h. Immunoblotting for total AP–MRAP and MRAP–AP with anti-Flag antibodies is shown in the left panels. As seen previously (**Figure 2A**), cytoplasmic

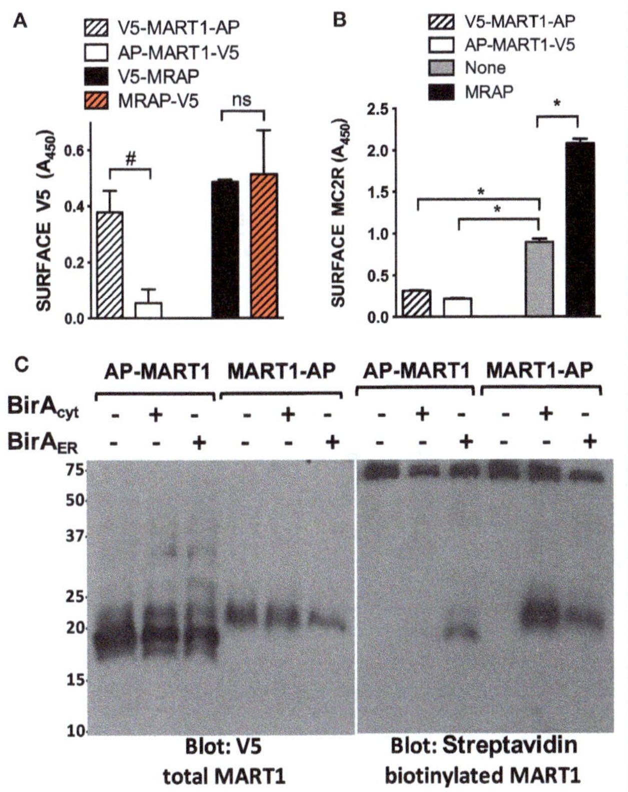

FIGURE 3 | Biotin labeling confirms single orientation of a control protein. **(A)** CHO cells were transfected with plasmids encoding MRAP or MART1 with AP and V5 epitopes at the N- or C-terminus as shown. The topology prediction programs TMHMM and HMMTOP predict that both unmodified and epitope-tagged versions of MART1 will assume an exclusively N_{exo} orientation whereas MRAPs are likely to assume both N_{exo} and N_{cyt} orientations. **(B)** Cells were transfected with plasmids encoding HA-tagged MC2 receptor and MRAP or MART1 as in **(A)** and surface receptor was quantified. Expression of tagged proteins on the plasma membrane was measured as described in Section "Materials and Methods." **(C)** Plasmids encoding MART1 tagged with AP at either the N- or C-terminus and V5 epitope at the opposite end were transfected into CHO cells stably expressing $BirA_{cyt}$ or $BirA_{ER}$. High MW bands seen in all lanes are endogenous biotinylated proteins. *$P < 0.05$; #$P < 0.1$.

BirA labeled the faster-moving non-glycosylated AP–MRAP band. Increased biotin labeling could be detected as early as 6 min after biotin supplementation and labeling continued over time; after 24 h, there was only a trace amount of a higher molecular weight biotin-labeled AP–MRAP (**Figure 5A**). This result does not support the idea that MRAP flips orientations after synthesis. In the case of MRAP–AP, a minor fraction of non-glycosylated biotin-labeled MRAP was visible but the proportion did not increase with time, indicating that MRAP does not gradually flip but rather that a small amount of N_{exo}/C_{cyt} MRAP does not become fully glycosylated (**Figure 5B**).

To characterize MRAP topology in its natural setting, we took advantage of the OS3 line of mouse adrenal cells that does not express MC2 receptors. ACTH responses were measured in parallel in OS3 and CHO cells transfected with the cAMP reporter CRE-luciferase with or without MC2 receptor and MRAP (**Figures 6A,B**). ACTH stimulated a 26-fold increase in the cAMP response in CHO cells expressing MRAP and MC2 receptor. Mock-transfected OS3 cells did not respond to ACTH, consistent with the reported absence of MC2 receptors (18). When the adrenal cells were transfected with MRAP and MC2 receptor, ACTH produced a striking 273-fold increase in cAMP reporter activity. OS3 cells must express MRAP, because MC2 receptors are functional when transfected alone. Interestingly, responses to forskolin were also exceptionally strong in OS3 cells. Forskolin acts directly on adenylyl cyclase and amplifies both basal and Gs-stimulated enzyme activity. Together, these findings suggest that adrenal OS3 cells have unusually efficient signal transduction at the G protein/adenylyl cyclase level.

We also explored MRAP orientation and the effects of MC2 receptor and ACTH (**Figures 6C,D**). OS3 cells and parallel cultures of CHO cells were transfected with BirA and AP-tagged MRAPs with or without MC2 receptors and incubated overnight with or without 10 nM ACTH. For reasons that are not clear, expression of AP–MRAP was higher when MC2 receptor was co-expressed and that of MRAP–AP was lower. ACTH had little effect. Biotin labeled the non-glycosylated AP–MRAP band, as predicted if topology does not change. In OS3 cells, there was a non-specific biotin-labeled protein at ~37 kDa that did not correspond to any MRAP band. MRAP–AP was weakly expressed in these cells and biotin-labeled species were partially obscured by the non-specific band.

Is the MRAP Protein Stable?

Having established that MRAP topology is stable, we examined the overall stability of the accessory protein. The stability of MRAP was estimated in CHO cells stably expressing Flag-tagged MRAP together with GFP or MC2 receptor. Cultures were treated for 4 h with the protein synthesis inhibitor cycloheximide (CHX), the proteasome inhibitor MG132 or both (**Figure 7A**). MRAP was quite labile, with little protein remaining 4 h after protein synthesis blockade. Surprisingly, MG132 by itself caused an enormous increase in the concentration of MRAP. On the other hand, MG132 did little to protect MRAP from degradation when CHX was present. A similar pattern was seen with the MC2 receptor, although the rate of degradation was slower (half-life between 3 and more than 8 h in different experiments) and effect of MG132 alone was much less marked. Mature MC2 receptor, which contains multiple sites for *N*-linked glycosylation (23, 24), ran as a broad band at high molecular weight, whereas immature core glycosylated and non-glycosylated receptor ran in more distinct bands close to the predicted molecular weight of 3xHA-hMC2 receptor, 37.3 kDa. **Figure 7B** shows a similar experiment demonstrating the rapidity of CHX and MG132 effects. The half-life of MRAP was estimated in similar experiments in which CHO cells were incubated with CHX from 0 to 5 h and MRAP levels were quantified densitometrically in immunoblots assuming first order kinetics. In most experiments, glycosylated MRAP was lost less rapidly than the non-glycosylated form, but this was not entirely consistent. The half-life of total MRAP averaged 1.7 ± 0.5 h ($n = 7$). The half-life of MRAP was short when it was transiently expressed with or without MC2 receptors in CHO cells but longer in adrenal OS3 cells, which grow less

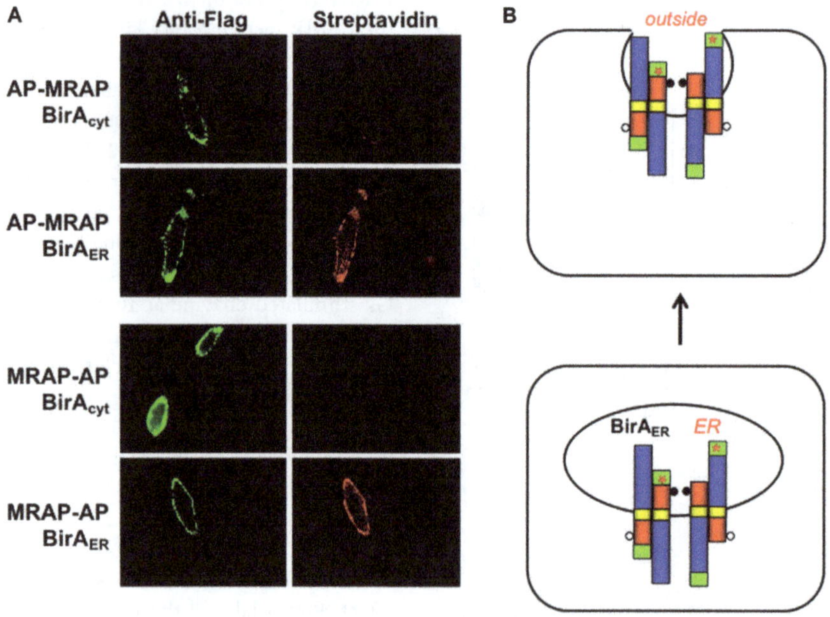

FIGURE 4 | Only ER-targeted BirA labels MRAP on the outer surface of the plasma membrane. **(A)** CHO cells stably expressing $BirA_{cyt}$ or $BirA_{ER}$ were grown on coverslips and transiently transfected with plasmids encoding AP–MRAP or MRAP–AP, each containing a Flag epitope in the C-terminal domain. Live cells were incubated with monoclonal anti-Flag epitope followed by Alexa488-labeled anti-mouse IgG (green) and Alexa555-labeled streptavidin (red), washed and imaged. Barely visible untransfected cells not expressing MRAPs demonstrate low background staining. **(B)** Schematic representation of N_{exo}/C_{cyt} and N_{cyt}/C_{exo} MRAPs before and after trafficking to the plasma membrane assuming that orientation does not change.

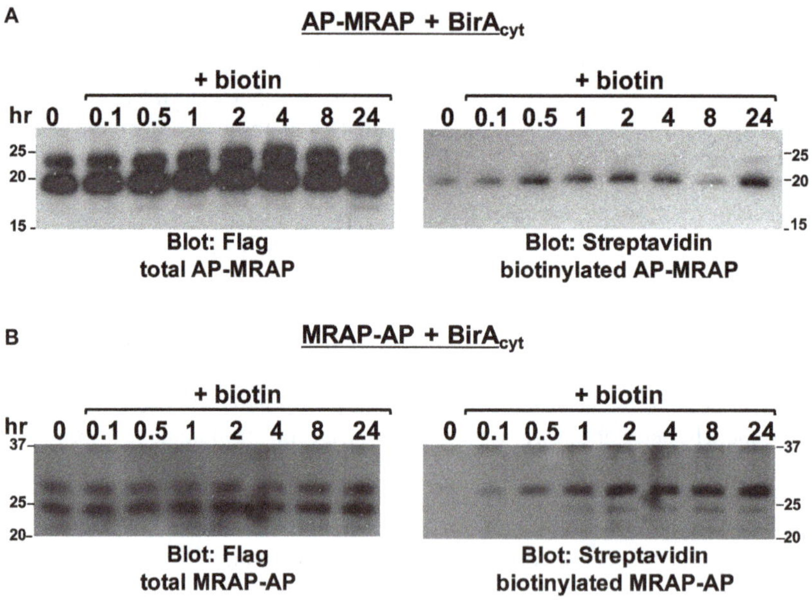

FIGURE 5 | Kinetics of biotin labeling. CHO cells were transfected with $BirA_{cyt}$ and either **(A)** AP–MRAP or **(B)** MRAP–AP, both containing Flag epitope. After overnight incubation in medium without added biotin, 2.5 μM biotin was added for the times shown. MRAPs were immunoprecipitated with anti-Flag antibody, resolved on SDS-PAGE and blotted with either anti-Flag antibody, to identify total MRAP, or HRP–streptavidin, to identify biotin-labeled protein.

rapidly than CHO cells (**Figure 7C**). To study turnover of MRAP on the plasma membrane, CHO cells were incubated for 1 h with protein synthesis or proteasome inhibitors and then either lysed or incubated with antibody to label cell surface MRAP selectively (**Figure 7D**). The effects of CHX and MG132 were not as extreme but clearly present when plasma membrane MRAP was isolated.

The use of a global protein synthesis inhibitor to study degradation of a particular protein is complicated by potential

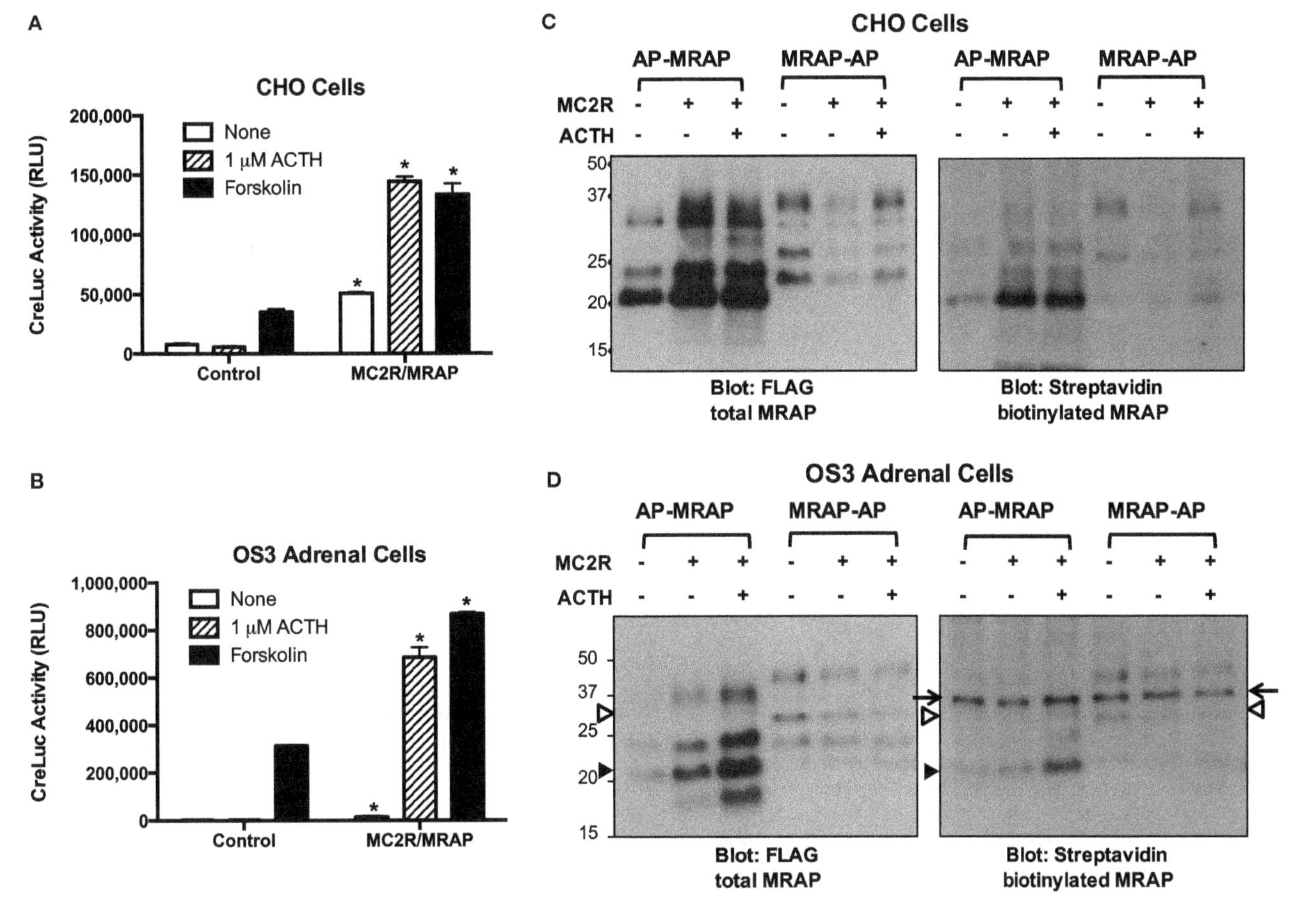

FIGURE 6 | MRAP orientation and function in CHO and adrenal cells. **(A)** CHO and **(B)** OS3 adrenal cells were transfected with CRE-luciferase without (control) or with MRAP and MC2 receptor. The day after transfection cells were incubated for 5 h with vehicle, 1 μM ACTH or 20 μM forskolin when luciferase activity, expressed as relative light units (RLU), was measured. Note different scales for responses of OS3 and CHO cells. **(C)** CHO and **(D)** OS3 adrenal cells were transfected with $BirA_{cyt}$ and AP–MRAP or MRAP–AP containing Flag epitope with or without MC2 receptor. Cultures were incubated overnight with or without 10 nM ACTH. Lysates were run on SDS-PAGE and blots were incubated with anti-Flag antibody to detect total MRAP or HRP–streptavidin to detect biotin-labeled MRAP. In **(D)**, the arrows point to a non-specific band, the solid arrowhead to non-glycosylated AP–MRAP, and the open arrowhead to glycosylated MRAP–AP. $^*P < 0.05$ vs. corresponding value in cells not expressing MC2R/MRAP.

effects on proteins other than the one under study. To avoid this problem, we studied cells stably expressing cytoplasmic BirA and then measured the amount of biotinylated-MRAP–AP at intervals after the removal of extracellular biotin with or without addition of CHX (**Figure 8**). Since biotin cannot be removed from a protein until it has been thoroughly degraded, this approach is conceptually equivalent to a radiolabeling pulse-chase experiment. For a low abundance protein, the method has the advantage of labeling only the protein of interest that can be concentrated on streptavidin beads prior to analysis. A limitation is the delay caused by the time required for washout of intracellular biotin. Following biotin withdrawal, total MRAP pools were quite stable over 20 h while normal synthesis and degradation were ongoing. The half-life of biotin-labeled MRAP was only 2.8 h, however, indicating that MRAP has a short half-life. In the presence of CHX, the corresponding values were 2.8 h for the total MRAP pool and 2.2 h for biotin-labeled MRAP. Because the half-lives measured by metabolic labeling and protein synthesis inhibition were strikingly similar, rapid turnover of MRAP was not an indirect effect of CHX.

In light of the effect of MG132, we investigated the possibility that MRAP itself undergoes ubiquitin-mediated degradation. In the canonical pathway ubiquitin is added to Lys residues and mouse MRAP has only four lysines, all located on the *N*-terminal side of the transmembrane helix in the juxtamembrane region. To test the importance of Lys to overall MRAP stability, we mutated these four residues to Arg (4K to R), retaining positive charge but removing lysine ε-amino groups that can be ubiquitylated. Arg-substituted MRAP was tagged with a V5 epitope on the *N*-terminus and a Flag epitope on the C-terminus, enabling analysis of its topology. Although (4K to R)MRAP was not expressed as highly as wild-type MRAP, it still assumed dual topology with both V5 and Flag epitopes on the plasma membrane (**Figure 9A**). Despite a lower level of MC2 receptor on the plasma membrane, cells expressing (4K to R)MRAP responded to ACTH with a cAMP increase equivalent to that supported by wild-type MRAP

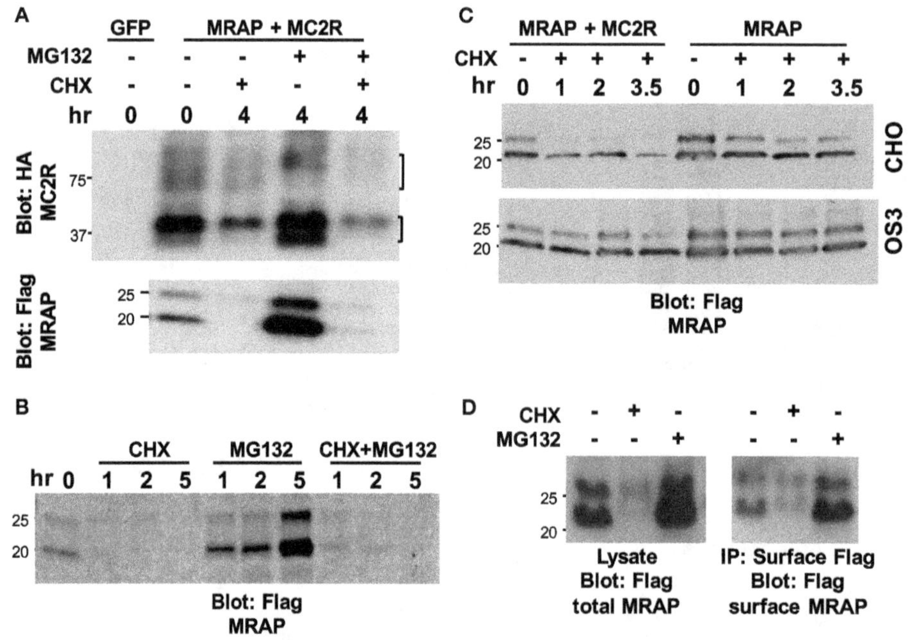

FIGURE 7 | Stability of MRAP and MC2 receptor. **(A)** CHO cells stably expressing Flag-tagged MRAP were transfected with either GFP or HA-tagged MC2 receptor and then incubated for 4 h with no drug, 10 μg/ml cycloheximide (CHX), 50 μM MG132, or both. Cell lysates were run on SDS-PAGE and blotted for either *(upper)* MC2 receptor or *(lower)* MRAP. Brackets on the right show glycosylated MC2 receptor and core and non-glycosylated receptor. **(B,D)** CHO cells stably expressing Flag-tagged MRAP were incubated with 10 μg/ml cycloheximide (CHX), 50 μM MG132, or both for **(B)** times shown or **(D)** 1 h. In **(B)**, cells were lysed and immunoprecipitation with anti-Flag antibody performed whereas in **(D)** cells were incubated for 15 min with1:1000 anti-Flag antibody and washed extensively before lysis and collection of Flag-labeled proteins on Protein A/G beads to isolate cell surface MRAP. **(C)** CHO and OS3 adrenal cells were transiently transfected with MRAP or MC2 receptor and MRAP, then incubated with 100 μg/ml cycloheximide for the times shown, lysed and blotted for MRAP.

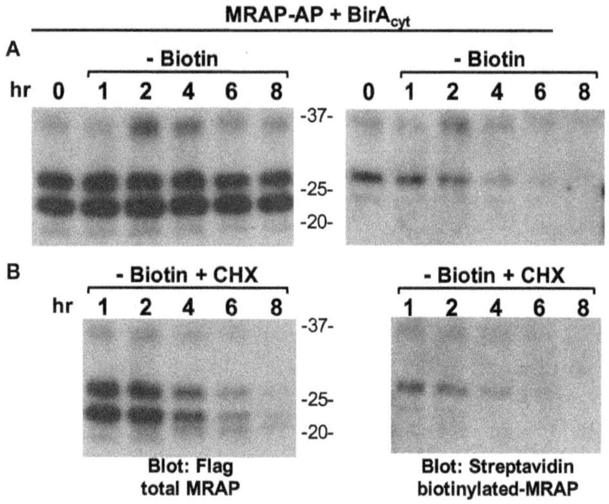

FIGURE 8 | Half-life of biotinylated MRAP is short with or without cycloheximide. **(A,B)** CHO cells stably expressing $BirA_{cyt}$ were transfected with MRAP–AP containing a Flag sequence, and incubated overnight in medium supplemented with biotin. Cells were then washed twice and incubated for 1–8 h in medium lacking biotin, **(A)** without or **(B)** with 10 μg/ml cycloheximide (CHX), when lysates were prepared and proteins resolved on SDS-PAGE and blots probed for either Flag epitope or biotin. The glycosylated form of MRAP–AP is labeled by cytoplasmic BirA.

(**Figure 9B**). MG132 by itself caused an enormous increase in (4K to R)MRAP concentration just as it did with wild-type. Replacing all of the MRAP Lys residues with Arg delayed MRAP degradation by at most threefold (**Figure 9C**).

We tested whether ubiquitin is directly added to MRAP lysines by co-expressing HA-ubiquitin with either wild-type or (4K to R)MRAP in CHO cells and incubating for 3 h with MG132 to allow accumulation of any ubiquitylated species. Co-immunoprecipitation and immunoblotting revealed that Flag-tagged MRAP undergoes ubiquitin modification (**Figure 10A**). Multiple ubiquitylated MRAP bands were observed and only one of them was lost in the Arg-substituted mutant, suggesting that ubiquitin is added to Lys and also to one of the amino acids less frequently ubiquitylated: the aminoterminal amino group, the hydroxyl group of Ser or Thr, or the sulfhydryl group of Cys (25). On average, ubiquitylated MRAP species totaled ~5% of total MRAP after incubation for 3 h with a proteasome inhibitor.

To rule out the possibility that MRAP ubiquitylation was occurring on one of the Lys residues in the Flag sequence, we tested AP–MRAP and AP-(4K to R)MRAP that contained the biotin acceptor peptide sequence but no epitope tag in cells expressing cytoplasmic BirA (**Figure 10B**). Once labeled with biotin, the AP tag has no lysine amino group available for ubiquitin addition. Once again, multiple ubiquitylated MRAP bands were observed and only one was lost in the Arg-substituted

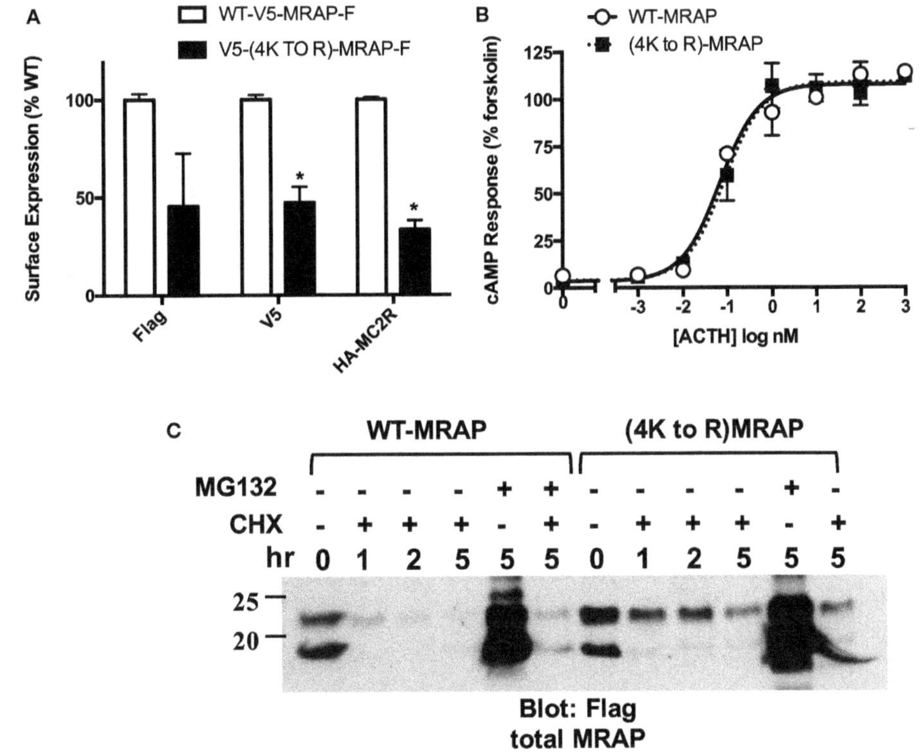

FIGURE 9 | Importance of MRAP Lys residues for function, orientation, and stability. CHO cells were transfected with no accessory protein, wild-type MRAP or (4K to R)MRAP with the four native Lys residues mutated to Arg. **(A)** Surface expression of the N-terminal V5 and C-terminal Flag epitopes of MRAP and (4K to R)MRAP, and surface expression of co-transfected HA-tagged MC2 receptor. Results are normalized to values with wild-type MRAP. **(B)** cAMP responses to ACTH in cells co-transfected with MC2 receptor and CRE-luciferase. **(C)** Cells expressing MRAP or (4K to R)MRAP were incubated for the times shown with 10 µg/ ml cycloheximide (CHX), 50 µM MG132 or both. Lysates were run on gels and blotted for Flag epitope. $^{*}P < 0.05$ vs. corresponding value in cells expressing wild-type MRAP.

mutant, suggesting that ubiquitin was added to MRAP at an atypical site.

The glycosylation status of various MRAP bands was analyzed in lysates of cells expressing HA-Ub and MRAP before and after enzymatic deglycosylation with PNGaseF. None of the ubiquitylated MRAP bands was lost following PNGaseF treatment, whereas the slower-migrating MRAP bands collapsed to the mobility of the faster-migrating non-glycosylated species (**Figure 11**).

DISCUSSION

The unusual antiparallel dimer structure of MRAP been described only for MRAP and its paralog MRAP2. These two proteins are evolutionarily ancient (26–28) and have retained features that result in dual topology, including highly conserved aminoterminal and transmembrane domains and basic residues in the juxtamembrane region (29). The experiments described here do not explain what advantages are conferred by the conserved MRAP structure but they do establish that MRAP topology is stable from the time of MRAP biosynthesis to the time of MRAP degradation.

It has been particularly difficult to study MRAP topology because each side of the protein faces each direction in the antiparallel homodimer. Many of the methods used to assign membrane orientation require the addition of bulky fluorescent proteins or enzymes that are themselves larger than MRAP. Biotin labeling avoids this issue but has other drawbacks. Analysis of biotin-labeling patterns depended on the ability to distinguish between N_{exo} and N_{cyt} MRAPs based on glycosylation. Protein glycosylation never reaches 100%, and in our experience the extent of MRAP glycosylation varies with MRAP species, epitope tags, and expression levels. In addition, some BirA activity appeared to remain in the cytoplasm when ER-targeted BirA was overexpressed. Finally, backgrounds on HRP–streptavidin blots tended to be high when low abundance proteins were being detected. Despite these limitations, some situations were unambiguous. Once it has left the ER and Golgi apparatus, MRAP cannot undergo further glycosylation. Once it has been biotinylated by cytoplasmic BirA, MRAP cannot be orientated with biotin facing the outside of the cell unless it flips. The important point is that changes in the orientation of MRAP were not observed in any of configurations examined.

When protein synthesis was blocked, MRAP protein levels declined with a half-life that varied in different experiments but averaged under 2 h. Use of biotin labeling to study MRAP stability was again instructive, confirming that rapid MRAP turnover was not an artifact of CHX treatment. Although it is not known how

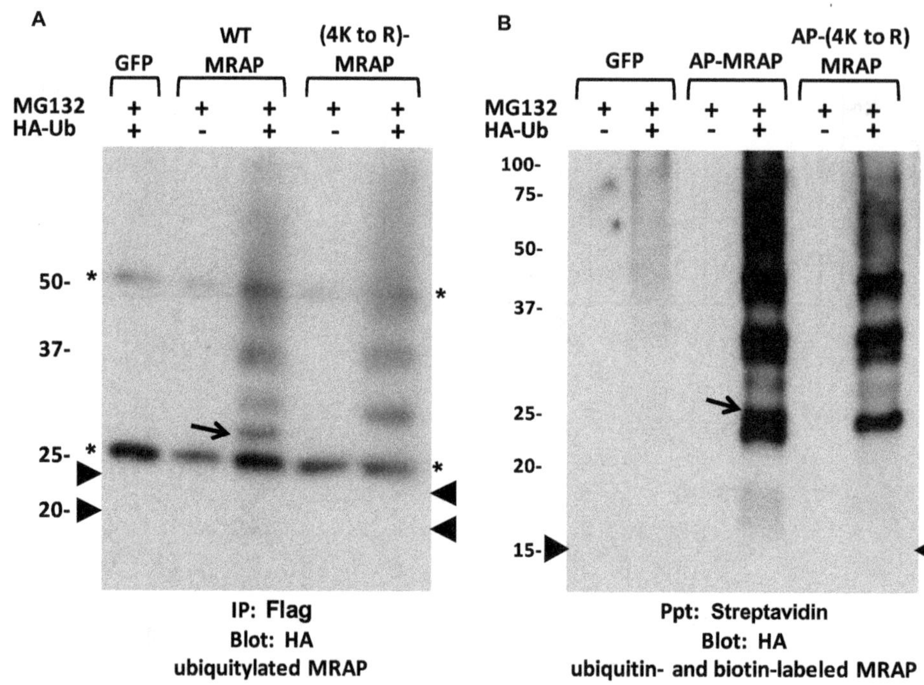

FIGURE 10 | MRAP is ubiquitylated. **(A)** CHO cells were transfected with plasmids encoding GFP, Flag-tagged MRAP or (4K to R)MRAP, with or without HA-labeled ubiquitin (HA-Ub). After overnight incubation, cells were treated for 3 h with 50 μM MG132. MRAP proteins were immunoprecipitated with anti-Flag antibody and resolved on SDS-PAGE; blots were probed for HA. Asterisks mark IgG bands and black arrowheads show the position of the two MRAP bands from a parallel gel blotted for Flag. **(B)** CHO cells stably expressing cytoplasmic BirA were transfected with plasmids encoding GFP or AP–MRAP or AP-(4K to R)MRAP, both lacking any epitope tag, with or without HA-ubiquitin (HA-Ub). After overnight incubation in biotin-supplemented media, 50 μM MG132 was added for 3 h. Biotin-labeled proteins were collected on streptavidin beads and resolved on gels; blots were probed for HA. The arrowhead shows the position of biotin-labeled non-glycosylated AP–MRAP found on a parallel gel probed with streptavidin. The red arrows point to bands present in WT but not Lys-substituted MRAP. AP–MRAPs without epitope tags run at lower MWs than their longer tagged counterparts.

quickly intracellular biotin declines when biotin is removed from the medium, this must happen quickly because biotin-labeled MRAP disappeared at roughly the same rate as total MRAP during protein synthesis blockade. A biotin-labeling approach has the potential to measure the half-life of any protein that can be modified by the addition of a biotin ligase acceptor peptide. It avoids the cost and risk of radioisotopes, is applicable for proteins with amino acid compositions that render them unsuitable for ^{35}S-Met/Cys labeling, and can be used for proteins expressed at low abundance because of the ease of enriching on streptavidin beads.

Despite the presence of an array of chaperones that assist with protein folding in the ER, it is believed that a sizable fraction of newly synthesized protein fails to fold or assemble correctly. The accumulation of misfolded proteins in the ER can have disastrous outcomes, preventing synthesis of other membrane or secretory proteins. Cells contain elaborate and essential systems to remove terminally misfolded proteins from the ER, a process termed ER-associated degradation or ERAD (30, 31). ERAD involves recognition of misfolded protein, retrotranslocation from the ER, polyubiquitylation, and proteasomal degradation. Proteins are deglycosylated prior to degradation.

The involvement of proteasomal pathways in MRAP degradation was investigated here. One puzzling finding was that MG132 caused a very striking increase in the amount of MRAP when protein synthesis was ongoing but provided almost no stabilization when protein synthesis was blocked. Assuming that MG132 effectively inhibited proteasome activity, the results indicate that an alternative pathway for MRAP degradation exists and is responsible for the majority of MRAP degradation. The ability of MG132 to increase MRAP may be explained if the proteasome inhibitor increases the efficiency of MRAP biosynthesis, perhaps by inducing molecular chaperones (32).

Although the results with MG132 suggest that proteasomal degradation is not the major pathway for MRAP turnover, ubiquitylated MRAP was detected following a 3-h incubation with MG132. One ubiquitylated MRAP band had a molecular weight 8–10 kDa higher than the comparable non-glycosylated MRAP band and was lost in Arg-substituted MRAP, indicating that it represents MRAP with a single ubiquitin added to a lysine. At least two heavier ubiquitylated MRAP bands were present in MRAP lacking any lysines and must, therefore, represent ubiquitylation at some other amino acid but based on their migration on gels, these did not form a classical ubiquitin ladder. Cooray et al. demonstrated that MGRN1, an E3 ubiquitin ligase implicated in MC1 receptor function, is present in adrenal fasciculata and capable of adding ubiquitin to the MC2 receptor. They did not detect ubiquitylation of human MRAP in HEK293 cells in the absence of

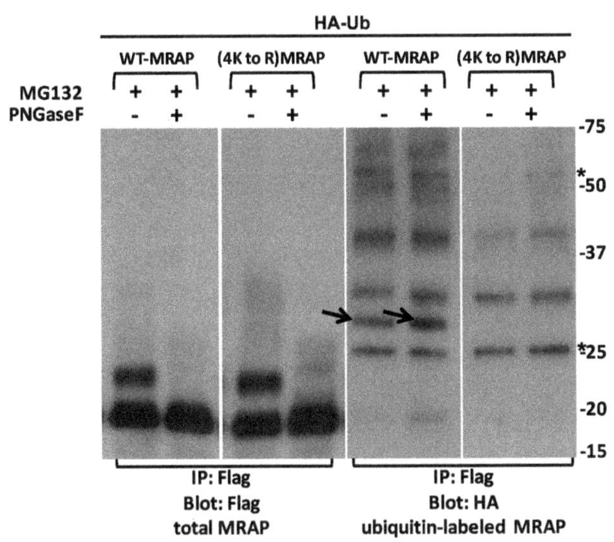

FIGURE 11 | Major ubiquitylated MRAP species are not glycosylated. CHO cells were transfected with HA-ubiquitin (HA-Ub) and wild-type or (4K to R)MRAPs, which contained Flag epitopes. After overnight incubation cultures were treated for 3 h with 50 μM MG132 when lysates were prepared. Flag-tagged proteins were immunoprecipitated and treated with or without PNGaseF, which collapsed the slower-running glycosylated MRAP and (4K to R)MRAP bands. Asterisks show IgG bands. With longer exposure, higher MW bands were visible in the anti-Flag blot but obscured by the major MRAP bands. Red arrows point to ubiquitin-labeled bands present in WT but not Lys-substituted MRAP.

a proteasome inhibitor (24). Taken together, published work and the experiments described here indicate that polyubiquitylation and proteasomal degradation do not account for most MRAP degradation.

The stability of MRAP may be of interest in tissues outside of the adrenal gland. MC2R mRNA is highly expressed in adrenal and testicular tissue, whereas MRAPα mRNA has a somewhat broader distribution with high levels in the adrenal gland and testes but substantial amounts in fat and brain, among other tissues (3, 7). To date, there is no information about the relative expression of the protein products of these genes. hMRAPα coprecipitates with all five melanocortin receptors (5) and has modest effects on signaling by MC1 and MC3–5 receptors (7), making it plausible that MRAP has a role outside of the adrenal cortex. Patients who have glucocorticoid deficiency due to mutations in MC2 receptors and those who have mutations in MRAP display rather similar phenotypes (33), but comparison of MC2 receptor and MRAP knockout mice may provide insight into non-adrenal actions of MRAP in the future. A paralog of MRAP termed MRAP2 is widely distributed and influences signaling by MC4 receptors (34, 35) and at least one receptor outside the melanocortin receptor family (36) to regulate energy metabolism.

Not only is it uncertain how many G protein-coupled receptors interact with MRAPs, it is also uncertain whether MRAP actions are limited to receptors. The work detailed above supports previous findings of an antiparallel homodimer structure for MRAP and indicates that partners in the MRAP dimer remain in a fixed orientation during trafficking and expression on the plasma membrane. The finding that MRAP turns over rapidly in CHO cells needs to be interpreted cautiously because of the heterologous cell system, protein overexpression, and likely imbalance of accessory protein and receptor. An important question that remains to be addressed is whether MC2 receptor and MRAP protein levels change on a rapid time scale *in vivo*. Fortunately, ever more powerful mass spectrometry techniques are being developed and information about the stability membrane signaling proteins in a native environment should be forthcoming in the near future.

AUTHOR CONTRIBUTIONS

ZM, LJ, SM, and PH designed and conducted experiments, and PH wrote the manuscript.

FUNDING

This research was supported by National Institute of Health grants DK19974 and DK67214.

REFERENCES

1. Liu H, Enyeart JA, Enyeart JJ. ACTH induces Cav3.2 current and mRNA by cAMP-dependent and cAMP-independent mechanisms. *J Biol Chem* (2010) 285:20040–50. doi:10.1074/jbc.M110.104190
2. Mountjoy KG, Robbins LS, Mortrud MT, Cone RD. The cloning of a family of genes that encode the melanocortin receptors. *Science* (1992) 257:1248–51. doi:10.1126/science.1325670
3. Metherell LA, Chapple JP, Cooray S, David A, Becker C, Ruschendorf F, et al. Mutations in MRAP, encoding a new interacting partner of the ACTH receptor, cause familial glucocorticoid deficiency type 2. *Nat Genet* (2005) 37:166–70. doi:10.1038/ng1501
4. Sebag JA, Hinkle PM. Melanocortin-2 receptor accessory protein MRAP forms antiparallel homodimers. *Proc Natl Acad Sci U S A* (2007) 104:20244–9. doi:10.1073/pnas.0708916105
5. Chan LF, Webb TR, Chung TT, Meimaridou E, Cooray SN, Guasti L, et al. MRAP and MRAP2 are bidirectional regulators of the melanocortin receptor family. *Proc Natl Acad Sci U S A* (2009) 106:6146–51. doi:10.1073/pnas.0809918106
6. Roy S, Rached M, Gallo-Payet N. Differential regulation of the human adrenocorticotropin receptor [melanocortin-2 receptor (MC2R)] by human MC2R accessory protein isoforms alpha and beta in isogenic human embryonic kidney 293 cells. *Mol Endocrinol* (2007) 21:1656–69. doi:10.1210/me.2007-0041
7. Kay EI, Botha R, Montgomery JM, Mountjoy KG. hMRAPa increases alphaMSH-induced hMC1R and hMC3R functional coupling and hMC4R constitutive activity. *J Mol Endocrinol* (2013) 50:203–15. doi:10.1530/JME-12-0221
8. Sebag JA, Hinkle PM. Opposite effects of the melanocortin-2 (MC2) receptor accessory protein MRAP on MC2 and MC5 receptor dimerization and trafficking. *J Biol Chem* (2009) 284:22641–8. doi:10.1074/jbc.M804413200
9. Roy S, Roy SJ, Pinard S, Taillefer LD, Rached M, Parent JL, et al. Mechanisms of melanocortin-2 receptor (MC2R) internalization and recycling in human embryonic kidney (hek) cells: identification of Key Ser/Thr (S/T) amino acids. *Mol Endocrinol* (2011) 25:1961–77. doi:10.1210/me.2011-0018
10. Malik S, Dolan TM, Maben ZJ, Hinkle PM. Adrenocorticotropic hormone (ACTH) responses require actions of the melanocortin-2 receptor accessory protein on the extracellular surface of the plasma membrane. *J Biol Chem* (2015) 290:27972–85. doi:10.1074/jbc.M115.668491

11. Sebag JA, Hinkle PM. Regions of melanocortin 2 (MC2) receptor accessory protein necessary for dual topology and MC2 receptor trafficking and signaling. *J Biol Chem* (2009) 284:610–8. doi:10.1074/jbc.M804413200
12. Mountjoy KG, Bird IM, Rainey WE, Cone RD. ACTH induces up-regulation of ACTH receptor mRNA in mouse and human adrenocortical cell lines. *Mol Cell Endocrinol* (1994) 99:R17–20. doi:10.1016/0303-7207(94)90160-0
13. Spiga F, Waite EJ, Liu Y, Kershaw YM, Aguilera G, Lightman SL. ACTH-dependent ultradian rhythm of corticosterone secretion. *Endocrinology* (2011) 152:1448–57. doi:10.1210/en.2010-1209
14. Liu Y, Smith LI, Huang V, Poon V, Coello A, Olah M, et al. Transcriptional regulation of episodic glucocorticoid secretion. *Mol Cell Endocrinol* (2013) 371:62–70. doi:10.1016/j.mce.2012.10.011
15. Xing Y, Parker CR, Edwards M, Rainey WE. ACTH is a potent regulator of gene expression in human adrenal cells. *J Mol Endocrinol* (2010) 45:59–68. doi:10.1677/JME-10-0006
16. Cooray SN, Chung TT, Mazhar K, Szidonya L, Clark AJ. Bioluminescence resonance energy transfer reveals the adrenocorticotropin (ACTH)-induced conformational change of the activated ACTH receptor complex in living cells. *Endocrinology* (2011) 152:495–502. doi:10.1210/en.2010-1053
17. Treier M, Staszewski LM, Bohmann D. Ubiquitin-dependent c-Jun degradation in vivo is mediated by the delta domain. *Cell* (1994) 78:787–98. doi:10.1016/S0092-8674(94)90502-9
18. Rae PA, Tsao J, Schimmer BP. Evaluation of receptor function in ACTH-responsive and ACTH-insensitive adrenal tumor cells. *Can J Biochem* (1979) 57:509–16. doi:10.1139/o79-064
19. Chepurny OG, Holz GG. A novel cyclic adenosine monophosphate responsive luciferase reporter incorporating a nonpalindromic cyclic adenosine monophosphate response element provides optimal performance for use in G protein coupled receptor drug discovery efforts. *J Biomol Screen* (2007) 12:740–6. doi:10.1177/1087057107301856
20. Zen KH, Consler TG, Kaback HR. Insertion of the polytopic membrane protein lactose permease occurs by multiple mechanisms. *Biochemistry* (1995) 34:3430–7. doi:10.1021/bi00010a035
21. Chen I, Howarth M, Lin W, Ting AY. Site-specific labeling of cell surface proteins with biophysical probes using biotin ligase. *Nat Methods* (2005) 2:99–104. doi:10.1038/nmeth735
22. Slavoff SA, Chen I, Choi YA, Ting AY. Expanding the substrate tolerance of biotin ligase through exploration of enzymes from diverse species. *J Am Chem Soc* (2008) 130:1160–2. doi:10.1021/ja076655i
23. Roy S, Perron B, Gallo-Payet N. Role of asparagine-linked glycosylation in cell surface expression and function of the human adrenocorticotropin receptor (melanocortin 2 receptor) in 293/FRT cells. *Endocrinology* (2010) 151:660–70. doi:10.1210/en.2009-0826
24. Cooray SN, Guasti L, Clark AJ. The E3 ubiquitin ligase Mahogunin ubiquitinates the melanocortin 2 receptor. *Endocrinology* (2011) 152:4224–31. doi:10.1210/en.2011-0147
25. Shimizu Y, Okuda-Shimizu Y, Hendershot LM. Ubiquitylation of an ERAD substrate occurs on multiple types of amino acids. *Mol Cell* (2010) 40:917–26. doi:10.1016/j.molcel.2010.11.033
26. Valsalan R, Krishnan A, Almen MS, Fredriksson R, Schioth HB. Early vertebrate origin of melanocortin 2 receptor accessory proteins (MRAPs). *Gen Comp Endocrinol* (2013) 188:123–32. doi:10.1016/j.ygcen.2013.01.004
27. Cortes R, Navarro S, Agulleiro MJ, Guillot R, Garcia-Herranz V, Sanchez E, et al. Evolution of the melanocortin system. *Gen Comp Endocrinol* (2014) 209:3–10. doi:10.1016/j.ygcen.2014.04.005
28. Dores RM, Garcia Y. Views on the co-evolution of the melanocortin-2 receptor, MRAPs, and the hypothalamus/pituitary/adrenal-interrenal axis. *Mol Cell Endocrinol* (2015) 408:12–22. doi:10.1016/j.mce.2014.12.022
29. Hinkle PM, Sebag JA. Structure and function of the melanocortin2 receptor accessory protein (MRAP). *Mol Cell Endocrinol* (2009) 300:25–31. doi:10.1016/j.mce.2008.10.041
30. Christianson JC, Ye Y. Cleaning up in the endoplasmic reticulum: ubiquitin in charge. *Nat Struct Mol Biol* (2014) 21:325–35. doi:10.1038/nsmb.2793
31. Ruggiano A, Foresti O, Carvalho P. Quality control: ER-associated degradation: protein quality control and beyond. *J Cell Biol* (2014) 204:869–79. doi:10.1083/jcb.201312042
32. Bush KT, Goldberg AL, Nigam SK. Proteasome inhibition leads to a heat-shock response, induction of endoplasmic reticulum chaperones, and thermotolerance. *J Biol Chem* (1997) 272:9086–92. doi:10.1074/jbc.272.14.9086
33. Chung TT, Chan LF, Metherell LA, Clark AJ. Phenotypic characteristics of familial glucocorticoid deficiency (FGD) type 1 and 2. *Clin Endocrinol (Oxf)* (2010) 72:589–94. doi:10.1111/j.1365-2265.2009.03663.x
34. Asai M, Ramachandrappa S, Joachim M, Shen Y, Zhang R, Nuthalapati N, et al. Loss of function of the melanocortin 2 receptor accessory protein 2 is associated with mammalian obesity. *Science* (2013) 341:275–8. doi:10.1126/science.1233000
35. Sebag JA, Zhang C, Hinkle PM, Bradshaw AM, Cone RD. Developmental control of the melanocortin-4 receptor by MRAP2 proteins in zebrafish. *Science* (2013) 341:278–81. doi:10.1126/science.1232995
36. Chaly AL, Srisai D, Gardner EE, Sebag JA. The Melanocortin Receptor Accessory Protein 2 promotes food intake through inhibition of the Prokineticin Receptor-1. *Elife* (2016) 5:e12397. doi:10.7554/eLife.12397

5

Glucocorticoid Regulation of Food-Choice Behavior in Humans: Evidence from Cushing's Syndrome

Scott J. Moeller[1,2], Lizette Couto[3,4], Vanessa Cohen[3,4], Yelena Lalazar[3,4], Iouri Makotkine[1], Nia Williams[1], Rachel Yehuda[1,2], Rita Z. Goldstein[1,2] and Eliza B. Geer[3,4]**

[1] Department of Psychiatry, Icahn School of Medicine at Mount Sinai, New York, NY, USA, [2] Department of Neuroscience, Icahn School of Medicine at Mount Sinai, New York, NY, USA, [3] Department of Medicine, Icahn School of Medicine at Mount Sinai, New York, NY, USA, [4] Department of Neurosurgery, Icahn School of Medicine at Mount Sinai, New York, NY, USA

***Correspondence:**
Scott J. Moeller
scott.moeller@mssm.edu;
Eliza B. Geer
eliza.geer@mssm.edu

The mechanisms by which glucocorticoids regulate food intake and resulting body mass in humans are not well-understood. One potential mechanism could involve modulation of reward processing, but human stress models examining effects of glucocorticoids on behavior contain important confounds. Here, we studied individuals with Cushing's syndrome, a rare endocrine disorder characterized by chronic excess endogenous glucocorticoids. Twenty-three patients with Cushing's syndrome (13 with active disease; 10 with disease in remission) and 15 controls with a comparably high body mass index (BMI) completed two simulated food-choice tasks (one with "explicit" task contingencies and one with "probabilistic" task contingencies), during which they indicated their objective preference for viewing high calorie food images vs. standardized pleasant, unpleasant, and neutral images. All participants also completed measures of food craving, and approximately half of the participants provided 24-h urine samples for assessment of cortisol and cortisone concentrations. Results showed that on the explicit task (but not the probabilistic task), participants with active Cushing's syndrome made fewer food-related choices than participants with Cushing's syndrome in remission, who in turn made fewer food-related choices than overweight controls. Corroborating this group effect, higher urine cortisone was negatively correlated with food-related choice in the subsample of all participants for whom these data were available. On the probabilistic task, despite a lack of group differences, higher food-related choice correlated with higher state and trait food craving in active Cushing's patients. Taken together, relative to overweight controls, Cushing's patients, particularly those with active disease, displayed a reduced vigor of responding for food rewards that was presumably attributable to glucocorticoid abnormalities. Beyond Cushing's, these results may have relevance for elucidating glucocorticoid contributions to food-seeking behavior, enhancing mechanistic understanding of weight fluctuations associated with oral glucocorticoid therapy and/or chronic stress, and informing the neurobiology of neuropsychiatric conditions marked by abnormal cortisol dynamics (e.g., major depression, Alzheimer's disease).

Keywords: Cushing's syndrome, choice behavior, decision-making, reward processing, glucocorticoids, cortisol, food craving

INTRODUCTION

Hypothalamic-pituitary-adrenal (HPA) axis activity is essential for ensuring body homeostasis and survival during stress. Stress initiates a cascade of neuroendocrine responses including secretion of corticotropin-releasing hormone (CRH) from the hypothalamus, which stimulates adrenocorticotrophic hormone (ACTH) secretion from pituitary corticotrophs, culminating in glucocorticoid (GC) secretion from the adrenal glands (Smith and Vale, 2006). This stress response precipitating the release of GCs has downstream effects on multiple regulatory systems such as appetite control (La Fleur, 2006), thereby helping to regulate eating and satiety (Uchoa et al., 2014). Chronic stress, which results in persistent excess GC exposure, has been associated with increased hepatic glucose production, decreased glucose transport and utilization, decreased protein synthesis, enhanced protein degradation in muscles, and adipose tissue expansion, culminating in obesity and insulin resistance (Nieuwenhuizen and Rutters, 2008; Lacroix et al., 2015). However, although GCs regulate food intake and resulting body mass, the mechanisms for these relationships in humans are not well-understood.

One potential mechanism of how GCs orchestrate eating behavior could involve reward processing (Adam and Epel, 2007). This hypothesis follows from research literatures that have examined modulation of reward processing via transiently (experimentally) increased cortisol (e.g., experimental administration of cortisol or laboratory stressors) or chronically enhanced cortisol (e.g., due to early life stress). Studies have reliably shown decreased *non-food* reward processing in individuals exposed to stress. For example, experimental administration of cortisol or laboratory stressors (e.g., cold pressors, watching aversive movie clips, or trying to solve unanswerable math problems) are associated with lower eagerness to receive task-related rewards or lower functional magnetic resonance imaging (fMRI) activity [e.g., during a card-guessing task or the anticipation phase of the monetary incentive delay (MID) tasks] in corticolimbic regions relevant to reward (e.g., striatum, amygdala, hippocampus, and/or medial prefrontal cortex) (Ossewaarde et al., 2011; Porcelli et al., 2012; Montoya et al., 2014). In addition, individuals characterized as highly stress-reactive (i.e., showing high cortisol reactivity and self-reported negative affect after a stress induction) showed diminished sensitivity to reward, but not punishment, under stress (Berghorst et al., 2013). Individuals who experienced childhood maltreatment or early life stress, relative to individuals who did not experience these stressors, also rated reward cues as being less pleasant and showed blunted fMRI response in the globus pallidus, a striatal dopaminergic region, to reward cues during a MID task (Dillon et al., 2009); showed less ventral striatal fMRI response to happy faces (Goff et al., 2013); and responded less to money as an incentive to improve task performance (Mueller et al., 2012). Results of studies examining the effects of stress on *food* reward have been less consistent. A large body of literature suggests that presence of stress typically elevates food reward and consumption, often for unhealthy foods with high caloric densities (Tomiyama et al., 2011; Groesz et al., 2012; Hoffman et al., 2012; Talbot et al., 2013; Tryon et al., 2013; Aschbacher et al., 2014; Ferreira de Sa et al., 2014; Pursey et al., 2014; Maier et al., 2015). However, one study in healthy individuals showed that stress was associated with decreased activation in the reward circuitry including the orbitofrontal cortex and putamen specifically during a food-choice procedure (i.e., when participants selected foods to be consumed later) (Born et al., 2010). Moreover, animal models (typically with the aim of examining a depressive phenotype) have shown that chronic administration of corticosterone or laboratory stress are associated with reduced eating behavior (Kvarta et al., 2015) or a diminished ability to establish preference for sweets (Mateus-Pinheiro et al., 2014).

A disease in humans characterized by excessive cortisol production is Cushing's syndrome (CS), which provides a unique model of chronic GC exposure (i.e., that is independent of precipitating chronic life stressors that could potentially have additional downstream functional consequences to cloud interpretations). CS is a rare endocrine disorder (1.2–2.4/million/year) characterized by chronic excess endogenous GCs due to an ACTH pituitary adenoma or a cortisol-producing adrenal adenoma (Lacroix et al., 2015); left untreated, CS results in increased mortality and multiple morbidities including obesity, diabetes, hypertension, cardiovascular disease, and overall lower health-related quality of life (Webb et al., 2008; Feelders et al., 2012; Carluccio et al., 2015). Individuals with CS also exhibit persistent neurocognitive impairments, including in memory and learning (Whelan et al., 1980; Martignoni et al., 1992; Mauri et al., 1993; Forget et al., 2000; Starkman et al., 2001, 2003; Leon-Carrion et al., 2009; Michaud et al., 2009; Pereira et al., 2010; Ragnarsson et al., 2012; Resmini et al., 2012); such deficits are quite anticipated in light of the wide distribution of GC receptors in brain areas (e.g., hippocampus, amygdala, and PFC) that are important for these respective executive functions (McEwen et al., 2016). Such deficits (e.g., in verbal memory) and associated improvement with treatment have been correlated with salivary or urinary cortisol concentrations (Grillon et al., 2004; Hook et al., 2007), supporting the idea that GC abnormalities underlie these deficits. More recently, and of greater importance for the current study, CS patients have also exhibited differences from controls in task-related decision-making (Crespo et al., 2014) and dispositional novelty-seeking (Dimopoulou et al., 2013). Such findings are consistent with a more general role of GCs in healthy individuals in potentially modulating risk-taking behavior during conditions of uncertainty (Coates and Herbert, 2008; Putman et al., 2010).

In the present study, we examined the effects of chronic GC exposure resulting from CS on laboratory food-choice tasks in which participants chose to view high-caloric food images vs. viewing standardized pleasant (e.g., smiling babies), unpleasant (e.g., disfigurement), or neutral (e.g., household objects) images; members of our team originally developed this task for use in cocaine addiction (i.e., evaluating choice for cocaine images) (Moeller et al., 2009). Given data suggesting that, on balance, chronic GC exposure is associated with blunted reward processing, we hypothesized that CS patients would choose to view fewer food-related and/or fewer pleasant-related images than a sample of healthy controls with similar body mass index (BMI). Moreover, given data suggesting that chronic GC exposure drives a metabolic memory that results in long-term mortality risk, cognitive and emotional impairments, and reduced quality of life even after normalization of cortisol levels (Tiemensma et al., 2010a,b; Geer et al., 2012; Pereira et al., 2012; Lambert et al., 2013; Andela et al., 2015; Pivonello et al., 2015), we further hypothesized that such blunted choice, although accentuated in CS participants with active disease, would also be present in CS in remission, who would show improved but not normalized reward processing.

METHODS

Participants

Participants included 23 patients with CS and 15 overweight healthy controls (OHC) with similar BMI (independent t-test: $p = 0.12$), such that results could be more plausibly attributed to differences in GCs between the groups, rather than to more general metabolic disturbances and food-seeking behaviors that often characterize obesity. Of these patients with CS, 13 were pre-surgery with active disease, and 10 were post-surgery with disease in remission; these groups were considered separately in all analyses reported below. All participants provided written informed consent, and the Mount Sinai Institutional Review Board approved the study procedures. Participants were required to be age 17 or older. Enrolled CS participants were those who were eligible for surgery within 3 months of test administration, or who had achieved endocrine remission from previous surgical treatment (range of time since endocrine remission was achieved in the treated cohort was 6–60 months). Exclusion criteria for both groups were pregnancy; untreated hypothyroidism; use of exogenous GCs, in the 1-week prior to testing (for the active CS and OHC cohorts); and being unable or unwilling to comply with the study procedures or give informed consent. Exclusion criteria for the OHC were underlying endocrine or metabolic disorders, history of alcohol abuse, or unstable weight.

Active CS participants had elevated cortisol levels, as measured by 24 h urine free cortisol (UFC) (see also **Table 1**), and normal or elevated plasma ACTH concentrations (if the participant had Cushing's disease: CD; $N = 22$), or low plasma ACTH (if the participant had adrenal CS; $N = 1$), as previously defined (Nieman et al., 2008). An MRI scan or inferior petrosal sinus sampling, which was indicated for 10 patients, confirmed pituitary source of CD. For CS participants studied after surgical treatment, endocrine remission was confirmed by resolution of CS features, 1–2 day post-operative hypocortisolemia (serum cortisol < 5 mcg/dL) and/or normal 24-h UFC after physiologic oral GC replacement had been discontinued, as previously defined (Nieman et al., 2015). Among all CS patients, two active patients were taking diabetes medications, five active and three remitted patients were taking psychiatric (including anti-anxiety, antidepressant, mood stabilizing, or sedating) medications, and one active patient was taking analgesic medications (for OHC, two participants were taking diabetes medications, and one was taking oral stimulant medication). Four remitted CS patients were taking physiologic oral hydrocortisone replacement (hydrocortisone 15–20 mg daily): two of these patients had required bilateral adrenalectomy in order to achieve endocrine remission after unsuccessful transsphenoidal surgery, and the remaining two were still transiently hypocortisolemic due to successful surgical treatment within the past 6 months. Two remitted patients, who underwent two transsphenoidal surgeries, developed hypopituitarism and were taking pituitary endocrine replacement, including physiologic levothyroxine in both and testosterone in one. All were ambulatory with normal renal function and no liver disease.

Table 1 provides demographics, self-reports, and clinical characteristics of the study sample, split by disease status (active CS, CS in remission, OHC). The groups did not differ on gender, age, race, childhood trauma, or trait impulsivity (Patton et al., 1995). However, there was a higher proportion medication usage in all CS patients than controls. Other group differences were between active CS patients vs. the other two groups: active CS patients had a higher BMI and more dysphoric symptoms, including higher scores on the Beck Depression Inventory (BDI) (Beck, 1996), the State-Trait Anxiety Inventory (STAI) (Spielberger et al., 1983), and the Perceived Stress Scale (PSS) (Cohen et al., 1983); such dysphoric symptoms are consistent with neuropsychiatric comorbidities commonly reported in this population (Pereira et al., 2010; Pivonello et al., 2015).

Picture Choice Tasks

Two picture choice tasks, which have been previously validated in cocaine addiction as extensively described elsewhere (Moeller et al., 2009, 2010, 2012a,b, 2013, 2014), were completed by all study participants at the Mount Sinai Clinical Research Unit in the morning after an overnight fast ≥8 h duration. The tasks—one with explicit contingencies and one with probabilistic contingencies—use standardized pleasant, unpleasant, and neutral images selected from the International Affective Picture System (IAPS) (Lang et al., 2008). For the current study, we incorporated images of food in lieu of cocaine, matched on size and ratio of human to non-human content. These food images depicted palatable "junk" foods (e.g., hamburgers, pizza, or ice cream), and people eating these foods. These two tasks assess complementary notions of choice as described below. **Table 2** provides the raw means and standard deviations of both choice tasks by study group.

Explicit Choice Task (Figure 1A)

Participants chose via continued button pressing between two fully-visible side-by-side images from different picture categories (pleasant, unpleasant, neutral, and food) [we note that a fifth picture category, blank (black) screens containing no image, was also included on this task, but these null images were not analyzed in this study to better equate behavior on the two tasks]. Choice for a desired image enlarged this chosen image to fully cover the screen, which participants could view for the trial duration of 5 s by continued button pressing; 0.5 s of non-response, however, returned the side-by-side image display. After each trial, a new trial with new images ensued. Button pressing (i.e., "working") for images was an important design feature of this task, meant to model "working" for a desired reward; from a behavioral economic perspective, choice on the explicit task can be thought to index breakpoint (i.e., preference for one category of image

TABLE 1 | Demographics, self-report measures, and clinical characteristics by study group.

	Statistical test	Active Cushing's (N = 13)	Cushing's in remission (N = 10)	Overweight controls (N = 15)
Gender (women/men)	$\chi^2_{(2, N=38)} = 3.86$	10/3	4/6	7/8
Medication (any) (yes/no)	$\chi^2_{(2, N=38)} = 13.07^*$	12/1[c]	7/3[c]	4/11[a,b]
Age (years)	$F_{(2, 35)} = 1.09$	42.1 ± 12.9	38.4 ± 16.5	34.4 ± 12.4
Race (White/non-White)	$\chi^2_{(2, N=38)} = 7.90$	12/1	10/0	9/6
Ethnicity (non-Hispanic, Hispanic)	$\chi^2(2, N = 38) = 1.23$	11/2	9/1	11/4
Body mass index (kg/m^2)	$F_{(2, 35)} = 4.85^*$	33.1 ± 4.6[b,c]	28.7 ± 2.9[a]	28.9 ± 4.2[a]
Barrett impulsiveness scale	$F_{(2, 35)} = 0.28$	58.9 ± 8.4	62.0 ± 10.7	59.7 ± 10.9
Childhood trauma questionnaire	$F_{(2, 35)} = 0.53$	40.3 ± 9.3	39.3 ± 15.5	45.5 ± 21.7
Perceived stress scale	$F_{(2, 35)} = 6.68^*$	47.0 ± 8.5[b,c]	36.5 ± 8.4[a]	36.4 ± 8.4[a]
Beck depression inventory	$F_{(2,34)} = 8.78^*$	23.7 ± 11.6[b,c]	12.2 ± 12.3[a]	6.7 ± 8.3[a]
State-trait anxiety inventory: state	$F_{(2, 34)} = 6.65^*$	30.5 ± 14.8[b,c]	16.0 ± 15.6[a]	12.9 ± 9.8[a]
State-trait anxiety inventory: trait	$F_{(2, 34)} = 8.50^*$	33.5 ± 12.9[b,c]	15.7 ± 14.7[a]	15.1 ± 11.6[a]
State food craving	$F_{(2, 35)} = 0.14$	42.4 ± 14.6	45.1 ± 11.2	43.1 ± 10.9
Trait food craving	$F_{(2, 35)} = 4.75^*$	136.8 ± 32.8[c]	114.9 ± 42.5	101.4 ± 15.4[a]
Urine free cortisol (μg/24 h)[d]	$F_{(2,21)} = 8.55^*$	279.0 ± 172.3[b,c]	54.7 ± 45.8[a]	81.0 ± 25.7[a]
Urine cortisone (μg/24 h)[d]	$F_{(2, 21)} = 6.31^*$	380.0 ± 210.5[c]	216.7 ± 146.1	140.7 ± 51.3[a]

Numbers are mean ± standard deviation.
**omnibus $p < 0.05$, with significant follow-up pairwise comparisons.*
[a]Differs significantly from active Cushing's patients.
[b]Differs significantly from Cushing's patients in remission.
[c]Differs from overweight controls.
[d]Sample sizes are 11, 3, and 10 for active Cushing's, Cushing's in remission, and overweight controls, respectively.

TABLE 2 | Descriptive statistics of choice behavior by study group.

	Active Cushing's (N = 13)	Cushing's in remission (N = 10)	Overweight controls (N = 15)
EXPLICIT TASK (TOTAL BUTTON PRESSES)			
A. Pleasant pictures	170.9 ± 147.1	243.8 ± 205.8	186.9 ± 135.2
B. Unpleasant pictures	6.9 ± 8.5	4.3 ± 8.9	36.3 ± 61.9
C. Neutral pictures	127.4 ± 129.6	147.9 ± 128.1	140.3 ± 104.2
D. Food pictures	132.3 ± 111.8	195.5 ± 164.2	207.1 ± 157.1
PROBABILISTIC TASK (TOTAL SELECTIONS)			
A. Pleasant pictures	20.2 ± 5.8	19.4 ± 5.3	18.5 ± 9.2
B. Unpleasant pictures	11.2 ± 7.6	11.1 ± 7.2	8.3 ± 5.4
C. Neutral pictures	17.5 ± 8.0	16.6 ± 5.7	8.9 ± 6.2
D. Food pictures	18.5 ± 9.4	24.1 ± 5.1	19.5 ± 8.8

Numbers are mean ± standard deviation, without correction for any covariates.

over another when there is a cost of effort expenditure) (e.g., Mackillop et al., 2010; Moeller et al., 2013). We summed the number of button presses (across 70 total trials), indexing vigor of responding, per picture category.

Probabilistic Choice Task (Figure 1B)

On each trial, participants chose via a single button press to view pictures hidden under flipped-over cards, arranged in four decks. Immediately after choosing from a particular "deck," an image was revealed that covered the entire screen for 2 s of passive viewing. The images were arranged probabilistically: each deck contained 26 (out of a total of 30) pictures from a particular category (e.g., pleasant), allowing pictures from other categories to be interspersed within each deck (two pictures from a secondary category, e.g., food; and one picture from each of the two remaining categories, e.g., unpleasant and neutral). After participants selected from a particular deck eight total times (corresponding to one task run), deck location of the four picture categories shifted. Thus, this task contained a "seeking" component, rather than a "working" component: throughout, participants needed to seek (and re-seek, once task contingencies changed) their preferred deck(s). In contrast to the explicit task, choice on the probabilistic task was meant to model more standard notions of choice; here, from a behavioral economic perspective, probabilistic choice can be thought to reflect intensity (i.e., preference for one category of image over another when there is no cost associated with the choice) (e.g., Mackillop et al., 2010; Moeller et al., 2013). We summed the total number of cards selected per picture category across four task runs.

Food Craving Questionnaires

State Food Craving

Current food craving was measured with the Food Craving Questionnaire-State [FCQ-S (Cepeda-Benito et al., 2000; Nijs et al., 2007)]. The FCQ-S consists of 15 items assessing: desire to eat, anticipation of positive reinforcement from eating, anticipation of negative reinforcement (reduction of negative affect) from eating, lack of control over eating, and

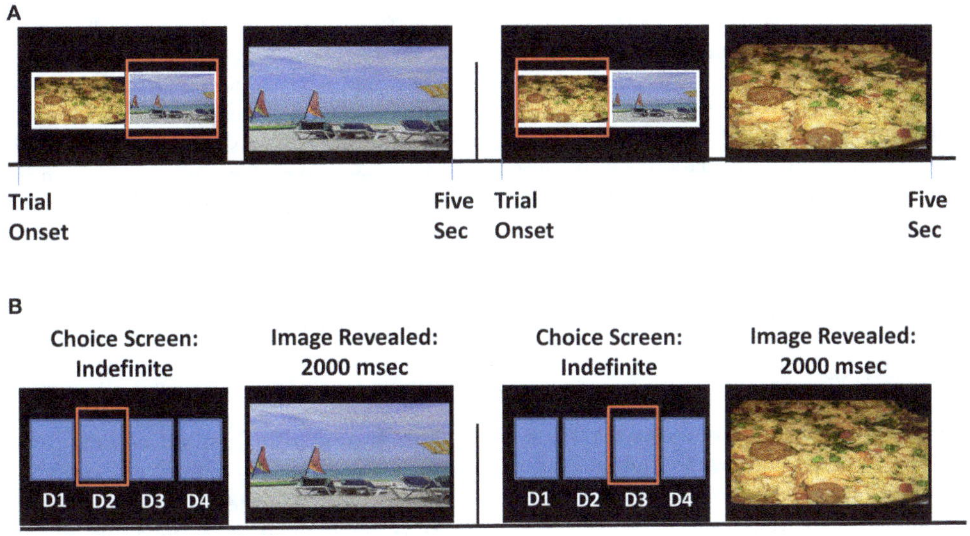

FIGURE 1 | Task schematics of the explicit and probabilistic food choice tasks. (A) The explicit task included training and one block, consisting of 70 trials. Two sample trials are displayed. Continuous button pressing for a given image (indicated by the red box) enlarged the corresponding image, for the 5-s trial duration; no response (for 0.5 s) after initial response returned the side-by-side display. **(B)** The probabilistic task included training and four task runs. In each trial within a run, participants pressed one of four buttons corresponding to their chosen deck (D1, D2, D3, or D4; also indicated by the red box).

(physiological) hunger; higher scores reflect stronger food craving. Participants respond, using a Likert-type scale, how much each item is true of them *right now*. Demonstrating applicability of this questionnaire to the current study, FCQ-S scores were increased after exposure to food images in "high cravers" of chocolate (Meule et al., 2012), and were correlated with increased attention allocation (that interfered with response inhibition) to food vs. neutral pictures (Meule et al., 2014a).

Trait Food Craving

Trait food craving was assessed with the Food Craving Questionnaire-Trait (FCQ-T) (Cepeda-Benito et al., 2000; Nijs et al., 2007). The FCQ-T consists of 39 items assessing: intentions/plans to eat, anticipation of positive reinforcement from eating, anticipation of negative reinforcement from eating, lack of control over eating, preoccupation with food, (physiological) hunger, emotions preceding or following food cravings or eating, environmental cues that may elicit food cravings, negative emotions including guilt experienced as a consequence of food cravings, and/or indulging such cravings; higher scores again indicate higher trait craving. Individuals are asked to respond, using a Likert-type scale, how much each item is true of them *in general*. Unlike the FCQ-S, and appropriately for a trait measure, the FCQ-T was unaffected by food deprivation (Meule et al., 2014b). In the current study, active CS had higher trait (but not state) food craving than OHC (**Table 1**).

Urine Cortisol and Cortisone Measures

Twenty-four hour UFC and cortisone were quantified by gas chromatography-mass spectroscopy (GC-MS) as previously described (Yehuda et al., 2009a,b). The limit of sensitivity is 2 ng, the inter-assay coefficients of variations are $<10\%$, and the normal range for UFC is 10–100 μg/24 h. As to be expected, these measures were highest in active CS (**Table 1**).

Statistical Analyses

Effects of Disease Status on Food Picture Choice

We analyzed both choice tasks using a 4 (Picture Type: pleasant, unpleasant, neutral, food) $\times$ 3 (Disease Status: active CS, CS in remission, OHC) mixed analysis of covariance (ANCOVA), with the total number of presses (explicit task) or selections (probabilistic task) entered as covariates in the appropriate model to control for individual differences in response frequency. Significant interactions were followed by paired (within-group) and independent (between-group) comparisons that similarly controlled for response frequency. For the latter, a core interest was in testing for between-group linear contrasts (i.e., stepwise patterns in the effects as a function of Disease Status). In all ANCOVAs and follow-up comparisons, $p < 0.05$ was considered significant.

Correlation Analyses

For both tasks, we examined associations between the food choice variables and the food vs. pleasant choice difference scores (food > pleasant) with the variables of interest specified below. The focus on this specific food > pleasant difference score follows from our prior results in individuals with cocaine use disorder, in which cocaine vs. pleasant (cocaine > pleasant) choice was particularly useful in predicting drug-relevant outcomes (Moeller et al., 2012a, 2013). Correlations were conducted across all participants and split by the three study groups. Due to the presence of some outliers across various measures, correlations were conducted using non-parametric (Spearman) analyses. In all correlational analyses, $p < 0.01$ was considered significant to protect against Type I error. After satisfying this initial criterion, however, we retained significant correlations if they achieved a significance level of $p < 0.05$ when accounting for covariates.

Between-task reliability and initial validity

Because these tasks were new to a CS population, and because they included a new image category (food), we tested for intercorrelations between the explicit and probabilistic task scores. To provide evidence of construct validity of these tasks in CS, we also examined correlations between the task variables with BMI and self-reported food craving (state and trait).

Associations with cortisol levels

To provide further attribution of our effects to GCs, we performed correlations between the two food-choice variables and the two food > pleasant choice scores with urine markers of cortisol inclusive of free cortisol and cortisone in the subsample of participants for whom these data were available.

Effects of Covariates

Because medication use, BMI, and dysphoric symptoms (i.e., state and trait anxiety, perceived stress, and depression symptoms) differed between the groups (**Table 1**), these variables were covaried in subsequent ANCOVAs or multiple regressions as appropriate. Note that food craving and urine cortisol/cortisone were considered dependent variables, not covariates.

RESULTS

Effects of Disease Status on Food Picture Choice

Results of the mixed 4 (Picture Type) × 3 (Disease Status) ANCOVAs revealed main effects of Picture Type [$F_{(3, 32)} > 36.50$, $p < 0.001$]: on both tasks, unpleasant choice was lowest, followed by neutral choice, and these were both lower than pleasant and food choice (all pairwise comparisons, $p < 0.01$). There were no main effects of Disease Status (both $p > 0.096$). Of greater interest, on the explicit task, the Picture Type × Disease Status interaction reached significance [$F_{(6, 64)} = 3.12$, $p = 0.010$] (**Figure 2A**). Planned linear contrast analyses showed that active CS participants made fewer food choices than CS participants in remission, who in turn made fewer food choices than OHC ($p = 0.021$); linear contrasts for the other picture categories did not reach significance (all $p > 0.074$), indicating specificity to food choice. Follow-up within-group comparisons showed that both active CS and CS in remission pressed for fewer food pictures than pleasant pictures (both $p < 0.012$) but not neutral pictures (both $p > 0.063$). OHC showed an opposite pattern of results, pressing for food pictures more than neutral pictures ($p = 0.003$) but not pleasant pictures ($p = 0.099$). These collective analyses suggest that CS patients displayed reduced vigor for responding to food reward, particularly in those with active disease. Because the Picture Type × Disease Status interaction did not reach significance on the probabilistic task [$F_{(6, 64)} = 1.18$, $p = 0.34$], no follow-up comparisons were performed.

Correlation Analyses

Between-Task Reliability and Initial Validity

Correlations did not reach significance at $p < 0.01$ across the whole sample. Nevertheless, after splitting the three groups, a positive correlation emerged between the food > pleasant choice variables on the two tasks in OHC ($r_s = 0.74$, $p = 0.001$) but not in either of the CS groups ($r_s < 0.39$, $p > 0.19$). In addition, higher food > pleasant choice, this time on the probabilistic task, positively correlated with higher state ($r_s = 0.82$, $p = 0.001$) and trait ($r_s = 0.79$, $p = 0.001$) food craving in active CS but not in CS in remission or OHC ($r_s < |0.38|$, $p > 0.28$) (**Figures 2B,C**). This correlation suggests that food-related choice on this task is a valid metric of the desire to eat, both currently and in general, in a CS patient population with active disease.

Associations with Cortisol Levels

Across all participants, food > pleasant choice on the explicit task negatively correlated with urine free cortisone (the higher the cortisone, the lower the food-related choice) ($r_s = -0.56$, $p = 0.004$) (**Figure 2D**). A similar trend was observed for UFC ($r_s = -0.42$, $p = 0.041$), which, although not reaching nominal significance, increases confidence in the cortisone effect.

Effects of Covariates

The Picture Type × Disease Status interaction remained significant after controlling for medication use ($p = 0.048$), BMI ($p = 0.018$), and dysphoric symptoms (state and trait anxiety, perceived stress, and depression symptoms: $p < 0.022$). In addition, results of multiple regression analyses controlling for these same covariates showed that correlations were still detected between the food > pleasant scores on both tasks in OHC ($p < 0.004$), between food > pleasant probabilistic choice with state ($p < 0.007$) and trait ($p < 0.032$) food craving in active CS, and between food > pleasant explicit choice and urine cortisone in all participants ($p < 0.025$). Thus, it is unlikely that these potential confounds drove the current results.

DISCUSSION

In this study, CS with active disease, CS with disease in remission, and OHC participants completed two behavioral tasks that tested the choice to view food pictures vs. non-food-related pleasant, unpleasant, and neutral pictures. We hypothesized that, as a model of chronic exposure to excessive GCs, individuals with CS (and especially those individuals with active disease) would make fewer food-related choices (and fewer pleasant-related choices) than OHC. Results supported the hypothesis that individuals with higher endogenous GC levels, independent of BMI, exhibited decreased food (but not pleasant) choice on the explicit (but not probabilistic) task.

The primary result of this study was that, when task contingencies were explicit (i.e., fully certain) and choice required working (continuously pressing buttons) to view the respective stimuli, individuals with active CS chose to view fewer food images than individuals with CS in remission, who in turn chose to view fewer food images than OHC; thus, CS patients, especially those with active disease, were less apt to *exert effort* to view

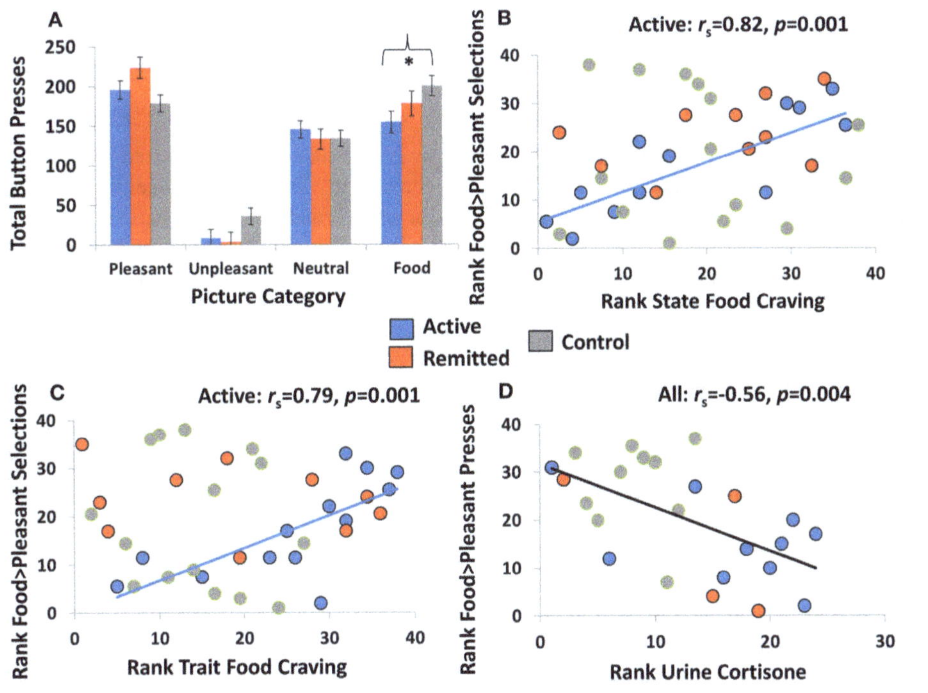

FIGURE 2 | Relevant choice task results and scatterplots showing associations between food-related choice with state food craving and cortisol. (A) Results of the explicit task showing total button presses (estimated marginal means) for each of the four picture categories (pleasant, unpleasant, neutral, and food) for individuals with active Cushing's syndrome (N = 13), individuals with Cushing's syndrome in remission (N = 10), and overweight comparison participants (N = 15). The asterisk indicates a significant linear contrast among the groups at $p < 0.05$, and error bars represent standard error of the mean. Note that results of the probabilistic choice are not shown, given the nonsignificant Picture Category × Diagnosis interactions (for descriptive statistics of this task, see **Table 2**). **(B,C)** In individuals with active Cushing's syndrome but not the other two study groups, higher probabilistic food choice (compared with probabilistic non-food pleasant choice) correlated with higher state and trait food craving. **(D)** Across all participants for whom urine cortisol markers were available (N = 24), higher explicit food choice (compared with explicit non-food pleasant choice) correlated with lower urine cortisone.

food cues. Although at first blush this decreased food choice may be unexpected given that individuals exposed to chronic stress or GCs often consume more calories and/or eat less healthfully (Tomiyama et al., 2011; Groesz et al., 2012; Hoffman et al., 2012; Talbot et al., 2013; Aschbacher et al., 2014), it is critical to note that the "control" group was also overweight (i.e., not differing from the overall CS group on BMI, which was a goal in our recruitment; see Methods). Moreover, our results are consistent with prior work showing that chronic excessive exposure to GCs, here attributable to active CS but potentially also generalizable to chronic stress or chronic GC administration, is associated with blunted reward sensitivity in human- (Dillon et al., 2009; Goff et al., 2013) and animal models (Mateus-Pinheiro et al., 2014; Kvarta et al., 2015). Because in the current study results were specific to the food-choice task that required "working," it is possible that active CS patients have a higher threshold for perceiving food as reinforcing, potentially needing to consume more to achieve the same hedonic effect. An important parallel can be made to addiction literature, whereby reduced drug sensitivity is associated with increased or uncontrolled drug use [e.g., whether because of putatively drug-mediated adaptations to dopamine neurotransmission in drug addiction (Volkow et al., 1997, 2010; Martinez et al., 2009; Peechatka et al., 2015) or because of genetics that elevate susceptibility to developing addiction later in life (Edenberg, 2007; de Wit and Phillips, 2012; Gubner et al., 2013)]. More broadly, our results support and extend prior research in CS on deficits in memory, learning, and decision-making (Whelan et al., 1980; Martignoni et al., 1992; Mauri et al., 1993; Forget et al., 2000; Starkman et al., 2001, 2003; Leon-Carrion et al., 2009; Michaud et al., 2009; Pereira et al., 2010; Ragnarsson et al., 2012; Resmini et al., 2012; Crespo et al., 2014); and that such neurocognitive deficits may be ameliorated, but not fully normalized, even after surgical remission (Tiemensma et al., 2010a,b; Geer et al., 2012; Pereira et al., 2012; Lambert et al., 2013; Andela et al., 2015; Pivonello et al., 2015).

In further analyses, we correlated our behavioral choice results with self-reported food craving and *in vivo* GC levels; these analyses, respectively, were meant to validate these food-choice tasks as a model of food reward in a CS population and to provide a putative neurobiological correlate of the food-choice results. For the latter (neurobiological correlate), and corroborating our main between-group analyses above, correlations emerged between food-related choice on the explicit task and urine GCs: across all participants, 24-h urine cortisone correlated with explicit food-related choice, with similar albeit nonsignificant effects emerging for UFC. The underlying mechanism of these effects, which requires testing in further studies, could involve

GC modulation of the dopamine system that alters the incentive salience of food cues (Borges et al., 2013; Yau and Potenza, 2013; Soares-Cunha et al., 2014). For the former (task validity), probabilistic (though not explicit) food-related choice positively correlated with state and trait food craving within active CS. Thus, although between-group effects in the current study were not observed on this probabilistic task, correlations with food craving help to validate these food-choice tasks as a model of food reward in active CS.

Limitations of this study include the following. First, the current study did not include a sample of normal-weight controls, and without this reference group we cannot definitively conclude whether results are primarily driven by decreased food-choice in CS, increased food-choice in OHC, or both. Future studies will need to include a normal-weight control group. Nevertheless, our paramount concern in this initial study was to equate the groups on BMI, which indeed was achieved for the full CS sample. Although a BMI group difference emerged when splitting the groups by disease status (**Table 1**), it is important to note that our results were robust to statistical correction for BMI, indicating that this variable did not drive our results. Second, urine cortisol markers were unavailable in half the study sample. However, effects with cortisone were indeed observed using a relatively strict statistical threshold, reducing the potential for spurious effects; and, more importantly, in our main analyses we found stepwise effects as a function of remission status on behavioral choice in the entire sample. Third, we did not obtain self-report ratings of preference for the food stimuli prior to their use in the current tasks. However, main effects of Picture Type indicated that these food images were indeed palatable, such that all participants chose them for viewing more often than neutral images or unpleasant images. Fourth, it is possible that demand characteristics or participants' task-related motivation could have contributed to the lower food-related choice in CS participants. However, if results were driven by demand characteristics associated with the desire to reduce food intake and lose weight, we strongly suspect that OHC participants would have been similarly motivated to avoid choosing food images. If results were driven by reduced task-related motivation in CS (e.g., due to anhedonia), one could anticipate that choice for non-food-related rewarding stimuli (here, pleasant images) would be reduced as well (Pizzagalli et al., 2009; Domschke et al., 2015; Fletcher et al., 2015), but this pattern of effects did not occur; moreover, dysphoric symptoms did not explain our findings.

In conclusion, chronic GC exposure from active CS was associated with reduced simulated food choice when compared with such choice in overweight individuals with intact GC functioning; CS patients in remission with remediated GC functioning showed an intermediate pattern of food choice, suggesting that that prior GC exposure may exert lasting effects on brain reward systems. Future studies can use neuroimaging and/or neurochemical approaches in CS, OHC, and (importantly) normal-weight controls to test for commonalities and/or differences in food choice and its neurobiological underpinnings among these study groups. Longitudinal designs can also test whether GC-mediated food-choices have downstream consequences, such as increasing risk for weight gain and/or cardiovascular events. More broadly, beyond illuminating neurocognitive sequelae of CS (and possibly chronic stress), our findings can also inform the neurobiology of elevated and/or dysregulated cortisol as seen in aging, major depressive disorder, and/or Alzheimer's disease (Pereira et al., 2012; Notarianni, 2013; Gupta and Morley, 2014; Du and Pang, 2015; Furtado and Katzman, 2015).

AUTHOR CONTRIBUTIONS

SM, RG, and EG designed research. LC, VC, and YL performed research. SM, IM, NW, RY, and EG analyzed data. SM and EG wrote the paper. All authors provided critical revisions of the paper.

ACKNOWLEDGMENTS

This study was supported by grants from the National Institute on Drug Abuse (to SM: K01DA037452), the National Institute of Diabetes and Digestive and Kidney Diseases (to EG: K23DK082617), and the Mount Sinai Clinical and Translational Science Awards (CTSA) Program (UL1TR000067). The content is solely the responsibility of the authors and does not necessarily represent the official views of the National Institutes of Health.

REFERENCES

1. Adam, T. C., and Epel, E. S. (2007). Stress, eating and the reward system. *Physiol. Behav.* 91, 449–458. doi: 10.1016/j.physbeh.2007.04.011
2. Andela, C. D., Scharloo, M., Pereira, A. M., Kaptein, A. A., and Biermasz, N. R. (2015). Quality of life (QoL) impairments in patients with a pituitary adenoma: a systematic review of QoL studies. *Pituitary* 18, 752–776. doi: 10.1007/s11102- 015-0636-7
3. Aschbacher, K., Kornfeld, S., Picard, M., Puterman, E., Havel, P. J., Stanhope, K., et al. (2014). Chronic stress increases vulnerability to diet-related abdominal fat, oxidative stress, and metabolic risk. *Psychoneuroendocrinology* 46, 14–22. doi: 10.1016/j.psyneuen.2014.04.003
4. Beck, A. T. (1996). *The Beck Depression Inventory (BDI-II)*. San Antonio, TX: The Psychological Corporation.
5. Berghorst, L. H., Bogdan, R., Frank, M. J., and Pizzagalli, D. A. (2013). Acute stress selectively reduces reward sensitivity. *Front. Hum. Neurosci.* 7:133. doi: 10.3389/fnhum.2013.00133
6. Borges, S., Coimbra, B., Soares-Cunha, C., Miguel Pêgo, J., Sousa, N., and João Rodrigues, A. (2013). Dopaminergic modulation of affective and social deficits induced by prenatal glucocorticoid exposure. *Neuropsychopharmacology* 38, 2068–2079. doi: 10.1038/npp.2013.108
7. Born, J. M., Lemmens, S. G., Rutters, F., Nieuwenhuizen, A. G., Formisano, E., Goebel, R., et al. (2010). Acute stress and food-related reward activation in the brain during food choice during eating in the absence of hunger. *Int. J. Obes. (Lond.)* 34, 172–181. doi: 10.1038/ijo.2009.221
8. Carluccio, A., Sundaram, N. K., Chablani, S., Amrock, L. G., Lambert, J. K., Post, K. D., et al. (2015). Predictors of quality of life in 102 patients with treated Cushing's disease. *Clin. Endocrinol. (Oxf.)* 82, 404–411. doi: 10.1111/cen. 12521
9. Cepeda-Benito, A., Gleaves, D. H., Fernandez, M. C., Vila, J., Williams, T. L., and Reynoso, J. (2000). The development and validation of Spanish

versions of the state and trait food cravings questionnaires. *Behav. Res. Ther.* 38, 1125–1138. doi: 10.1016/S0005-7967(99)00141-2

10. Coates, J. M., and Herbert, J. (2008). Endogenous steroids and financial risk taking on a London trading floor. *Proc. Natl. Acad. Sci. U.S.A.* 105, 6167–6172. doi: 10.1073/pnas.0704025105
11. Cohen, S., Kamarck, T., and Mermelstein, R. (1983). A global measure of perceived stress. *J. Health Soc. Behav.* 24, 385–396. doi: 10.2307/2136404
12. Crespo, I., Esther, G. M., Santos, A., Valassi, E., Yolanda, V. G., De Juan-Delago, M., et al. (2014). Impaired decision-making and selective cortical frontal thinning in Cushing's syndrome. *Clin. Endocrinol. (Oxf.)* 81, 826–833. doi: 10.1111/cen.12564
13. de Wit, H., and Phillips, T. J. (2012). Do initial responses to drugs predict future use or abuse? *Neurosci. Biobehav. Rev.* 36, 1565–1576. doi: 10.1016/j.neubiorev.2012.04.005
14. Dillon, D. G., Holmes, A. J., Birk, J. L., Brooks, N., Lyons-Ruth, K., and Pizzagalli, D. A. (2009). Childhood adversity is associated with left basal ganglia dysfunction during reward anticipation in adulthood. *Biol. Psychiatry* 66, 206–213. doi: 10.1016/j.biopsych.2009.02.019
15. Dimopoulou, C., Ising, M., Pfister, H., Schopohl, J., Stalla, G. K., and Sievers, C. (2013). Increased prevalence of anxiety-associated personality traits in patients with Cushing's disease: a cross-sectional study. *Neuroendocrinology* 97, 139–145. doi: 10.1159/000338408
16. Domschke, K., Zwanzger, P., Rehbein, M. A., Steinberg, C., Knoke, K., Dobel, C., et al. (2015). Magnetoencephalographic correlates of emotional processing in major depression before and after pharmacological treatment. *Int. J. Neuropsychopharmacol.* doi: 10.1093/ijnp/pyv093. [Epub ahead of print].
17. Du, X., and Pang, T. Y. (2015). Is dysregulation of the HPA-axis a core pathophysiology mediating co-morbid depression in neurodegenerative diseases? *Front. Psychiatry* 6:32. doi: 10.3389/fpsyt.2015.00032
18. Edenberg, H. J. (2007). The genetics of alcohol metabolism: role of alcohol dehydrogenase and aldehyde dehydrogenase variants. *Alcohol Res. Health* 30, 5–13.
19. Feelders, R. A., Pulgar, S. J., Kempel, A., and Pereira, A. M. (2012). The burden of Cushing's disease: clinical and health-related quality of life aspects. *Eur. J. Endocrinol.* 167, 311–326. doi: 10.1530/EJE-11-1095
20. Ferreira de Sa, D. S., Schulz, A., Streit, F. E., Turner, J. D., Oitzl, M. S., Blumenthal, T. D., et al. (2014). Cortisol, but not intranasal insulin, affects the central processing of visual food cues. *Psychoneuroendocrinology* 50, 311–320. doi: 10.1016/j.psyneuen.2014.09.006
21. Fletcher, K., Parker, G., Paterson, A., Fava, M., Iosifescu, D., and Pizzagalli, D. A. (2015). Anhedonia in melancholic and non-melancholic depressive disorders. *J. Affect. Disord.* 184, 81–88. doi: 10.1016/j.jad.2015.05.028
22. Forget, H., Lacroix, A., Somma, M., and Cohen, H. (2000). Cognitive decline in patients with Cushing's syndrome. *J. Int. Neuropsychol. Soc.* 6, 20–29. doi: 10.1017/s1355617700611037
23. Furtado, M., and Katzman, M. A. (2015). Examining the role of neuroinflammation in major depression. *Psychiatry Res.* 229, 27–36. doi: 10.1016/j.psychres.2015.06.009
24. Geer, E. B., Shen, W., Strohmayer, E., Post, K. D., and Freda, P. U. (2012). Body composition and cardiovascular risk markers after remission of Cushing's disease: a prospective study using whole-body MRI. *J. Clin. Endocrinol. Metab.* 97, 1702–1711. doi: 10.1210/jc.2011-3123
25. Goff, B., Gee, D. G., Telzer, E. H., Humphreys, K. L., Gabard-Durnam, L., Flannery, J., et al. (2013). Reduced nucleus accumbens reactivity and adolescent depression following early-life stress. *Neuroscience* 249, 129–138. doi: 10.1016/j.neuroscience.2012.12.010
26. Grillon, C., Smith, K., Haynos, A., and Nieman, L. K. (2004). Deficits in hippocampus-mediated Pavlovian conditioning in endogenous hypercortisolism. *Biol. Psychiatry* 56, 837–843. doi: 10.1016/j.biopsych.2004.09.003
27. Groesz, L. M., McCoy, S., Carl, J., Saslow, L., Stewart, J., Adler, N., et al. (2012). What is eating you? Stress and the drive to eat. *Appetite* 58, 717–721. doi: 10.1016/j.appet.2011.11.028
28. Gubner, N. R., McKinnon, C. S., Reed, C., and Phillips, T. J. (2013). Accentuating effects of nicotine on ethanol response in mice with high genetic predisposition to ethanol-induced locomotor stimulation. *Drug Alcohol Depend.* 127, 108–114. doi: 10.1016/j.drugalcdep.2012.06.015
29. Gupta, D., and Morley, J. E. (2014). Hypothalamic-pituitary-adrenal (HPA) axis and aging. *Compr. Physiol.* 4, 1495–1510. doi: 10.1002/cphy.c130049
30. Hoffman, G. J., Lee, J., and Mendez-Luck, C. A. (2012). Health behaviors among Baby Boomer informal caregivers. *Gerontologist* 52, 219–230. doi: 10.1093/geront/gns003
31. Hook, J. N., Giordani, B., Schteingart, D. E., Guire, K., Giles, J., Ryan, K., et al. (2007). Patterns of cognitive change over time and relationship to age following successful treatment of Cushing's disease. *J. Int. Neuropsychol. Soc.* 13, 21–29. doi: 10.1017/s1355617707070051
32. Kvarta, M. D., Bradbrook, K. E., Dantrassy, H. M., Bailey, A. M., and Thompson, S. M. (2015). Corticosterone mediates the synaptic and behavioral effects of chronic stress at rat hippocampal temporoammonic synapses. *J. Neurophysiol.* 114, 1713–1724. doi: 10.1152/jn.00359.2015
33. La Fleur, S. E. (2006). The effects of glucocorticoids on feeding behavior in rats. *Physiol. Behav.* 89, 110–114. doi: 10.1016/j.physbeh.2006.01.028
34. Lacroix, A., Feelders, R. A., Stratakis, C. A., and Nieman, L. K. (2015). Cushing's syndrome. *Lancet* 386, 913–927. doi: 10.1016/S0140-6736(14)61375-1
35. Lambert, J. K., Goldberg, L., Fayngold, S., Kostadinov, J., Post, K. D., and Geer, E. B. (2013). Predictors of mortality and long-term outcomes in treated Cushing's disease: a study of 346 patients. *J. Clin. Endocrinol. Metab.* 98, 1022–1030. doi: 10.1210/jc.2012-2893
36. Lang, P. J., Bradley, M. M., and Cuthbert, B. N. (2008). *International Affective Picture System (IAPS): Affective Ratings of Pictures and Instruction Manual.* Technical Report A-8, Gainsville, FL, University of Florida.
37. Leon-Carrion, J., Atutxa, A. M., Mangas, M. A., Soto-Moreno, A., Pumar, A., Leon- Justel, A., et al. (2009). A clinical profile of memory impairment in humans due to endogenous glucocorticoid excess. *Clin. Endocrinol. (Oxf.)* 70, 192–200. doi: 10.1111/j.1365-2265.2008.03355.x
38. Mackillop, J., Miranda, R. Jr., Monti, P. M., Ray, L. A., Murphy, J. G., Rohsenow, D. J., et al. (2010). Alcohol demand, delayed reward discounting, and craving in relation to drinking and alcohol use disorders. *J. Abnorm. Psychol.* 119, 106–114. doi: 10.1037/a0017513
39. Maier, S. U., Makwana, A. B., and Hare, T. A. (2015). Acute stress impairs self-control in goal-directed choice by altering multiple functional connections within the brain's decision circuits. *Neuron* 87, 621–631. doi: 10.1016/j.neuron.2015.07.005
40. Martignoni, E., Costa, A., Sinforiani, E., Liuzzi, A., Chiodini, P., Mauri, M., et al. (1992). The brain as a target for adrenocortical steroids: cognitive implications. *Psychoneuroendocrinology* 17, 343–354. doi: 10.1016/0306-4530(92) 90040-E
41. Martinez, D., Greene, K., Broft, A., Kumar, D., Liu, F., Narendran, R., et al. (2009). Lower level of endogenous dopamine in patients with cocaine dependence: findings from PET imaging of D(2)/D(3) receptors following acute dopamine depletion. *Am. J. Psychiatry* 166, 1170–1177. doi: 10.1176/appi.ajp.2009.08121801
42. Mateus-Pinheiro, A., Patrício, P., Alves, N. D., Machado-Santos, A. R., Morais, M., Bessa, J. M., et al. (2014). The Sweet Drive Test: refining phenotypic characterization of anhedonic behavior in rodents. *Front. Behav. Neurosci.* 8:74. doi: 10.3389/fnbeh.2014.00074
43. Mauri, M., Sinforiani, E., Bono, G., Vignati, F., Berselli, M. E., Attanasio, R., et al. (1993). Memory impairment in Cushing's disease. *Acta Neurol. Scand.* 87, 52–55. doi: 10.1111/j.1600-0404.1993.tb04075.x
44. McEwen, B. S., Nasca, C., and Gray, J. D. (2016). Stress effects on neuronal structure: hippocampus, amygdala, and prefrontal cortex. *Neuropsychopharmacology* 41, 3–23. doi: 10.1038/npp.2015.171
45. Meule, A., Lutz, A. P., Vögele, C., and Kübler, A. (2014a). Impulsive reactions to food-cues predict subsequent food craving. *Eat. Behav.* 15, 99–105. doi: 10.1016/j.eatbeh.2013.10.023
46. Meule, A., Skirde, A. K., Freund, R., Vögele, C., and Kübler, A. (2012). High-calorie food-cues impair working memory performance in high and low food cravers. *Appetite* 59, 264–269. doi: 10.1016/j.appet.2012.05.010
47. Meule, A., Teran, C. B., Berker, J., Grundel, T., Mayerhofer, M., and Platte, P. (2014b). On the differentiation between trait and state food craving: half-year retest-reliability of the Food Cravings Questionnaire-Trait-reduced (FCQ-T-r) and the Food Cravings Questionnaire-State (FCQ-S). *J. Eat. Disord.* 2:25. doi: 10.1186/s40337-014-0025-z
48. Michaud, K., Forget, H., and Cohen, H. (2009). Chronic glucocorticoid hypersecretion in Cushing's syndrome exacerbates cognitive aging. *Brain Cogn.* 71, 1–8. doi: 10.1016/j.bandc.2009.02.013
49. Moeller, S. J., Beebe-Wang, N., Woicik, P. A., Konova, A. B., Maloney, T., and Goldstein, R. Z. (2013). Choice to view cocaine images predicts concurrent and prospective drug use in cocaine addiction. *Drug Alcohol Depend.* 130,

178–185. doi: 10.1016/j.drugalcdep.2012.11.001

50. Moeller, S. J., Hajcak, G., Parvaz, M. A., Dunning, J. P., Volkow, N. D., and Goldstein, R. Z. (2012a). Psychophysiological prediction of choice: relevance to insight and drug addiction. *Brain* 135, 3481–3494. doi: 10.1093/brain/aws252
51. Moeller, S. J., Konova, A. B., Parvaz, M. A., Tomasi, D., Lane, R. D., Fort, C., et al. (2014). Functional, structural, and emotional correlates of impaired insight in cocaine addiction. *JAMA Psychiatry* 71, 61–70. doi: 10.1001/jamapsychiatry.2013.2833
52. Moeller, S. J., Maloney, T., Parvaz, M. A., Alia-Klein, N., Woicik, P. A., Telang, F., et al. (2010). Impaired insight in cocaine addiction: laboratory evidence and effects on cocaine-seeking behaviour. *Brain* 133, 1484–1493. doi: 10.1093/brain/awq066
53. Moeller, S. J., Maloney, T., Parvaz, M. A., Dunning, J. P., Alia-Klein, N., Woicik, P. A., et al. (2009). Enhanced choice for viewing cocaine pictures in cocaine addiction. *Biol. Psychiatry* 66, 169–176. doi: 10.1016/j.biopsych.2009.02.015
54. Moeller, S. J., Tomasi, D., Woicik, P. A., Maloney, T., Alia-Klein, N., Honorio, J., et al. (2012b). Enhanced midbrain response at 6-month follow-up in cocaine addiction, association with reduced drug-related choice. *Addict. Biol.* 17, 1013–1025. doi: 10.1111/j.1369-1600.2012.00440.x
55. Montoya, E. R., Bos, P. A., Terburg, D., Rosenberger, L. A., and van Honk, J. (2014). Cortisol administration induces global down-regulation of the brain's reward circuitry. *Psychoneuroendocrinology* 47, 31–42. doi: 10.1016/j.psyneuen.2014.04.022
56. Mueller, S. C., Hardin, M. G., Korelitz, K., Daniele, T., Bemis, J., Dozier, M., et al. (2012). Incentive effect on inhibitory control in adolescents with early-life stress: an antisaccade study. *Child Abuse Negl.* 36, 217–225. doi: 10.1016/j.chiabu.2011.10.010
57. Nieman, L. K., Biller, B. M., Findling, J. W., Murad, M. H., Newell-Price, J., Savage, M. O., et al. (2015). Treatment of Cushing's syndrome: an endocrine society clinical practice guideline. *J. Clin. Endocrinol. Metab.* 100, 2807–2831. doi: 10.1210/jc.2015-1818
58. Nieman, L. K., Biller, B. M., Findling, J. W., Newell-Price, J., Savage, M. O., Stewart, P. M., et al. (2008). The diagnosis of Cushing's syndrome: an endocrine society clinical practice guideline. *J. Clin. Endocrinol. Metab.* 93, 1526–1540. doi: 10.1210/jc.2008-0125
59. Nieuwenhuizen, A. G., and Rutters, F. (2008). The hypothalamic-pituitary-adrenal-axis in the regulation of energy balance. *Physiol. Behav.* 94, 169–177. doi: 10.1016/j.physbeh.2007.12.011
60. Nijs, I. M., Franken, I. H., and Muris, P. (2007). The modified trait and state food-cravings questionnaires: development and validation of a general index of food craving. *Appetite* 49, 38–46. doi: 10.1016/j.appet.2006.11.001
61. Notarianni, E. (2013). Hypercortisolemia and glucocorticoid receptor-signaling insufficiency in Alzheimer's disease initiation and development. *Curr. Alzheimer Res.* 10, 714–731. doi: 10.2174/15672050113109990137
62. Ossewaarde, L., Qin, S., Van Marle, H. J., van Wingen, G. A., Fernández, G., and Hermans, E. J. (2011). Stress-induced reduction in reward-related prefrontal cortex function. *Neuroimage* 55, 345–352. doi: 10.1016/j.neuroimage.2010.11.068
63. Patton, J. H., Stanford, M. S., and Barratt, E. S. (1995). Factor structure of the Barratt impulsiveness scale. *J. Clin. Psychol.* 51, 768–774.
64. Peechatka, A. L., Whitton, A. E., Farmer, S. L., Pizzagalli, D. A., and Janes, A. C. (2015). Cigarette craving is associated with blunted reward processing in nicotine-dependent smokers. *Drug Alcohol Depend.* 155, 202–207. doi: 10.1016/j.drugalcdep.2015.07.015
65. Pereira, A. M., Tiemensma, J., and Romijn, J. A. (2010). Neuropsychiatric disorders in Cushing's syndrome. *Neuroendocrinology* 92(Suppl. 1), 65–70. doi: 10.1159/000314317
66. Pereira, A. M., Tiemensma, J., Romijn, J. A., and Biermasz, N. R. (2012). Cognitive impairment and psychopathology in patients with pituitary diseases. *Neth. J. Med.* 70, 255–260.
67. Pivonello, R., Simeoli, C., De Martino, M. C., Cozzolino, A., De Leo, M., Iacuaniello, D., et al. (2015). Neuropsychiatric disorders in Cushing's syndrome. *Front. Neurosci.* 9:129. doi: 10.3389/fnins.2015.00129
68. Pizzagalli, D. A., Holmes, A. J., Dillon, D. G., Goetz, E. L., Birk, J. L., Bogdan, R., et al. (2009). Reduced caudate and nucleus accumbens response to rewards in unmedicated individuals with major depressive disorder. *Am. J. Psychiatry* 166, 702–710. doi: 10.1176/appi.ajp.2008.08081201
69. Porcelli, A. J., Lewis, A. H., and Delgado, M. R. (2012). Acute stress influences neural circuits of reward processing. *Front. Neurosci.* 6:157. doi: 10.3389/fnins.2012.00157
70. Pursey, K. M., Stanwell, P., Callister, R. J., Brain, K., Collins, C. E., and Burrows, T. L. (2014). Neural responses to visual food cues according to weight status: a systematic review of functional magnetic resonance imaging studies. *Front. Nutr.* 1:7. doi: 10.3389/fnut.2014.00007
71. Putman, P., Antypa, N., Crysovergi, P., and van der Does, W. A. (2010). Exogenous cortisol acutely influences motivated decision making in healthy young men. *Psychopharmacology (Berl.)* 208, 257–263. doi: 10.1007/s00213-009-1725-y
72. Ragnarsson, O., Berglund, P., Eder, D. N., and Johannsson, G. (2012). Long- term cognitive impairments and attentional deficits in patients with Cushing's disease and cortisol-producing adrenal adenoma in remission. *J. Clin. Endocrinol. Metab.* 97, E1640–E1648. doi: 10.1210/jc.2012-1945
73. Resmini, E., Santos, A., Gómez-Anson, B., Vives, Y., Pires, P., Crespo, I., et al. (2012). Verbal and visual memory performance and hippocampal volumes, measured by 3-Tesla magnetic resonance imaging, in patients with Cushing's syndrome. *J. Clin. Endocrinol. Metab.* 97, 663–671. doi: 10.1210/jc.2011-2231
74. Smith, S. M., and Vale, W. W. (2006). The role of the hypothalamic-pituitary-adrenal axis in neuroendocrine responses to stress. *Dialogues Clin. Neurosci.* 8, 383–395.
75. Soares-Cunha, C., Coimbra, B., Borges, S., Carvalho, M. M., Rodrigues, A. J., and Sousa, N. (2014). The motivational drive to natural rewards is modulated by prenatal glucocorticoid exposure. *Transl. Psychiatry* 4, e397. doi: 10.1038/tp.2014.45
76. Spielberger, C. D., Gorsuch, R. L., Lushene, R., Vagg, P. R., and Jacobs, G. A. (1983). *Manual for the State-Trait Anxiety Inventory.* Palo Alto, CA: Consulting Psychologists Press.
77. Starkman, M. N., Giordani, B., Berent, S., Schork, M. A., and Schteingart, D. E. (2001). Elevated cortisol levels in Cushing's disease are associated with cognitive decrements. *Psychosom. Med.* 63, 985–993. doi: 10.1097/00006842-200111000- 00018
78. Starkman, M. N., Giordani, B., Gebarski, S. S., and Schteingart, D. E. (2003). Improvement in learning associated with increase in hippocampal formation volume. *Biol. Psychiatry* 53, 233–238. doi: 10.1016/S0006-3223(02)01750-X
79. Talbot, L. S., Maguen, S., Epel, E. S., Metzler, T. J., and Neylan, T. C. (2013). Posttraumatic stress disorder is associated with emotional eating. *J. Trauma. Stress* 26, 521–525. doi: 10.1002/jts.21824
80. Tiemensma, J., Biermasz, N. R., Middelkoop, H. A., van der Mast, R. C., Romijn, J. A., and Pereira, A. M. (2010a). Increased prevalence of psychopathology and maladaptive personality traits after long-term cure of Cushing's disease. *J. Clin. Endocrinol. Metab.* 95, E129–E141. doi: 10.1210/jc.2010-0512
81. Tiemensma, J., Kokshoorn, N. E., Biermasz, N. R., Keijser, B. J., Wassenaar, M. J., Middelkoop, H. A., et al. (2010b). Subtle cognitive impairments in patients with long-term cure of Cushing's disease. *J. Clin. Endocrinol. Metab.* 95, 2699–2714. doi: 10.1210/jc.2009-2032
82. Tomiyama, A. J., Dallman, M. F., and Epel, E. S. (2011). Comfort food is comforting to those most stressed: evidence of the chronic stress response network in high stress women. *Psychoneuroendocrinology* 36, 1513–1519. doi: 10.1016/j.psyneuen.2011.04.005
83. Tryon, M. S., Carter, C. S., Decant, R., and Laugero, K. D. (2013). Chronic stress exposure may affect the brain's response to high calorie food cues and predispose to obesogenic eating habits. *Physiol. Behav.* 120, 233–242. doi: 10.1016/j.physbeh.2013.08.010
84. Uchoa, E. T., Aguilera, G., Herman, J. P., Fiedler, J. L., Deak, T., and de Sousa, M. B. (2014). Novel aspects of glucocorticoid actions. *J. Neuroendocrinol.* 26, 557–572. doi: 10.1111/jne.12157
85. Volkow, N. D., Wang, G. J., Fowler, J. S., Logan, J., Gatley, S. J., Hitzemann, R., et al. (1997). Decreased striatal dopaminergic responsiveness in detoxified cocaine-dependent subjects. *Nature* 386, 830–833. doi: 10.1038/ 386830a0
86. Volkow, N. D., Wang, G. J., Tomasi, D., Telang, F., Fowler, J. S., Pradhan, K., et al. (2010). Methylphenidate attenuates limbic brain inhibition after cocaine-cues exposure in cocaine abusers. *PLoS ONE* 5:e11509. doi: 10.1371/journal.pone.0011509
87. Webb, S. M., Badia, X., Barahona, M. J., Colao, A., Strasburger, C. J., Tabarin, A., et al. (2008). Evaluation of health-related quality of life in patients with Cushing's syndrome with a new questionnaire. *Eur. J. Endocrinol.* 158, 623–630. doi: 10.1530/EJE-07-0762

88. Whelan, T. B., Schteingart, D. E., Starkman, M. N., and Smith, A. (1980). Neuropsychological deficits in Cushing's syndrome. *J. Nerv. Ment. Dis.* 168, 753–757. doi: 10.1097/00005053-198012000-00008

89. Yau, Y. H., and Potenza, M. N. (2013). Stress and eating behaviors. *Minerva Endocrinol.* 38, 255–267.

90. Yehuda, R., Bierer, L. M., Andrew, R., Schmeidler, J., and Seckl, J. R. (2009a). Enduring effects of severe developmental adversity, including nutritional deprivation, on cortisol metabolism in aging Holocaust survivors. *J. Psychiatr. Res.* 43, 877–883. doi: 10.1016/j.jpsychires.2008.12.003

91. Yehuda, R., Bierer, L. M., Sarapas, C., Makotkine, I., Andrew, R., and Seckl, J. R. (2009b). Cortisol metabolic predictors of response to psychotherapy for symptoms of PTSD in survivors of the World Trade Center attacks on September 11, 2001. *Psychoneuroendocrinology* 34, 1304–1313. doi: 10.1016/j.psyneuen.2009.03.018

6

PRKACA: The Catalytic Subunit of Protein Kinase A and Adrenocortical Tumors

Annabel S. Berthon, Eva Szarek and Constantine A. Stratakis *

Section on Endocrinology and Genetics, Program on Developmental Endocrinology and Genetics and Pediatric Endocrinology Inter-Institute Training Program, Eunice Kennedy Shriver National Institute of Child Health and Human Development, National Institutes of Health, Bethesda, MD, USA

***Correspondence:** Constantine A. Stratakis, Section on Endocrinology and Genetics, Program on Developmental Endocrinology and Genetics and Pediatric Endocrinology Inter-Institute Training Program, Eunice Kennedy Shriver National Institute of Child Health and Human Development, National Institutes of Health, 10 Center Drive, Building 10, NIH-Clinical Research Center, Room 1-3330, MSC1103, Bethesda MA 20892, USA stratakc@mail.nih.gov*

Cyclic-AMP (cAMP)-dependent protein kinase (PKA) is the main effector of cAMP signaling in all tissues. Inactivating mutations of the *PRKAR1A* gene, coding for the type 1A regulatory subunit of PKA, are responsible for Carney complex and primary pigmented nodular adrenocortical disease (PPNAD). *PRKAR1A* inactivation and PKA dysregulation have been implicated in various types of adrenocortical pathologies associated with ACTH-independent Cushing syndrome (AICS) from PPNAD to adrenocortical adenomas and cancer, and other forms of bilateral adrenocortical hyperplasias (BAH). More recently, mutations of *PRKACA*, the gene coding for the catalytic subunit C alpha (Cα), were also identified in the pathogenesis of adrenocortical tumors. *PRKACA* copy number gain was found in the germline of several patients with cortisol-producing BAH, whereas the somatic Leu206Arg (c.617A>C) recurrent *PRKACA* mutation was found in as many as half of all adrenocortical adenomas associated with AICS. *In vitro* analysis demonstrated that this mutation led to constitutive Cα activity, unregulated by its main partners, the PKA regulatory subunits. In this review, we summarize the current understanding of the involvement of *PRKACA* in adrenocortical tumorigenesis, and our understanding of PKA's role in adrenocortical lesions. We also discuss potential therapeutic advances that can be made through targeting of *PRKACA* and the PKA pathway.

Keywords: adrenal cortex, adenoma, *PRKACA*, PKA, Cushing syndrome

Introduction

The adrenal cortex is divided into three concentric zones: the outermost zone named *zona glomerulosa*, the centrally located *zona fasciculata* and the innermost, *zona reticularis* involved in the production of mineralocorticoids, glucocorticoids, and androgens, respectively (Blake et al., 2008; Mcnicol, 2013). Thus, adrenal dysfunction leads to several hormonal syndromes due to the hypo- or hyper-secretion of one or more adrenal hormones.

In this review, we focus on Cushing's syndrome (CS) resulting from overproduction of cortisol from adrenocortical tumors (ACT). CS leads to central obesity and metabolic abnormalities and several other manifestations including moon face, buffalo hump, striae, and opportunistic infections (Newell-Price et al., 2006). Severe and prolonged hypercortisolism could lead to increased morbidity and mortality, due to sepsis, cardiovascular, and other complications (Plotz et al., 1952; Arnaldi et al., 2012). Hypersecretion of cortisol can be due to either an excess of pituitary or ectopic adrenocorticotropin hormone (ACTH) secretion or adrenocortical tumors

(ACT) secreting cortisol autonomously; the latter form of CS is known as "ACTH-independent CS" (AICS).

Cortisol-producing ACTs include bilateral adrenocortical hyperplasias (BAH), adrenocortical adenomas (ACA) and cancer (ACC). BAHs account for 10–15% of AICS and are classified in two subtypes: macronodular (nodules >1 cm) and micronodular (nodules <1 cm) (Lacroix, 2009; Duan et al., 2014). Macronodular hyperplasia, previously known as massive macronodular adrenocortical disease (MMAD) or ACTH-independent macronodular adrenocortical hyperplasia (AIMAH), has been recently renamed as primary macronodular hyperplasia (PMAH) after the discovery of intra-adrenal ACTH production (Lacroix, 2013; Louiset et al., 2013). PMAH is typically diagnosed in the fifth and sixth decade of life; subclinical CS is common in this disease (Duan et al., 2014), despite the fact that macroscopically, the adrenal glands are massively enlarged with a combined weight reach from 60 to 200 g.

Micronodular hyperplasias include a pigmented form named primary pigmented nodular adrenocortical disease (PPNAD), which is typically diagnosed at a younger age. PPNAD is the most common endocrine lesion of Carney complex (CNC), occurring in more than 60% of CNC patients (Almeida and Stratakis, 2010). Grossly, PPNAD is associated with normal to slightly enlarged adrenal glands (4.3–17 g) with a large number of yellow to brown-black micro-nodules (0.1–0.3 mm in size) due to lipofuscin accumulation (responsible for the pigmentation) (Stratakis and Boikos, 2007; Stratakis, 2008).

Unilateral ACTs, ACAs account for 90% of adrenal CS (Newell-Price et al., 2006; Bertagna et al., 2009). Clinically, these tumors arise at any age, with a slight female predominance. The presentation ranges from subclinical to overt CS. Macroscopically, the average ACA ranges in size from 1.5 cm to 6 cm and weighs between 10 and 40 g. In contrast to ACAs, ACCs are rare and account for few cases of adrenal CS (Wajchenberg et al., 2000). They arise sporadically, mostly around the fourth and fifth decade of life; ACCs typically weigh more than 100 g, tend to be adherent to other tissues, or invade adjacent structures.

cAMP Signaling, *PRKAR1A* Defects, and Adrenocortical Tumors

In normal physiology, cAMP signaling plays an essential role in the regulation of cortisol secretion under the control of the hypothalamic-pituitary-adrenal axis (**Figure 1**). Hypothalamic corticotropin-releasing hormone (CRH) secretion stimulates ACTH secretion from the pituitary gland, both acting through their respective G-protein coupled receptor (GPCR). ACTH binds to the melanocortin-2 receptor (MC2R) in *zona fasciculata* cells, leading to the activation of adenylate cyclase, which ensures the conversion of adenosine triphosphate (ATP) to cyclic adenosine monophosphate (cAMP). cAMP activates its main intracellular mediators, EPAC (Exchange Protein Activated by cAMP), and a serine/threonine kinase called cAMP-dependent protein kinase A (PKA) (Bossis and Stratakis, 2004). The protein kinase A (PKA) holoenzyme is a heterotetramer that consists of two regulatory subunits each binding to one catalytic subunit (Bossis and Stratakis, 2004). Four regulatory (RIα, RIβ, RIIα, and RIIβ) and four catalytic (Cα, Cβ, Cγ, and Prkx) subunits have been described (Almeida and Stratakis, 2011). In order to activate PKA cAMP interacts with the regulatory subunit of PKA leading to a conformational change permitting the release of the catalytic subunits. The free catalytic subunits phosphorylate downstream targets such as cAMP response element-binding protein (CREB), which induce the transcription of target genes, such as those involved in cortisol synthesis (**Figure 1**) (Christenson et al., 1999; Manna et al., 2009). The intracellular cAMP is hydrolysed by specific phosphodiesterases (PDEs), and the two regulatory and catalytic subunits of PKA are reassembled in order to return to their inactive state (Stratakis and Boikos, 2007).

Several lines of evidence support cAMP's role in the development of cortisol-producing ACTs (Stratakis, 2014a). In McCune-Albright syndrome (MAS), which is caused by mutations in the *GNAS* gene that encodes the stimulatory subunit α of the G protein (Weinstein et al., 1991), ACAs or, more frequently, BAH are common. In CNC, inactivating mutations of the *PRKAR1A* gene (encoding the RIα subunit of PKA) (Kirschner et al., 2000a,b) lead to PPNAD. Mutations of the *PRKAR1A* gene have also been identified in sporadic cases of PPNAD (not associated with CNC), as well as in ACAs (Groussin et al., 2002; Bertherat et al., 2003). In addition, a number of *in vitro* and transgenic mouse studies have demonstrated that *PRKAR1A* is an adrenocortical tumor suppressor gene and its inactivation leads to ACTH-independent cortisol secretion (Sahut-Barnola et al., 2010; Almeida and Stratakis, 2011).

PRKACA Genetic Defects Lead to Tumors of the Adrenal Cortex

In an initial cohort of 10 cortisol-producing ACAs associated with overt AICS, the Leu206Arg (c.617A>C) *PRKACA* recurrent mutation was identified in 70% of these cases; with one ACA having another *PRKACA* defect, Leu199_Cys200insTrp (Beuschlein et al., 2014). Both of these mutations affect residues that are highly conserved across species from invertebrates to humans suggesting the major role played by these amino acids is in protein function (Beuschlein et al., 2014; Goh et al., 2014). Dalmazi and collaborators have also identified two additional mutations: the insertion Cys200_Gly201insVal (c.600_601insGTG) and the missense Ser213Arg (c.639C>G) associated with 12 base pair duplication Leu212_Lys214insIleIleLeuArg (c.638_640insATTATCCTGAGG), in respectively 13.4% (3/22) and 4.5% (1/22) of their cortisol-producing ACA cohort (Di Dalmazi et al., 2014b). Recently, four independent projects of exome sequencing of cortisol-producing ACA development (Cao et al., 2014; Goh et al., 2014; Kubota et al., 2014; Sato et al., 2014) led to confirmation of *PRKACA*'s role in the pathogenesis of this neoplasm. The Leu206Arg variant has been identified at a frequency that ranges from 14.2 to 65.5% of cortisol-producing ACA depending on the studies (Beuschlein et al., 2014; Cao et al., 2014; Di Dalmazi et al., 2014a; Goh et al., 2014; Nakajima et al., 2014; Sato et al., 2014). No *PRKACA* mutations were found

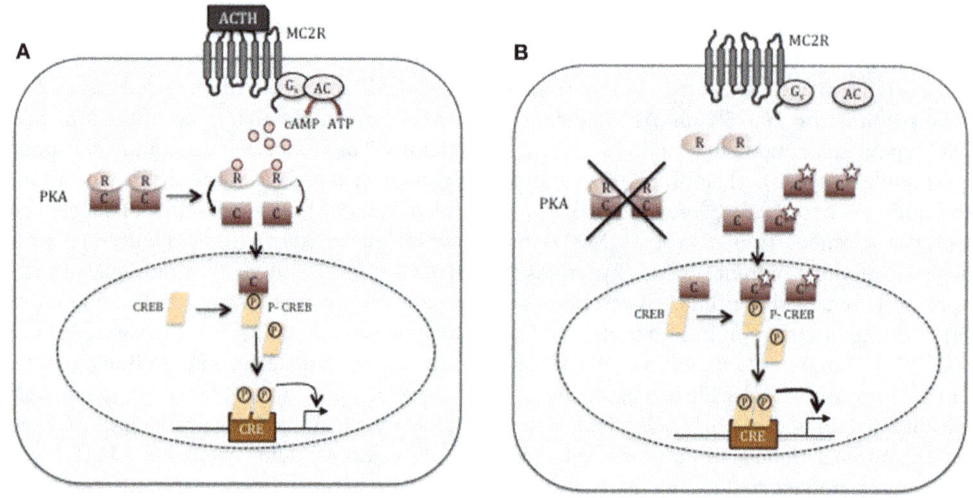

FIGURE 1 | cAMP signaling. (A) In normal adrenocortical cells, ACTH binds to its G-coupled receptor, MC2R. This leads to the activation of adenylate cyclase (AC), which convert ATP into cAMP. cAMP then binds the regulatory (R) subunit of PKA, inducing the release of the catalytic subunit (C). The catalytic subunit phosphorylates its downstream target such as CREB, which in turn induces the expression of genes involved in cortisol synthesis. **(B)** In adrenocortical adenoma cells producing cortisol autonomously with *PRKACA* mutations (star), the catalytic (C) subunit of PKA is unable to interact with the regulatory subunit (R). The unregulated *PRKACA* may now mediate its serine-threonine kinase activity without any restrains.

either in 1600 in-house exomes or in the 1000 Genomes Project data set or in blood of patients harboring *PRKACA* mutations in tumors. The Leu206Arg substitution likely alters the function of the Cα subunit at the heterozygote state, since both the wild type and mutant alleles were expressed in the tumor tissue (Beuschlein et al., 2014; Goh et al., 2014).

Functional Analysis of *PRKACA* Mutations

PRKACA encodes the most highly expressed catalytic PKA isoform in the human adrenal and the functional consequences of two mutant variants have been predicted using different modeling approaches based on mouse PKA crystal structure (Beuschlein et al., 2014; Cao et al., 2014; Goh et al., 2014; Sato et al., 2014). In the absence of cAMP, the regulatory subunit fits into a highly conserved hydrophobic cleft in the catalytic subunit formed by Leu206 and Leu199. Therefore, the substitution from the small hydrophobic leucine to a large positively charge hydrophilic arginine in position 206 should abolish the interaction between the catalytic and regulatory subunit leading then to cAMP-independent PKA activation (**Figure 1**) (Beuschlein et al., 2014; Cao et al., 2014; Goh et al., 2014; Sato et al., 2014). Similar consequences are predicted for each one of the pathogenic *PRKACA* variants that have been identified so far in ACAs (Di Dalmazi et al., 2014a).

The activating effect of the novel *PRKACA* mutations in ACA predicted by what is known about the structural biology of the PKA tetramer has been validated by *in vitro* experiments in HEK293 cells for the most frequent variant, Leu206Arg (Beuschlein et al., 2014; Cao et al., 2014; Goh et al., 2014; Sato et al., 2014). The expression of Leu206Arg *PRKACA* increases the PKA activity and the level of CREB phosphorylation at Ser133 in basal conditions compared to the wild type *PRKACA* in two independent studies; the Leu206Arg did not interfere with the catalytic activity (Beuschlein et al., 2014; Cao et al., 2014; Goh et al., 2014). In contrast with cells transfected with the wild-type sequence, the Leu206Arg is not responsive to cAMP stimulation and its activity is not reduced by the co-expression with excess wild-type regulatory subunit (Beuschlein et al., 2014). The absence of interaction between this variant and the regulatory subunit was confirmed by FRET and co-immunoprecipitation experiments (Beuschlein et al., 2014; Goh et al., 2014; Sato et al., 2014). Altogether, these results demonstrated that the Leu206Arg mutant protein is constitutively active. Consistent with these conclusions, basal PKA activity in ACA with *PRKACA* mutations compared to those without mutations is increased (Beuschlein et al., 2014; Cao et al., 2014). Similarly, Goh and collaborators demonstrated by immunohistochemistry a higher staining of the phosphorylation of CREB at Ser133 in 8 *PRKACA* mutant ACA vs. 5 ACA without identified mutations (Goh et al., 2014). However, Sato and collaborators did not find any differences in phosphorylation level of CREB by Western blot (Sato et al., 2014).

Clinical Phenotype Associated with *PRKACA* Mutations

In total, the *PRKACA* gene has now been sequenced in 854 ACTs and no mutations have been found in cortisol-producing ACCs, non-secreting ACAs, androgen-secreting ACAs, aldosterone-producing ACAs, and adrenal oncocytomas. Thus, the overall frequency of the *PRKACA* hotspot mutation is 38.2% and it has been identified in cortisol-producing adenomas only (**Table 1**). One study described a predominance of *PRKACA* mutations in females (Cao et al., 2014). Patients harboring tumors with *PRKACA* mutations were diagnosed with CS at younger ages (45.3 ± 13.5 vs. 52.5 ± 11.9 years) (Goh et al., 2014). In five studies including both overt and subclinical CS (Beuschlein et al., 2014; Di Dalmazi et al., 2014b; Goh et al., 2014; Nakajima et al.,

TABLE 1 | Frequency of copy number gain (CNG) including *PRKACA* gene and *PRKACA* mutations in adrenocortical tumors.

References	Cortisol-producing ACA	Cortisol-producing ACA with over CS	Cortisol-producing BAH	Cortisol-producing ACC	Non-secreting ACA	Aldosterone-producing ACA	Androgen-producing ACA	Adrenocortical oncocytoma
Beuschlein et al., 2014	22.2% mutations (22/99)	37% mutations (22/59[a])	1.75% CNG (5/35[b])	0% (0/42)	0% (0/20)	0% (0/20)	–	–
Cao et al., 2014	65.5% p.Leu206Arg (57/87)	NA	0% (0/13 PMAH)	0% (0/16)	–	–	–	0% (0/3)
Goh et al., 2014	23.6% p.Leu206Arg (57/87)	35% p.Leu206Arg (10/28)	–	0% (0/8)	–	–	–	–
Di Dalmazi et al., 2014b	32.3% mutations (22/68[c])	34.3% mutations (22/64[c])	0% (0/8)	0% (0/5)	–	–	–	–
Nakajima et al., 2014	14.2% p.Leu206Arg (3/21)	23% p.Leu206Arg (3/13)	–	–	0% (0/32)	–	0% (0/4)	–
Sato et al., 2014	52.3% p.Leu206Arg (34/65)	57.1% p.Leu206Arg (32/56)	–	–	–	–	–	–
Total	38.2% (151/395)	40%(89/220)	8.9% CNG (5/56)	0% (0/71)	0% (0/52)	0% (0/53)	0% (0/4)	0% (0/3)

[a]*21/59 harboring p.Leu206Arg and 1/59 with Leu199_Cys200insTrp.*
[b]*31 PPNAD + 2 iMAD+ 2 PMAH.*
[c]*18/22 harboring p.Leu206Arg; 3/22 Cys200_Gly201insVal; 1/22 Ser213Arg+Leu212_Lys214insIle-Ile-Leu-Arg*

2014; Sato et al., 2014), *PRKACA* mutations are significantly associated with overt CS and higher serum cortisol level after 1 mg of dexamethasone, increased urinary free cortisol and midnight cortisol levels compared to patients without mutations (Beuschlein et al., 2014). These results highlight a direct link between *PRKACA* mutations and cortisol production, which is expected knowing the physiological function of PKA. In accordance with this observation, no *PRKACA* mutations have been found in subclinical CS patients in three independent studies (Beuschlein et al., 2014; Di Dalmazi et al., 2014b; Nakajima et al., 2014). However, Gao et al. and Sato et al. have found 11% (3/27) and 22% (2/9) of *PRKACA* mutations, respectively, at position 206 in subclinical CS patients (**Table 1**) (Goh et al., 2014; Sato et al., 2014). The term subclinical CS is used to describe cortisol-secreting tumors in patients without any typical symptoms of CS. However, its usage can vary between investigators and countries; this may explain the differences observed between these studies. Interestingly, in transcriptomic data from 25 wild-type ACA and 11 mutant ACA, 232 genes are differentially expressed and pathway analysis demonstrates an enrichment in "biosynthesis and metabolism of steroid and cholesterol" and "response to chemical stimulus" (Cao et al., 2014). This is in accordance with the essential role of PKA in the control of cortisol secretion.

PRKACA and other Defects in ACAs

Altogether these results demonstrate that *PRKACA* mutations constitutively activate PKA leading to cortisol-producing adenomas, thereby suggesting that *PRKACA* is a main contributor to adrenocortical tumorigenesis. By whole-exome sequencing analysis, even if the number of exonic mutations is generally low, *PRKACA* is not the only oncogene mutated in cortisol-producing tumors. Activating mutations have also been identified in *CTNNB1* and *GNAS* genes at lower frequency (Cao et al., 2014; Goh et al., 2014; Sato et al., 2014). Importantly, *PRKACA* mutations were never found in association with other mutations. This suggests that the identified activating mutations may be mutually exclusive confirming the driver role played by Cα subunits in the development of cortisol-producing ACA. Interestingly, Goh and collaborators sequenced both ACA and ACC and were able to divide the ACA into two groups based on genetic results (Goh et al., 2014). Five out of 22 ACA are genetically closer to 3 ACC even if their Weiss score is 0 or 1, without any histological evidence of carcinoma. These findings are consistent with a progressive model of tumors forming in the adrenal cortex in the sequence hyperplasia-adenoma-carcinoma (Berthon et al., 2010; Stratakis, 2014b). However, the second ACA group, which included the ACA with *PRKACA* mutations, appears to have a distinct tumorigenesis mechanism. This is supported by the observation of three studies that tumors with mutations in *PRKACA* were significantly smaller than the non-mutant ones (Di Dalmazi et al., 2014b; Goh et al., 2014; Sato et al., 2014). Similarly, the weight of the sporadic ACT harboring *PRKAR1A* mutations is lower (11.2 ± 0.8 vs. 23.4 ± 12.05 g) (Bertherat et al., 2003). Therefore, PKA activation through constitutive activation of Cα subunit or RIα loss-of-function drastically increases cortisol secretion but has a limited impact on cell proliferation and tumor growth. Most recently, genomic duplication of the locus of *PRKACB* encoding for the Cβ catalytic subunit have also been described in a patient with CNC without CS (Forlino et al., 2014). It is possible that this reflects different roles of the two main catalytic subunits of PKA, with regards to their function in the adrenal cortex.

PRKACA Copy Number Gain and Bilateral Adrenocortical Hyperplasia

Comparative genomic hybridization of 35 BAH with overt CS demonstrated copy number gain at chr19p locus that included *PRKACA* gene in 5 patients (Beuschlein et al., 2014; Stratakis, 2014a; Carney et al., 2015). The defect was present in the germline and there were no *PRKACA* coding sequence mutations. Two patients, a mother and a son, included in this study the same duplication and both presented with BAH (Beuschlein et al., 2014; Carney et al., 2015); this is the only case of inheritance in the cohort. Other duplications at this locus have not been found in 24 cortisol-producing ACAs (Carney et al., 2015). Interestingly, the histological phenotype of these five patients has been published and 3 of them looked like PPNAD. This phenotype is comparable with PKA activation through *PRKAR1A* inactivation or PDEs mutations causing PPNAD (Almeida and Stratakis, 2010). However, the two remaining patients did not have PPNAD but diffuse adrenal cortex hyperplasia with nodules (Carney et al., 2015). This demonstrates that the same genetic alteration can lead to different histological phenotypes. It also demonstrates that differences in *PRKACA* gains and, thus, functional "dosage" have different effects on the histology of the adrenal cortex (Stratakis, 2014a). Whereas somatic mutations that lead to overactivity cause ACAs (Stratakis, 2014a), germline defects cause BAH depending on genetic dosage (Lodish et al., 2015).

Is Cα a new Therapeutic Target for Cushing Syndrome?

PRKACA mutations have been described in almost 40% of cortisol-producing ACA and are therefore, the most frequent genetic alteration in these tumors (**Table 1**). Beyond the importance of PKA in adrenal, its involvement in genetic diseases like CNC and cancers has been demonstrated (Caretta and Mucignat-Caretta, 2011). The ability to inhibit its constitutive activation through chemical components is a major challenge due to its critical role on cell function. Two inhibitors H89 and KT5720 have successfully decreased PKA activity induced by the transfection of Leu206Arg variant in HEK293 cells (Sato et al., 2014). These two inhibitors have been extensively used to better understand the role of PKA, however, their lack of specificity has been well established (Lochner and Moolman, 2006; Murray, 2008). Most of the inhibitors targeted the ATP-binding site but this was problematic due to the high percentage of identity of this domain among the Ser/Thr kinases family responsible to the low specificity of these inhibitors (Sapio et al., 2014). Moreover, these inhibitors cannot be used for activating *PRKACA* mutations. Better understanding of PKA function permits the development of substrate-competitive inhibitors, which would be more specific as there is diverse substrate-binding domain. The PKA inhibitor (PKI) is an endogenous thermostable peptide that interacts with the catalytic domain and is able to inhibit Leu206Arg variant *in vitro* (Cao et al., 2014). However, its main disadvantage preventing its use for clinical application is its weak permeability and its susceptibility to proteases. The discovery of new PKA inhibitors is desirable and can be helpful in the treatment of cortisol-producing ACA but also others cancers.

Conclusions

The discovery of somatic mutations in *PRKACA* is one additional proof of the central role of cAMP-PKA pathway in the development of cortisol-producing ACA. The high frequency of mutations (approximately 40%) and the even higher presence of PKA function alterations (Bimpaki et al., 2009), suggest that perhaps other components of the pathway may also be found mutated in the future. However, as *PRKACA* is ubiquitously expressed, its mutations may also be found in other tissues with PKA-dependent tumorigenesis. Future analysis and use of animal models will provide useful information to help answer this, and other, questions.

Acknowledgments

This work was supported by the intramural program of the Eunice Kennedy Shriver National Institute of Child Health & Human Development, National Institutes of Health (NIH).

References

1. Almeida, M. Q., and Stratakis, C. A. (2010). Carney complex and other conditions associated with micronodular adrenal hyperplasias. *Best Pract. Res. Clin. Endocrinol. Metab.* 24, 907–914. doi: 10.1016/j.beem.2010.10.006
2. Almeida, M. Q., and Stratakis, C. A. (2011). How does cAMP/protein kinase A signaling lead to tumors in the adrenal cortex and other tissues? *Mol. Cell. Endocrinol.* 336, 162–168. doi: 10.1016/j.mce.2010.11.018
3. Arnaldi, G., Mancini, T., Tirabassi, G., Trementino, L., and Boscaro, M. (2012). Advances in the epidemiology, pathogenesis, and management of Cushing's syndrome complications. *J. Endocrinol. Invest.* 35, 434–448. doi: 10.1007/BF03345431
4. Bertagna, X., Guignat, L., Groussin, L., and Bertherat, J. (2009). Cushing's disease. *Best pract. Res. Clin. Endocrinol. Metab.* 23, 607–623. doi: 10.1016/j.beem.2009.06.001
5. Bertherat, J., Groussin, L., Sandrini, F., Matyakhina, L., Bei, T., Stergiopoulos, S., et al. (2003). Molecular and functional analysis of PRKAR1A and its locus (17q22-24) in sporadic adrenocortical tumors: 17q losses, somatic mutations, and protein kinase A expression and activity. *Cancer Res.* 63, 5308–5319.
6. Berthon, A., Sahut-Barnola, I., Lambert-Langlais, S., De Joussineau, C., Damon- Soubeyrand, C., Louiset, E., et al. (2010). Constitutive beta-catenin activation induces adrenal hyperplasia and promotes adrenal cancer development. *Hum. Mol. Genet.* 19, 1561–1576. doi: 10.1093/hmg/ddq029
7. Beuschlein, F., Fassnacht, M., Assie, G., Calebiro, D., Stratakis, C. A.,

Osswald, A., et al. (2014). Constitutive activation of PKA catalytic subunit in adrenal Cushing's syndrome. *N. Engl. J. Med.* 370, 1019–1028. doi: 10.1056/NEJMoa1310359

8. Bimpaki, E. I., Nesterova, M., and Stratakis, C. A. (2009). Abnormalities of cAMP signaling are present in adrenocortical lesions associated with ACTH- independent Cushing syndrome despite the absence of mutations in known genes. *Eur. J. Endocrinol.* 161, 153–161. doi: 10.1530/EJE-09-0027
9. Blake, M. A., Holalkere, N. S., and Boland, G. W. (2008). Imaging techniques for adrenal lesion characterization. *Radiol. Clin. North Am.* 46, 65–78, vi. doi: 10.1016/j.rcl.2008.01.003
10. Bossis, I., and Stratakis, C. A. (2004). Minireview: PRKAR1A: normal and abnormal functions. *Endocrinology* 145, 5452–5458. doi: 10.1210/en.2004-0900 Cao, Y., He, M., Gao, Z., Peng, Y., Li, Y., Li, L., et al. (2014). Activating hotspot L205R mutation in PRKACA and adrenal Cushing's syndrome. *Science* 344, 913–917. doi: 10.1126/science.1249480
11. Caretta, A., and Mucignat-Caretta, C. (2011). Protein kinase a in cancer. *Cancers* 3, 913–926. doi: 10.3390/cancers3010913
12. Carney, J. A., Lyssikatos, C., Lodish, M. B., and Stratakis, C. A. (2015). Germline PRKACA amplification leads to Cushing syndrome caused by 3 adrenocortical pathologic phenotypes. *Hum. Pathol.* 46, 40–49. doi: 10.1016/j.humpath.2014.09.005
13. Christenson, L. K., Johnson, P. F., Mcallister, J. M., and Strauss, J. F. III. (1999). CCAAT/enhancer-binding proteins regulate expression of the human steroidogenic acute regulatory protein (StAR) gene. *J. Biol. Chem.* 274, 26591–26598. doi: 10.1074/jbc.274.37.26591
14. Di Dalmazi, G., Berr, C. M., Fassnacht, M., Beuschlein, F., and Reincke, M. (2014a). Adrenal function after adrenalectomy for subclinical hypercortisolism and Cushing's syndrome: a systematic review of the literature. *J. Clin. Endocrinol. Metab.* 99, 2637–2645. doi: 10.1210/jc.2014-1401
15. Di Dalmazi, G., Kisker, C., Calebiro, D., Mannelli, M., Canu, L., Arnaldi, G., et al. (2014b). Novel somatic mutations in the catalytic subunit of the protein kinase A as a cause of adrenal Cushing's syndrome: a European multicentric study. *J. Clin. Endocrinol. Metab.* 99, E2093–E2100. doi: 10.1210/jc.2014-2152
16. Duan, K., Gomez Hernandez, K., and Mete, O. (2014). Clinicopathological correlates of adrenal Cushing's syndrome. *J. Clin. Pathol.* 68, 175–186. doi: 10.1136/jclinpath-2014-202612
17. Forlino, A., Vetro, A., Garavelli, L., Ciccone, R., London, E., Stratakis, C. A., et al. (2014). PRKACB and Carney complex. *N. Engl. J. Med.* 370, 1065–1067. doi: 10.1056/NEJMc1309730
18. Goh, G., Scholl, U. I., Healy, J. M., Choi, M., Prasad, M. L., Nelson-Williams, C., et al. (2014). Recurrent activating mutation in PRKACA in cortisol-producing adrenal tumors. *Nat. Genet.* 46, 613–617. doi: 10.1038/ng.2956
19. Groussin, L., Jullian, E., Perlemoine, K., Louvel, A., Leheup, B., Luton, J. P., et al. (2002). Mutations of the PRKAR1A gene in Cushing's syndrome due to sporadic primary pigmented nodular adrenocortical disease. *J. Clin. Endocrinol. Metab.* 87, 4324–4329. doi: 10.1210/jc.2002-020592
20. Kirschner, L. S., Carney, J. A., Pack, S. D., Taymans, S. E., Giatzakis, C., Cho, Y. S., et al. (2000a). Mutations of the gene encoding the protein kinase A type I-alpha regulatory subunit in patients with the Carney complex. *Nat. Genet.* 26, 89–92. doi: 10.1038/79238
21. Kirschner, L. S., Sandrini, F., Monbo, J., Lin, J. P., Carney, J. A., and Stratakis, C.
22. A. (2000b). Genetic heterogeneity and spectrum of mutations of the PRKAR1A gene in patients with the carney complex. *Hum. Mol. Genet.* 9, 3037–3046. doi: 10.1093/hmg/9.20.3037
23. Kubota, Y., Mitsukawa, N., Uchida, M., Uchida, Y., Akita, S., Hasegawa, M., et al. (2014). Low-level mesodermal somatic mutation mosaicism: late-onset craniofacial and cervical spinal hyperostoses. *Am. J. Med. Genet. A* 164A, 741–747. doi: 10.1002/ajmg.a.36310
24. Lacroix, A. (2009). ACTH-independent macronodular adrenal hyperplasia. *Best Pract. Res. Clin. Endocrinol. Metab.* 23, 245–259. doi: 10.1016/j.beem.2008.10.011
25. Lacroix, A. (2013). Heredity and cortisol regulation in bilateral macronodular adrenal hyperplasia. *N. Engl. J. Med.* 369, 2147–2149. doi: 10.1056/NEJMe1312792
26. Lochner, A., and Moolman, J. A. (2006). The many faces of H89: a review.
27. *Cardiovasc. Drug Rev.* 24, 261–274. doi: 10.1111/j.1527-3466.2006.00261.x Lodish, M. B., Yuan, B., Levy, I., Braunstein, G. D., Lyssikatos, C., Salpea, P., et al.
28. (2015). Germline *PRKACA* amplification cases variable phenotypes that may
29. depend on the extent of the genomic defect: molecular mechanisms and clinical presentations. *Eur. J. Endocrinol.* 172, 803–811. doi: 10.1530/EJE-14-1154
30. Louiset, E., Duparc, C., Young, J., Renouf, S., Tetsi Nomigni, M., Boutelet, I., et al. (2013). Intraadrenal corticotropin in bilateral macronodular adrenal hyperplasia. *N. Engl. J. Med.* 369, 2115–2125. doi: 10.1056/NEJMoa1215245
31. Manna, P. R., Dyson, M. T., and Stocco, D. M. (2009). Regulation of the steroidogenic acute regulatory protein gene expression: present and future perspectives. *Mol. Hum. Reprod.* 15, 321–333. doi: 10.1093/molehr/gap025
32. Mcnicol, A. M. (2013). Diagnostic and molecular aspects of adrenal cortical tumors. *Semin. Diagn. Pathol.* 30, 197–206. doi: 10.1053/j.semdp.2013.07.001 Murray, A. J. (2008). Pharmacological PKA inhibition: all may not be what it seems. *Science signaling* 1:re4. doi: 10.1126/scisignal.122re4
33. Nakajima, Y., Okamura, T., Gohko, T., Satoh, T., Hashimoto, K., Shibusawa, N., et al. (2014). Somatic mutations of the catalytic subunit of cyclic AMP-dependent protein kinase (PRKACA) gene in Japanese patients with several adrenal adenomas secreting cortisol [Rapid Communication]. *Endocr. J.* 61, 825–832. doi: 10.1507/endocrj.EJ14-0282
34. Newell-Price, J., Bertagna, X., Grossman, A. B., and Nieman, L. K. (2006). Cushing's syndrome. *Lancet* 367, 1605–1617. doi: 10.1016/S0140-6736(06)68699-6
35. Plotz, C. M., Knowlton, A. I., and Ragan, C. (1952). The natural history of Cushing's syndrome. *Am. J. Med.* 13, 597–614. doi: 10.1016/0002-9343(52)90027-2
36. Sahut-Barnola, I., De Joussineau, C., Val, P., Lambert-Langlais, S., Damon, C., Lefrancois-Martinez, A. M., et al. (2010). Cushing's syndrome and fetal features resurgence in adrenal cortex-specific Prkar1a knockout mice. *PLoS Genet.* 6:e1000980. doi: 10.1371/journal.pgen.1000980
37. Sato, Y., Maekawa, S., Ishii, R., Sanada, M., Morikawa, T., Shiraishi, Y., et al. (2014). Recurrent somatic mutations underlie corticotropin-independent Cushing's syndrome. *Science* 344, 917–920. doi: 10.1126/science.1252328
38. Sapio, L., Di Michela, F., Illiano, M., Esposito, A., Chiosi, E., Spina, A., et al. (2014). Targeting protein kinase A in cancer therapy: update. *EXCLI J.* 13, 843–855.
39. Stratakis, C. A., and Boikos, S. A. (2007). Genetics of adrenal tumors associated with Cushing's syndrome: a new classification for bilateral adrenocortical hyperplasias. *Nat. Clin. Pract. Endocrinol.Metab.* 3, 748–757. doi: 10.1038/ncpendmet0648
40. Stratakis, C. A. (2008). Cushing syndrome caused by adrenocortical tumors and hyperplasias (corticotropin- independent Cushing syndrome). *Endocr. Dev.* 13, 117–132. doi: 10.1159/000134829
41. Stratakis, C. A. (2014a). E pluribus unum? The main protein kinase A catalytic subunit (PRKACA), a likely oncogene, and cortisol-producing tumors. *J. Clin. Endocrinol. Metab.* 99, 3629–3633. doi: 10.1210/jc.2014-3295
42. Stratakis, C. A. (2014b). Adrenal cancer in 2013: time to individualize treatment for adrenocortical cancer? *Nat. Rev. Endocrinol.* 10, 76–78. doi: 10.1038/nrendo.2013.263
43. Wajchenberg, B. L., Albergaria Pereira, M. A., Medonca, B. B., Latronico, A. C., Campos Carneiro, P., Alves, V. A., et al. (2000). Adrenocortical carcinoma: clinical and laboratory observations. *Cancer* 88, 711–736.
44. Weinstein, L. S., Shenker, A., Gejman, P. V., Merino, M. J., Friedman, E., and Spiegel, A. M. (1991). Activating mutations of the stimulatory G protein in the McCune-Albright syndrome. *N. Engl. J. Med.* 325, 1688–1695. doi: 10.1056/NEJM199112123252403

7

The Role of ACTH and Corticosteroids for Sepsis and Septic Shock

Djillali Annane*[1,2]

[1] General Intensive Care Unit, Raymond Poincaré Hospital (AP-HP), Garches, France, [2] Laboratory of Infection and Inflammation, U1173, University of Versailles Saint-Quentin-en-Yvelines University, INSERM, Garches, France

Correspondence:
Djillali Annane
djillali.annane@aphp.fr

Sepsis is a common disorder associated with high morbidity and mortality. It is now defined as an abnormal host response to infection, resulting in life-threatening dysfunction of organs. There is evidence from *in vitro* and *in vivo* experiments in various animal models and in patients that endotoxin or sepsis may directly and indirectly alter the hypothalamic–pituitary–adrenal response to severe infection. These alterations may include necrosis or hemorrhage or inflammatory mediator-mediated decreased ACTH synthesis, steroidogenesis, cortisol delivery to tissues, clearance from plasma, and decreased sensitivity of tissues to cortisol. Disruption of the hypothalamic–pituitary–adrenal axis may translate in patients with sepsis into cardiovascular and other organ dysfunction, and eventually an increase in the risk of death. Exogenous administration of corticosteroids at moderate dose, i.e., <400 mg of hydrocortisone or equivalent for >96 h, may help reversing sepsis-associated shock and organ dysfunction. Corticosteroids may also shorten the duration of stay in the ICU. Except for increased blood glucose and sodium levels, treatment with corticosteroids was rather well tolerated in the context of clinical trials. The benefit of treatment on survival remains controversial. Based on available randomized controlled trials, the likelihood of survival benefit is greater in septic shock versus sepsis patients, in sepsis with acute respiratory distress syndrome or with community-acquired pneumonia versus patients without these conditions, and in patients with a blunted cortisol response to 250 μg of ACTH test versus those with normal response.

Keywords: sepsis, nitric oxide, cytokines, hypothalamic–pituitary–adrenal axis, stress response

Sepsis places a burden on health-care systems worldwide due to an annual incidence of about 100 per 100,000 inhabitants (1) and mortality rates between 15 and 40% (when shock is present) in the short term and up to 80% at 5 years (2). Moreover, roughly half of survivors may present with progressive decline in cognitive function (2, 3).

Sepsis is defined as an abnormal host response to infection, resulting in life-threatening dysfunction of organs (4). Host response to stress was originally described by Selye (5). The so-called general adaptation syndrome typically includes an early alarm phase, followed by a phase of resistance, and then a phase of exhaustion, which may result in death. Host response to stress relies on three major systems: the hypothalamic–pituitary–adrenal (HPA) axis, the autonomic nervous system, and the immune system (6). A correct balance between activation of these systems allows controlling infection while maintaining cardiovascular and metabolic homeostasis. A typical neuroendocrine response to stress includes (i) immediate increased secretion of catecholamines from the sympathetic nervous system and adrenal medulla, release of corticotrophin-releasing hormone (CRH) and vasopressin from parvocellular neurons into the portal circulation, and secretion of oxytocin from the neural lobe of the pituitary, (ii) 5–10 s later, secretion of corticotrophin (ACTH) by anterior pituitary cells, (iii) followed a few seconds later by decreased secretion of pituitary gonadotropins and increased secretion of prolactin and growth hormone (in primates), and of renin and glucagon from the kidneys and pancreas, respectively, and (iv) a few minutes later, increased plasma levels of glucocorticoids and inhibition of gonadal steroids secretion. Any imbalance between neuroendocrine and immune responses favoring a proinflammatory state may trigger organ dysfunction and progression of infection to sepsis.

This review will summarize current knowledge on HPA axis and disruption during sepsis and the potential role of treatment with corticosteroids.

ACTIVATION OF THE HYPOTHALAMIC–PITUITARY–ADRENAL AXIS DURING SEPSIS

During stress, the HPA axis is mainly activated by CRH-independent pathways, involving immune mediators. The hypothalamus and pituitary glands are protected from exogenous or endogenous toxic molecules by the blood–brain barrier (BBB). Invading pathogens are identified by various cells, including epithelial, endothelial, and immune cells, thanks to danger molecule associated patterns (DAMP) they express on their surface or cytosol (7). Subsequently, these cells produce factors promoting recruitment of additional cells and destruction and clearance of pathogens. Among them, proinflammatory cytokines, such as tumor necrosis factor (TNF), interleukin (IL)-1 and -6, and anti-inflammatory cytokines, such as IL-4 and -10, may contribute activating the HPA axis.

Activation of the Hypothalamic–Pituitary Axis

At the Hypothalamic–Pituitary Axis Level

There are three main routes for immune mediators to reach the hypothalamus and/or the pituitary gland. First, terminal nerve endings of autonomic nervous afferent fibers express pathogens or DAMP and receptors for many mediators (8). Then, sensing pathogens or related DAMP in tissues results in hypothalamic signaling *via* autonomic nuclei in the brainstem, which have projections to the hypothalamus, for example, between the locus ceruleus and the arcuate nucleus, and other structures of the limbic system as well. Then, efferent fibers, particularly of the vagus nerve, contribute to the attenuation of inflammation and in resuming homeostasis (9). Corticotrophin-releasing hormone is released upon acetylcholine stimulation of muscarinic receptor, an effect that is prevented by non-specific nitric oxide (NO) blockade (10). Second, inflammatory mediators released in blood from tissues can reach the portal circulation in the median eminence, located outside the BBB, *via* the anterior hypophyseal arteries. They are carried onto the brain structures, expressing receptors for these mediators, either through areas lacking a BBB, i.e., the circumventricular organs or across it using specific transporters (11, 12). Third, systemic inflammation may cause breakdown to the BBB, facilitating blood-borne cytokines traffic to deep brain structures (13–16). Among the various factors that contribute to the disruption of tight junctions or swelling of the BBB, the complement system, particularly C5a anaphylatoxin expressed both by astrocytes and endothelial cells, may play a key role (17).

Dendritic and microglial cells may produce immune molecules. In animals, peripheral administration of endotoxin yielded expression of IL-1 (18) and TNF (19). Similarly, in patients with septic shock, postmortem examination suggested overexpression of IL-1 and TNF in hypothalamic nuclei (20). Different cytokines in different brain regions induce different brain responses. For example, IL-1 and TNF are likely the two main mediators of the so-called sickness behavior, whereas IL-6 may have no apparent direct effect on behavior (21). Experiments in animals suggest that TNF- and IL-1-induced release of corticosterone is CRH-dependent mechanism (22, 23), whereas IL-6 may stimulate adrenal function by both CRH-dependent and -independent mechanisms (24). IL-1-related activation of the HPA axis is mainly dependent on brain endothelial cells and is independent of hematopoietic cells and perivascular macrophages (25).

At the Adrenal Gland Level

Tumor necrosis factor is produced in adrenal tissues by resident macrophages and by adrenocortical cells, particularly in the fasciculate and reticular layers (26). The presence within the adrenals of TNF and of its receptors suggests that this cytokine plays a role in adrenal function, even though experiments found variably stimulatory (27, 28) or inhibitory (26, 29) effects of TNF on steroidogenesis. Similarly, IL-1 and its receptor are also produced in adrenal tissues and may contribute to steroidogenesis at least partly by regulating prostaglandins pathways (30). Toll-like receptors (TLR) types 2 and 4 are expressed in human's adrenal cortex (31). TLR2 or TLR4 knockout mice showed impaired glucocorticoid response to LPS (32, 33). Recent data suggested that these DAMP molecules expressed by immune cells recruited in adrenal tissues play a major role in the local immune-adrenal crosstalk (34).

Mechanisms of Disrupted Hypothalamic–Pituitary–Adrenal Axis in Sepsis

Irreversible Damage to Neuroendocrine Cells

Sepsis is infrequently associated with necrosis or hemorrhage within the HPA axis. The venous drainage of the adrenals being limited, sepsis-associated massive increase in arterial blood flow to these glands results in enlarged glands (**Table 1**) (35). Then, adrenal necrosis and hemorrhage have been reported as a consequence of sepsis for more than a century (36, 37). Predisposing factors of the Waterhouse–Friderichsen syndrome include renal failure, disseminated intravascular coagulopathy, and treatment with anticoagulants or tyrosine kinase inhibitors. Ischemic lesions and hemorrhage have also been described within the hypothalamus or pituitary gland (38).

TABLE 1 | Mechanism explaining hypothalamic–pituitary–adrenal axis disruption in sepsis.

HPA axis level	Main mechanisms	Precipitating factors
Hypothalamus	Necrosis or hemorrhage	Anticoagulants, brisk variations in blood pressure, high dose of vasopressors Coagulopathy, severe hypoxia, hyperglycemia
	Decreased CRH/AVP synthesis/release	Treatment with corticosteroids, psychoactive drugs Increased brain levels of proinflammatory cytokines (mainly TNF and IL-1) Hypercortisolemia
Pituitary gland	Necrosis or hemorrhage	Anticoagulants, brisk variations in blood pressure, high dose of vasopressors Coagulopathy, severe hypoxia, hyperglycemia
	Decreased ACTH synthesis/release	Treatment with corticosteroids, psychoactive drugs, anti-infective drugs, megestrol acetate medroxyprogesterone Increased blood levels of proinflammatory cytokines (mainly TNF and IL-1) Coagulopathy, severe hypoxia, hypercortisolemia
Adrenals	Necrosis or hemorrhage	Anticoagulants, brisk variations in blood pressure, high dose of vasopressors Coagulopathy, severe hypoxia
	Decreased steroidogenesis	
	Depletion of lipid droplets	Cholesterol-lowering drugs
	Decreased expression of scavenger receptor B1	Proinflammatory mediators
	Enzymes inhibition	Aminoglutethimide, ketoconazole, fluconazole, etomidate, dexmedetomidine Proinflammatory mediators
	Decreased sensitivity of ACTH receptors	Circulating and adrenals proinflammatory mediators (e.g., corticostatins)
Tissue resistances	Decreased cortisol delivery to tissues	Proinflammatory mediators, liver failure, severe denutrition
	Accelerated glucose clearance	Phenobarbital, phenytoin, rifampin
	Decreased binding capacity and affinity of glucocorticoid receptor	Proinflammatory mediators

HPA, hypothalamic–pituitary–adrenal.

Altered CRH/ACTH Synthesis

Hypothalamic/pituitary stimulation by cytokines, particularly IL-1, induced a biphasic response with initial proportional increase followed by progressive decline in anterior pituitary ACTH concentrations (39, 40). Sepsis is associated in animals (41, 42) and in humans (20) with marked overexpression of the inducible isoform of NO synthase (iNOS) in hypothalamic nuclei that is partly triggered by TNF and IL-1. Subsequent abundant release of NO may cause apoptosis of neurons and glial cells in the neighborhood. In both rodents and humans, sepsis decreased ACTH synthesis, though its secretagogues remained unaltered (43). Then, the suppression in ACTH synthesis following sepsis may be mediated by NO (11).

ACTH synthesis can also be inhibited by various treatments (44). Opioids are the main component of patients' sedation regimen in ICU worldwide. In animals, depending on dose, timing, and duration, opioids have been shown to variably stimulate or inhibit the CRH/ACTH axis, whereas in humans, they predominantly inhibited it (45). In animals, sepsis is associated with early marked increase in ACTH levels that returned to baseline values around 72 h (46). Clinical studies have found ACTH levels to be significantly lower in critically ill patients (47, 48) and particularly in septic shock (48) than in controls. However, altered ACTH synthesis in response to metyrapone was observed in roughly half of septic shock, and very occasionally in patients without sepsis (48).

Altered Steroidogenesis

The adrenals storage of cortisol is very limited. Therefore, adequate response to stress relies almost entirely on cortisol synthesis. The normal HPA axis response to sepsis remains unknown. Cortisol production rate is increased in critically ill patients (47). The main finding in this study was an average 50% reduction in cortisol clearance from plasma, mainly resulting from a loss in cortisol inactivation through suppressed liver and renal cortisol to cortisone shuttle. About half of septic-shock patients have decreased cortisol synthesis (48). Following administration of metyrapone, 60% of septic shock had 11β deoxycortisol concentrations <7 μg/dl, suggesting decreased cortisol synthesis. The alteration may occur at various steps in the cortisol synthesis chain. First, histological examination of the adrenal cortex of both animals and humans with sepsis found marked depletion in lipid droplets, suggesting deficiency in esterified cholesterol storage (49). This loss in lipid droplets is likely mediated by annexin A1 and formyl peptide receptors (50). In normal conditions, both increased plasma ACTH concentrations and depletion in adrenal cholesterol stores upregulate adrenals scavenger receptor B1 (SRB1), an HDL receptor, which captures esterified cholesterol from blood (51). SRB1-mediated cholesterol uptake is considered an essential protective mechanism against endotoxin (52). Then, sepsis-induced deficiency, in SRB1 expression by the adrenal cortex, was associated with increased mortality (53). Second, a number of environmental factors may inhibit adrenal steroidogenesis (54). Steroidogenesis may be inhibited at various enzymatic steps by drugs, including P-450 aromatase, hydroxysteroid dehydrogenase, or mitochondrial cytochrome P-450-dependent enzymes (44). In critically ill patients, etomidate, which inhibits the last enzymatic step in cortisol synthesis, increased the risk of adrenal insufficiency, 4–6 h (OR 19.98; 95% CI 3.95–101.11) and 12 h (OR 2.37; 95% CI 1.61–3.47) post-dosing (55). This effect was associated with organ dysfunction, but the ultimate effects on mortality remained unclear. Finally, inflammatory mediators, such as corticostatins, may bind to ACTH receptors in the adrenal cortex, thus preventing ACTH stimulation of cortisol synthesis (56).

Tissues Resistance to Glucocorticoids

A number of factors may prevent cortisol bioactivity in tissues. First, cortisol clearance may be accelerated, particularly following administration of various drugs, for example, psychoactive drugs (barbiturates, phenytoin) or antibiotics (rifampicin) (52). Second, sepsis is often associated with marked reduction in corticosteroid-binding globulin (CBG) and albumin (48, 57). On the one hand, the reduction in cortisol carriers increased free cortisol concentrations in plasma. On the other hand, cortisol bound to CBG is specifically released at the level of inflamed tissues, *via* neutrophils elastase-dependent mechanisms (58, 59). Thus, the net effect of sepsis-associated reduced CBG and albumin levels is reduced cortisol delivery to local sites of inflammation. Third, at tissue levels, T-helper 2 cell-derived cytokines, for example, IL-2 or IL-4, may inactivate cortisol to cortisone by upregulating the 11β-hydroxysteroid dehydrogenase (11β-HSD) type 2 enzyme (60). Finally, downregulation of the glucocorticoid receptor (GR)-α is a well-known complication of sepsis (61). The decrease in GR binding and affinity may be at least partly related to exaggerated release of NO in tissues (62). Sepsis may also cause alteration in the translocation of the GR-α (63). The loss in the dimerization of the GR-α caused resistance to glucocorticoids and lethality in septic animals (64).

CORTICOSTEROIDS FOR SEPSIS AND SEPTIC SHOCK

Corticosteroids have been used for more than 60 years in the management of patients with severe infections. There is a strong rationale (as described earlier) for exogenous administration of glucocorticoids in sepsis. Nevertheless, their use in practice still remains controversial. There is a general agreement that corticosteroids improve sepsis-associated comorbidities, such as shock, organ dysfunction, and length of hospital stay. Their effects on survival and on the risk of secondary infections are controversial.

Corticosteroids Improve Cardiovascular Function

Corticosteroids contribute to restoring effective blood volume, notably *via* sodium and water retention by binding to mineralocorticoid receptors in the kidney. They also contribute to restoring systemic vascular resistance. First, increase in sodium and water content in a vessel's interstitium results in increased stiffness of the vessel wall. Second, corticosteroids enhance vascular contractile (65) and blood pressure (66) responses to α-1 agonists. This effect occurs within minutes following corticosteroid administration and is likely a non-genomic effect *via* modulation of the α-1 agonists' receptors second messenger (65) and ATP-sensitive potassium channels (67). The endothelial GR is crucial for preventing prolonged activation of NO and NF-κB, following sepsis (68). Thus, prolonged improvement in vascular responsiveness to corticosteroids is likely a genomic transrepressive effect. Patients with septic shock and blunted response to 250 μg ACTH bolus, i.e., increase in total cortisol of <9 μg/dl, have more depressed systemic vascular resistance and a greater effect of hydrocortisone bolus on blood pressure response to norepinephrine than patients with intact HPA axis (65). Corticosteroids also improved microcirculation and tissue perfusion in septic shock (69). This effect may be mediated by upregulation of endothelial NO synthase *via* activation of the mitogen-activated protein kinase and protein Akt pathway (70).

A recent systematic review found 12 trials (n = 1561 patient) and reported the effects of corticosteroids on shock reversal (weaned off vasopressor therapy) by 1 week (71). In this review, the relative risk (RR) of having shock reversed by day 7 was 1.31 (95% CI 1.14–1.51; P value = 0.0001, random effects model), in favor of corticosteroids.

Corticosteroids Decrease Organ Failure

There is strong evidence that corticosteroids attenuate inflammation in various organs in sepsis. For example, they have been shown to dramatically decrease NF-κB activity in peripheral immune cells (72) or in the lung (73). Corticosteroids have been shown to inhibit iNOS activation in the renal cortex, preventing hypoxic injuries and restoring an adequate oxygen delivery to oxygen balance (74). They also improve glomerular function (75), free water clearance, and sodium renal excretion (76). Corticosteroids may attenuate sepsis-associated brain inflammation particularly by preventing the breakdown of the BBB (77, 78). A total of eight trials (n = 1132 patients) (71) reported a dramatic reduction in the number and degree of severity of failing organs, with a mean reduction in the SOFA score – a measure of organ dysfunction (79) – of −1.53 (−2.04 to −1.03; P value < 0.00001), in favor of corticosteroids. Corticosteroids also reduced ICU length of stay by −1.68 days (−3.27 to −0.09; P value = 0.04) and −2.19 days (95% CI −3.93 to −0.46; P value = 0.01), in ICU survivors (71).

Corticosteroid Tolerance

Secondary Infections

Corticosteroids shift the recruitment of T cells from T-helper type 1 to T-helper type 2 and thus to favor the production of anti-inflammatory cytokines. Data from 19 trials (n = 2567 patients) found that the RR for superinfection was 1.02 (0.87–1.20; P value = 0.81) (71). Corticosteroids may blunt febrile response to infection and alter leukocyte count and most inflammatory biomarkers. Thus, it may become difficult to recognize secondary infections in corticosteroid-treated patients. In practice, physicians should systematically screen on a daily basis any potential source of infection and draw samples for bacterial culture.

Metabolic Complications

Corticosteroids induce hyperglycemia by stimulating neoglucogenesis, glycogenolysis, and by insulin resistance in skeletal muscles and adipocytes. In septic shock, corticosteroids are associated with hyperglycemia (P value < 0.00001) and hypernatremia (P value < 0.00001) (71). As compared with bolus administration, continuous infusion of corticosteroids may ease the control of glycemia in sepsis (79). However, preventing hyperglycemia by intensive insulin therapy did not improve morbidity or mortality (80).

Acquired Neuromyopathy

Myopathy is a common complication of prolonged or acute exposure to corticosteroids, particularly high doses of fluorinated derivatives (e.g., dexamethasone). They induce myonecrosis, diffuse atrophy of fibers, cumulated sarcoplasmic glycogen vesicles, myofibril disorganization, and selective depletion of thick myosin filaments (81, 82). Upregulation of the calpain pathway suggests that altered calcium metabolism and/or increased proteolysis may contribute to corticosteroid muscle toxicity (82). The risk of myopathy associated with corticosteroids may be potentiated by hyperglycemia, hypoxia, or non-depolarizing neuromuscular drugs.

Other Complications

In theory, corticosteroids may be associated with psychotic disorders or gastroduodenal bleeding. In practice, data from 19 trials ($n = 2382$) found that the RR of gastroduodenal bleeding was of 1.24 (95% CI 0.92–1.67; P value = 0.15) (71). ICU studies variably found that exposure to systemic corticosteroids increased (83) or not (84) the risk of transition to delirium. Corticosteroid weaning may be associated with psychiatric manifestations, including depressive state and apathy.

Corticosteroids' Effects on Survival

Most experiments, in both small and large animals, based on endotoxin challenges or live bacteria-induced sepsis, found survival benefit from various doses and durations of corticosteroids (85). At least 33 trials have evaluated corticosteroids for severe infection with or without septic shock (71). Data from 27 trials ($n = 3176$ patients) found a RR of dying at 28 days of 0.87 (0.76–1.00, P value = 0.05). The survival benefit was more remarkable (P value = 0.01) in 22 trials of prolonged (>96 h) treatment with a moderate (<400 mg daily of hydrocortisone or equivalent) dose of corticosteroids. In this Cochrane review, meta-regression found a significant dose effect of corticosteroids, i.e., the lower the dose, the lower the RR of dying. This review also suggested that septic shock, ARDS, or community-acquired pneumonia were more likely to draw a survival benefit. Finally, data from eight trials ($n = 583$ patients), reporting subgroups based on the response to 250 µg ACTH test, found a RR of dying of 0.88 (0.88–1.02, P value = 0.09), in favor of corticosteroids. Depending on trial selection and definition of outcomes, different meta-analyses variably found (86), or did not find (87, 88), survival benefit from corticosteroids. Current international guidelines recommend restricting the use of hydrocortisone to vasopressor-dependent septic shock (89).

CONCLUSION

There are numerous experimental and clinical data establishing the paramount importance of an appropriate activation of the HPA axis to respond to severe infection. Similarly, experiments in animals and clinical observations strongly support the role of an inadequate HPA axis response in the physiopathology and outcome of sepsis. In most animal studies, corticosteroid administration consistently protected against lethal sepsis. In contrast, clinical trials in sepsis found much less consistency in survival benefits from corticosteroids, though most trials demonstrated faster resolution in shock and organ dysfunction. Thus, physicians should consider corticosteroids mainly in septic shock who do not respond rapidly to fluid therapy and vasopressors. Trials also consistently found that corticosteroids should be given at doses of 200 mg of hydrocortisone equivalent per day for at least 3 days at full dose.

AUTHOR CONTRIBUTIONS

DA is the sole author and is responsible for the whole content.

REFERENCES

1. Moss M. Epidemiology of sepsis: race, sex, and chronic alcohol abuse. *Clin Infect Dis* (2005) 41(Suppl 7):S490–7. doi:10.1086/432003
2. Iwashyna TJ, Ely EW, Smith DM, Langa KM. Long-term cognitive impairment and functional disability among survivors of severe sepsis. *JAMA* (2010) 304:1787–94. doi:10.1001/jama.2010.1553
3. Annane D, Sharshar T. Cognitive decline after sepsis. *Lancet Respir Med* (2015) 3:61–9. doi:10.1016/S2213-2600(14)70246-2
4. Singer M, Deutschman CS, Seymour CW, Shankar-Hari M, Annane D, Bauer M, et al. The third international consensus definition for sepsis and septic shock (sepsis 3). *JAMA* (2016) 315:1–10. doi:10.1001/jama.2016.0287
5. Selye H. A syndrome produced by diverse nocuous agents. *Nature* (1936) 138:32. doi:10.1038/138032a0
6. Chrousos GP. The hypothalamic-pituitary-adrenal axis and immune-mediated inflammation. *N Engl J Med* (1995) 322(20):1351–62.
7. Annane D, Bellissant E, Cavaillon JM. Septic shock. *Lancet* (2005) 365:63–78. doi:10.1016/S0140-6736(04)17667-8
8. Kenney MJ, Ganta CK. Autonomic nervous system and immune system interactions. *Compr Physiol* (2014) 4:1177–200. doi:10.1002/cphy.c130051
9. Borovikova LV, Ivanova S, Zhang M, Yang H, Botchkina GI, Watkins LR, et al. Vagus nerve stimulation attenuates the systemic inflammatory response to endotoxin. *Nature* (2000) 405:458–62. doi:10.1038/35013070
10. Karanth S, Lyson K, McCann SM. Effects of cholinergic agonists and antagonists on interleukin-2-induced corticotropin-releasing hormone release from the mediobasal hypothalamus. *Neuroimmunomodulation* (1999) 6:168–74. doi:10.1159/000026378
11. McCann SM, Kimura M, Karanth S, Yu WH, Mastronardi CA, Rettori V. The mechanism of action of cytokines to control the release of hypothalamic and pituitary hormones in infection. *Ann NY Acad Sci* (2000) 917:4–18. doi:10.1111/j.1749-6632.2000.tb05368.x
12. Koenig JI. Presence of cytokines in the hypothalamic-pituitary axis. *Prog Neuroendocrinoimmunol* (1991) 4:143–53.
13. Deng X, Wang X, Andersson R. Endothelial barrier resistance in multiple organs after septic and nonseptic challenges in the rat. *J Appl Physiol* (1985) 78:2052–61.
14. Papadopoulos MC, Lamb FJ, Moss RF, Davies DC, Tighe D, Bennett ED. Faecal peritonitis causes oedema and neuronal injury in pig cerebral cortex. *Clin Sci (Lond)* (1999) 96:461–6. doi:10.1042/cs0960461
15. Sharshar T, Carlier R, Bernard F, Guidoux C, Brouland JP, Nardi O, et al. Brain lesions in septic shock: a magnetic resonance imaging study. *Intensive Care Med* (2007) 33:798–806. doi:10.1007/s00134-007-0598-y
16. Stubbs DJ, Yamamoto AK, Menon DK. Imaging in sepsis-associated encephalopathy – insights and opportunities. *Nat Rev Neurol* (2013) 9:551–61. doi:10.1038/nrneurol.2013.177
17. Gasque P, Singhrao SK, Neal JW, Gotze O, Morgan BP. Expression of the receptor for complement C5a (CD88) is up-regulated on reactive astrocytes, microglia, and endothelial cells in the inflamed human central nervous system. *Am J Pathol* (1997) 150:31–41.
18. van Dam AM, Brouns M, Louisse S, Berkenbosch F. Appearance of interleukin-1 in macrophages and in ramified microglia in the brain of endotoxin-treated

rats: a pathway for the induction of non-specific symptoms of sickness? *Brain Res* (1992) 588:291–6. doi:10.1016/0006-8993(92)91588-6
19. Gatti S, Bartfai T. Induction of tumor necrosis factor-alpha mRNA in the brain after peripheral endotoxin treatment: comparison with interleukin-1 family and interleukin-6. *Brain Res* (1993) 624:291–4. doi:10.1016/0006-8993(93)90090-A
20. Sharshar T, Gray F, Lorin de la Grandmaison G, Hopkinson NS, Ross E, Dorandeu A, et al. Apoptosis of neurons in cardiovascular autonomic centres triggered by inducible nitric oxide synthase after death from septic shock. *Lancet* (2003) 362:1799–805. doi:10.1016/S0140-6736(03)14899-4
21. Dantzer R, O'Connor JC, Freund GG, Johnson RW, Kelley KW. From inflammation to sickness and depression: when the immune system subjugates the brain. *Nat Rev Neurosci* (2008) 9:46–56. doi:10.1038/nrn2297
22. Bernardini R, Kamilaris TC, Calogero AE, Johnson EO, Gomez MT, Gold PW, et al. Interactions between tumor necrosis factor-alpha, hypothalamic corticotropin-releasing hormone, and adrenocorticotropin secretion in the rat. *Endocrinology* (1990) 126:2876–81. doi:10.1210/endo-126-6-2876
23. Sapolsky R, Rivier C, Yamamoto G, Plotsky P, Vale W. Interleukin-1 stimulates the secretion of hypothalamic corticotropin-releasing factor. *Science* (1987) 238:522–4. doi:10.1126/science.2821621
24. Bethin KE, Vogt SK, Muglia LJ. Interleukin-6 is an essential, corticotropin-releasing hormone-independent stimulator of the adrenal axis during immune system activation. *Proc Natl Acad Sci U S A* (2000) 97:9317–22. doi:10.1073/pnas.97.16.9317
25. Matsuwaki T, Eskilsson A, Kugelberg U, Jönsson JI, Blomqvist A. Interleukin-1β induced activation of the hypothalamus-pituitary-adrenal axis is dependent on interleukin-1 receptors on non-hematopoietic cells. *Brain Behav Immun* (2014) 40:166–73. doi:10.1016/j.bbi.2014.03.015
26. Jaattela M, Ilvesmaki V, Voutilainen R, Stenman UH, Saksela E. Tumor necrosis factor as a potent inhibitor of adrenocorticotropin-induced cortisol production and steroidogenic P450 enzyme gene expression in cultured human fetal adrenal cells. *Endocrinology* (1991) 128:623–9. doi:10.1210/endo-128-1-623
27. Darling G, Goldstein DS, Stull R, Gorschboth CM, Norton JA. Tumor necrosis factor: immune endocrine interaction. *Surgery* (1989) 106:1155–60.
28. Mikhaylova IV, Kuulasmaa T, Jääskeläinen J, Voutilainen R. Tumor necrosis factor-alpha regulates steroidogenesis, apoptosis, and cell viability in the human adrenocortical cell line NCI-H295R. *Endocrinology* (2007) 148:386–92. doi:10.1210/en.2006-0726
29. Jaattela M, Carpen O, Stenman UH, Saksela E. Regulation of ACTH induced steroidogenesis in human fetal adrenals by rTNF. *Mol Cell Endocrinol* (1990) 68:R31–6. doi:10.1016/0303-7207(90)90196-F
30. Engström L, Rosén K, Angel A, Fyrberg A, Mackerlova L, Konsman JP, et al. Systemic immune challenge activates an intrinsically regulated local inflammatory circuit in the adrenal gland. *Endocrinology* (2008) 149:1436–50. doi:10.1210/en.2007-1456
31. Bornstein SR, Schumann RR, Rettori V, McCann SM, Zacharowski K. Toll-like receptor 2 and toll-like receptor 4 expression in human adrenals. *Horm Metab Res* (2004) 36:470–3. doi:10.1055/s-2004-825750
32. Bornstein SR, Zacharowski P, Schumann RR, Barthel A, Tran N, Papewalis C, et al. Impaired adrenal stress response in toll-like receptor 2-deficient mice. *Proc Natl Acad Sci U S A* (2004) 101:16695–700. doi:10.1073/pnas.0407550101
33. Zacharowski K, Zacharowski PA, Koch A, Baban A, Tran N, Berkels R, et al. Toll-like receptor 4 plays a crucial role in the immune-adrenal response to systemic inflammatory response syndrome. *Proc Natl Acad Sci U S A* (2006) 103:6392–7. doi:10.1073/pnas.0601527103
34. Kanczkowski W, Alexaki VI, Tran N, Großklaus S, Zacharowski K, Martinez A, et al. Hypothalamo-pituitary and immune-dependent adrenal regulation during systemic inflammation. *Proc Natl Acad Sci U S A* (2013) 110:14801–6. doi:10.1073/pnas.1313945110
35. Jung B, Nougaret S, Chanques G, Mercier G, Cisse M, Aufort S, et al. The absence of adrenal gland enlargement during septic shock predicts mortality: a computed tomography study of 239 patients. *Anesthesiology* (2011) 115:334–43. doi:10.1097/ALN.0b013e318225cfd7
36. Waterhouse R. A case of suprarenal apoplexy. *Lancet* (1911) 1:576.
37. Friderichsen C. Nebennierenapoplexie bei kleinen Kindern. *Jahrb f Kinderheilk* (1918) 87:109.
38. Sharshar T, Annane D, Lorin de la Grandmaison G, Brouland JP, Hopkinson NS, Gray F. The neuropathology of septic shock. *Brain Pathol* (2004) 14:21–33. doi:10.1111/j.1750-3639.2004.tb00494.x
39. Mélik Parsadaniantz S, Levin N, Lenoir V, Roberts JL, Kerdelhué B. Human interleukin 1 beta: corticotropin releasing factor and ACTH release and gene expression in the male rat: *in vivo* and *in vitro* studies. *J Neurosci Res* (1994) 37:675–82. doi:10.1002/jnr.490370602
40. Parsadaniantz SM, Batsché E, Gegout-Pottie P, Terlain B, Gillet P, Netter P, et al. Effects of continuous infusion of interleukin 1 beta on corticotropin-releasing hormone (CRH), CRH receptors, proopiomelanocortin gene expression and secretion of corticotropin, beta-endorphin and corticosterone. *Neuroendocrinology* (1997) 65:53–63. doi:10.1159/000127164
41. Wong ML, Rettori V, al-Shekhlee A, Bongiorno PB, Canteros G, McCann SM, et al. Inducible nitric oxide synthase gene expression in the brain during systemic inflammation. *Nat Med* (1996) 2:581–4. doi:10.1038/nm0596-581
42. Brunetti L, Volpe AR, Ragazzoni E, Preziosi P, Vacca M. Interleukin-1 beta specifically stimulates nitric oxide production in the hypothalamus. *Life Sci* (1996) 58:L373–7. doi:10.1016/0024-3205(96)00238-X
43. Polito A, Sonneville R, Guidoux C, Barrett L, Viltart O, Mattot V, et al. Changes in CRH and ACTH synthesis during experimental and human septic shock. *PLoS One* (2011) 6(11):e25905. doi:10.1371/journal.pone.0025905
44. Bornstein SM. Predisposing factors for adrenal insufficiency. *N Engl J Med* (2009) 360:2328–39. doi:10.1056/NEJMra0804635
45. Vuong C, Van Uum SH, O'Dell LE, Lutfy K, Friedman TC. The effects of opioids and opioid analogs on animal and human endocrine systems. *Endocr Rev* (2010) 31:98–132. doi:10.1210/er.2009-0009
46. Cortés-Puch I, Hicks CW, Sun J, Solomon SB, Eichacker PQ, Sweeney DA, et al. Hypothalamic-pituitary-adrenal axis in lethal canine *Staphylococcus aureus* pneumonia. *Am J Physiol Endocrinol Metab* (2014) 307:E994–1008. doi:10.1152/ajpendo.00345.2014
47. Boonen E, Vervenne H, Meersseman P, Andrew R, Mortier L, Declercq PE, et al. Reduced cortisol metabolism during critical illness. *N Engl J Med* (2013) 368:1477–88. doi:10.1056/NEJMoa1214969
48. Annane D, Maxime V, Ibrahim F, Alvarez JC, Abe E, Boudou P. Diagnosis of adrenal insufficiency in severe sepsis and septic shock. *Am J Respir Crit Care Med* (2006) 174:1319–26. doi:10.1164/rccm.200509-1369OC
49. Polito A, Lorin de la Grandmaison G, Mansart A, Louiset E, Lefebvre H, Sharshar T, et al. Human and experimental septic shock are characterized by depletion of lipid droplets in the adrenals. *Intensive Care Med* (2010) 36:1852–8. doi:10.1007/s00134-010-1987-1
50. Buss NA, Gavins FN, Cover PO, Terron A, Buckingham JC. Targeting the annexin 1-formyl peptide receptor 2/ALX pathway affords protection against bacterial LPS-induced pathologic changes in the murine adrenal cortex. *FASEB J* (2015) 29:2930–42. doi:10.1096/fj.14-268375
51. Wang N, Weng W, Breslow JL, Tall AR. Scavenger receptor BI (SR-BI) is up-regulated in adrenal gland in apolipoprotein A-I and hepatic lipase knock-out mice as a response to depletion of cholesterol stores. *In vivo* evidence that SR-BI is a functional high density lipoprotein receptor under feedback control. *J Biol Chem* (1996) 271(35):21001–4.
52. Cai L, Ji A, de Beer FC, Tannock LR, van der Westhuyzen DR. SR-BI protects against endotoxemia in mice through its roles in glucocorticoid production and hepatic clearance. *J Clin Invest* (2008) 118:364–75. doi:10.1172/JCI31539
53. Gilibert S, Galle-Treger L, Moreau M, Saint-Charles F, Costa S, Ballaire R, et al. Adrenocortical scavenger receptor class B type I deficiency exacerbates endotoxic shock and precipitates sepsis-induced mortality in mice. *J Immunol* (2014) 193:817–26. doi:10.4049/jimmunol.1303164
54. Harvey PW. Adrenocortical endocrine disruption. *J Steroid Biochem Mol Biol* (2016) 155:199–206. doi:10.1016/j.jsbmb.2014.10.009
55. Bruder EA, Ball IM, Ridi S, Pickett W, Hohl C. Single induction dose of etomidate versus other induction agents for endotracheal intubation in critically ill patients. *Cochrane Database Syst Rev* (2015) 1:CD010225. doi:10.1002/14651858
56. Tominaga T, Fukata J, Naito Y, Nakai Y, Funakoshi S, Fujii N, et al. Effects of corticostatin-I on rat adrenal cells *in vitro*. *J Endocrinol* (1990) 125:287–92. doi:10.1677/joe.0.1250287
57. Beishuizen A, Thijs LG, Vermes I. Patterns of corticosteroid binding globulin and the free cortisol index during septic shock and multitrauma. *Intensive Care Med* (2000) 27:1584–91. doi:10.1007/s001340101073
58. Pemberton PA, Stein PE, Pepys MB, Potter JM, Carrell RW. Hormone binding globulins undergo serpin conformational change in inflammation. *Nature* (1988) 336:257–8. doi:10.1038/336257a0

59. Hammond GL, Smith CL, Paterson NA, Sibbald WJ. A role for corticosteroid-binding globulin in delivery of cortisol to activated neutrophils. *J Clin Endocrinol Metab* (1990) 71:34–9. doi:10.1210/jcem-71-1-34
60. Rook G, Baker R, Walker B, Honour J, Jessop D, Hernandez-Pando R, et al. Local regulation of glucocorticoid activity in sites of inflammation. Insights from the study of tuberculosis. *Ann N Y Acad Sci* (2000) 917:913–22. doi:10.1111/j.1749-6632.2000.tb05457.x
61. Stith RD, McCallum RE. Down regulation of hepatic glucocorticoid receptors after endotoxin treatment. *Infect Immun* (1983) 40:613–21.
62. Galigniana MD, Piwien-Pilipuk G, Assreuy J. Inhibition of glucocorticoid receptor binding by nitric oxide. *Mol Pharmacol* (1999) 55:317–23.
63. Kamiyama K, Matsuda N, Yamamoto S, Takano K, Takano Y, Yamazaki H, et al. Modulation of glucocorticoid receptor expression, inflammation, and cell apoptosis in septic guinea pig lungs using methylprednisolone. *Am J Physiol Lung Cell Mol Physiol* (2008) 295:L998–1006. doi:10.1152/ajplung.00459.2007
64. Kleiman A, Hübner S, Rodriguez Parkitna JM, Neumann A, Hofer S, Weigand MA, et al. Glucocorticoid receptor dimerization is required for survival in septic shock via suppression of interleukin-1 in macrophages. *FASEB J* (2012) 26:722–9. doi:10.1096/fj.11-192112
65. Liu J, Haigh RM, Jones CT. Enhancement of noradrenaline-induced inositol polyphosphate formation by glucocorticoids in rat vascular smooth muscle cells. *J Endocrinol* (1992) 133:405–11. doi:10.1677/joe.0.1330405
66. Annane D, Bellissant E, Sebille V, Lesieur O, Mathieu B, Raphael JC, et al. Impaired pressor sensitivity to noradrenaline in septic shock patients with and without impaired adrenal function reserve. *Br J Clin Pharmacol* (1998) 46:589–97. doi:10.1046/j.1365-2125.1998.00833.x
67. d'Emmanuele di Villa Bianca R, Lippolis L, Autore G, Popolo A, Marzocco S, Sorrentino L, et al. Dexamethasone improves vascular hyporeactivity induced by LPS *in vivo* by modulating ATP-sensitive potassium channels activity. *Br J Pharmacol* (2003) 140:91–6. doi:10.1038/sj.bjp.0705406
68. Goodwin JE, Feng Y, Velazquez H, Sessa WC. Endothelial glucocorticoid receptor is required for protection against sepsis. *Proc Natl Acad Sci U S A* (2013) 110:306–11. doi:10.1073/pnas.1210200110
69. Büchele GL, Silva E, Ospina-Tascón GA, Vincent JL, De Backer D. Effects of hydrocortisone on microcirculatory alterations in patients with septic shock. *Crit Care Med* (2009) 37:1341–7. doi:10.1097/CCM.0b013e3181986647
70. Hafezi-Moghadam A, Simoncini T, Yang Z, Limbourg FP, Plumier JC, Rebsamen MC, et al. Acute cardiovascular protective effects of corticosteroids are mediated by non-transcriptional activation of endothelial nitric oxide synthase. *Nat Med* (2002) 8:473–9. doi:10.1038/nm0502-473
71. Annane D, Bellissant E, Bollaert PE, Briegel J, Keh D, Kupfer Y. Corticosteroids for treating sepsis. *Cochrane Database Syst Rev* (2015) 12:CD002243. doi:10.1002/14651858
72. van Leeuwen HJ, van der Bruggen T, van Asbeck BS, Boereboom FT. Effect of corticosteroids on nuclear factor-kappaB activation and hemodynamics in late septic shock. *Crit Care Med* (2001) 29:1074–7. doi:10.1097/00003246-200105000-00041
73. Meduri GU, Muthiah MP, Carratu P, Eltorky M, Chrousos GP. Nuclear factor kappaB- and glucocorticoid receptor alpha-mediated mechanisms in the regulation of systemic and pulmonary inflammation during sepsis and acute respiratory distress syndrome. Evidence for inflammation-induced target tissue resistance to glucocorticoids. *Neuroimmunomodulation* (2005) 12:321–38. doi:10.1159/000091126
74. Johannes T, Mik EG, Klingel K, Dieterich HJ, Unertl KE, Ince C. Low-dose dexamethasone-supplemented fluid resuscitation reverses endotoxin-induced acute renal failure and prevents cortical microvascular hypoxia. *Shock* (2009) 31:521–8. doi:10.1097/SHK.0b013e318188d198
75. Rinaldi S, Adembri C, Grechi S, DE Gaudio R. Low-dose hydrocortisone during severe sepsis: effects on microalbuminuria. *Crit Care Med* (2006) 34:2334–9. doi:10.1097/01.CCM.0000233872.04706.BB
76. Laviolle B, Annane D, Fougerou C, Bellissant E. Gluco- and mineralocorticoid biological effects of a 7-day treatment with low doses of hydrocortisone and fludrocortisone in septic shock. *Intensive Care Med* (2012) 38:1306–14. doi:10.1007/s00134-012-2585-1
77. Forster C, Burek M, Romero IA, Weksler B, Couraud PO, Drenckhahn D. Differential effects of hydrocortisone and TNFalpha on tight junction proteins in an in vitro model of the human blood-brain barrier. *J Physiol* (2008) 586:1937–49. doi:10.1113/jphysiol.2007.146852
78. Kashiwamura Y, Sano Y, Abe M, Shimizu F, Haruki H, Maeda T, et al. Hydrocortisone enhances the function of the blood-nerve barrier through the up-regulation of claudin-5. *Neurochem Res* (2011) 36:849–55. doi:10.1007/s11064-011-0413-6
79. Loisa P, Parviainen I, Tenhunen J, Hovilehto S, Ruokonen E. Effect of mode of hydrocortisone administration on glycemic control in patients with septic shock: a prospective randomized trial. *Crit Care* (2007) 11:R21. doi:10.1186/cc5696
80. Annane D, Cariou A, Maxime V, Azoulay E, D'honneur G, Timsit JF, et al. Corticosteroid treatment and intensive insulin therapy for septic shock in adults: a randomized controlled trial. *JAMA* (2010) 303:341–8. doi:10.1001/jama.2010.2
81. Lacomis D, Giulani M, van Cott A, Kramer D. Acute myopathy of intensive care – clinical, electromyographic and pathologic aspects. *Ann Neurol* (1996) 40:645–54. doi:10.1002/ana.410400415
82. Schakman O, Kalista S, Barbé C, Loumaye A, Thissen JP. Glucocorticoid-induced skeletal muscle atrophy. *Int J Biochem Cell Biol* (2013) 45:2163–72. doi:10.1016/j.biocel.2013.05.036
83. Schreiber MP, Colantuoni E, Bienvenu OJ, Neufeld KJ, Chen KF, Shanholtz C, et al. Corticosteroids and transition to delirium in patients with acute lung injury. *Crit Care Med* (2014) 42:1480–6. doi:10.1097/CCM.0000000000000247
84. Wolters AE, Veldhuijzen DS, Zaal IJ, Peelen LM, van Dijk D, Devlin JW, et al. Systemic corticosteroids and transition to delirium in critically ill patients. *Crit Care Med* (2015) 43:e585–8. doi:10.1097/CCM.0000000000001302
85. Annane D. Corticosteroids for severe sepsis: an evidence-based guide for physicians. *Ann Intensive Care* (2011) 1(1):7. doi:10.1186/2110-5820-1-7
86. Moran JL, Graham PL, Rockliff S, Bersten AD. Updating the evidence for the role of corticosteroids in severe sepsis and septic shock: a Bayesian meta-analytic perspective. *Crit Care* (2010) 14:R134. doi:10.1186/cc9182
87. Kalil AC, Sun J. Low-dose steroids for septic shock and severe sepsis: the use of Bayesian statistics to resolve clinical trial controversies. *Intensive Care Med* (2011) 37:420–9. doi:10.1007/s00134-010-2121-0
88. Volbeda M, Wetterslev J, Gluud C, Zijlstra JG, van der Horst IC, Keus F. Glucocorticosteroids for sepsis: systematic review with meta-analysis and trial sequential analysis. *Intensive Care Med* (2015) 41:1220–34. doi:10.1007/s00134-015-3899-6
89. Dellinger RP, Levy MM, Rhodes A, Annane D, Gerlach H, Opal SM, et al. Surviving sepsis campaign: international guidelines for management of severe sepsis and septic shock, 2012. *Intensive Care Med* (2013) 39:165–228. doi:10.1007/s00134-012-2769-8

8

Effect of Novel Melanocortin Type 2 Receptor Antagonists on the Corticosterone Response to ACTH in the Neonatal Rat Adrenal Gland *In Vivo* and *In Vitro*

Nasha K. Nensey*[1,2], *Jonathan Bodager*[1,2], *Ashley L. Gehrand*[2] and *Hershel Raff*[1,2]

[1] Department of Medicine, Medical College of Wisconsin, Milwaukee, WI, USA, [2] Endocrine Research Laboratory, Aurora St. Luke's Medical Center, Aurora Research Institute, Milwaukee, WI, USA

***Correspondence:**
Hershel Raff
hraff@mcw.edu

Stress-induced increases in neonatal corticosterone demonstrate a unique shift from ACTH independence to ACTH dependence between postnatal day 2 (PD2) and day 8 (PD8) in newborn rats. This shift could be due to the binding of a bioactive, non-immunoreactive plasma ligand to the adrenocortical melanocortin 2 receptor (MC2R) (ACTH receptor). A potent MC2R antagonist would be useful to evaluate this phenomenon in the neonate. Therefore, we investigated the acute corticosterone response to $ACTH_{(1-39)}$ injection in rat pups pretreated with newly developed MC2R antagonists (GPS1573 and GPS1574), which have not been tested *in vivo*. The doses used *in vivo* were based on their *in vitro* potency, with GP1573 being more potent than GPS1574. GPS1573 (PD2 and PD8), GPS1574 (PD2 only), or vehicle were injected intraperitoneally (ip) 10 min before baseline sampling. Then, 0.001 mg/kg of $ACTH_{(1-39)}$ was injected ip, and subsequent blood samples obtained for the measurement of plasma corticosterone. Pretreatment of PD2 pups with GPS1573 demonstrated augmentation, rather than inhibition, of the corticosterone response to ACTH. In PD8 pups, pretreatment with 0.1 mg/kg GPS1573, but not 4 mg/kg, augmented the corticosterone response to ACTH. Pretreatment with GPS1574 attenuated the plasma corticosterone response to ACTH at 30 min in PD2 pups. The activity of these two compounds *in vivo* do not match their potency *in vitro*, with GPS1573 leading to a small augmentation of the corticosterone response to ACTH *in vivo* while GPS1574 resulted in inhibition.

Keywords: ACTH, MC2R, corticosterone, adrenal cortex, antagonist

INTRODUCTION

Development of the neonatal hypothalamic–pituitary–adrenal (HPA) axis is critical for normal maturation of the lung, closing of the patent ductus arteriosus, and improving vasoconstrictor responses to catecholamines, as well as for stress-induced increases in blood glucose and blood pressure (1–3). In light of the increasing rate of premature births in the United States, it is important to understand the mechanisms of steroidogenesis and HPA axis maturation in the premature and full-term neonate (4). The neonatal rat model of human prematurity serves as a useful tool in studying the development of the HPA axis because the rat is an altricial animal. The full-term, newborn rat is immature compared to a full-term human neonate (5, 6). The primary glucocorticoid in the neonatal rat, corticosterone, is secreted from the zona fasciculata of the adrenal cortex in response to ACTH binding and activation of the melanocortin 2 receptor (MC2R) (7, 8). The binding of ACTH to MC2R leads to an increase in intracellular cyclic adenosine monophosphate (cAMP), causing activation of protein kinase A (PKA), and subsequent increase in movement of free cholesterol across the mitochondrial membrane into the cytosol (7–10). This transport of free cholesterol, mediated by the steroidogenic acute regulatory protein (StAR), is the rate-limiting step of steroidogenesis (11).

We have previously shown that on postnatal day 2 (PD2), rat pups exposed to hypoxic stress demonstrate an increase in corticosterone without an appreciable increase in immunoassayable ACTH and adrenal cAMP (12, 13). This phenomenon could be due to larger posttranslational products of POMC activating the MC2R receptor (14), which are not necessarily detected in our ACTH immunoassay. Although difficult to study without completely eliminating potential confounders, there are data suggesting that premature infants born at <32 weeks can mount a cortisol response without the large increase in plasma ACTH found in infants born >32 weeks gestational age (15). As stated earlier, the newborn rat is useful as a model of human prematurity (5, 6).

By postnatal day 8 (PD8), pups show an increase in corticosterone with the classic increase in immunoassayable ACTH and adrenal cAMP (12, 13, 16). The ability of the PD2 adrenal gland to respond to stress without a detectable increase in immunoreactive ACTH could be due to a bioactive, non-immunoreactive form of ACTH or another POMC product that can bind to and activate the adrenocortical MC2R. If the corticosterone response to stress in PD2 pups can be blocked by antagonizing the MC2R, it would suggest that a bioactive form of ACTH (not measured by immunoassay) is working through the MC2R in PD2 pups.

GPS1573 (Nle-P-f-R-w-F-K-A-V-G-K-K-R-R NH_2) and GPS1574 [Nle-(E-f-R-w-F-K)-A-V-G-K-K-R-R NH_2] are newly described, potent ($IC_{50} = 66 \pm 23$ and 260 ± 1 nM, respectively), and dose-dependent antagonists of ACTH-stimulated MC2R activity *in vitro* (17). Note that the structures of the two compounds are similar except that GPS1574 has a ring structure. However, they have not been studied *in vivo*. The primary goal of the present study is to investigate the effect of GPS1573 and GPS1574 *in vitro* (adrenal cells) and *in vivo* (neonatal rats) in order to set the stage for its use in evaluating the role of endogenous ACTH in the neonatal adrenal stress response. We hypothesize that these MC2R antagonists are effective in adrenal cells from neonatal rats *in vitro*. Furthermore, we hypothesize that in the neonatal rat, GPS1573 and GPS1574, when given at a 100- to 4000-fold higher dose and 4000- to 8000-fold higher dose, respectively, than exogenous $ACTH_{(1-39)}$, will attenuate the adrenocortical corticosterone response to ACTH.

MATERIALS AND METHODS

Animal Treatment and Experimental Protocol

The animal protocol was approved by the Institutional Animal Care and Use Committee of Aurora Health Care. Timed-pregnant Sprague-Dawley rats at 14–17 gestational days ($N = 45$) were obtained from Harlan Sprague Dawley (Indianapolis, IN, USA), maintained on a standard diet, and had water available *ad libitum* in a controlled environment (0600–1800 hours lights on). Dams were allowed to deliver and care for their pups without interference until experimentation. The MC2R antagonists GPS1573 and GPS1574 were synthesized by Genepep (St. Jean de Védas, France) and reconstituted, as described previously (17).

Adrenal Cell Preparation and GPS1573 and GPS1574 *In Vitro*

Adrenal cells from rats ($N = 11$ adults, 46 PD2 pups, and 26 PD8 pups) were dispersed and studied as previously described (18, 19). Briefly, rats were killed by decapitation, and both adrenal glands were removed and cleaned of surrounding fat. Only adult adrenal glands were decapsulated prior to cell dispersion. After a 90-min type I collagenase treatment and washing, viable cells were plated in a 96-well microtiter plate (10,000 cells/well) and pretreated for 1 h with (a) no antagonist (b) 750 nM GPS1573, or (c) 750-nM GPS1574 at 37°C in 10% CO_2 (balance room air). After pretreatment, rat $ACTH_{(1-39)}$ (Bachem) was added to cell suspensions at appropriate concentrations and incubated for 1 h. Medium was removed and immediately assayed for corticosterone (20).

GPS1573 and GPS1574 Studies in the Neonatal Rat *In Vivo*

Rat pups were randomly assigned to experimental groups on the morning of the experiment. Then, rat pups were removed from the dams and placed in a small cage with adequate bedding, where they were allowed free range of motion and room to huddle. A variable control heating pad (Moore Medical, Farmington, CT, USA) was placed beneath the bedding and kept at the lowest setting required to maintain body temperature in normoxic rats at these ages (13, 21). After 10 min, rat pups were removed from the cage and quickly weighed.

In the GPS1573 studies, pups (both sexes; $N = 252$) were studied at PD2 ($N = 96$) and PD8 ($N = 156$) because these ages span the critical time during which the neonatal rat's adrenal response to hypoxia shifts from immunoreactive ACTH independent to ACTH dependent (13, 16). Pups were injected intraperitoneally (ip) with either vehicle (10 μl/kg body wt of isotonic saline) or GPS1573 (diluted in isotonic saline) in low or high dose (0.1 or 4.0 mg/kg body wt, respectively). We chose to give GPS1573 ip because (a) it is a small peptide amenable to proper absorption by this route, (b) ACTH injections given ip are effective, and (c) subcutaneous injection was ineffective (data not shown).

In the GPS1574 studies, pups (both sexes, $N = 42$) were only studied at PD2, with the 60-min time point omitted because of drug's limited supply, the data from the 60-min time point with GPS1573 described above, higher necessary dose based on the *in vitro* studies [current experiments and Ref. (17)], and its expense. GPS1574 was given at a dose of 4 or 8 mg/kg ip. Otherwise, the experiments were performed as described for GPS1573.

Ten minutes after GPS1573 or GPS1574 injection, a subset of pups was quickly decapitated and trunk blood was collected (baseline, time 0). Immediately after the baseline collection,

1 μg/kg (0.001 mg/kg) of porcine ACTH (Sigma Chemical, St. Louis, MO, USA) was injected ip, as described (22–24). Subsets of pups were decapitated at 15, 30, or 60 min (GPS1573 only) post-injection. In another group of pups ($N = 163$), the vehicle for ACTH injection (isotonic saline) was injected ip 10 min after GPS1573 or GPS1574 administration, and blood collected as described above. Trunk blood was collected in EDTA tubes (1 pup/sample), processed to plasma, and stored frozen (−20°C). Plasma corticosterone was measured by immunoassay, as described previously (MP Biomedicals, Orangeburg, NJ, USA) (25).

Statistical Analyses

Corticosterone data were analyzed by two-way ANOVA. *Post hoc* analysis was performed by Holm–Sidak multiple range test ($P < 0.05$) (SigmaPlot 11.0). Data are presented as mean ± SEM.

RESULTS

GPS1573 and GPS1574 *In Vitro*

Figure 1 shows the corticosterone response to ACTH in dispersed adrenal cells of rat pups (PD2 and PD8) and adults treated with GPS1573 and GPS1574. The cells from adult adrenal glands showed significant inhibition of the corticosterone response to ACTH *in vitro*, with GPS1573 being more potent than GPS1574. A similar response was observed in PD2 pup adrenal cells, as previously described for adult rats (17). In PD8 pup adrenal cells, however, there was equivalent inhibition between GPS1573 and GPS1574, compared to vehicle control.

GPS1573 *In Vivo*

The plasma corticosterone responses to exogenous ACTH in PD2 pups pretreated with either vehicle (for GPS1573) or the low or high dose of GPS1573 are shown in **Figure 2**. Baseline plasma corticosterone responses (10 min after injection of GPS1573) ranged from 30.4 ± 3.7 to 45.7 ± 8.7 ng/ml and were not different from our previously published baseline data without an injection 10 min before sampling (23, 24). PD2 pups pretreated with vehicle did not show an increase in corticosterone in response to ACTH at 15 min but did have an increase in corticosterone at 30 min (166.0 ± 17.1 ng/ml) and 60 min (137.2 ± 43.5 ng/ml). After pretreatment with the low dose of GPS1573, compared to vehicle, the PD2 pups showed a significantly augmented plasma corticosterone response at 15 min (67.8 ± 7.9 ng/ml) and 60 min (200.0 ± 23.6 ng/ml). When pretreated with the high dose of GPS1573, PD2 pups demonstrate an even greater augmentation of the corticosterone response at 15 min (115.5 ± 11.0 ng/ml), when compared to pretreatment with low dose or vehicle.

The plasma corticosterone responses to exogenous ACTH in PD8 pups pretreated with either vehicle (for GPS1573) or the low or high dose of GPS1573 are shown in **Figure 3**. Baseline plasma corticosterone responses (10 min after injection of GPS1573) ranged from 22.8 ± 3.7 to 25.7 ± 2.9 ng/ml and were not different from our previously published baseline data, without an injection 10 min before sampling (23, 24). The plasma corticosterone response to ACTH in PD8 pups was less than PD2 pups. In fact, there was no significant increase in corticosterone in response to ACTH in PD8 pups. Compared to vehicle, PD8 pups pretreated with the low dose of GPS1573 showed an augmentation of the plasma corticosterone response to ACTH at 15 min (45.8 ± 2.6 ng/ml), 30 min (54.5 ± 3.7 ng/ml), and 60 min (50.4 ± 6.5 ng/ml). The corticosterone response to ACTH in PD8 pups pretreated with the high dose of GPS1573 was not different than vehicle at 15 min (34.3 ± 4.5 ng/ml) and 30 min (36.0 ± 6.0 ng/ml) but was less than the low dose of GPS1573 at 60 min (40.4 ± 5.9 ng/ml).

We also evaluated a time control in which pups were pretreated with GPS1573 and then injected with vehicle for ACTH (**Table 1**). For the most part, there were no statistically significant changes in plasma corticosterone. It is important to note that baseline plasma corticosterone concentrations were similar to those in our prior studies without ip injection prior to baseline (23, 24). However, there was a small increase in plasma corticosterone at 15 min in PD2 pups pretreated with the high dose of GPS1573 and at 30 min in PD8 pups pretreated with the low dose of GPS1573.

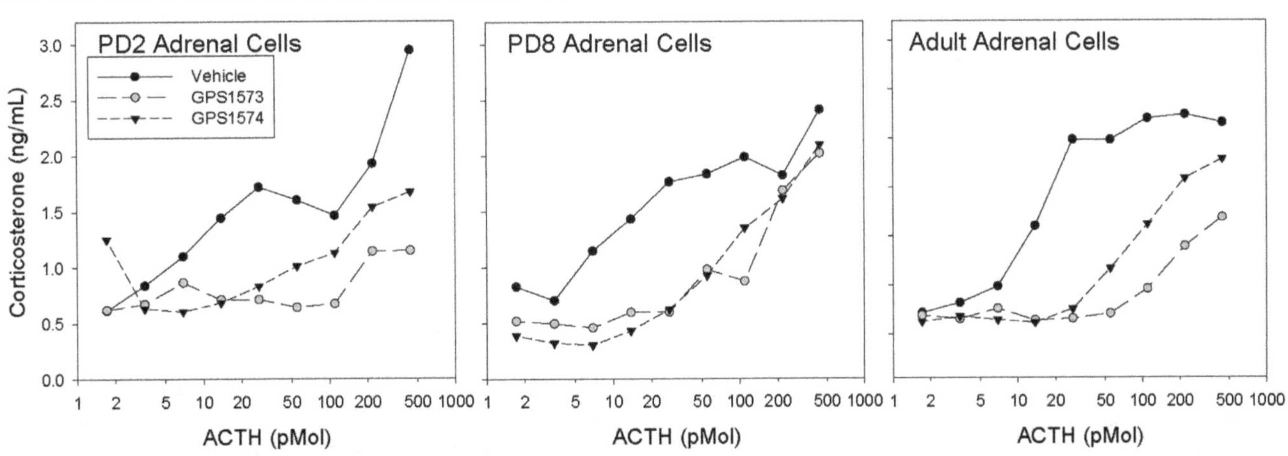

FIGURE 1 | Corticosterone responses to ACTH *in vitro* in adrenal cells from rats of different ages. Cells were pretreated with vehicle, GPS1573, or GPS1574 (750 nM). Each point is the mean of two replicates.

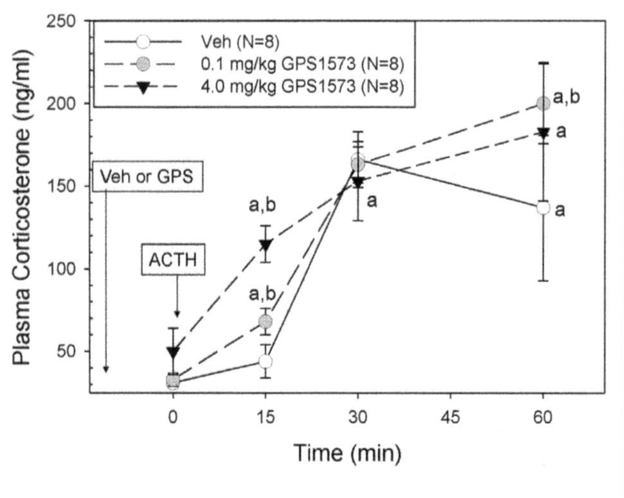

FIGURE 2 | Plasma corticosterone response to ACTH injection in postnatal 2 (PD2) rats pretreated with the low and high doses of GPS1573. PD2 pups were injected with vehicle and low or high dose of GPS1573 (0.1 or 4.0 mg/kg body wt ip, respectively). Ten minutes later, baseline samples were obtained, and then porcine ACTH (0.001 mg/kg) was injected ip. [a]Significantly different from baseline (0 min). [b]Significantly different from vehicle ($P < 0.05$). Data are presented as means ± SE. *N* values (number of pups) for each mean are shown in the figure label.

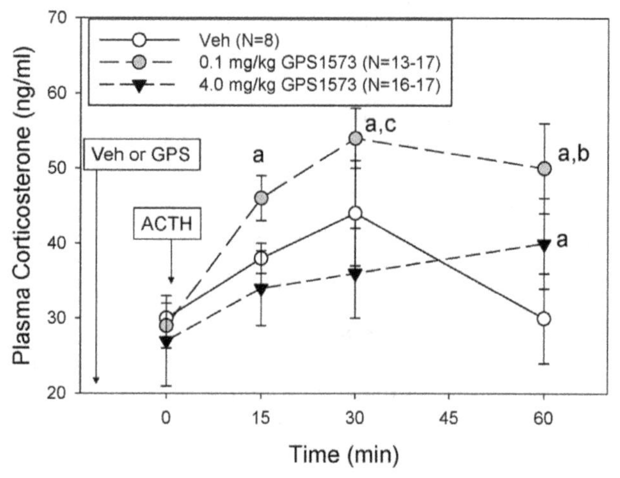

FIGURE 3 | Plasma corticosterone response to ACTH injection in postnatal 8 (PD8) rats pretreated with the low and high doses of GPS1573. PD8 pups were injected with vehicle and low or high dose of GPS1573 (0.1 or 4.0 mg/kg body wt ip, respectively). Ten minutes later, baseline samples were obtained, and then porcine ACTH (0.001 mg/kg) was injected ip. [a]Significantly different from baseline (0 min). [b]Significantly different from vehicle ($P < 0.05$). [c]Significantly different from 4.0 mg/kg. Data are presented as means ± SE. Note the *y*-axis range is lower than **Figure 2** (PD2 pups). *N* values (number of pups) for each mean are shown in the figure label.

GPS1574 *In Vivo*

Although we originally planned to only evaluate GPS1573 because of its higher potency *in vitro* (17), which was confirmed by our *in vitro* studies, the lack of inhibition with GPS1573 described above led us to do a limited number of new *in vivo* experiments with the apparently less potent GPS1574. We limited the GPS1574 study to PD2 (an age we are most interested in) through 30 min because of the need to use a higher dose of this very expensive drug, which was in limited supply and because the peak response to ACTH injection was at 30 min. As **Figure 4** demonstrates, there was no inhibition at 15 min after ACTH administration, but a dose-dependent inhibition at 30 min was seen after ACTH injection. The time control for GPS1574 (saline injection rather than ACTH) did not reveal any changes in corticosterone (data not shown) and had baseline serum corticosterone concentrations similar to our previous studies without injection before baseline sampling.

DISCUSSION

This study evaluated the corticosterone response to exogenous ACTH injection in neonatal rats pretreated with potent, *in vitro* MC2R antagonists, which have not previously been tested *in vivo* (17). We hypothesized that these compounds would attenuate the adrenocortical MC2R, thereby resulting in a lower corticosterone response to ACTH in PD2 and PD8 rats. If these antagonists were effective *in vivo*, it would allow us to evaluate the possibility that stress-induced increases in corticosterone at PD2 that are independent of increases in immunoreactive plasma ACTH could be explained by binding of a non-immunoreactive corticotrophic ligand to the adrenocortical MC2R (12, 13, 16, 21). We chose to study neonatal rats based on previous studies (23, 24). Additionally, we are currently unable to study these compounds in adult rats because of the very large quantities of the GPS compounds needed, the compounds' expense, and their limited supply.

Although the limited GPS1574 *in vivo* studies were performed after the responses to GPS1573 were ascertained, we will first discuss the GPS1574 data. GPS1574 resulted in an attenuated corticosterone response at 30 min after ACTH injection. We studied GPS1574 at a dose 4000- and 8000-fold higher than the exogenous ACTH dose. We were unable to use an even higher dose because of the limited supply of this compound. With the assumption that these GPS compounds are absorbed in a manner similar to ACTH, we calculated the plasma concentration of the GPS compounds to be at least 10- to 20-fold higher than the peak plasma ACTH concentration after injection. It is possible that these drugs are not as well absorbed as $ACTH_{(1-39)}$ and/or that they are metabolized much more readily than $ACTH_{(1-39)}$, perhaps requiring even higher doses ip. These preliminary results show promise for a more comprehensive analysis of this compound at much higher doses.

GPS1573, given *in vivo* at a 4000-fold higher dose of exogenous ACTH, did not antagonize the adrenal response to ACTH at either age. Rather, we demonstrated that pretreatment with GPS1573 augmented the corticosterone response to ACTH stimulation *in vivo*. In PD2 pups, the low dose of GPS1573 significantly augmented the corticosterone response to ACTH at 15 and 60 min compared to vehicle while the high dose demonstrated an even greater augmentation at 15 min compared to

TABLE 1 | Plasma corticosterone (nanogram per milliliter) response to vehicle (for ACTH injections) after pretreatment of PD2 and PD8 pups with the low dose (0.1 μg/kg) or high dose (4 μg/kg) of GPS1573.

Age	Dose	Time (min)			
		Baseline	15	30	60
PD2	Low (*N* = 5–6)	25.7 ± 7.0	49.4 ± 16.6	37.1 ± 10.3	42.0 ± 7.7
	High (*N* = 7)	41.0 ± 9.6	67.4 ± 6.2[a]	25.4 ± 4.9	29.0 ± 9.4
PD8	Low (*N* = 5)	17.0 ± 4.1	24.6 ± 3.4	41.2 ± 4.4[a,b]	30.3 ± 11.5
	High (*N* = 11–12)	16.4 ± 2.6	21.0 ± 3.2	14.5 ± 3.2	15.7 ± 2.9

[a]*Different from baseline.*
[b]*Different from high dose within PD8.*

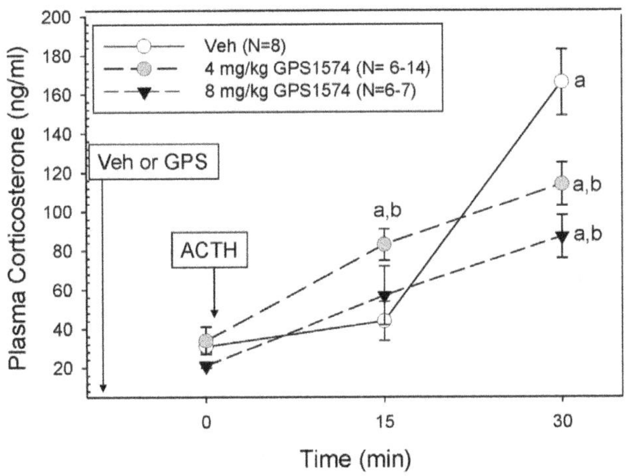

FIGURE 4 | Plasma corticosterone response to ACTH injection in postnatal 2 (PD2) rats pretreated with GPS1574. Pups were injected with vehicle or GPS1574 (4 or 8 mg/kg body wt ip, respectively). Ten minutes later, baseline samples were obtained, and then porcine ACTH (0.001 mg/kg) was injected ip. [a]Significantly different from baseline (0 min). [b]Significantly different from vehicle ($P < 0.05$). Data are presented as means ± SE. *N* values (number of pups) for each mean are shown in the figure label.

vehicle and low dose. In PD8 pups, pretreatment with the low dose of GPS1573 showed significant augmentation compared to vehicle at 60 min while pretreatment with the high dose showed no significant increase in corticosterone at any time point. GPS1573 did not consistently act as an agonist *per se*, with only small increases in corticosterone in response to ACTH vehicle (saline) at two time points.

This leads us to conclude that although GPS1573 acts as a competitive antagonist *in vitro* in adrenal cells from PD2, PD8, and adult cells, pretreatment with it *in vivo* results in an augmentation of the response to the natural ligand for the MC2R (ACTH). A similar phenomenon has been shown for nuclear (intracellular) receptors (26).

What could explain the effect demonstrated for a G-protein coupled receptor like the MC2R? First, it could be that the IC_{50} of GPS1573 is too high to be effective *in vivo*, despite the fact that we gave it at a 4000-fold higher dose than ACTH. The data from GPS1574 do not corroborate this notion since it has a higher IC_{50} *in vitro* but was effective *in vivo*. It is also possible that GPS1573 acts as an antagonist *in vitro* but is a biasing agonist *in vivo*. That is, *in vivo*, rather than blocking the receptor, it actually augments G-protein coupled transduction when ACTH binds to the MC2R (27, 28). This phenomenon could also be attributable to GPS1573 triggering a non-specific sympathetic nervous system-induced increase in the sensitivity of the adrenal cortex to ACTH (22, 29–36). Another possibility is that GPS1573 is inactivated shortly after being injected or that it has a very short half-life *in vivo*.

Potential drawbacks of our study design include the route of administration of GPS1573 and GPS1574. We chose ip administration *a priori*, since these antagonists are small compounds, and we have previously shown that ip ACTH injection is effective in stimulating corticosteronogenesis (22–24). We performed a few pilot studies with subcutaneous injection, which were ineffective (data not shown). However, an alternate route of administration (e.g., intravenous or intramuscular) may be more effective. It is also possible that these compounds would have been more effective *in vivo* in postpubertal rats. Alternate controllers of neonatal steroidogenesis, including postganglionic sympathetic input described above, have been proposed; however, the current study avoids these confounders by injecting ACTH rather than using stress as a stimulus to ACTH (22–24).

In conclusion, it appears that high dose of GPS1574 has potential as a competitive antagonist of ACTH *in vivo*. However, GPS1573 seems to act like a biasing agonist *in vivo* when given before an ACTH injection even though it is not consistently an agonist when given alone. The differences in behavior between these two compounds *in vivo* may be related to the ring structure of GPS1574.

AUTHOR CONTRIBUTIONS

NN, JB, AG, and HR all contributed substantially to the design and performance of the experiments and assays, writing and editing of the manuscript, approval of the final version, and agreement to account for all aspects of the work.

ACKNOWLEDGMENTS

The authors thank Barbara Jankowski and Brian Hoeynck for their expert technical assistance. This study was funded, in part, by the Aurora Research Institute and by the NHLBI T35 Summer Research Training Grant.

REFERENCES

1. Watterberg KL, Gerdes JS, Gifford KL, Lin HM. Prophylaxis against early adrenal insufficiency to prevent chronic lung disease in premature infants. *Pediatrics* (1999) **104**(6):1258–63. doi:10.1542/peds.104.6.1258
2. Morales P, Rastogi A, Bez ML, Akintorin SM, Pyati S, Andes SM, et al. Effect of dexamethasone therapy on the neonatal ductus arteriosus. *Pediatr Cardiol* (1998) **19**(3):225–9. doi:10.1007/s002469900290
3. Deruelle P, Houfflin-Debarge V, Magnenant E, Jaillard S, Riou Y, Puech F, et al. Effects of antenatal glucocorticoids on pulmonary vascular reactivity in the ovine fetus. *Am J Obstet Gynecol* (2003) **189**(1):208–15. doi:10.1067/mob.2003.444
4. Martin JA, Hamilton BE, Sutton PD, Ventura SJ, Menacker F, Kirmeyer S, et al. Births: final data for 2005. *Natl Vital Stat Rep* (2007) **56**(6):1–103.
5. Romijn HJ, Hofman MA, Gramsbergen A. At what age is the developing cerebral cortex of the rat comparable to that of the full-term newborn human baby? *Early Hum Dev* (1991) **26**(1):61–7. doi:10.1016/0378-3782(91)90044-4
6. Sheldon RA, Chuai J, Ferriero DM. A rat model for hypoxic-ischemic brain damage in very premature infants. *Biol Neonate* (1996) **69**(5):327–41. doi:10.1159/000244327
7. Gallo-Payet N, Payet MD. Mechanism of action of ACTH: beyond cAMP. *Microsc Res Tech* (2003) **61**(3):275–87. doi:10.1002/jemt.10337
8. Gallo-Payet N, Battista MC. Steroidogenesis-adrenal cell signal transduction. *Compr Physiol* (2014) **4**(3):889–964. doi:10.1002/cphy.c130050
9. Raff H, Findling JW. A physiologic approach to diagnosis of the Cushing syndrome. *Ann Intern Med* (2003) **138**(12):980–91. doi:10.7326/0003-4819-138-12-200306170-00010
10. Richards JS. New signaling pathways for hormones and cyclic adenosine 3',5'-monophosphate action in endocrine cells. *Mol Endocrinol* (2001) **15**(2):209–18. doi:10.1210/mend.15.2.0606
11. Stocco DM, Clark BJ. The role of the steroidogenic acute regulatory protein in steroidogenesis. *Steroids* (1997) **62**(1):29–36. doi:10.1016/S0039-128X(96)00155-9
12. Chintamaneni K, Bruder ED, Raff H. Effects of age on ACTH, corticosterone, glucose, insulin, and mRNA levels during intermittent hypoxia in the neonatal rat. *Am J Physiol Regul Integr Comp Physiol* (2013) **304**(9):R782–9. doi:10.1152/ajpregu.00073.2013
13. Bruder ED, Kamer KJ, Guenther MA, Raff H. Adrenocorticotropic hormone and corticosterone responses to acute hypoxia in the neonatal rat: effects of body temperature maintenance. *Am J Physiol Regul Integr Comp Physiol* (2011) **300**(3):R708–15. doi:10.1152/ajpregu.00708.2010
14. Karpac J, Ostwald D, Bui S, Hunnewell P, Shankar M, Hochgeschwender U. Development, maintenance, and function of the adrenal gland in early postnatal proopiomelanocortin-null mutant mice. *Endocrinology* (2005) **146**(6):2555–62. doi:10.1210/en.2004-1290
15. Bagnoli F, Mori A, Fommei C, Coriolani G, Badii S, Tomasini B. ACTH and cortisol cord plasma concentrations in preterm and term infants. *J Perinatol* (2013) **33**(7):520–4. doi:10.1038/jp.2012.165
16. Bruder ED, Taylor JK, Kamer KJ, Raff H. Development of the ACTH and corticosterone response to acute hypoxia in the neonatal rat. *Am J Physiol Regul Integr Comp Physiol* (2008) **295**(4):R1195–203. doi:10.1152/ajpregu.90400.2008
17. Bouw E, Huisman M, Neggers SJ, Themmen AP, van der Lely AJ, Delhanty PJ. Development of potent selective competitive-antagonists of the melanocortin type 2 receptor. *Mol Cell Endocrinol* (2014) **394**(1–2):99–104. doi:10.1016/j.mce.2014.07.003
18. Jasper MS, Engeland WC. Splanchnicotomy increases adrenal sensitivity to ACTH in nonstressed rats. *Am J Physiol* (1997) **273**(2 Pt 1):E363–8.
19. Bruder ED, Nagler AK, Raff H. Oxygen-dependence of ACTH-stimulated aldosterone and corticosterone synthesis in the rat adrenal cortex: developmental aspects. *J Endocrinol* (2002) **172**(3):595–604. doi:10.1677/joe.0.1720595
20. Wilkinson CW, Shinsako J, Dallman MF. Daily rhythms in adrenal responsiveness to adrenocorticotropin are determined primarily by the time of feeding in the rat. *Endocrinology* (1979) **104**(2):350–9. doi:10.1210/endo-104-2-350
21. Guenther MA, Bruder ED, Raff H. Effects of body temperature maintenance on glucose, insulin, and corticosterone responses to acute hypoxia in the neonatal rat. *Am J Physiol Regul Integr Comp Physiol* (2012) **302**(5):R627–33. doi:10.1152/ajpregu.00503.2011
22. Raff H, Lee JJ, Widmaier EP, Oaks MK, Engeland WC. Basal and adrenocorticotropin-stimulated corticosterone in the neonatal rat exposed to hypoxia from birth: modulation by chemical sympathectomy. *Endocrinology* (2004) **145**(1):79–86. doi:10.1210/en.2003-1130
23. Bodager J, Gessert T, Bruder ED, Gehrand A, Raff H. Adrenocortical sensitivity to ACTH in neonatal rats: correlation of corticosterone responses and adrenal cAMP content. *Am J Physiol Regul Integr Comp Physiol* (2014) **307**(3):R347–53. doi:10.1152/ajpregu.00125.2014
24. Johnson K, Bruder ED, Raff H. Adrenocortical control in the neonatal rat. *Physiol Rep* (2013) **1**(3):e00054. doi:10.1002/phy2.54
25. Raff H, Jacobson L, Cullinan WE. Elevated corticosterone and inhibition of ACTH responses to CRH and ether in the neonatal rat: effect of hypoxia from birth. *Am J Physiol Regul Integr Comp Physiol* (2003) **285**(5):R1224–30. doi:10.1152/ajpregu.00259.2003
26. Wardell SE, Kazmin D, McDonnell DP. Research resource: transcriptional profiling in a cellular model of breast cancer reveals functional and mechanistic differences between clinically relevant SERM and between SERM/estrogen complexes. *Mol Endocrinol* (2012) **26**(7):1235–48. doi:10.1210/me.2012-1031
27. Reversi A, Rimoldi V, Marrocco T, Cassoni P, Bussolati G, Parenti M, et al. The oxytocin receptor antagonist atosiban inhibits cell growth via a "biased agonist" mechanism. *J Biol Chem* (2005) **280**(16):16311–8. doi:10.1074/jbc.M409945200
28. Wisler JW, Xiao K, Thomsen AR, Lefkowitz RJ. Recent developments in biased agonism. *Curr Opin Cell Biol* (2014) **27**:18–24. doi:10.1016/j.ceb.2013.10.008
29. Ehrhart-Bornstein M, Bornstein SR, Gonzalez-Hernandez J, Holst JJ, Waterman MR, Scherbaum WA. Sympathoadrenal regulation of adrenocortical steroidogenesis. *Endocr Res* (1995) **21**(1–2):13–24. doi:10.3109/07435809509030417
30. Ehrhart-Bornstein M, Haidan A, Alesci S, Bornstein SR. Neurotransmitters and neuropeptides in the differential regulation of steroidogenesis in adrenocortical-chromaffin co-cultures. *Endocr Res* (2000) **26**(4):833–42. doi:10.3109/07435800009048606
31. Ehrhart-Bornstein M, Hinson JP, Bornstein SR, Scherbaum WA, Vinson GP. Intraadrenal interactions in the regulation of adrenocortical steroidogenesis. *Endocr Rev* (1998) **19**(2):101–43. doi:10.1210/edrv.19.2.0326
32. Bruder ED, Henderson LM, Raff H. Adrenal lipid profiles of chemically sympathectomized normoxic and hypoxic neonatal rats. *Horm Metab Res* (2006) **38**(12):807–11. doi:10.1055/s-2006-956183
33. Engeland WC. Functional innervation of the adrenal cortex by the splanchnic nerve. *Horm Metab Res* (1998) **30**(6–7):311–4. doi:10.1055/s-2007-978890
34. Schinner S, Bornstein SR. Cortical-chromaffin cell interactions in the adrenal gland. *Endocr Pathol* (2005) **16**(2):91–8. doi:10.1385/EP:16:2:091
35. Seidler FJ, Slotkin TA. Adrenomedullary function in the neonatal rat: responses to acute hypoxia. *J Physiol* (1985) **358**:1–16. doi:10.1113/jphysiol.1985.sp015536
36. Walker CD. Chemical sympathectomy and maternal separation affect neonatal stress responses and adrenal sensitivity to ACTH. *Am J Physiol* (1995) **268**(5 Pt 2):R1281–8.

9

Regulation of StAR by the N-terminal Domain and Coinduction of SIK1 and TIS11b/Znf36l1 in Single Cells

*Jinwoo Lee[1,2], Tiegang Tong[1], Haichuan Duan[3], Yee Hoon Foong[1], Ibrahim Musaitif[1], Takeshi Yamazaki[4] and Colin Jefcoate[1,2,3,5]**

[1] Department of Cell and Regenerative Biology, University of Wisconsin, Madison, WI, USA, [2] Endocrinology and Reproductive Physiology Program, University of Wisconsin, Madison, WI, USA, [3] Molecular and Cellular Pharmacology, University of Wisconsin, Madison, WI, USA, [4] Graduate School of Integrated Arts and Sciences, Hiroshima University, Higashi-Hiroshima, Japan, [5] Molecular and Environmental Toxicology Center, University of Wisconsin, Madison, WI, USA

***Correspondence:**
Colin Jefcoate
jefcoate@wisc.edu

The cholesterol transfer function of steroidogenic acute regulatory protein (StAR) is uniquely integrated into adrenal cells, with mRNA translation and protein kinase A (PKA) phosphorylation occurring at the mitochondrial outer membrane (OMM). The StAR C-terminal cholesterol-binding domain (CBD) initiates mitochondrial intermembrane contacts to rapidly direct cholesterol to Cyp11a1 in the inner membrane (IMM). The conserved StAR N-terminal regulatory domain (NTD) includes a leader sequence targeting the CBD to OMM complexes that initiate cholesterol transfer. Here, we show how the NTD functions to enhance CBD activity delivers more efficiently from StAR mRNA in adrenal cells, and then how two factors hormonally restrain this process. NTD processing at two conserved sequence sites is selectively affected by StAR PKA phosphorylation. The CBD functions as a receptor to stimulate the OMM/IMM contacts that mediate transfer. The NTD controls the transit time that integrates extramitochondrial StAR effects on cholesterol homeostasis with other mitochondrial functions, including ATP generation, inter-organelle fusion, and the major permeability transition pore in partnership with other OMM proteins. PKA also rapidly induces two additional StAR modulators: salt-inducible kinase 1 (SIK1) and Znf36l1/Tis11b. Induced SIK1 attenuates the activity of CRTC2, a key mediator of StAR transcription and splicing, but only as cAMP levels decline. TIS11b inhibits translation and directs the endonuclease-mediated removal of the 3.5-kb StAR mRNA. Removal of either of these functions individually enhances cAMP-mediated induction of StAR. High-resolution fluorescence *in situ* hybridization (HR-FISH) of StAR RNA reveals asymmetric transcription at the gene locus and slow RNA splicing that delays mRNA formation, potentially to synchronize with cholesterol import. Adrenal cells may retain slow transcription to integrate with intermembrane NTD activation. HR-FISH resolves individual 3.5-kb StAR mRNA molecules *via* dual hybridization at the 3′- and

Abbreviations: 3′EU, oligomer set targeting extended 3′UTR; AMG, aminoglutethimide; CBD, cholesterol-binding domain; CTD, C-terminal domain; CHX, cycloheximide; FISH, fluorescence *in situ* hybridization; HR-FISH, high-resolution fluorescence *in situ* hybridization; IMM, inner mitochondrial membrane; N-SIM, Nikon's structured illumination microscope; NTD, N-terminal domain; OMM, outer mitochondrial membrane; PKA, protein kinase A; p-RNA, primary RNA; sp-RNA, spliced primary RNA; SIK1, salt-inducible kinase 1; StAR, steroidogenic acute regulatory protein.

5′-ends and reveals an unexpectedly high frequency of 1:1 pairing with mitochondria marked by the matrix StAR protein. This pairing may be central to translation-coupled cholesterol transfer. Altogether, our results show that adrenal cells exhibit high-efficiency StAR activity that needs to integrate rapid cholesterol transfer with homeostasis and pulsatile hormonal stimulation. StAR NBD, the extended 3.5-kb mRNA, SIK1, and Tis11b play important roles.

Keywords: StAR, Sik1, Tis11b, fluorescence *in situ* hybridization, PCR

INTRODUCTION

Steroidogenic acute regulatory protein (StAR) functions as a key determinant of steroidogenesis by transferring cholesterol from the outer mitochondrial membrane (OMM) to Cyp11a1 in the inner mitochondrial membrane (IMM) (1–4). Cyp11a1 metabolizes this cholesterol in the adrenal mitochondria very rapidly such that accumulation only occurs when constraints are placed on this turnover. The Cyp11a1 inhibitor aminoglutethimide (AMG) causes the accumulation of 3–5 cholesterol molecules per Cyp11a1 and increased cholesterol–Cyp11a1 complex formation (5). Turnover is driven by NADPH generated from the Krebs cycle (isocitrate dehydrogenase), but highest potency is achieved with succinate dehydrogenase linked to the ATP-dependent NADH/NADPH transhydrogenase (NNT) (6). CYP11a1 not only depends on the shuttling of ferredoxin between the flavoprotein reductase and CYP11a1 (7) but also competes with electron transfer to IMM Cyp11b1 (8).

The role of StAR has been definitively established through transgenic deletion of its gene in mice, which reproduces the pathology of human adrenal lipidemic hyperplasia (ALH) (9, 10). This role extends to testis Leydig cells and multiple cell types in the ovary. Mutations that cause the human disease are concentrated in the cholesterol-binding domain (CBD) rather than the N-terminal domain (NTD) (11). One mutation (R182) resolves cholesterol exchange activity to optimal levels when steroidogenic activity is deficient (12, 13). The NTD retains the net positive charge common to mitochondrial import sequences, but with appreciable helical content and dual cleavage sites that are atypical for mitochondrial target sequences. NTD modulatory activity is suggested by the involvement of the 30–62 sequences in the binding of StAR to VDAC2, which then facilitates both cholesterol transfer and NTD cleavage (14). Deletion of the NTD (N-47 mouse), while clearly establishing cholesterol transfer activity for the CBD alone, equally establishes a major modulatory role for the NTD that is tissue-dependent (15). StAR functions without the NTD to mediate linkage to lipid droplets (16, 17), including in a reconstituted system employing rat adrenal mitochondria (18).

Steroidogenic acute regulatory protein activity under hormonal control is mediated by phosphorylation at S-194 in the CBD, by cAMP and protein kinase A (PKA) in fasciculate cells, and by Ca-dependent kinases in glomerulosa cells (19, 20). StAR activity is inhibited by cholesterol sulfate such that cholesterol sulfatase can enhance activity (21). The large number of cholesterol molecules transferred per each molecule of transiting StAR implicates the controlled generation of OMM/IMM contacts by receptor-like activity derived from the CBD (1). StAR, or STARD1, was the first member of a family that was identified based on the CBD sequence and structure. Forms D1 and D3 differ in their N-terminal targeting to mitochondria and to late endosomes, respectively; D4, D5, and D6 differ in their carrier specificity for cholesterol derivatives (22). The phosphatidylcholine exchange protein (STARD2) also functions at the mitochondria but with a partnering enzyme, Acot13 (23). Cholesterol transfer into the adrenal cortex mitochondria *in vivo* depends on continuous translation of the 37-kDa StAR pre-protein with concomitant phosphorylation by PKA. Inhibition with cycloheximide (CHX) halts adrenocorticotropic hormone (ACTH)-stimulated steroidogenesis within 5 min, while accumulating cholesterol in the OMM remains inaccessible to IMM Cyp11a1 (24–26). This intermembrane cholesterol barrier in the adrenal mitochondria caused by CHX treatment is readily breached by mild mitochondrial disruption, including the elevation of Ca^{2+}. Such artificial transfer also removes succinate-initiated NNT support for this CHX-sensitive Cyp11a1 activity (6).

The NTD and the timing of the conserved IMM processing link StAR activity to other processes. PBR/TSPO associates with abundant VDAC1 to control OMM/IMM contacts at cholesterol-rich regions (27), including through the formation of a transmembrane complex (28). Participation of the mitochondrial permeability transition pore (MPFP) is a common feature of these processes. PAP7/ACBD3, which partners with TSPO, is a suppressor of SREBP forms, thus representing a link to cholesterol and fatty acid homeostasis (29). GTP enhances the *in vitro* mitochondrial uptake of cholesterol *via* GTPase activity in partnership with Ca (30). GTPases, such as Mfn2 and Opa1, which mediate the continuous dynamics of inter-mitochondrial fusion and fission, play pivotal roles in cAMP-stimulated cholesterol transfer (31). Mitochondrial fusion with the ER through sigma receptor sites has also been implicated (14). MAPK phosphorylation of StAR (S-232) stimulates StAR activity while slowing N-terminal cleavage (32).

In addition to NTD intervention, StAR activity is restricted at the mRNA level by the salt-inducible kinase (SIK1) (33) and the RNA-binding protein Znf36l1/Tis11b (34) which are each rapidly induced by cAMP. A critical feature of StAR mRNA is its alternative polyadenylation (1.6- and 3.5-kb StAR mRNA), which introduces an extra 2 kb of 3′UTR, facilitating additional regulation of mRNA stability and translation (34). Here, we have used the high-resolution fluorescence *in situ* hybridization method (HR-FISH) (35, 36) to image primary (p-RNA) and spliced StAR transcripts (sp-RNA) at the StAR gene loci in Y-1 and MA-10 cells (37, 38). Y-1 adrenal cells are distinguished by a proportion of basally active loci that produce cytoplasmic mRNA sufficient to mediate peak activation of steroidogenesis by PKA. Activation of individual cells by Br-cAMP increases StAR transcripts at the gene loci, where we have resolved primary and spliced transcripts before observing increased mRNA in the cytoplasm and specific positioning at the mitochondria.

The need for continuous translation places particular demands on the hormonal stimulation of transcription. StAR transcription depends on multiple promoter sites within 300 bp of the transcription start site, including SF1, CREB, GATA4, and AP1, which are further supplemented by newly synthesized C/EBP and NF4a1/Nurr77 (39, 40). CREB activity, which is essential, is activated by PKA-mediated phosphorylation at S133, which mediates synergistic recruitment of the histone acetyl transferase CBP and the coactivators of the CRTC/TORC family (38, 41–43). PKA deactivates the repressor kinases SIK1 and SIK2, which otherwise maintain CRTC2 in an inactive phosphorylated state. Merely inhibiting SIK is sufficient to stimulate the expression of StAR and most steroidogenic genes in Y-1 cells (33, 41). SIK1 is rapidly induced in adrenal cells *in vivo* and in cultured Y-I cells by PKA at an early stage of increased StAR expression (41, 42). Importantly, PKA also inhibits activity through S577 phosphorylation, and thus, this increase does not impact StAR until PKA activity declines (38). Br-cAMP also rapidly stimulates Znf36l1/Tis11b, which binds to specific dual AU-rich elements in the extended 3′UTR. This homodimer complex recruits ribonucleases to selectively degrade the 3.5-kb StAR mRNA. Here, we show that removal of TIS11b enhances the potency of Br-cAMP as a stimulant of StAR expression. Another cAMP-sensitive protein, Akap1, may work with TIS11b to position StAR mRNA at the mitochondria *via* elements in the extended 3′UTR (44).

The work presented here provides evidence that mRNA generation, mitochondrial positioning, translation, and N-terminal targeting of new StAR proteins may be coordinated to match organizational steps involving cholesterol transfer across the mitochondrial membranes, consistent with an integrated CHX-sensitive mechanism.

MATERIALS AND METHODS

Cell Culture and DNA Vector Transfection

The MA-10 mouse Leydig tumor cell line (a gift of Dr. Mario Ascoli) was derived from the Leydig tumor M5480P (45). Y-1 mouse adrenocortical tumor cells were expanded from a subclone obtained from Dr. Bernard Schimmer (University of Toronto) with a lower passage number than those available from ATCC. Cells were grown according to previously described method (34). DNA vectors were transfected using TransIt-LT1 (Mirus Bio) and Lipofectamine 2000 (Invitrogen) according to the manufacturers' protocols.

siRNA Transfection and shRNA Cell Line Generation

ON-TARGETplus SMARTpool siRNA sequences against mouse *TIS11b*, along with non-target siRNA sequences, were purchased from Dharmacon, Inc. (Lafayette, CO, USA). They were transiently transfected into MA-10 cells using the DharmaFECT 1 reagent according to the manufacturer's protocol. siRNA-transfected samples were prepared according to a previously described method (34). The GeneClip™ U1 Hairpin Cloning system was used to express short hairpin RNAs (shRNAs) in MA-10 and Y-1 cells. Stable cell lines were generated using a positive selection marker, neomycin. The U1 promoter was previously employed with success to knock down the target genes in these cell lines.

Western Blot Analysis

Protein samples were prepared and assayed according to a previously described method (34). Protein bands were visualized using ECL reagent and Hyperfilm (Amersham Biosciences, Arlington Heights, IL, USA).

Real-time RT-PCR

Primer design and cDNA synthesis were performed according to previously described methods (34, 37). q-PCR was performed using a BioRad CFX96TM Real-Time PCR Detection System. The q-PCR protocol was carried out as follows: initial denaturation at 95°C for 3 min, followed by 40 cycles of 10 s at 95°C, 30 s at 55°C, and 10 s at 95°C. Fluorescence signals were recorded at each extension step at 55°C. A melting curve analysis was then performed from 65 to 95°C at increments of 0.5°C for 5 s to assess amplicon specificity.

Northern Blot Analysis

Total RNA was isolated using a QIAGEN RNeasy Mini kit per the manufacturer's instructions. Approximately 10 μg of total RNA was resolved by electrophoresis in a 1% (weight/volume) agarose–formaldehyde–formamide denaturing gel and transferred to a Hybond-N+ membrane (Amersham Biosciences) for approximately 16 h *via* the capillary method. RNA on the membrane was immobilized with a UV Stratalinker 1800 in auto mode (1900 J × 100 for 30 s). The membrane was then prehybridized at 65°C for 1 h in QuickHyb hybridization solution (Stratagene). Hybridization was performed at 65°C for 2 h in QuickHyb with a 0.9-kb mouse StAR cDNA probe that was radiolabeled with [α-^{32}P]dCTP (PerkinElmer, Norwalk, CT, USA; 3000 Ci/mmol) using a Ready-To-Go DNA-labeling kit (Amersham Biosciences). The membrane was exposed overnight and scanned using a phosphorimager (Molecular Dynamics, Sunnyvale, CA, USA) (34).

High-Resolution Fluorescence *In Situ* Hybridization

The term HR-FISH has been employed to distinguish the use of a probe set consisting of 40 fluorescent 20mers. The RNA probe sets for StAR were generated using the Stellaris probe designer (http://www.biosearchtech.com/stellarisdesigner/). Samples were prepared according to a previously described method (37). Freshly prepared p-RNA (Quasar-570, Biosearch Technology), sp-RNA (Quasar-570, Biosearch Technology), and 3″ EU (Quasar-570, Biosearch Technology) probe sets and antibodies for StAR and TIS11B were used. Clean coverslips were placed over the samples to prevent the hybridization solution [10% dextran sulfate (Sigma), 10% deionized formamide (Ambion), 2× SSC] from drying during the incubation. Samples were incubated in a dark humidified chamber at 37°C overnight. After a 30-min wash in wash buffer, samples were incubated in DAPI nuclear stain (wash buffer with 5 ng/ml DAPI) to counterstain the nuclei for 30 min. For combined FISH, an extra wash step was needed for the secondary antibody. Samples were processed according to a previously described method (37).

Image Acquisition and Analysis

To detect and visualize p-RNA, sp-RNA, and mRNA, we used an Olympus wide-field fluorescence microscope (Model IX81) and the Nikon's structured illumination microscope (N-SIM) to obtain higher resolution images.

Olympus IX81

Images were captured by Olympus IX81 motorized inverted microscope equipped with a Hamamatsu Orca2 camera. Images were obtained with 0.2 µm spacing with the 100× oil objective and projected onto a single plane or 3D image. At least 30 *Z*-sections at 0.2 µm intervals were taken to cover the entire thickness of the cell. The exposure times ranged from 0.2 s (nuclear loci) to 4 s (cytoplasmic mRNA). The exposure time increases not only sensitivity approximately proportionately but also the background. Comparisons are made at the same exposure times. The target size is much smaller than the image due to the dispersion of the fluorescent light from the target. Loci have multiple clustered RNA molecules either p-RNA or sp-RNA. These terms have been used rather than pre-mRNA and mRNA to emphasize the absence of information on RNA processing. We term this fluorescent cluster the RNA locus, which elsewhere has been shown to overlap with the gene (DNA) locus. p-RNA and sp-RNA at the RNA are separate in the images. Captured images were deconvoluted with Slidebook 5.0 software (Intelligent Imaging Innovations, Inc.) for further analysis.

Nikon's Structured Illumination Microscope

Super-resolution imaging was performed with an N-SIM microscope system (Nikon) equipped with a SR Apo TIRF 100× 1.49 N.A. oil immersion objective and an iXon3 camera (Andor Technology). 3D-SIM image stacks were acquired with a *Z*-distance of 0.2 µm, covering the entire thickness of the cell (about 6 µm) using laser power setting 40%. The camera settings were configured as follows: format for capture, no binning; exposure time, 50–200 ms (one frame recommended); readout mode, EM gain 10 MHz 14-bit; gain multiplier, 20–200 ms (max 300); conversion gain. 5.1× 15 raw images per plane were acquired and computationally reconstructed using the reconstruction slice system from NIS-Elements software (Nikon).

Data Analysis

Statistical significance was determined using Student's *t*-test or ANOVA; $P < 0.05$ was considered statistically significant; $^*P < 0.05$, $^{**}P < 0.01$, and $^{***}P < 0.001$. Data were analyzed using PRISM software (San Diego, CA, USA).

RESULTS

N-Terminal Modulation of StAR in Mouse Cell Lines

Steroidogenic acute regulatory protein activity is dependent on co-translational phosphorylation prior to N-terminal processing. This process leads to the inhibition of cholesterol metabolism within 5 min in primary rat adrenal cells or *in vivo* (1). In MA-10 cells, StAR is barely detectable until cells undergo 60 min of stimulation by Br-cAMP. To test whether PKA phosphorylation at S-194 affects this processing, we substantially elevated StAR protein levels *via* the transfection of StAR dUTR prior to the addition of Br-cAMP (**Figure 1A**). After 30 min of stimulation, extensive new active phosphorylation of p37 was evident, although less than half of this p37 was processed to p30, and scarcely any of the third products, p32, was detectable. In the absence of vector-derived StAR, appreciable amounts of p37, p32, and p30 were generated after 60 min of stimulation by Br-cAMP in proportions similar to those seen with the vector. Again, phosphorylation was appreciable for p30 but was scarcely detectable for p32.

Evidently, transfected StAR is phosphorylated and cleaved at the mitochondria at very similar rates to those observed for endogenous StAR. Mature p30 and, in particular, p32 are phosphorylated at much lower levels, indicating that the PKA targeting of S-194 impacts these cleavage reactions. Phosphorylation occurs outside the mitochondria and therefore before predominant cleavage by the IMM proteases. Either S-194 phosphorylation enhances removal of the processed forms in the matrix or slows their formation.

This N-terminal processing is very consistent across species and adrenal cell lines. The commonly used COS-1 transfection model (monkey kidney line), however, demonstrates a substantial deficiency in the rate of cleavage compared to Y-1 and MA-10 cells (**Figure 1B**).

N-Terminal Modulation of StAR in Primary Bovine Adrenal Cells

Bovine adrenal cortex tissue is the best source of information regarding human adrenal mechanisms. The electron transfer activity of purified Cyp11a1 and its partnering ferredoxin was established in bovine adrenal tissue (7). Cultured primary bovine adrenal cortex (BAC) cells, which predominantly express cortisol, are stimulated fourfold by ACTH (47). Inhibition of protein synthesis by CHX has no effect on mitochondrial cholesterol accumulation but prevents increases in both cholesterol–Cyp11a1 complex formation and metabolism (**Figure 2A**).

N-terminal domain sequences are highly conserved across species (**Figure 2B**), including the two major cleavage products. These have been characterized by mass spectrometry for bovine StAR and found to have masses of 27,503 and 25,906 Da (48). The major cleavage products in BAC cells match those observed in MA-10 cells and with vector expression in COS-1 cells.

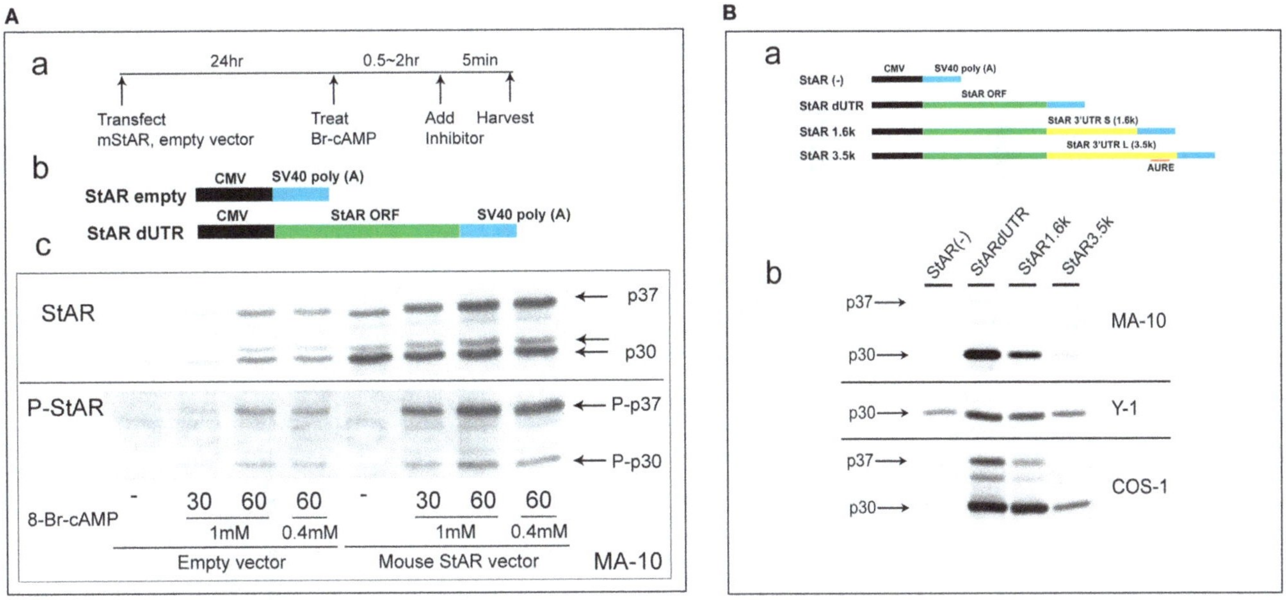

FIGURE 1 | Characterization of N-terminal sequence changes in the 3′UTR of mouse StAR mRNA. (A) Design for the transfection of MA-10 cells with dUTR–StAR and stimulation by Br-cAMP (a). Diagram showing empty vector and StAR expression vector (StAR dUTR) (b). Comparison of the N-terminal cleavage and phosphorylation of natively expressed and transfected StAR dUTR. Each is stimulated for 0, 30, and 60 min (c). **(B)** Diagram showing empty vector and StAR expression vectors with different 3′UTRs (a). Effects of StAR 3′UTR on basal expression in StAR cDNA constructs. Western blot of StAR protein in MA-10, Y-1, and COS-1 cells transfected with these vectors (b) (46).

Single and combinatorial mutation of the A (M30) and B (M28) sites in the bovine sequence reveals a complex additive cleavage process; however, mutation in COS-1 cells did not affect StAR activity (without PKA activation). Removal of site A prevents the formation of p30 but results in a concomitant increase in p35, indicating that this cleavage form is an intermediate during the generation of p30 (**Figure 2C**). Mutation of site B decreases p30 and removes p28 while revealing a major product with a mobility that is intermediate between p28 and p30 (p29). Mutation of B exerts no effect on p35. We envisage p29 as the major precursor to p28. Dual mutation confirms an additive response, further establishing the independence of the two pathways.

In primary BAC cells, p37 pro-StAR is cleaved into two products with different sizes, lower (28 kDa) and higher (30 kDa), each of which can be divided into four further species in 2D gels based on pI (20). In culture, PKA activation in either glomerulosa or fasciculate BAC appreciably increases the total amount of newly cleaved products within minutes. The low-pI p28 and p30 phosphorylated forms are increased by 5- to 10-fold (**Figure 2D**). In glomerular cells, the same pattern is observed after stimulation with angiotensin and K+, which both increase intracellular Ca and calmodulin kinase levels. Aldosterone synthesis responds proportionately (dibutyl cA > angiotensin > K+) (20). The close correlation between the appearance of N-terminal cleavage and PKA phosphorylation suggests that these intermediate NTD products contribute to cholesterol transfer. The dual p28 and p30 products resolved by pI indicate further posttranslational modification in addition to phosphorylation at S-194. S-232 phosphorylation delivered by MAPK represents one possibility (32).

Y-1 Cells Exhibit Higher Basal StAR Expression and an Acute Response That Is Limited to 15 min

Y-1 adrenal cells, like their primary counterparts and in contrast to MA-10 cells, possess sufficient basal mRNA to mediate maximum steroidogenesis within 15 min without a corresponding increase in mRNA. This basal expression has been observed utilizing a combination of q-PCR and HR-FISH microscopy, described in detail elsewhere (37). The locations for q-PCR target probes in the StAR primary transcript (p-RNA) and spliced transcripts (sp-RNA/mRNA) are shown in **Figure 3A. Figure 3B** indicates the presence of both p-RNA and sp-RNA/mRNA at a ratio of 1:4 under basal conditions. In both cell types, the ratio of q-PCR at early (E7-S) and late (E7-L) sites in the 3′UTR is close to 1:1, indicating complete transcription of the 3′UTR and formation of the 3.5-kb form at a far great frequency than the 1.6-kb form (**Figure 3C**). The much higher p-RNA levels in Y-1 cells compared to MA-10 cells indicate active synthesis under basal conditions. Stimulation by Br-cAMP reveals a fourfold rise in both the early and late introns (1 and 6), but no increase in either exon 7 or spliced transcripts consistent with the approximately 30-min delay in elongation and splicing reported previously for Y-1 and MA-10 cells (37, 38).

We examined changes at the nuclear loci using HR-FISH. The HR-FISH probe locations on the StAR primary transcript

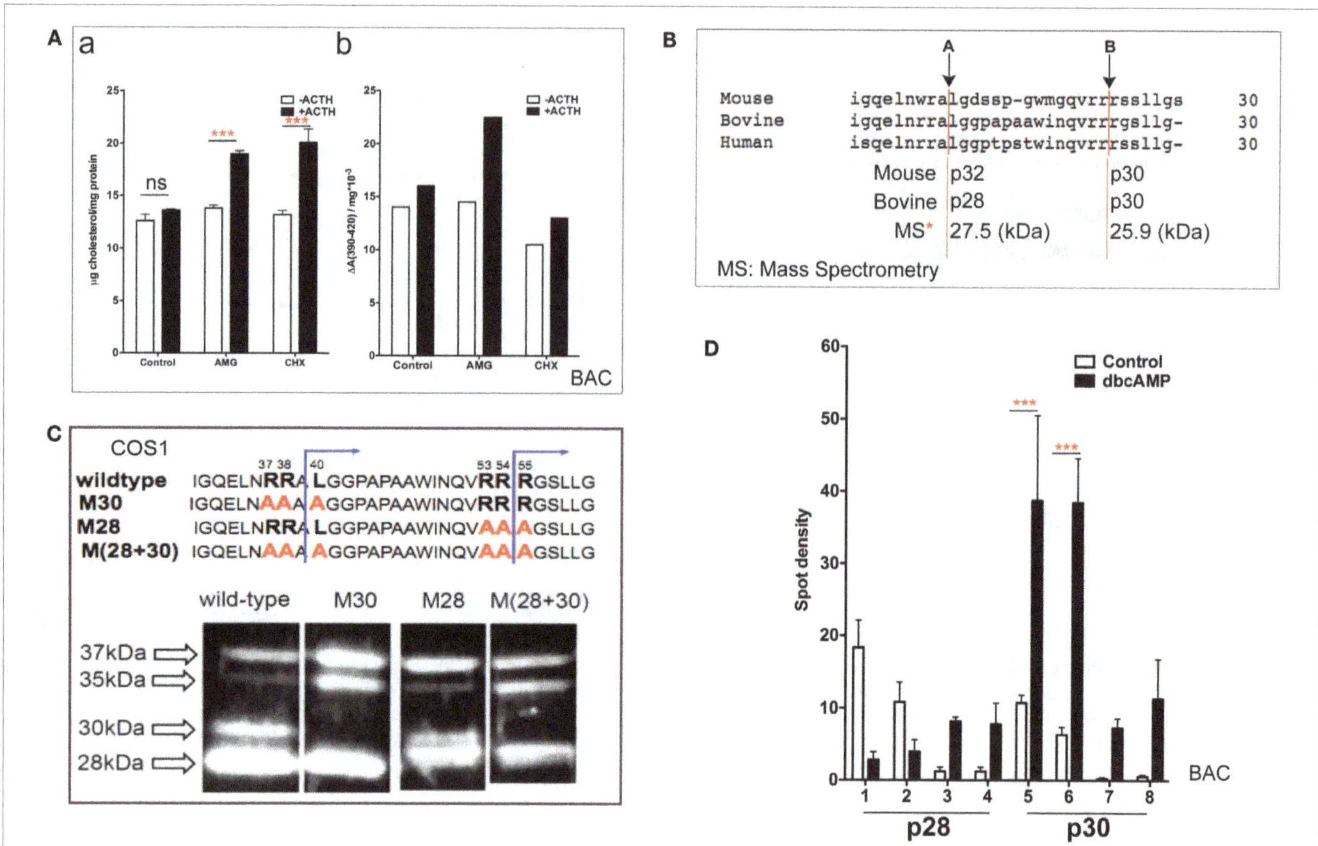

FIGURE 2 | NTD cleavage in COS-1 cells parallels changes in primary bovine adrenal cells. (A) Effects of aminoglutethimide (0.5 mM) and cycloheximide (0.2 mM) on cholesterol transfer in ACTH-stimulated cultured bovine adrenal cells (47) are shown in (a) mitochondrial cholesterol and (b) determination of cholesterol–CYP11A1 complex. Data are represented as mean ± SEM, ***$P < 0.001$. **(B)** Multispecies sequence comparison of StAR NTD that shares conserved MMP cleavage sites A and B. The typically used mouse and bovine identification of products is compared to the average M.W determined by mass spectrometry for bovine products. **(C)** Mutation of conserved cleavage sites (M28, M30) in the NTD of bovine StAR. The blue lines indicate the predicted cleavage sites for the production of the 30- and 28-kDa form of StAR. Expression of CMV bovine StAR vectors in COS-1 cells. Effects of mutations as observed by immunoblotting for StAR (48). **(D)** 2D gel determinations of NTD cleavage products in BAC cells (20). Decreases (p28, #1–2) and increases (p28, #3–4; p30, #5–6) of NTD cleavage products are shown in response to dibutryl cAMP. Data are represented as mean ± SEM, ***$P < 0.001$.

(p-RNA) and spliced form are shown in **Figure 3D**. The dual presence of p-RNA and sp-RNA at the two StAR loci in Y-1 cells after 60-min stimulation with Br-cAMP is shown in **Figure 3E**. Elsewhere, we have shown that spliced and unspliced transcripts can be resolved at these loci with N-SIM ultrahigh-resolution microscopy. Separation in MA-10 cells varies from 100 to 300 nm (38). **Figure 3F** shows that p-RNA and sp-RNA are detectable at low levels in association with the loci in most adrenal cells, although they are undetectable in MA-10 cells. Cytoplasmic mRNA is also appreciable, corresponding to higher levels than those observed in MA-10 cells, even after 60 min of stimulation. There are significant increases for both p-RNA and sp-RNA in approximately half of the loci after 15 min, but no increases in cytoplasmic mRNA.

High-resolution fluorescence *in situ* hybridization confirms the q-PCR basal expression of StAR. Thus, in contrast to MA-10 testis cells, HR-FISH imaging of Y-1 cells reveals p-RNA and sp-RNA at the loci, although at much lower levels than those observed after 60 min of stimulation. Variable levels of expression can be seen at the loci in each cell, representing different numbers of transcripts. Some cells have only one active locus, and some have no active loci, corresponding to the asymmetric activation of StAR loci and the asynchronous responses of individual cells as previously reported for MA-10 cells (37, 38). Importantly, mRNA is visible in the cytoplasm under basal conditions with this greater experimental sensitivity. Following a 15-min stimulation by Br-cAMP that induces maximum steroidogenesis in Y-1 cells (1), the intensity of p-RNA expression at the loci increases. However, the increase in sp-RNA is modest, consistent with the q-PCR results (**Figure 3B**), indicating no increase in cytoplasmic mRNA, despite maximal steroidogenesis.

Y-1 Cells Share Undergo Early Onset Slow Splicing and Delayed Rapid Splicing Phases

q-PCR analyses of Br-cAMP stimulation through 120 min (**Figure 4A**) indicate that both early and extended sites on the 3′UTR only increase after 30 min, although with comparable

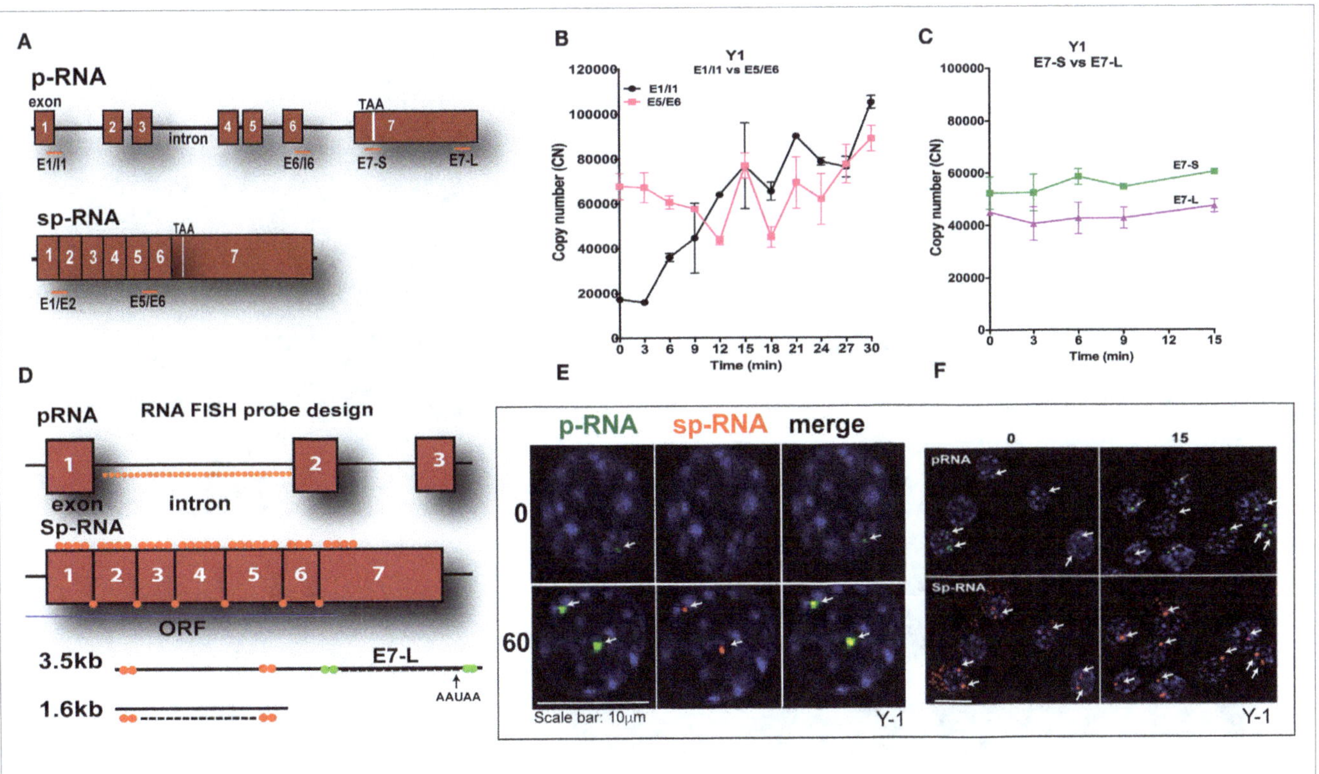

FIGURE 3 | PCR determination of acute activation of StAR transcription in Y-1 adrenal cells. **(A)** Design of PCR primers for StAR p-RNA and sp-RNA/mRNA. **(B)** PCR time course for Y-1 cells [p-RNA (E1/I1) versus sp-RNA (E5/E6)] (0–30 min every 3 min). **(C)** PCR time course for E7-S and E7-L (0–15 min). **(D)** HR-FISH 20-mer fluorescent probes for StAR p-RNA and sp-RNA/mRNA. **(E)** Co-expression of p-RNA and sp-RNA at StAR loci in Y-1 cells after 60 min of stimulation. **(F)** Locus changes and cytoplasmic mRNA in Y-1 cells under basal conditions and after acute activation for 15 min (p-RNA versus sp-RNA) (sensitivity is high for mRNA detection).

copy numbers for the E5 and E6 spliced RNA. In **Figure 4B**, the images of StAR loci in multiple cells reveal that as stimulation progresses, more loci per cell become active for both p-RNA and sp-RNA, again mirroring the q-PCR results. The intensities of p-RNA and sp-RNA at the loci also increase as stimulation progresses. In **Figure 4C**, the images of typical nuclei indicate that levels of p-RNA and sp-RNA are not comparable until 60 min of stimulation. This is consistent with the delay in splicing identified from the q-PCR analyses.

Figure 4D diagrams different optical slices taken at various cellular depths. The StAR loci are always positioned close to the nuclear midline, whereas the cytoplasmic mRNA is largely distributed at lower levels. To determine the proportions and distribution of the 1.6- and 3.5-kb StAR mRNA forms, we used both sp-RNA probes and an additional set, targeting an 800-bp sequence at the 3′ end of the 3.5-kb mRNA UTR (3′EU probes). **Figure 4E** indicates that cytoplasmic 3.5-kb mRNA exhibits dual labeling. These probes extensively overlap at the loci, which appear strongly yellow. **Figure 4F** shows the measurement of the nucleus, locus, and individual messages. The length of the diameter of Y-1 cell is approximately 5–10 μm. The length of a diffraction-limited mRNA dot is about 0.2 μm. The juxtaposition of the two probes on the 3.5-kb mRNA is evident for approximately 60% of mRNA particles (**Figure 4G**). The size distribution is consistent with a single mRNA species (37). However, equal numbers of mRNAs are singly hybridized either by sp-RNA or 3′EU. Single 3′EU hybridization should represent incomplete binding to the 3.5-kb mRNA, similar to single sp-RNA hybridization. Detection of the 1.6-kb mRNA form is evidenced by the enrichment of such binding in lower *Z*-slices.

The mitochondria uniformly express the StAR protein in the inner matrix (38). Interestingly, after 60 min of stimulation, approximately half of StAR sp-RNA hybridization, which is predominantly represented by the 3.5-kb mRNA form, pairs with StAR proteins (**Figure 4H**). StAR mRNA is expected to position on polyribosomes attached to the OMM (**Figure 4I**). Adrenal mitochondria have a diameter of approximately 0.5 μm (15).

SIK1 Is Induced Rapidly *via* Expression of the 4.4-kb mRNA but Prior to the Increase in Protein Levels

CRTC2 activation, which is essential for StAR transcription, is suppressed by SIK1 and SIK2 in adrenal cells. Each shares a conserved mechanism of control, but SIK2 is predominantly constitutive and located in the cytoplasm, whereas SIK1 in highly inducible by PKA. SIK1 is regulated through dual phosphorylation at T182 by LKB1 in the catalytic domain and by PKA at SIK577 in the C-terminal region (43) (**Figure 5A**). After Br-cAMP stimulation, SIK1 p-RNA increases to a steady

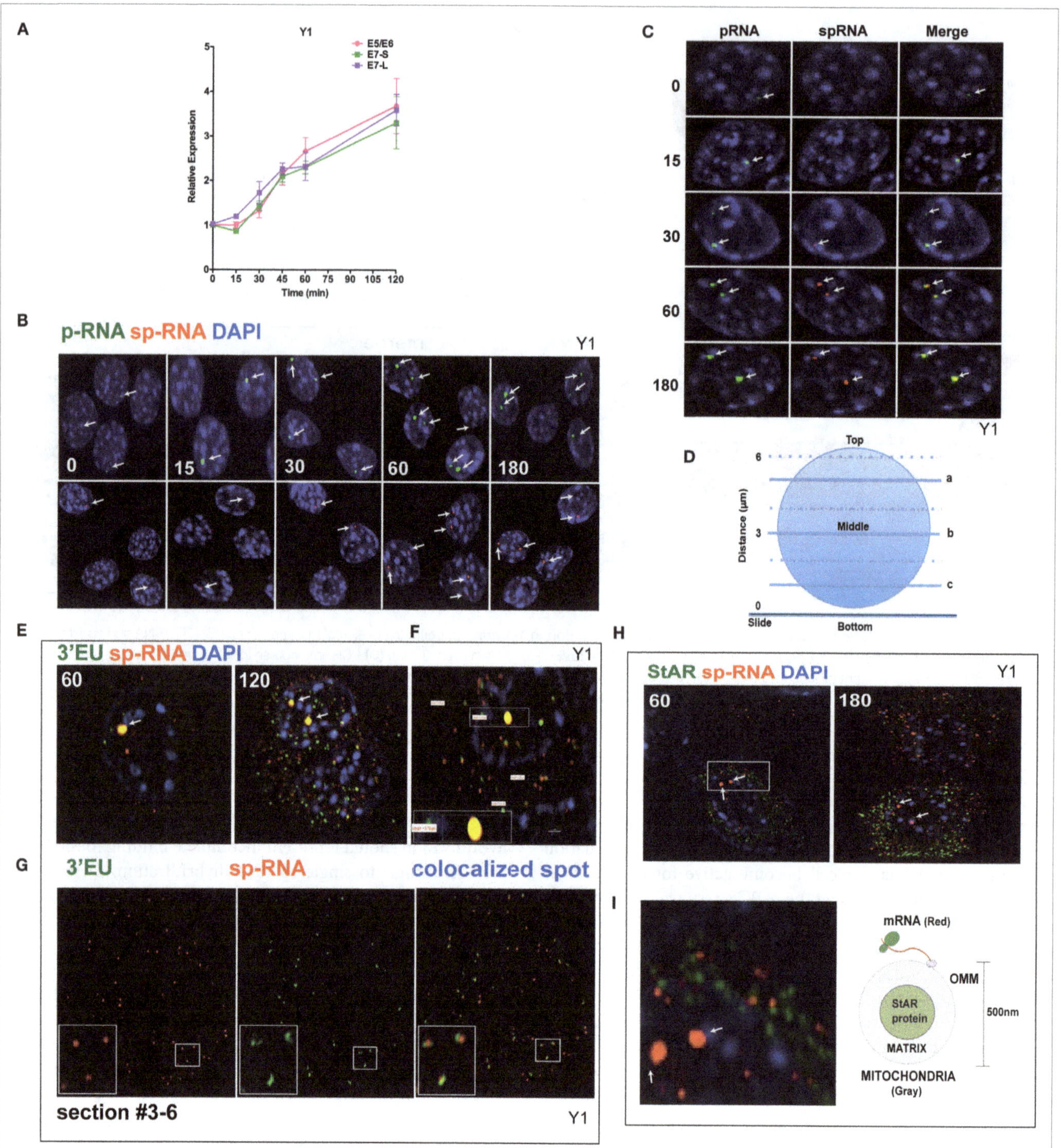

FIGURE 4 | Spatiotemporal regulation of StAR mRNA in Y-1 cells. (A) Time course of 0–120 min for the stimulation of StAR RNA as determined by q-PCR to detect the 3′UTR (E7-S, E7-L) and translated sequence (E5/E6). **(B)** p-RNA and sp-RNA at StAR loci in multiple cells; sensitivity is sufficient to detect RNA concentrated at loci but not cytoplasmic mRNA. Lower expression of mRNA requires a higher sensitivity setting for the microscope. **(C)** Loci in representative nuclei (0–180 min). p-RNA, sp-RNA, and merged. **(D)** Nuclear positioning for *Z*-sections a, b, and c. The positioning of sp-RNA versus 3′EU HR-FISH probes. StAR loci are found near the nuclear midline; cytoplasmic StAR mRNA is primarily observed between slice b and the adherent plasma membrane (37). **(E)** *Z*-projections of HR-FISH for StAR RNA at high sensitivity (N-SIM microscope) after stimulation for 60 and 120 min (dual addition of 3′EU and sp-RNA). StAR loci (yellow, due to probe overlap), sp-RNA (red), and 3′EU (green) visualize cytoplasmic mRNA. DAPI (blue) visualizes nuclear DNA. **(F)** Measurements of the nucleus, locus, and individual message. Scale bar, 1 μm. **(G)** N-SIM mRNA images after 120 min in the lower portion of the cell (slice c) with dual labeling by sp-RNA and 3′EU. Enlargement resolution of dual labeling with StAR mRNA and sp-RNA or 3′EU. **(H)** HR-FISH of StAR mRNA (sp-RNA) and immunochemistry of StAR proteins after 60 and 180 min of stimulation employing N-SIM microscopy. The StAR protein is present in the matrix of all Y-1 mitochondria (38). **(I)** Enlarged region after 60 min of stimulation showing the pairing of StAR mRNA and mitochondrial matrix-localized StAR proteins. Diagram of the spatial relationship between matrix proteins and OMM-associated StAR mRNA.

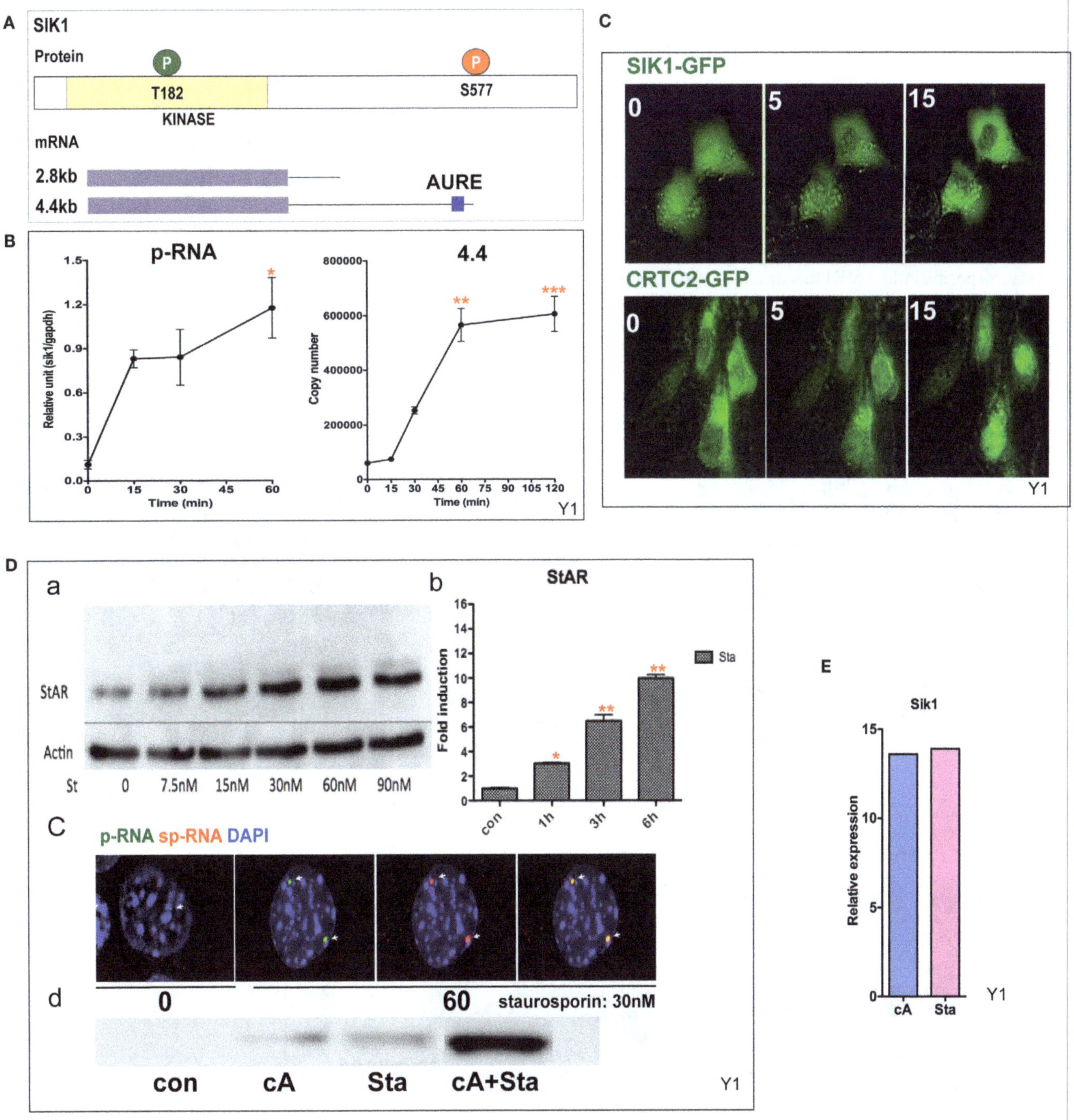

FIGURE 5 | Induction and mobilization of SIK1 in Y-1 cells. **(A)** Diagram of SIK1 protein kinase sites; T182/LKB, S577 PKA. Short and long mRNAs differing in terms of their 3′UTR. **(B)** Stimulation of SIK1 p-RNA and long mRNA (4.4 kb) by Br-cAMP. Data are represented as mean ± SEM, $^{*}P < 0.05$, $^{**}P < 0.01$, and $^{***}P < 0.001$. **(C)** Br-cAMP (1 mM) affects the relocation of SIK1–GFP (initially nuclear) and CRTC2–GFP (initially cytoplasmic) (38). **(D)** Induction by the SIK1 inhibitor staurosporine; concentration (a), time-dependence (b), stimulation of RNA and sp-RNA at the gene loci after 60 min (c), and synergy lowering the E50 for each (d). **(E)** Br-cAMP and staurosporine induce SIK1 to a similar extent, suggesting that SIK1 exhibits feedback control.

state within 15 min, while the 4.4-kb mRNA form that contains the extended 3′UTR exhibits a delay of 15 min but reaches a steady state after 60 min (**Figure 5B**). The q-PCR primers for the translated sequence, which quantify both mRNA forms, indicate that mRNA transcription responses follow the same time course (not shown). This 4.4-kb form, like the 3.5-kb StAR mRNA form, contains AU-rich elements. The SIK2 form with high basal expression responds minimally to Br-cAMP [Ref. (38, 49), p. 502]. After the inhibition of SIK2 when PKA is activated, CRTC2 is dephosphorylated by cytoplasmic phosphatases and then migrates into the nucleus (38). This relocation is stimulated by ACTH within the same time frame *in vivo* (49). The two proteins complete their exchange within 15 min (**Figure 5C**). As noted earlier, some StAR loci require between 15 and 60 min for initiation. We found no evidence for significant asynchrony in CRTC2 or SIK1 transfer, indicating that the availability of CRTC2 and SIK1 is not a cause of asynchrony.

Staurosporine, although a general kinase inhibitor, potently inhibits SIK forms and induces StAR by 10-fold within 6 h (EC50 = 15 nM). Br-cAMP and staurosporine demonstrate effective synergy, lowering the EC50 for each (**Figure 5D**). Br-cAMP and staurosporine induce SIK1 to a similar extent, suggesting that SIK1 exhibits feedback control (**Figure 5E**). This inhibition of the SIK forms does not affect CREB phosphorylation. The slower staurosporine induction of StAR transcription compared to Br-cAMP should reflect additional PKA contributions, including CREB S133 phosphorylation.

SIK1 Completely Blocks StAR Transcription in Y-1 Cells When PKA Sites Are Blocked by Mutations

Mutation at SIK1-S577 prevents the inhibition of SIK1 and also induces the complete relocation of SIK1 to the nuclear speckles and prevents PKA-mediated export to the cytoplasm (**Figure 6A**). We have previously shown that nuclear SIK-S577A does not slow the initial transfer of CRTC2-GFP to the nucleus but eventually limits the extent of transfer. Surprisingly, CRTC2

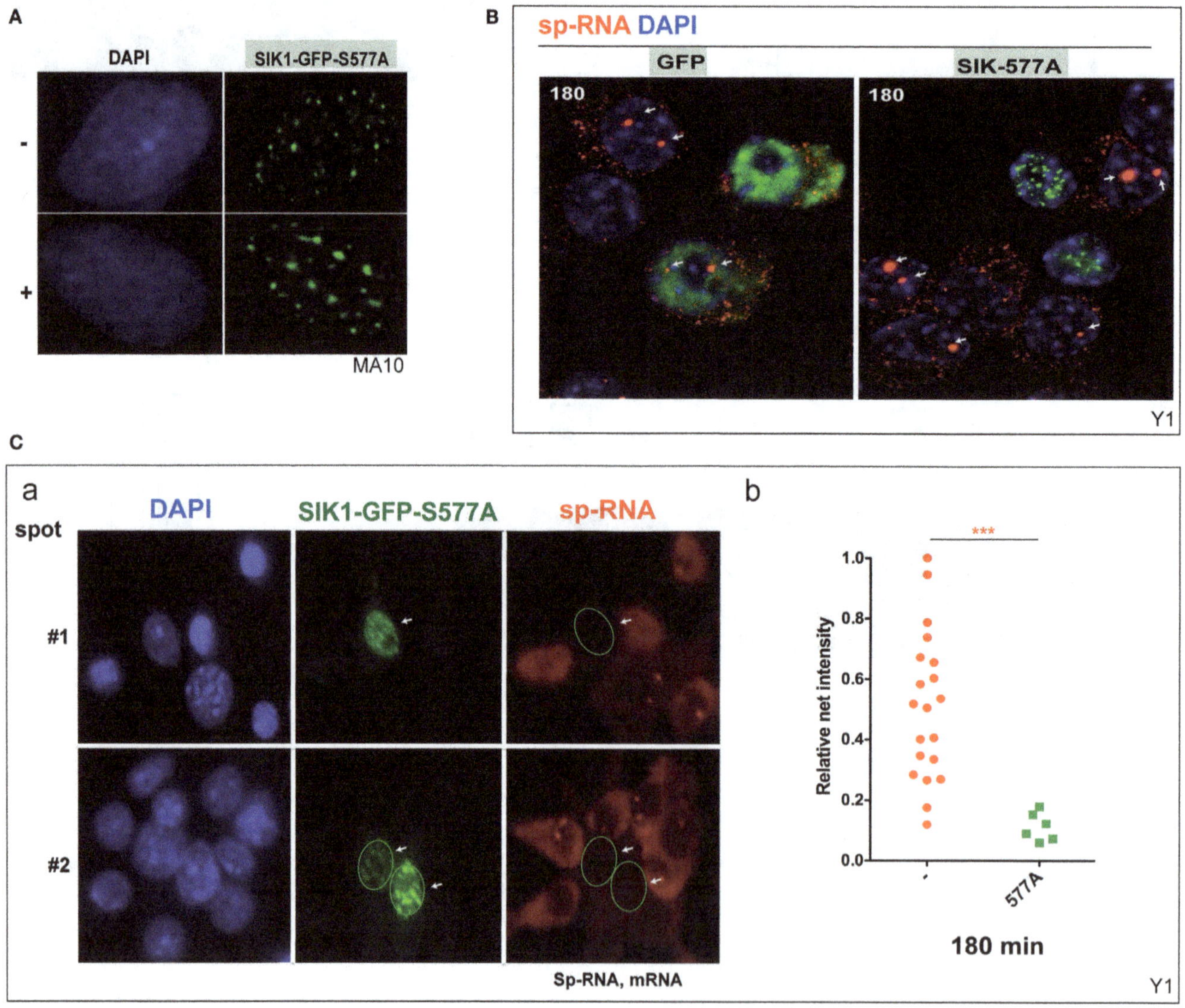

FIGURE 6 | Inhibition of basal and induced expression of StAR by PKA-resistant SIK1–S577A–GFP. (A) Nuclear location of SIK1–S577A–GFP with and without Br-cAMP. **(B)** Suppression of Br-cAMP induction (180 min) of StAR RNA at the loci or in the cytoplasm in cells that transfected with SIK1–S577A–GFP versus GFP. **(C)** Quantitative expression in transfected Y-1 cells versus neighboring untransfected cells (a, image #1 and image #2). Associated mRNA intensity in 20 transfected cells versus 6 adjacent untransfected cells (b).

and SIK1–S577A co-localize in these nuclear speckles before CRTC2 is eventually phosphorylated by SIK1 and reverts to its cytoplasmic localization (38).

We show that the stimulation of Y-1 cells by Br-cAMP for 180 min is completely prevented in cells that express SIK1–S577–GFP, but not the control GFP vector (**Figure 6B**). StAR expression was undetectable in Y-1 cells expressing SIK1–S577A–GFP, but expression was normal in cells lacking the inhibitory vector or expressing the GFP control vector. We have quantitated the impact on acute expression and expression after 180 min of stimulation (**Figure 6C**).

StAR Is Selectively Targeted by Znf36l1/Tis11b in the 3′UTR of the 3.5-kb mRNA

The Zn-finger protein Znf36l1/Tis11b binds as a dimer to the extended 3′UTR of the 3.5-kb form of StAR through a TATTTATT sequence that forms a homodimer with Tis11b (**Figure 7A**). Based on this element, TIS11b targets a variety of regulatory proteins, including VEGF (50) (**Figure 7B**). This target sequence is conserved in the extended region of the StAR 3′UTR at equivalent positions surrounding the polyadenylation site for both mice and humans (**Figure 7C**). CMV–StAR expression vectors differing only in their 3′UTR sequence were co-expressed with a TIS11b expression vector in MA-10 cells. StAR protein levels are most extensively decreased with the full 3′UTR sequence. Similar results were obtained with Y-1 cells. Co-expression of TIS11b specifically decreases expression of the extended 3′UTR that contains the TIS11b recognition element. This loss of the StAR protein is matched by the loss of StAR mRNA (**Figure 7D**).

StAR 3.5-kb mRNA Is Suppressed by the Expression of Tis11b in Y-1 and MA-10 Cells. Deletion of TIS11b *via* Long-term shRNA Expression

Tis11b is highly induced by Br-cAMP in MA-10 and Y-1 cells (**Figure 8A**). We tested the effects of TIS11b on StAR expression in MA-10 and Y-1 cells *via* the transient introduction of siRNA and shRNA and the generation of cell lines expressing a CMV-promoted shRNA vector. Tis11b levels were reduced by the transfection of siRNA, 24 h prior to the addition of Br-cAMP (**Figure 8B**). The near complete suppression of TIS11b selectively increases StAR 3.5-kb mRNA levels by approximately 50% without altering 1.6-kb mRNA levels (**Figure 8C**).

Tis11b was equivalently suppressed in Y-1 and MA-10 cells following the permanent expression of shRNA (versus scrambled shRNA) targeting the Tis11b sequence. This process differs from direct siRNA in that it requires significant cell amplification following the selection process. Passage number affects the PKA response characteristics. TIS11b suppression equally affected both the 3.5- and 1.6-kb forms at all doses of Br-cAMP in both Y-1 and MA-10 cells (**Figures 8D,E**). The effects of Tis11b suppression correspond to a 5- to 10-fold increase in the EC50 for Br-cAMP in each line (**Figures 8F,G**).

Nuclear versus Cytoplasmic Distribution of TIS11b

Separation of the nuclei and cytoplasm in each cell line revealed that appreciable amounts of TIS11b were present

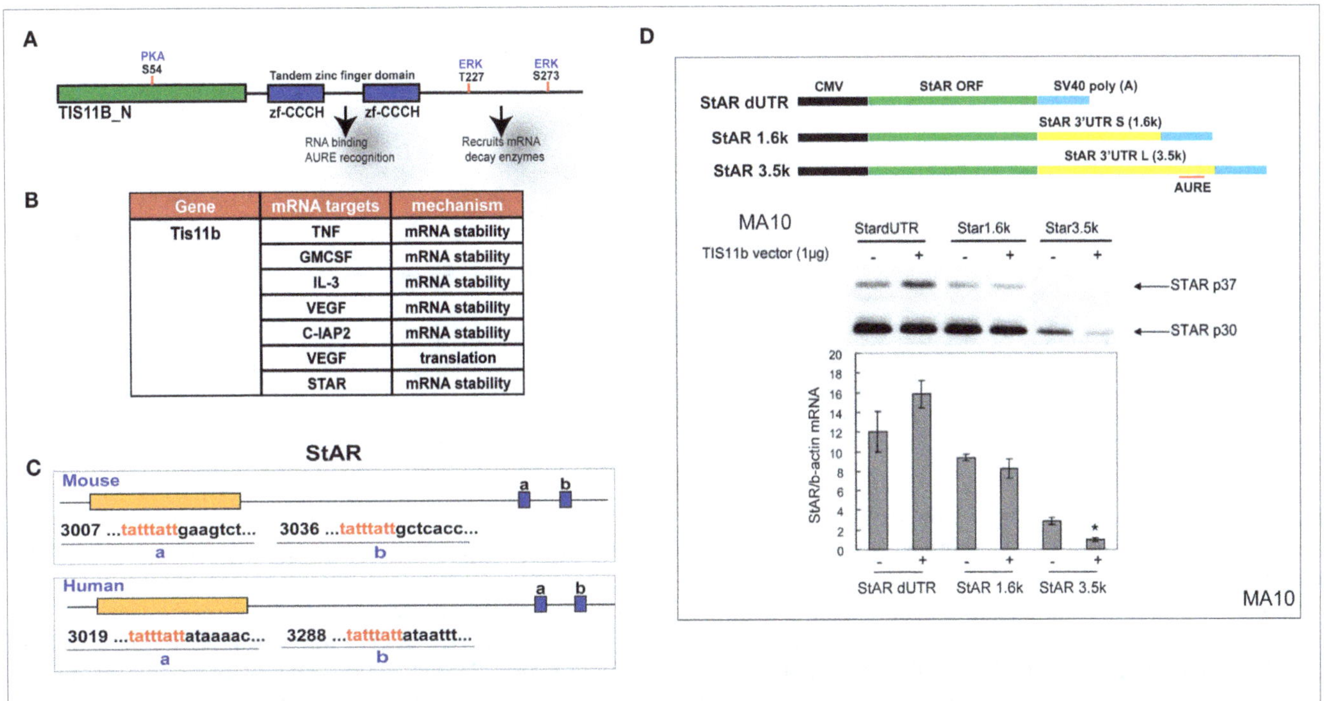

FIGURE 7 | Selective targeting of extended StAR 3′UTR by transfected TIS11b/Znf36l1. (A) The structure of TIS11b/Znf36li with RNA binding Zn-finger domains and kinase sites. **(B)** Other genes exhibiting RNA target sites (TATTTATT) (51). **(C)** Tis11b targeted sequences are conserved in mouse and human StAR 3′UTRs, specifically the terminal cleavage/polyadenylation site. **(D)** The impact of TIS11b on StAR mRNA and protein expression according to terms of the 3′UTR length: CMV–StAR vectors; StAR protein expression (immunoblot) and mRNA (q-PCR relative to actin) with and without Tis11b transfection (34).

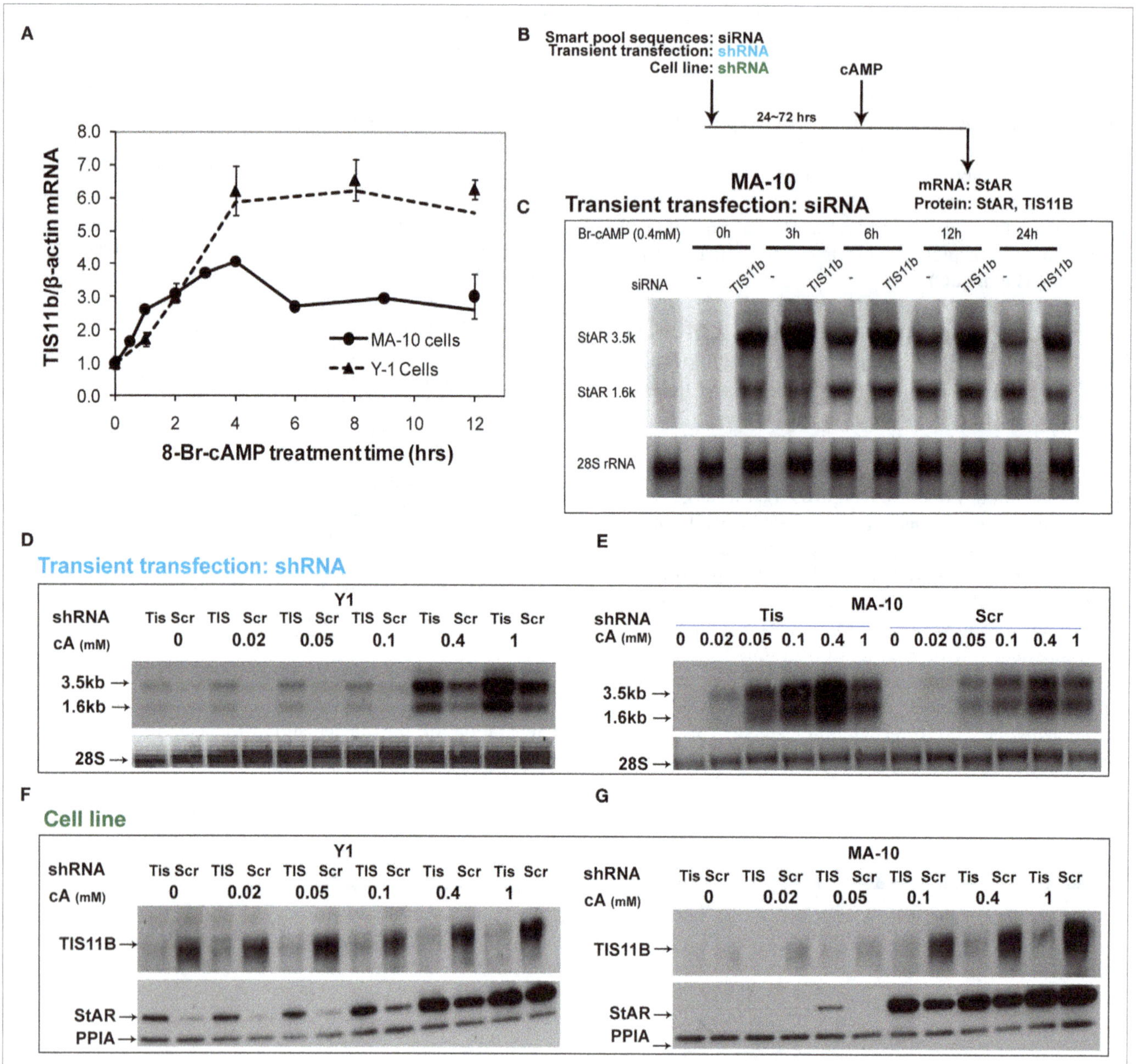

FIGURE 8 | Suppressive effects of Tis11b in both Y-1 and MA-10 cells. (A) Induction of TIS11b in Y-1 and MA-10 cells by 1 mM Br-cAMP, measured by q-PCR (34). **(B)** Schematic for the suppression of TIS11b using siRNA and shRNA in the indicated cell lines. **(C)** Time course for the selective stimulation of 3.5-kb StAR mRNA following the suppression of Tis11b (34). **(D,E)** Effects of Tis11b (shRNA) suppression on the dose–response stimulation of StAR mRNA levels. **(F,G)** Effects of Tis11b (cell line) suppression on the dose–response stimulation of Tis11b mRNA and StAR protein levels.

in both fractions and that expression in both the nuclear and cytoplasmic fractions was increased by the application of Br-cAMP (**Figure 9A**). Examination of MA-10 cells by immunohistochemistry showed that TIS11b was predominantly present in nuclear speckles under basal conditions but then increased in the cytoplasm following stimulation by Br-cAMP with a half-life of approximately 60 min and peak cytoplasmic levels after 3–6 h. We also created a TIS11b–GFP fusion protein. Unlike native Tis11b, the fusion protein does not exhibit net transfer into the nucleus, even under basal conditions (not shown) (**Figure 9B**). Analysis of StAR sp-RNA in the nuclei and cytoplasm of cells expressing Tis11b–GFP indicated suppression at both the StAR loci and in the cytoplasm. Expression is maintained in cells expressing the GFP control (**Figure 9C**). **Figure 9D** illustrates the quantitation of mRNA in cells that individually express either or neither of the GFP vectors. The efficacy of Tis11b–GFP is evident. Finally, we show the modulation of StAR control of cholesterol availability *via* the N-terminal StAR regulatory domain, SIK1, and TIS11b (**Figure 10**).

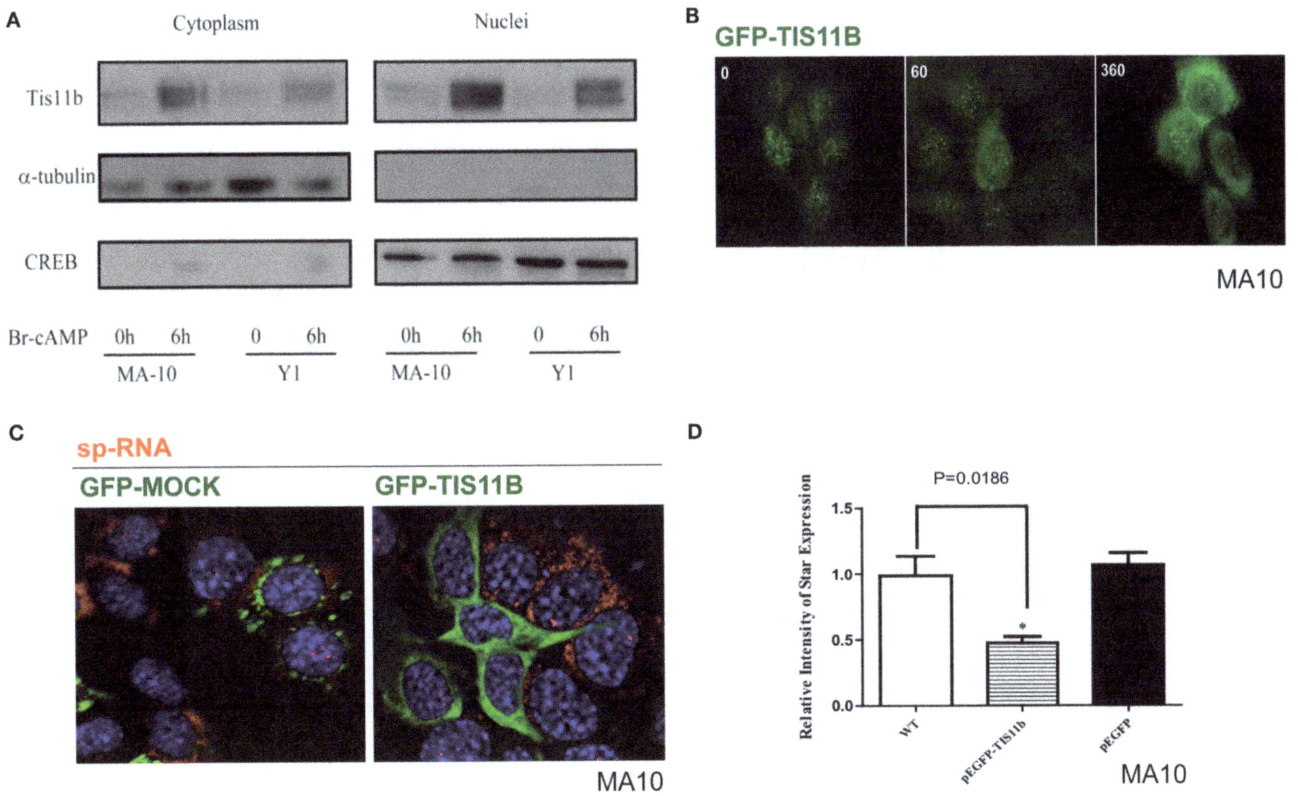

FIGURE 9 | Nuclear/cytoplasmic distribution of Tis11b and activity. (A) TIS11b protein expression in the nuclei and cytoplasm of Y-1 and MA-10 cells under basal conditions and after stimulation (6 h/400 μM Br-cAMP). **(B)** Effects of stimulation time on TIS11b immunohistochemistry in MA-10 cells. **(C)** Stimulation of StAR sp-RNA/mRNA in MA-10 cells transfected with either mock CMV–GFP or CMV–Tis11b–GFP. **(D)** Quantitation of StAR sp-RNA/mRNA in MA-10 cells transfected with either mock CMV–GFP or CMV–Tis11b–GFP.

DISCUSSION

Previous work to elucidate the mechanism of mitochondrial cholesterol transfer has largely focused on the COS-1 model, in which StAR CBD is transfected with a functioning mitochondrial Cyp11a1 system (11, 52). In this model, the StAR CBD is sufficient to obtain maximum cholesterol transfer, including when this domain anchored to the OMM. NT sequences that result in rapid CBD import attenuate activity, consistent with primary CBD activity on the OMM and low activity derived from transit to the IMM. However, these definitive findings raise questions concerning the much more potent activity observed in adrenal cells. In COS-1 cells, p37 StAR import and processing are similar to Y-1 cells (**Figure 1B**) but are far slower. Therefore, p37 is resident for longer periods of time at the OMM, shifting greater weight onto the OMM steps. Even in MA-10 cells, CYP11a1 levels are modest compared to primary adrenal cells, thus demanding less of the StAR transfer process. In Y-1 cells, more rapid StAR import delivers results in much more rapid cholesterol transfer with very low levels of StAR expression, including a notably lower proportion of OMM p37. This paper addresses the role of the NTD in increasing the potency of StAR and decreasing the inadvertent side effects of cytoplasmic StAR (53). The rapid removal of StAR and glucocorticoids is a component of this NTP activity, which is an important feature of ACTH physiology (54). Here, we provide an update regarding two acute cAMP-mediated responses in adrenal cells that antagonize the StAR mechanism.

Under physiological conditions, ACTH stimulates cholesterol transfer activity in adrenal cells, not only at low StAR mRNA levels but also through a coordinated translation/phosphorylation mechanism (47). CHX inhibition results in cholesterol reaching the OMM, but with a distribution that provides minimal access to IMM Cyp11a1 (**Figure 2A**). This initial dependence on StAR CBD activity in the OMM suggests that a first step involves the redistribution of cholesterol to sites where transfer occurs to the IMM, albeit at a suboptimal rate for adrenal cells. Inter-mitochondrial membrane and ER membrane fusion processes appear to be important for this process (31, 52) as well as proteins, such as TSPO, the sigma receptor, and various VDAC forms (28). A relationship with the IMM Ca-sensitive permeability complex, which is regulated by TSPO/VDAC1, appears likely (27). Membrane cross-linking experiments have identified various intermembrane complexes (28), although typically under conditions where mitochondrial integrity has not been a point of focus. Here, we note the importance of this integrity because contacts and cholesterol transfer readily occur even when perturbations result in the retention of Krebs cycle activity. We have previously suggested that low levels of succinate depend on

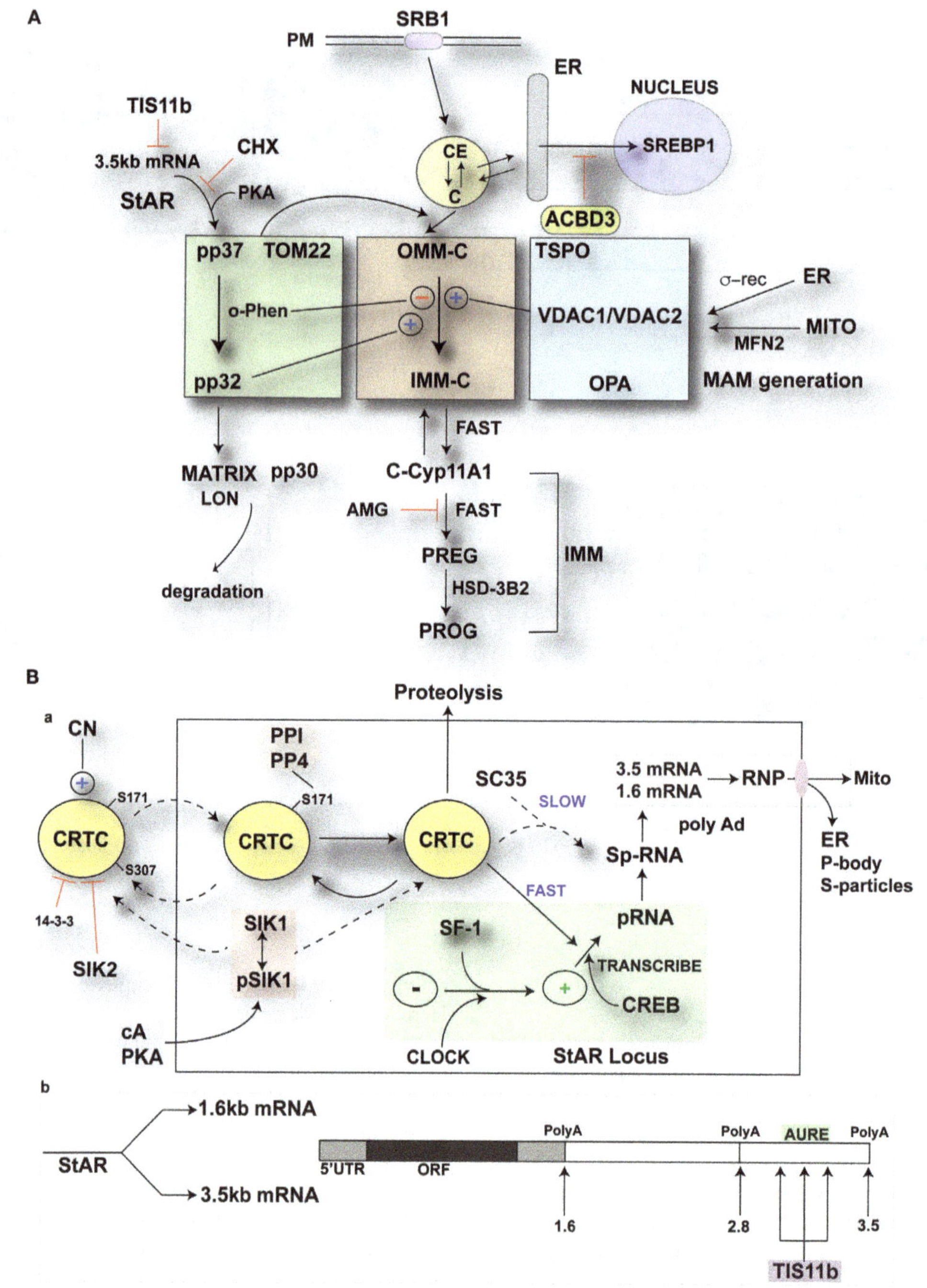

FIGURE 10 | Modulation of StAR control of cholesterol availability *via* the N-terminal StAR regulatory domain, SIK1, and TIS11b. (A) Modulation of the cholesterol transfer activity of the C-terminal StAR domain by the N-terminal regulatory domain. Three functional compartments are distinguishable: green: StAR transfer from OMM cholesterol-binding activity and transfer of pp37 from the OMM to the IMM, where proteolytic processing occurs with possible supplemental activity in adrenal cells. Brown: cholesterol transfer at sites of membrane contact, possibly directed by mPTP modulation. Blue: factors modulating the partnership between StAR and cholesterol, including VDACs, TSPO, GTPases (OPA1, MFN2), and the activation effects of membrane fusion (ER, inter-into). **(B)** (a) schematic detailing the activities of SIK1 and CRTC2 in mediating the effects of cAMP and PKA on StAR mRNA expression in comparison to Tis11b and (b) modulation of StAR mRNA availability to the mitochondria by SIK1/CRTC2 (transcription and splicing) and Znf36l1/Tis11b (regulation of 3.5-kb StAR mRNA location/3′UTR processing).

mitochondrial integrity and ATP generation to support NADPH generation by NNT (8).

The deletion of 47 amino acids from the StAR NTD largely restores corticosterone synthesis to StAR-ko mice, but only with a compensating rise in cytoplasmic cholesterol. This increase alone should enhance mitochondrial uptake. In contrast, N-47 StAR is completely ineffective in Leydig cells where no such compensation occurs (15). The presence of cytoplasmic StAR that exerts effective cholesterol transfer activity (55) redirects cholesterol to other sites and activities (53). The C-terminal domain (CTD) alone works with sufficient ACTH to overstimulate SR-B1/HSL to activate homeostasis directed by the SREBP and LXR forms (56).

The HR-FISH approach presented here shows individual StAR 3.5-kb mRNA molecules paired with single mitochondria (**Figure 4I**). StAR-mediated cholesterol transfer into adrenal mitochondria is a co-translational process as evidenced by the rapid inhibition induced by CHX. Close access of StAR mRNA to the mitochondria is necessary. StAR mRNA 5′-3′ dual hybridization, size analyses, and counts per cell in terms of q-PCR copy numbers indicate that nearly all StAR mRNA was imaged in the 3.5-kb form. NTD, targeting the import process, determines the key spatiotemporal aspects of this process. Rigorous MS analyses of the intermediate StAR forms revealed two conserved cleavage sites. Metalloprotease cleavage enzymes (MMPs) on the inside of the IMM generate intermembrane StAR with either BAC or rodent sequences. We propose that the first cleavage (A) is an activation step (p30/p32 likely refers to same cleavage site), while the second cleavage inactivates and perhaps moves the StAR core to LON-directed clearance sites in the matrix (53). Site A cleavage exposes a hydrophobic sequence in an intermediate form that has been recognized as being at least dually modified in 2D gels (1, 32). Interaction of the p30/p32 forms with VDAC2 has been linked to the cholesterol transfer process (14). Potent inhibition of this MMP cleavage in Y-1 cells by o-phenanthroline selectively intervenes in this process without affecting mitochondrial Cyp11a1 activity (1).

High-resolution fluorescence *in situ* hybridization analyses of StAR expression at the gene loci established that slow splicing of StAR p-RNA attenuates mRNA during acute stimulation and ultradian oscillations. Prolonged effects of stress or diurnal changes are necessary to increase StAR mRNA.

cAMP also rapidly induces SIK1, which decreases the transcription of StAR. The ready entry of SIK1 into the nucleus and the susceptibility of CRTC2 to direct inhibition there through S-171 phosphorylation represent a rapid mechanism to minimize StAR p-RNA accumulation (41, 57). SIK1 induction through a 4.4-kb labile mRNA that is induced by CREB/CRTC2 activation also introduces rapid feedback inhibition. SIK1 becomes active as cAMP and PKA activity decline, thus releasing the inhibitory dephosph-S577 form. SIK inhibition alone is nearly as effective as cAMP in producing both transcription and splicing at the StAR loci (**Figure 5D**). We expect that the high levels of SIK1 during the rapid cAMP decline after the application of pulsatile stimuli will contribute to the non-genomic decline of StAR p-RNA (54).

TIS11b exclusively targets the terminal segment of the 3.5-kb mRNA through the formation of homodimers at conserved AU-rich sites in the extended 3′UTR. This control mechanism, likely targeting the mitochondria (44), provide an explanation for the near-exclusive initial formation of the 3.5-kb mRNA, although this form is less stable, and the 1.6-kb form is an equivalent source of protein (46). Tis11b may target nuclear StAR p-RNA and 3.5-kb mRNA prior to conversion to the 1.6-kb mRNA form. Interestingly, Tis11b mRNA is also expressed with a long 3′UTR that contains the homodimer recognition element, thus allowing self-regulation. Tis11b, the SIK forms, and CRTC2 can function coordinately through the shared and competitive binding of their phosphorylated forms to cytoplasmic 14–3–3.

Highlights for StAR Regulation in Adrenal Cells

Adrenocorticotropic hormone stimulation of cholesterol metabolism requires continuous translation and phosphorylation of p37 StAR. The CBD generates substantial activity through the redistribution of cholesterol at the OMM aided by other OMM proteins, including TSPO and VDAC1. Peak glucocorticoid formation is achieved with low basal levels of the 3.5-kb mRNA form, which individually pairs with single mitochondria. Cholesterol transfer may be enhanced by conserved site A NTD cleavage by IMM metalloproteases and terminated by site B cleavage. StAR 3.5-kb mRNA formation is slowed by a pause in elongation, slow splicing, and the intervention of TIS11b through sites at the end of the 3′UTR. Dephosphorylated CRTC assumes control of transcription and splicing at StAR gene loci, where p-RNA and sp-RNA have been spatially separated by HR-FISH. The inhibition of SIK forms alone replicates the PKA activation of StAR expression in adrenal cells. cAMP-mediated induction of SIK1 by ACTH attenuates StAR through migration into nuclear sites shared with CRTC2, once ACTH levels and cAMP decline during physiological pulses.

AUTHOR CONTRIBUTIONS

We thank members of Jefocate lab as well as TY for NTD work.

ACKNOWLEDGMENTS

The MA-10 cell line was a generous gift from Professor Mario Ascoli. This study was financially supported by the NIH (RO1 DK074819, RO1 DK090249).

REFERENCES

1. Artemenko IP, Zhao D, Hales DB, Hales KH, Jefcoate CR. Mitochondrial processing of newly synthesized steroidogenic acute regulatory protein (StAR), but not total StAR, mediates cholesterol transfer to cytochrome P450 side chain cleavage enzyme in adrenal cells. *J Biol Chem* (2001) 276:46583–96. doi:10.1074/jbc.M107815200
2. Caron KM, Ikeda Y, Soo SC, Stocco DM, Parker KL, Clark BJ. Characterization of the promoter region of the mouse gene encoding the steroidogenic acute regulatory protein. *Mol Endocrinol* (1997) 11:138–47. doi:10.1210/mend.11.2.9880
3. Clark BJ, Wells J, King SR, Stocco DM. The purification, cloning, and expression of a novel luteinizing hormone-induced mitochondrial protein in MA-10 mouse Leydig tumor cells. Characterization of the steroidogenic acute regulatory protein (StAR). *J Biol Chem* (1994) 269:28314–22.
4. Kiriakidou M, McAllister JM, Sugawara T, Strauss JF III. Expression of steroidogenic acute regulatory protein (StAR) in the human ovary. *J Clin Endocrinol Metab* (1996) 81:4122–8. doi:10.1210/jc.81.11.4122
5. Jefcoate CR, Simpson ER, Boyd GS, Brownie AC, Orme-Johnson WH. The detection of different states of the P-450 cytochromes in adrenal mitochondria: changes induced by ACTH. *Ann N Y Acad Sci* (1973) 212:243–61. doi:10.1111/j.1749-6632.1973.tb47600.x

6. Yamazaki T, Kowluru R, McNamara BC, Jefcoate CR. P450scc-dependent cholesterol metabolism in rat adrenal mitochondria is inhibited by low concentrations of matrix Ca2+. *Arch Biochem Biophys* (1995) 318:131–9. doi:10.1006/abbi.1995.1213
7. Hanukoglu I, Jefcoate CR. Mitochondrial cytochrome P-450scc. Mechanism of electron transport by adrenodoxin. *J Biol Chem* (1980) 255:3057–61.
8. Yamazaki T, McNamara BC, Jefcoate CR. Competition for electron transfer between cytochromes P450scc and P45011 beta in rat adrenal mitochondria. *Mol Cell Endocrinol* (1993) 95:1–11. doi:10.1016/0303-7207(93)90023-D
9. Caron KM, Soo SC, Wetsel WC, Stocco DM, Clark BJ, Parker KL. Targeted disruption of the mouse gene encoding steroidogenic acute regulatory protein provides insights into congenital lipoid adrenal hyperplasia. *Proc Natl Acad Sci U S A* (1997) 94:11540–5. doi:10.1073/pnas.94.21.11540
10. Chen X, Baker BY, Abduljabbar MA, Miller WL. A genetic isolate of congenital lipoid adrenal hyperplasia with atypical clinical findings. *J Clin Endocrinol Metab* (2005) 90:835–40. doi:10.1210/jc.2004-1323
11. Sahakitrungruang T, Soccio RE, Lang-Muritano M, Walker JM, Achermann JC, Miller WL. Clinical, genetic, and functional characterization of four patients carrying partial loss-of-function mutations in the steroidogenic acute regulatory protein (StAR). *J Clin Endocrinol Metab* (2010) 95:3352–9. doi:10.1210/jc.2010-0437
12. Baker BY, Yaworsky DC, Miller WL. A pH-dependent molten globule transition is required for activity of the steroidogenic acute regulatory protein, StAR. *J Biol Chem* (2005) 280:41753–60. doi:10.1074/jbc.M510241200
13. Barbar E, Lehoux JG, Lavigne P. Toward the NMR structure of StAR. *Mol Cell Endocrinol* (2009) 300:89–93. doi:10.1016/j.mce.2008.12.007
14. Prasad M, Kaur J, Pawlak KJ, Bose M, Whittal RM, Bose HS. Mitochondria-associated endoplasmic reticulum membrane (MAM) regulates steroidogenic activity via steroidogenic acute regulatory protein (StAR)-voltage-dependent anion channel 2 (VDAC2) interaction. *J Biol Chem* (2015) 290:2604–16. doi:10.1074/jbc.M114.605808
15. Sasaki G, Ishii T, Jeyasuria P, Jo Y, Bahat A, Orly J, et al. Complex role of the mitochondrial targeting signal in the function of steroidogenic acute regulatory protein revealed by bacterial artificial chromosome transgenesis in vivo. *Mol Endocrinol* (2008) 22:951–64. doi:10.1210/me.2007-0493
16. Arakane F, Sugawara T, Nishino H, Liu Z, Holt JA, Pain D, et al. Steroidogenic acute regulatory protein (StAR) retains activity in the absence of its mitochondrial import sequence: implications for the mechanism of StAR action. *Proc Natl Acad Sci U S A* (1996) 93:13731–6. doi:10.1073/pnas.93.24.13731
17. Manna PR, Cohen-Tannoudji J, Counis R, Garner CW, Huhtaniemi I, Kraemer FB, et al. Mechanisms of action of hormone-sensitive lipase in mouse Leydig cells: its role in the regulation of the steroidogenic acute regulatory protein. *J Biol Chem* (2013) 288:8505–18. doi:10.1074/jbc.M112.417873
18. Lin Y, Hou X, Shen WJ, Hanssen R, Khor VK, Cortez Y, et al. SNARE-mediated cholesterol movement to mitochondria supports steroidogenesis in rodent cells. *Mol Endocrinol* (2016) 30:234–47. doi:10.1210/me.2015-1281
19. Dyson MT, Kowalewski MP, Manna PR, Stocco DM. The differential regulation of steroidogenic acute regulatory protein-mediated steroidogenesis by type I and type II PKA in MA-10 cells. *Mol Cell Endocrinol* (2009) 300:94–103. doi:10.1016/j.mce.2008.11.029
20. Elliott ME, Goodfriend TL, Jefcoate CR. Bovine adrenal glomerulosa and fasciculata cells exhibit 28.5-kilodalton proteins sensitive to angiotensin, other agonists, and atrial natriuretic peptide. *Endocrinology* (1993) 133:1669–77. doi:10.1210/endo.133.4.8404608
21. Sugawara T, Fujimoto S. The potential function of steroid sulphatase activity in steroid production and steroidogenic acute regulatory protein expression. *Biochem J* (2004) 380:153–60. doi:10.1042/bj20031379
22. Letourneau D, Lefebvre A, Lavigne P, LeHoux JG. The binding site specificity of STARD4 subfamily: breaking the cholesterol paradigm. *Mol Cell Endocrinol* (2015) 408:53–61. doi:10.1016/j.mce.2014.12.016
23. Kang HW, Wei J, Cohen DE. PC-TP/StARD2: of membranes and metabolism. *Trends Endocrinol Metab* (2010) 21:449–56. doi:10.1016/j.tem.2010.02.001
24. Krueger RJ, Orme-Johnson NR. Acute adrenocorticotropic hormone stimulation of adrenal corticosteroidogenesis. Discovery of a rapidly induced protein. *J Biol Chem* (1983) 258:10159–67.
25. Pon LA, Hartigan JA, Orme-Johnson NR. Acute ACTH regulation of adrenal corticosteroid biosynthesis. Rapid accumulation of a phosphoprotein. *J Biol Chem* (1986) 261:13309–16.
26. Privalle CT, Crivello JF, Jefcoate CR. Regulation of intramitochondrial cholesterol transfer to side-chain cleavage cytochrome P-450 in rat adrenal gland. *Proc Natl Acad Sci U S A* (1983) 80:702–6. doi:10.1073/pnas.80.3.702
27. Fan J, Campioli E, Midzak A, Culty M, Papadopoulos V. Conditional steroidogenic cell-targeted deletion of TSPO unveils a crucial role in viability and hormone-dependent steroid formation. *Proc Natl Acad Sci U S A* (2015) 112:7261–6. doi:10.1073/pnas.1502670112
28. Rone MB, Midzak AS, Issop L, Rammouz G, Jagannathan S, Fan J, et al. Identification of a dynamic mitochondrial protein complex driving cholesterol import, trafficking, and metabolism to steroid hormones. *Mol Endocrinol* (2012) 26:1868–82. doi:10.1210/me.2012-1159
29. Chen Y, Patel V, Bang S, Cohen N, Millar J, Kim SF. Maturation and activity of sterol regulatory element binding protein 1 is inhibited by acyl-CoA binding domain containing 3. *PLoS One* (2012) 7:e49906. doi:10.1371/journal.pone.0049906
30. Kowluru R, Yamazaki T, McNamara BC, Jefcoate CR. Metabolism of exogenous cholesterol by rat adrenal mitochondria is stimulated equally by physiological levels of free Ca2+ and by GTP. *Mol Cell Endocrinol* (1995) 107:181–8. doi:10.1016/0303-7207(94)03441-U
31. Duarte A, Poderoso C, Cooke M, Soria G, Cornejo Maciel F, Gottifredi V, et al. Mitochondrial fusion is essential for steroid biosynthesis. *PLoS One* (2012) 7:e45829. doi:10.1371/journal.pone.0045829
32. Duarte A, Castillo AF, Podesta EJ, Poderoso C. Mitochondrial fusion and ERK activity regulate steroidogenic acute regulatory protein localization in mitochondria. *PLoS One* (2014) 9:e100387. doi:10.1371/journal.pone.0100387
33. Takemori H, Kanematsu M, Kajimura J, Hatano O, Katoh Y, Lin XZ, et al. Dephosphorylation of TORC initiates expression of the StAR gene. *Mol Cell Endocrinol* (2007) 26(5–266):196–204. doi:10.1016/j.mce.2006.12.020
34. Duan H, Cherradi N, Feige JJ, Jefcoate C. cAMP-dependent posttranscriptional regulation of steroidogenic acute regulatory (STAR) protein by the zinc finger protein ZFP36L1/TIS11b. *Mol Endocrinol* (2009) 23:497–509. doi:10.1210/me.2008-0296
35. Raj A, Tyagi S. Detection of individual endogenous RNA transcripts in situ using multiple singly labeled probes. *Methods Enzymol* (2010) 472:365–86. doi:10.1016/S0076-6879(10)72004-8
36. Raj A, van den Bogaard P, Rifkin SA, van Oudenaarden A, Tyagi S. Imaging individual mRNA molecules using multiple singly labeled probes. *Nat Methods* (2008) 5:877–9. doi:10.1038/nmeth.1253
37. Lee J, Foong YH, Musaitif I, Tong T, Jefcoate C. Analysis of specific RNA in cultured cells through quantitative integration of q-PCR and N-SIM single cell FISH images: application to hormonal stimulation of StAR transcription. *Mol Cell Endocrinol* (2016) 429:93–105. doi:10.1016/j.mce.2016.04.001
38. Lee J, Tong T, Takemori H, Jefcoate C. Stimulation of StAR expression by cAMP is controlled by inhibition of highly inducible SIK1 via CRTC2, a co-activator of CREB. *Mol Cell Endocrinol* (2015) 408:80–9. doi:10.1016/j.mce.2015.01.022
39. Daems C, Di-Luoffo M, Paradis E, Tremblay JJ. MEF2 cooperates with forskolin/cAMP and GATA4 to regulate star gene expression in mouse MA-10 Leydig cells. *Endocrinology* (2015) 156:2693–703. doi:10.1210/en.2014-1964
40. Manna PR, Dyson MT, Stocco DM. Role of basic leucine zipper proteins in transcriptional regulation of the steroidogenic acute regulatory protein gene. *Mol Cell Endocrinol* (2009) 302:1–11. doi:10.1016/j.mce.2008.12.009
41. Jefcoate CR, Lee J, Cherradi N, Takemori H, Duan H. cAMP stimulation of StAR expression and cholesterol metabolism is modulated by co-expression of labile suppressors of transcription and mRNA turnover. *Mol Cell Endocrinol* (2011) 336:53–62. doi:10.1016/j.mce.2010.12.006
42. Spiga F, Liu Y, Aguilera G, Lightman SL. Temporal effect of adrenocorticotrophic hormone on adrenal glucocorticoid steroidogenesis: involvement of the transducer of regulated cyclic AMP-response element-binding protein activity. *J Neuroendocrinol* (2011) 23:136–42. doi:10.1111/j.1365-2826.2010.02096.x
43. Takemori H, Okamoto M. Regulation of CREB-mediated gene expression by salt inducible kinase. *J Steroid Biochem Mol Biol* (2008) 108:287–91. doi:10.1016/j.jsbmb.2007.09.006
44. Grozdanov PN, Stocco DM. Short RNA molecules with high binding affinity to the KH motif of A-kinase anchoring protein 1 (AKAP1): implications for the regulation of steroidogenesis. *Mol Endocrinol* (2012) 26:2104–17. doi:10.1210/me.2012-1123

45. Ascoli M. Characterization of several clonal lines of cultured Leydig tumor cells: gonadotropin receptors and steroidogenic responses. *Endocrinology* (1981) 108:88–95. doi:10.1210/endo-108-1-88
46. Duan H, Jefcoate CR. The predominant cAMP-stimulated 3 x 5 kb StAR mRNA contains specific sequence elements in the extended 3′UTR that confer high basal instability. *J Mol Endocrinol* (2007) 38:159–79. doi:10.1677/jme.1.02153
47. DiBartolomeis MJ, Jefcoate CR. Characterization of the acute stimulation of steroidogenesis in primary bovine adrenal cortical cell cultures. *J Biol Chem* (1984) 259:10159–67.
48. Yamazaki T, Matsuoka C, Gendou M, Izumi S, Zhao D, Artemenko I, et al. Mitochondrial processing of bovine adrenal steroidogenic acute regulatory protein. *Biochim Biophys Acta* (2006) 1764:1561–7. doi:10.1016/j.bbapap.2006.08.016
49. Evans AN, Liu Y, Macgregor R, Huang V, Aguilera G. Regulation of hypothalamic corticotropin-releasing hormone transcription by elevated glucocorticoids. *Mol Endocrinol* (2013) 27:1796–807. doi:10.1210/me.2013-1095
50. Ciais D, Cherradi N, Bailly S, Grenier E, Berra E, Pouyssegur J, et al. Destabilization of vascular endothelial growth factor mRNA by the zinc-finger protein TIS11b. *Oncogene* (2004) 23:8673–80. doi:10.1038/sj.onc.1207939
51. Baou M, Jewell A, Murphy JJ. TIS11 family proteins and their roles in posttranscriptional gene regulation. *J Biomed Biotechnol* (2009) 2009:634520. doi:10.1155/2009/634520
52. Bose HS, Lingappa VR, Miller WL. Rapid regulation of steroidogenesis by mitochondrial protein import. *Nature* (2002) 417:87–91. doi:10.1038/417087a
53. Bahat A, Perlberg S, Melamed-Book N, Isaac S, Eden A, Lauria I, et al. Transcriptional activation of LON gene by a new form of mitochondrial stress: a role for the nuclear respiratory factor 2 in StAR overload response (SOR). *Mol Cell Endocrinol* (2015) 408:62–72. doi:10.1016/j.mce.2015.02.022
54. Spiga F, Walker JJ, Gupta R, Terry JR, Lightman SL. 60 YEARS OF NEUROENDOCRINOLOGY: glucocorticoid dynamics: insights from mathematical, experimental and clinical studies. *J Endocrinol* (2015) 226:T55–66. doi:10.1530/JOE-15-0132
55. Arakane F, King SR, Du Y, Kallen CB, Walsh LP, Watari H, et al. Phosphorylation of steroidogenic acute regulatory protein (StAR) modulates its steroidogenic activity. *J Biol Chem* (1997) 272:32656–62. doi:10.1074/jbc.272.51.32656
56. Manna PR, Slominski AT, King SR, Stetson CL, Stocco DM. Synergistic activation of steroidogenic acute regulatory protein expression and steroid biosynthesis by retinoids: involvement of cAMP/PKA signaling. *Endocrinology* (2014) 155:576–91. doi:10.1210/en.2013-1694
57. Yoon YS, Lee MW, Ryu D, Kim JH, Ma H, Seo WY, et al. Suppressor of MEK null (SMEK)/protein phosphatase 4 catalytic subunit (PP4C) is a key regulator of hepatic gluconeogenesis. *Proc Natl Acad Sci U S A* (2010) 107:17704–9. doi:10.1073/pnas.1012665107

10

Effects of Chronic ACTH Excess on Human Adrenal Cortex

*Xavier Bertagna**

Service des Maladies Endocriniennes et Métaboliques, Centre de Référence des Maladies Rares de la Surrénale, Faculté de Médecine Paris Descartes, Université Paris 5, Hôpital Cochin, Paris, France

***Correspondence:**
Xavier Bertagna
xavier.bertagna@aphp.fr

Chronic ACTH excess leads to chronic cortisol excess, without escape phenomenon, resulting in Cushing's syndrome. Excess adrenal androgens also occur: in females, they will overcompensate the gonadotrophic loss, inducing high testosterone; in males, they will not compensate it, inducing low testosterone. Chronic ACTH excess leads to chronic adrenal mineralocorticoid excess and low aldosterone levels: after an acute rise, aldosterone plasma levels resume low values after a few days when ACTH is prolonged. Two other mineralocorticoids in man, cortisol and 11 deoxycorticosterone (DOC), at the zona fasciculata, will not escape the long-term effect of chronic ACTH excess and their secretion rates will remain elevated in parallel. Over all, the concomitant rise in cortisol and 11 DOC will more than compensate the loss of aldosterone, and eventually create a state of chronic mineralocorticoid excess, best evidenced by the accompanying suppression of the renin plasma levels, a further contribution to the suppression of aldosterone secretion. Prolonged *in vivo* stimulation with ACTH leads to an increase in total adrenal protein and RNA synthesis. Cell proliferation is indicated by an increase in total DNA the resulting adrenocortical hyperplasia participates in the amplified response of the chronically stimulated gland, and the weight of each gland can be greatly increased. The growth-stimulatory effect of ACTH *in vivo* most likely proceeds through the activation of a local and complex network of autocrine growth factors and their own receptors; a number of compounds, including non-ACTH proopiomelanocortin peptides such as γ3-MSH, have been shown to exert some adrenocortical growth effect.

Keywords: adrenal, ACTH excess, Cushing's syndrome, cortisol, androgens, mineralocorticoids, adrenal cortex growth

INTRODUCTION

The pituitary–adrenal axis is a central actor in Endocrinology. Through it, the fine tuning of corticosteroids secretion is maintained, from fetal to adult life, under basal and stressful conditions, with immediate and/or long-term consequences. Altered ACTH secretion induces catastrophic clinical situations: adrenal insufficiency on the one hand, Cushing's syndrome on the other hand. Both are debilitating conditions that severely alter the quality of life, create multiple complications, and, ultimately may lead to premature death. Besides ACTH-dependent Cushing's syndrome, there are many situations where ACTH is chronically oversecreted. This review will examine the effects of chronic ACTH excess on adrenal cortex in man, and concentrate on steroid secretion and adrenal cortex growth.

Rare and particular situations will also be addressed.

THE VARIOUS SITUATIONS IN MAN WITH CHRONIC ACTH EXCESS

The many situations that are associated with chronic ACTH excess in man are presented in **Table 1**. Depending on the «quality» of the original adrenal cortex they can be artificially distinguished in three different groups.

There Are Three Situations Where the Adrenal Cortex Is Originally, Functionally, and Anatomically Normal

- Healthy volunteers administered with exogenous ACTH or its synthetic analog Cortrosyn ($ACTH_{1-24}$).
- Patients with ACTH-dependent Cushing's syndrome, either Cushing's disease or the ectopic ACTH secretion syndrome. Excess ACTH is chronically produced by a pituitary or a non-pituitary tumor and acts on a basically normal adrenal cortex.
- Patients with the syndrome of general resistance to glucocorticoids.

These three situations allow measuring the effects of chronic ACTH excess on both corticosteroid secretions and adrenal cortex growth.

There Are Two Situations Where the Adrenal Cortex Has, Congenital or Acquired, Intrinsic Steroidogenic Defects

- The various types of congenital adrenal hyperplasias (CAHs) associated with altered cortisol synthesis.
- Treatment of ACTH-dependent Cushing's syndrome with anticortisolic drugs that inhibit steroidogenesis (metyrapone, ketoconazole, etomidate, aminoglutethimide, LCI699).

TABLE 1 | Conditions with chronic ACTH excess in man.

Normal adrenal cortex[a]
ACTH/Cortrosyn administration to normal volunteers
ACTH-dependent Cushing's syndrome
Cushing's disease; ectopic ACTH secretion syndrome
General resistance to glucocorticoids
Abnormal adrenal cortex: disorders of steroid synthesis[b]
Congenital adrenal hyperplasia
21 Hydroxylase-, 11 hydroxylase-, 17 hydroxylase deficiencies
Inhibitors of adrenal steroidogenesis
Metyrapone, ketoconazole, etomidate, aminoglutethimide, LCI699
Abnormal adrenal cortex: «missing» adrenal glands
Acquired destruction
Addison's disease
Bilateral adrenalectomy
Adrenolytic drugs (*o,p'*DDD)
Congenital developmental defects

[a]*Model to study both the functional and anatomical effects of chronic ACTH excess.*
[b]*Model to study the anatomical effects of chronic ACTH excess.*

In both situations, chronic ACTH excess is an adapted response to chronic cortisol deprivation. They preclude studying the effects of chronic ACTH excess on corticosteroid secretions. Still the effects on adrenocortical growth can be evaluated in a pertinent fashion.

In the Last Situations, the Adrenal Cortex Is Simply—And Anatomically—Missing or Compromised

- Bilateral adrenalectomy, usually for ACTH-dependent Cushing's syndrome.
- Adrenolytic treatments (*o,p'*DDD) of ACTH-dependent Cushing's syndrome.
- Acquired adrenal destructions (infections, hemorrhagies, autoimmune, bilateral metastases…).
- Congenital developmental defects (genetic syndromes).

Evidently, none of these situations help to study the «adrenal» effects of chronic ACTH excess. They would be, however, adapted to study the non-adrenal effects of chronic ACTH—and proopiomelanocortin (POMC)-related peptides excess. Indeed, by opposition with the sole situation where ACTH itself—or its synthetic analog Cortrosyn—are exogenously administered to healthy volunteers, all other situations with chronic excess of endogenous ACTH are accompanied by parallel excess of other non-ACTH POMC-derived peptides.

CHRONIC ACTH EXCESS IN MAN AND CORTICOSTEROID SECRETION

Cortisol

Chronic ACTH Excess Leads to Chronic Cortisol Excess

Experiments in healthy volunteers, more than half a century ago, have shown the effects of repeated ACTH administrations (1, 2).

- When the same dose of ACTH is exogenously administered daily in man, a stepwise increase in daily cortisol secretion is observed over the days [see Figure 8 in Ref. (1)].
- This «amplifying» phenomenon has now a molecular explanation: adrenocortical cells exposed to ACTH *in vitro* acquire an increased number of ACTH receptors (MC2R) and an increased rate of protein Gs expression (3–6).
- Through the cAMP pathway the binding of ACTH and the transducing apparatus are both amplified, explaining the higher sensitivity and the greater response potential of chronically stimulated cells.
- No escape phenomenon is observed, although the cortisol oversecretion tends to plateau after several days.
- Over a wide range, the cortisol response is proportional to the dose of administered ACTH.

In patients with ACTH-dependent Cushing's syndrome, chronic excess of endogenous ACTH also leads to chronic cortisol excess. Interestingly in many patients with Cushing's disease, cortisol excess is associated with «normal» ACTH plasma values compared with those seen in the morning in normal subjects (7, 8). These values are considered «abnormally» normal or «inappropriate» in face of the hypercortisolism that should normally totally suppress ACTH secretion. Furthermore, these levels remain constant over the day, with no circadian variation, and ACTH acts on hyperresponsive adrenocortical cells; indeed, acute ACTH stimulation of the hyperplastic adrenals in Cushing's disease patients triggers a much higher and more lasting response than would be observed in normal subjects given the same dose [see Figure 2 in Ref. (2)].

Chronic ACTH excess in case of non-pituitary tumors (the ectopic ACTH secretion syndrome) has the exact same consequences on cortisol secretion. Because ACTH plasma levels are often higher in these patients, they also have—in general—higher cortisol oversecretion (8).

In the syndrome of general resistance to cortisol, the glucocorticoid receptor type 2 is mutated with a loss of function. It is an autosomal dominant familial disease (9–11). All cells and tissues have lost their normal sensitivity to cortisol. At the hypothalamic–pituitary level, it is felt as an apparent lack of cortisol, which—naturally—induces an adapted response with chronic increase in ACTH secretion (12). This natural human situation offers a privileged model to observe the response of a perfectly normal adrenal cortex to chronic ACTH excess: unsurprisingly chronic cortisol excess is observed, but without the clinical features of Cushing's syndrome. Together with cortisol, other ACTH-dependent corticosteroids, androgens dehydroepiandrosterone (DHEA), and mineralocorticoids deoxycorticosterone (DOC) are oversecreted by the zona fasciculata (see further).

A state of chronic and acquired general resistance to cortisol can be artificially created in Cushing's disease patients chronically treated with RU486 (Mifepristone). The drug is an antagonist to the glucocorticoid receptor type 2, the acute administration of which triggers an immediate pituitary ACTH retort in normal subjects (13, 14). As expected, under long-term RU486 administration some clinical peripheral features of the Cushing's syndrome are ameliorated such as hyperglycemia (15); as expected also, in the patients with Cushing's disease, the hypothalamic–pituitary–adrenal axis is stimulated (by the "apparent" cortisol deprivation) and ACTH is acutely and/or chronically increased further with plasma levels raising up *ca.* three times above their baseline initial values (16, 17). In the SEISMIC study, several patients developed high blood pressure, edema, and hypokelmia suggestive of a state of chronic hypermineralocorticism (17). All ACTH-dependent corticosteroids presumably increase in parallel: cortisol, the clinical impact of which remains blunted at the glucocorticoid receptor by the drug; but also adrenal androgens and DOC, the actions of which are not opposed at their respective androgen and mineralocorticoid receptors (for both DOC and cortisol) and which may thus induce serious clinical features: possibly hyperandogenism in women; hypertension and hypokalemia in both sexes (18).

Adrenocortical Androgens

Chronic ACTH Excess Leads to Chronic Adrenal Androgens Excess with Contrasted Impacts in Females and Males

Adrenal androgens are produced by the zona fasciculata/reticularis, and—as cortisol—are under the same—and dominant if not exclusive—control of ACTH and the cAMP pathway. Acute administration to healthy volunteers induces abrupt increase in circulating adrenal androgens (19). The situation has been particularly studied in Cushing's disease patients. The specific adrenal androgen DHEA sulfate (DHEAS) is chronically increased both in males and females (20). Thus DHEA, DHEAS, and Δ-4-androstenedione are elevated in Cushing's disease patients (21–23). Yet, the impact of chronic ACTH excess upon the overall androgenic status is contrasted between females and males:

- In both females and males, chronic excess of androgens, and cortisol, both lead to suppressed gonadotroph function directly at the hypothalamic–pituitary levels.
- In females, because the pituitary gonadotrophic function normally accounts for only half of the total circulating androgens, the excess adrenal androgens will eventually overcompensate the gonadotrophic loss and induce an overall excess of circulating androgens: their peripheral transformation to testosterone and dihydrotestosterone may lead to a moderate state of androgen excess in females with its clinical impact: hirsutism, infertility [see Figure 3 in Ref. (22)].
- In males, because the pituitary gonadotrophic/gonadal function normally accounts for the vast majority of circulating androgens (*ca.* 90%), the excess of adrenal androgens will not compensate that which has been lost due to the cortisol-induced suppression of the gonadotrophic/gonadal function. The overall circulating androgens will eventually be abnormally low (testosterone), with a clinical impact: decreased sexual activity, infertility (24).

In a way similar to that observed with cortisol, chronic increase in adrenal androgens will be observed in other situations with chronic ACTH excess such as the ectopic ACTH secretion syndrome, and the general resistance to glucocorticoids. In the latter situation, as evoked earlier, excess androgens in females may be the dominant symptom that should alert on the diagnosis in the absence of «Cushing's» features; it may provoke precocious puberty in children (12).

In patients with Cushing's disease treated with the antiglucocorticoid RU486, the inescapable rise in ACTH secretion will—theoretically—increase further the state of hyperandrogenism in females and this should be a major drawback for the use of this compound .... Surprisingly, there is no report on the clinical or hormonal androgen status of women in the SEISMIC study (17).

Dissociation between cortisol and adrenal androgens is observed, however, in the particular situation of patients resuming normal corticotroph function after long-term ACTH excess. After successful pituitary surgery in Cushing's disease patients, DHEAS remains suppressed for months or years after plasma cortisol has normalized (21).

Mineralocorticoids

Chronic ACTH Excess Leads to Chronic Adrenal Mineralocorticoid Excess and Low Aldosterone Levels

It has long been known that acute ACTH administration to man leads to immediate aldosterone secretion; yet this effect is only transient and is not maintained when ACTH is prolonged over periods of time, and aldosterone plasma levels resume low values after a few days (25, 26).

Yet this "escape" phenomenon on aldosterone will not prevent the establishment of a state of chronic mineralocorticoid excess, for two reasons:

- This "escape" will *only concern aldosterone*, at the zona glomerulosa. Its exact mechanism is not entirely understood: it is suggested that increased concentrations of cortisol in the adrenal cortex directly inactivates the last steps of aldosterone synthesis in the ZG (27); there is also evidence that initial ZG cells undergo a differentiation process toward cortisol producing cells (28).
- Two other mineralocorticoids in man, cortisol and 11 DOC, at the zona fasciculata, will not escape the long-term effect of chronic ACTH excess and their secretion rates will remain elevated in parallel (29).

Over all, the concomitant rise in cortisol and DOC, even though each of these molecules is intrinsically less potent than aldosterone at the mineralocorticoid receptor, will more than compensate the loss of aldosterone, and eventually create a state of chronic mineralocorticoid excess, best evidenced by the accompanying suppression of the renin plasma levels, a further—if not exclusive—contribution to the suppression of aldosterone secretion (30). This general mineralocorticoid effect is in correlation with the level of ACTH excess: its clinical consequences (high blood pressure, hypokalemic alkalosis) are more frequent in patients with the ectopic ACTH secretion syndrome than in those with Cushing's disease (31).

As expected, patients with the syndrome of general resistance to glucocorticoids have parallel increases in cortisol and DOC, and hypokalemic hypertension may be another—sometime predominant—clinical presentation in these patients, as reported in the first published cases (9).

These complications may also occur in patients with Cushing's disease treated by RU486 (Mifepristone). The drug induces a further increase in cortisol and probably DOC (this latter steroid rarely if ever measured in these patients!), which both can interact, without any opposition, at the mineralocorticoid receptor (18), and see **Figure 1**.

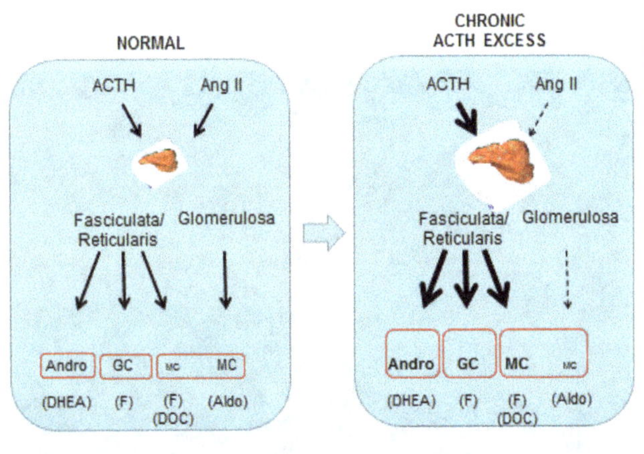

FIGURE 1 | Schematic overview of the comparative effects of normal and prolonged ACTH excess in man on adrenal cortical steroids at the zona glomerulosa and the zona fasciculata/reticularis.

CHRONIC ACTH EXCESS IN MAN AND ADRENAL CORTEX GROWTH

The central role of ACTH on the adrenal cortex trophicity has long been known. Hypophysectomy results in adrenal cortex atrophy that is restored by the sole administration of ACTH (32). Thus, *in vivo*, ACTH is the predominant if not the exclusive trophic factor for the adrenals. More recently, various animal models, which eliminate ACTH or its receptor (MC2R) in transgenic mice, have confirmed the central role of ACTH to maintain normal adrenal cortex growth (33–35). Prolonged *in vivo* stimulation with chronic ACTH administration or oversecretion eventually leads to an increase in total adrenal protein and RNA synthesis. Cell proliferation is indicated by an increase in total DNA (32) the resulting adrenocortical hyperplasia participates in the amplified response of the chronically stimulated gland, and the weight of each gland can be greatly increased.

The exact mechanism whereby ACTH promotes adrenocortical growth still is complex and remains partially understood, since *in vitro* studies show a paradoxical negative effect of ACTH on adrenocortical cell proliferation (36) The growth-stimulatory effect of ACTH *in vivo* most likely proceeds through the activation of a local and complex network of autocrine growth factors and their own receptors; a number substances, including non-ACTH POMC peptides such as γ3-MSH, have been shown to exert some adrenocortical growth effect (28).

In ACTH-dependent Cushing's syndrome, chronic ACTH excess leads to bilateral adrenal hyperplasia: both adrenals are enlarged, their weight is increased in comparison with normal glands, and the histological appearance shows diffuse widening of the fasciculata/reticularis zona (**Figure 2**). This hyperplasia is typically homogeneous and rather symmetrical. In some cases however, it may be asymmetrical, and/or one or the two glands may bear nodular zones or authentic nodules embedded within the diffuse hyperplasia. Today, CT-Scan allows to see the adrenal hyperplasia *in vivo* in patients with ACTH-dependent Cushing's syndrome, and to observe its fate after the suppression of ACTH, that is after successful pituitary surgery: the two enlarged glands and the nodules progressively shrink and can even become atrophic until normal ACTH secretion is spontaneously restored, which may take months or years (37, 38). In parallel to these anatomical changes, baseline cortisol and its response to the acute stimulation by ACTH is suppressed, and progressively resume

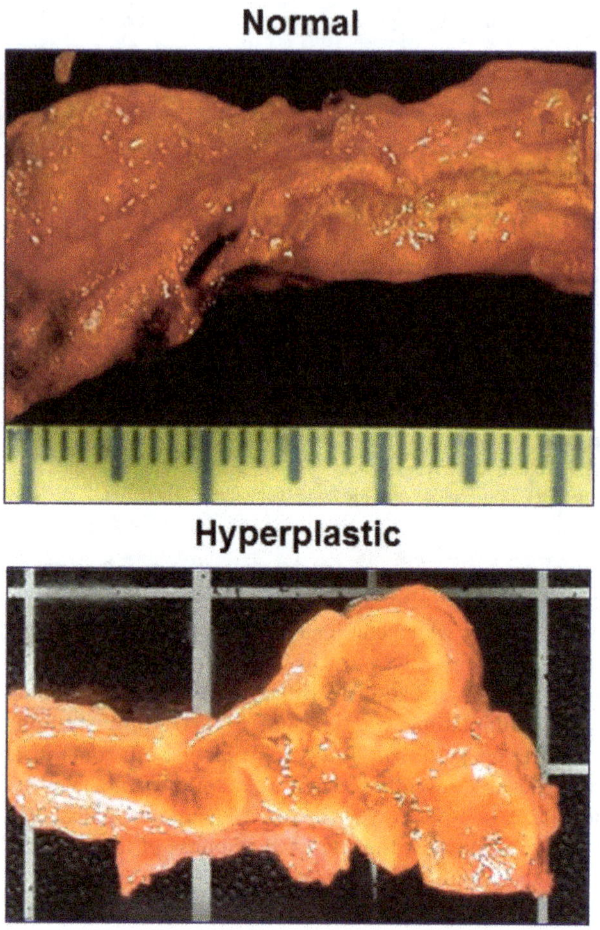

FIGURE 2 | Comparing the macroscopic aspect of normal adrenals and those of a Cushing's disease patient.

over months or years. As already mentioned, cortisol response is restored more rapidly than androgen response.

A rather similar presentation is observed in patients with CAH: both glands are enlarged, and become smaller under glucocorticoid administration (**Figure 3**).

Some studies seem to demonstrate that chronic ACTH excess also favors the appearance of adrenocortical nodules, and it has been suggested that some of them ultimately become autonomous (i.e., ACTH-independent). Yet, it is common observation that suppression of chronic ACTH excess, in Cushing's or CAH patients, reduces both the hyperplastic and nodular parts of the enlarged glands (**Figure 3**).

Interestingly, the growth promoting effect of chronic ACTH excess can be exerted also at distance, on adrenal rests:

- Testicular adrenal rests may develop as local tumors which impinge the normal spermatogenesis, and may become cause of infertility in poorly controlled male patients with CAH (39). There is some evidence that lowering ACTH plasma levels may shrink these tumors which, in contrast with the normal testicular tissue, are loaded with the MC2R (40). The close phenotype shared by TART and fetal adrenals, including classical markers of adrenal steroidogenesis, highly favors the hypothesis that TART develops from an original adrenal cortical cell type.
- In Cushing's disease patients, particularly those treated by "total" bilateral adrenalectomy, a large increase in ACTH secretion can be triggered. It may play a role in the growth of adrenal rests, locally (adrenal extrusions that have escaped the surgeon tools!), but also at distance, in the testis, and many other places (41, 42).

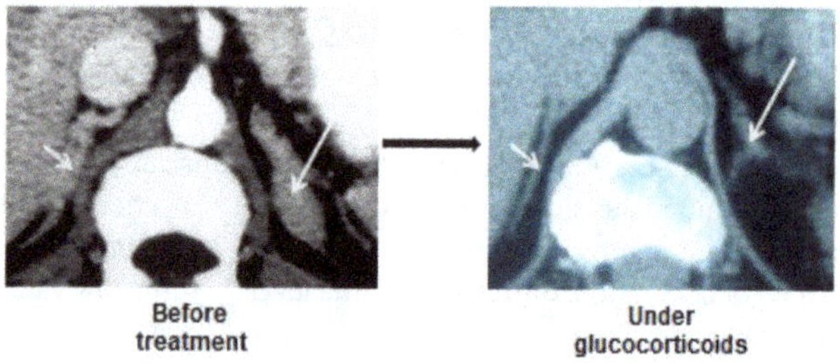

FIGURE 3 | CT-scan images of enlarged and nodular adrenal glands in a patient with 21 hydroxylase deficiency. Regression under ACTH suppression by large doses of glucocorticoids.

RARE AND PARTICULAR SITUATIONS

Mimicking Chronic ACTH Excess

There are several pathological conditions where pituitary ACTH is actually suppressed and cortisol is oversecreted in response to molecular phenomenon which occur directly at the adrenal level, and, somehow, mimick chronic ACTH excess:

- ACTH may be produced locally by tumoral adrenal cells, and its autocrine action may participate in cortisol oversecretions in cases of bilateral macronodular adrenal hyperplasia (43).
- In the absence of ACTH, its signaling pathway may be nevertheless overactivated and generate excess of corticosteroid secretion: adrenocortical tumors which express illegitimate G-protein coupled receptors (44, 45), activated mutated MC2R (46), mutated PRKAR1A in the Carney complex (47, 48), and mutated PKACa in adrenocortical adenomas (49).
- It has also been suggested auto antibodies acting at the ACTH receptor might be responsible for excess cortisol secretion in some cases of Wulffraat (50). Yet little confirmation has been obtained since the original paper.

It is interesting to observe that all these situations eventually result in the overactivation of the cAMP signaling pathway, and always occur in benign tumors. They concur with the idea that chronic ACTH excess, or chronic activation of its signaling pathway at the same time may have some growth effect but also a differentiation action.

When "Normal" ACTH Is Too Much!

In the syndrome of apparent mineralocorticoid excess, the loss of function of 11 hydroxysteroid dehydrogenase type II, particularly at the kidney, locally enhances the mineralocorticoid action of cortisol (51).

In the glucocorticoid-remediable aldosteronism, gene rearrangement induces the "ectopic" expression of the Aldo synthase gene within the ZF cells and thus provokes the oversecretion of aldosterone under the action of ACTH (52).

In these two situations, the HPA axis and cortisol secretion are normal. Yet, it drives a state of "apparent" or "real" mineralocorticoid excess, and the treatment option is indeed to suppress ACTH secretion.

Non-ACTH POMC Peptides

As mentioned earlier, ACTH is part of a larger polypeptide precursor, POMC the enzymatic processing of which liberates ACTH itself and a number of other "non-ACTH" POMC-derived peptides. Among these peptides, the lipotropins (beta- and gamma-lipotropins) exert a definitive action on the melanocytes in man, and are responsible, together with ACTH, for skin hyperpigmentation that is observed in all situations of excess endogenous ACTH secretion. Beta-endorphin is an opioid peptide, which is a processing product of POMC. It circulates in blood, in parallel with the ACTH that is secreted by normal or tumoral pituitary or non-pituitary corticotroph cells. Yet, even at extremely high plasma values, circulating beta-endorphin has no known actions in man, and does not exert any analgesic action (53). The analgesic effect of beta-endorphin is entirely due to that which is produced locally in the brain by a set of POMC-expressing neurons: the circulating beta-endorphin does not cross the blood–brain barrier.

Experimental evidence suggest that non-ACTH N-terminal POMC peptides may exert a growth effect on the adrenal cortex (54, 55). The small peptide N-$POMC_{1-28}$, which bears two intramolecular disulfide bridges, is responsible for this action which has also been described in the human adreno cortical tumors cells NCI-H295 (56). Yet the receptor for the N-$POMC_{1-28}$ peptide remains elusive (55).

Chronic Stress and Pseudo-Cushing

Pseudo-Cushing corresponds to these situations in man where an authentic hypercortisolism is biologically present (increased urinary cortisol, abnormal response to dexamethasone suppression test) and may be confused with "endogenous" Cushing's disease. Yet, in Pseudo-Cushing there is no pituitary adenoma; the ACTH excess is thought to be "functional," driven by the overactivity of the hypothalamus and oversecretion of corticotrophin-releasing hormone under chronic stress, severe depression, intense physical activity, and anorexia nervosa (57).

AUTHOR CONTRIBUTIONS

The author confirms being the sole contributor of this work and approved it for publication.

REFERENCES

1. Liddle GW, Island D, Rinfret AP, Forsham PH. Factors enhancing the response of the human adrenal to corticotropin: is there an adrenal growth factor? *J Clin Endocrinol Metab* (1954) 14:839–58. doi:10.1210/jcem-14-8-839
2. Liddle GW. Regulation of adrenocortical function in man. In: Christy NP, editor. *The Human Adrenal Cortex*. New York: Harper and Row Publisher (1971). p. 41–68.
3. Penhoat A, Jaillard C, Saez JM. Corticotropin positively regulates its own receptors and cAMP response in cultured bovine adrenal cells. *Proc Natl Acad Sci U S A* (1989) 86:4978–81. doi:10.1073/pnas.86.13.4978
4. Begeot M, Langlois D, Penhoat A, Saez JM. Variations in guanine-binding proteins (Gs, Gi) in cultured bovine adrenal cells. Consequences on the effects of phorbol and cholera-toxin-induced cAMP production. *Eur J Biochem* (1988) 174:317–21. doi:10.1111/j.1432-1033.1988.tb14100.x
5. Mountjoy KG, Robbins LS, Mortrud MT, Cone RD. The cloning of a family of genes that encode the melanocortin receptors. *Science* (1992) 257:1248–51. doi:10.1126/science.1325670
6. Penhoat A, Lebrethon MC, Bégeot M, Saez JM. Regulation of ACTH receptor mRNA and binding sites by ACTH and angiotensin II in cultured human and bovine adrenal fasciculata cells. *Endocr Res* (1995) 21(1–2):157–68. doi:10.3109/07435809509030431
7. Kuhn JM, Proeschel MF, Seurin DJ, Bertagna XY, Luton JP, Girard FL. Comparative assessment of ACTH and lipotropin plasma levels in the diagnosis and follow-up of patients with Cushing's syndrome: a study of 210 cases. *Am J Med* (1989) 86(6 Pt 1):678–84. doi:10.1016/0002-9343(89)90443-9
8. Bertagna X, Guignat L, Raux-Demay MC, Guilhaume B, Girard F. Cushing's disease. 3rd ed. In: Melmed S, editor. *The Pituitary*. London, UK: Academic Press (2011). p. 533–617.
9. Vingerhoeds AC, Thijssen JH, Schwarz F. Spontaneous hypercortisolism without Cushing's syndrome. *J Clin Endocrinol Metab* (1976) 43(5):1128–33. doi:10.1210/jcem-43-5-1128
10. Chrousos GP, Vingerhoeds A, Brandon D, Eil C, Pugeat M, DeVroede M, et al. Primary cortisol resistance in man. A glucocorticoid receptor-mediated disease. *J Clin Invest* (1982) 69(6):1261–9. doi:10.1172/JCI110565
11. Malchoff DM, Brufsky A, Reardon G, McDermott P, Javier EC, Bergh CH, et al. A mutation of the glucocorticoid receptor in primary cortisol resistance. *J Clin Invest* (1993) 91(5):1918–25. doi:10.1172/JCI116410
12. Charmandari E, Kino T, Ichijo T, Chrousos GP. Generalized glucocorticoid resistance: clinical aspects, molecular mechanisms, and implications of a rare genetic disorder. *J Clin Endocrinol Metab* (2008) 93(5):1563–72. doi:10.1210/jc.2008-0040
13. Bertagna X, Bertagna C, Luton JP, Husson JM, Girard F. The new steroid analog RU 486 inhibits glucocorticoid action in man. *J Clin Endocrinol Metab* (1984) 59(1):25–8. doi:10.1210/jcem-59-1-25
14. Gaillard RC, Riondel A, Muller AF, Herrmann W, Baulieu EE. RU 486: a steroid with antiglucocorticosteroid activity that only disinhibits the human pituitary-adrenal system at a specific time of day. *Proc Natl Acad Sci U S A* (1984) 81(12):3879–82. doi:10.1073/pnas.81.12.3879
15. Fleseriu M, Biller BM, Findling JW, Molitch ME, Schteingart DE, Gross C, et al. Mifepristone, a glucocorticoid receptor antagonist, produces clinical and metabolic benefits in patients with Cushing's syndrome. *J Clin Endocrinol Metab* (2012) 97(6):2039–49. doi:10.1210/jc.2011-3350
16. Bertagna X, Bertagna C, Laudat MH, Husson JM, Girard F, Luton JP. Pituitary-adrenal response to the antiglucocorticoid action of RU 486 in Cushing's syndrome. *J Clin Endocrinol Metab* (1986) 63(3):639–43. doi:10.1210/jcem-63-3-639
17. Fleseriu M, Findling JW, Koch CA, Schlaffer SM, Buchfelder M, Gross C. Changes in plasma ACTH levels and corticotroph tumor size in patients with Cushing's disease during long-term treatment with the glucocorticoid receptor antagonist mifepristone. *J Clin Endocrinol Metab* (2014) 99(10):3718–27. doi:10.1210/jc.2014-1843
18. Castinetti F, Fassnacht M, Johanssen S, Terzolo M, Bouchard P, Chanson P, et al. Merits and pitfalls of mifepristone in Cushing's syndrome. *Eur J Endocrinol* (2009) 160(6):1003–10. doi:10.1530/EJE-09-0098

19. Reisch N, Slawik M, Zwermann O, Beuschlein F, Reincke M. Genetic influence of an ACTH receptor promoter polymorphism on adrenal androgen secretion. *Eur J Endocrinol* (2005) 153(5):711–5. doi:10.1530/eje.1.02015
20. Barbetta L, Dall'Asta C, Re T, Colombo P, Travaglini P, Ambrosi B. Androgen secretion in ectopic ACTH syndrome and in Cushing's disease: modifications before and after surgery. *Horm Metab Res* (2001) 33(10):596–601. doi:10.1055/s-2001-17906
21. Yamaji T, Ishibashik M, Sekihara H, Itabashi A, Yanaihara T. Serum dehydroepiandrosterone sulfate in Cushing's syndrome. *J Clin Endocrinol Metab* (1984) 1984:1164–8. doi:10.1210/jcem-59-6-1164
22. Halpin DM, Burrin JM, Joplin GF. Serum testosterone levels in women with Cushing's disease. *Acta Endocrinol (Copenh)* (1990) 122(1):71–5.
23. Smals AG, Kloppenborg PW, Benraad TJ. Plasma testosterone profiles in Cushing's syndrome. *J Clin Endocrinol Metab* (1977) 45(2):240–5. doi:10.1210/jcem-45-2-240
24. Luton JP, Thieblot P, Valcke JC, Mahoudeau JA, Bricaire H. Reversible gonadotropin deficiency in male Cushing's disease. *J Clin Endocrinol Metab* (1977) 45(3):488–95.
25. Gaillard RC, Riondel AM, Favrod-Coune CA, Vallotton MB, Muller AF. Aldosterone escape to chronic ACTH administration in man. *Acta Endocrinol (Copenh)* (1983) 103(1):116–24.
26. Rauh W, Levine LS, Gottesdiener K, New MI. Mineralocorticoids, salt balance and blood pressure after prolonged ACTH administration in juvenile hypertension. *Klin Wochenschr* (1978) 56(Suppl 1):161–7. doi:10.1007/BF01477468
27. Bird IM, Pasquarette MM, Rainey WE, Mason JI. Differential control of 17 alpha hydroxylase and 3-beta hydroxyl dehydrogenase expression in human adrenocortical H295R cells. *J Clin Endocrinol Metab* (1996) 81:2171–8. doi:10.1210/jcem.81.6.8964847
28. Gallo-Payet N. Adrenal and extra-adrenal functions of ACTH. *J Mol Endocrinol* (2016) 56(4):T135–56. doi:10.1530/JME-15-0257
29. Kater CE, Biglieri EG, Brust N, Chang B, Hirai J, Irony I. Stimulation and suppression of the mineralocorticoid hormones in normal subjects and adrenocortical disorders. *Endocr Rev* (1989) 10(2):149–64. doi:10.1210/edrv-10-2-149
30. Oelkers W. Prolonged ACTH infusion suppresses aldosterone secretion in spite of high renin activity. *Acta Endocrinol (Copenh)* (1985) 108:91–7.
31. Schambelan M, Slaton PE Jr, Biglieri EG. Mineralocorticoid production in hyperadrenocorticism. Role in pathogenesis of hypokalemic alkalosis. *Am J Med* (1971) 51(3):299–303. doi:10.1016/0002-9343(71)90264-6
32. Gill GN. ACTH regulation of the adrenal cortex. In: Gill GN, editor. *Pharmacology of Adrenal Cortical Hormones*. New York: Pergamon (1979). p. 35–66.
33. Chida D, Nakagawa S, Nagai S, Sagara H, Katsumata H, Imaki T, et al. Melanocortin 2 receptor is required for adrenal gland development, steroidogenesis, and neonatal gluconeogenesis. *Proc Natl Acad Sci U S A* (2007) 104:18205–10. doi:10.1073/pnas.0706953104
34. Coll AP, Challis BG, Yeo GS, Snell K, Piper SJ, Halsall D, et al. The effects of proopiomelanocortin deficiency on murine adrenal development and responsiveness to adrenocorticotropin. *Endocrinology* (2004) 145:4721–7. doi:10.1210/en.2004-0491
35. Karpac J, Ostwald D, Bui S, Hunnewell P, Shankar M, Hochgeschwender U. Development, maintenance, and function of the adrenal gland in early postnatal proopiomelanocortin-null mutant mice. *Endocrinology* (2005) 146:2555–62. doi:10.1210/en.2004-1290
36. Hornsby PJ. The mechanism of action of ACTH in the adrenal cortex. In: Cooke BA, King RJB, Van Der Molen HJ, editors. *Hormones and Their Actions, Part II*. Amsterdam: Elsevier Science Publishers BV (Biomedical Division) (1988). p. 193–210.
37. Imaki T, Naruse M, Takano K. Adrenocortical hyperplasia associated with ACTH-dependent Cushing's syndrome: comparison of the size of adrenal glands with clinical and endocrinological data. *Endocr J* (2004) 51(1):89–95. doi:10.1507/endocrj.51.89
38. Albiger NM, Occhi G, Sanguin F, Iacobone M, Casarrubea G, Ferasin S, et al. Adrenal nodules in patients with Cushing's disease: prevalence, clinical significance and follow-up. *J Endocrinol Invest* (2011) 34:204–9. doi:10.3275/7349
39. Ahmad IC, Yilmaz TF, Kocakoç E. Doppler ultrasonography and magnetic resonance imaging findings of testicular adrenal rest tissue in a patient with 11 β hydroxilase deficiency. Case report. *Med Ultrason* (2014) 16(4):383–5.
40. Lottrup G, Nielsen JE, Skakkebaek NE, Juul A, Rajpert-De Meyts E. Abundance of DLK1, differential expression of CYP11B1, CYP21A2 and MC2R, and lack of INSL3 distinguish testicular adrenal rest tumours from Leydig cell tumours. *Eur J Endocrinol* (2015) 172(4):491–9. doi:10.1530/EJE-14-0810
41. Baranetsky NG, Zipser RD, Goebelsmann U, Kurman RJ, March CM, Morimoto I, et al. Adrenocorticotropin-dependent virilizing paraovarian tumors in Nelson's syndrome. *J Clin Endocrinol Metab* (1979) 49(3):381–6. doi:10.1210/jcem-49-3-381
42. Carpenter PC, Wahner HW, Salassa RM, Duick DS. Demonstration of steroid-producing gonadal tumors by external scanning with the use of NP-59. *Mayo Clin Proc* (1979) 54(5):332–4.
43. Louiset E, Duparc C, Young J, Renouf S, Tetsi Nomigni M, Boutelet I, et al. Intraadrenal corticotropin in bilateral macronodular adrenal hyperplasia. *N Engl J Med* (2013) 369(22):2115–25. doi:10.1056/NEJMoa1215245
44. Lacroix A, Bolté E, Tremblay J, Dupré J, Poitras P, Fournier H, et al. Gastric inhibitory polypeptide-dependent cortisol hypersecretion – a new cause of Cushing's syndrome. *N Engl J Med* (1992) 327(14):974–80. doi:10.1056/NEJM199210013271402
45. Reznik Y, Allali-Zerah V, Chayvialle JA, Leroyer R, Leymarie P, Travert G, et al. Food-dependent Cushing's syndrome mediated by aberrant adrenal sensitivity to gastric inhibitory polypeptide. *N Engl J Med* (1992) 327(14):981–6. doi:10.1056/NEJM199210013271403
46. Swords FM, Baig A, Malchoff DM, Malchoff CD, Thorner MO, King PJ, et al. Impaired desensitization of a mutant adrenocorticotropin receptor associated with apparent constitutive activity. *Mol Endocrinol* (2002) 16(12):2746–53. doi:10.1210/me.2002-0099
47. Kirschner LS, Carney JA, Pack SD, Taymans SE, Giatzakis C, Cho YS, et al. Mutations of the gene encoding the protein kinase A type I-alpha regulatory subunit in patients with the Carney complex. *Nat Genet* (2000) 26(1):89–92. doi:10.1038/79238
48. Groussin L, Jullian E, Perlemoine K, Louvel A, Leheup B, Luton JP, et al. Mutations of the PRKAR1A gene in Cushing's syndrome due to sporadic primary pigmented nodular adrenocortical disease. *J Clin Endocrinol Metab* (2002) 87(9):4324–9. doi:10.1210/jc.2002-020592
49. Beuschlein F, Fassnacht M, Assié G, Calebiro D, Stratakis CA, Osswald A, et al. Constitutive activation of PKA catalytic subunit in adrenal Cushing's syndrome. *N Engl J Med* (2014) 370(11):1019–28. doi:10.1056/NEJMoa1310359
50. Wulffraat NM, Drexhage HA, Wiersinga WM, van der Gaag RD, Jeucken P, Mol JA. Immunoglobulins of patients with Cushing's syndrome due to pigmented adrenocortical micronodular dysplasia stimulate in vitro steroidogenesis. *J Clin Endocrinol Metab* (1988) 66(2):301–7. doi:10.1210/jcem-66-2-301
51. Stewart PM, Corrie JE, Shackleton CH, Edwards CR. Syndrome of apparent mineralocorticoid excess. A defect in the cortisol-cortisone shuttle. *J Clin Invest* (1988) 82(1):340–9.
52. Lifton RP, Dluhy RG, Powers M, Rich GM, Cook S, Ulick S, et al. A chimaeric 11 beta-hydroxylase/aldosterone synthase gene causes glucocorticoid-remediable aldosteronism and human hypertension. *Nature* (1992) 355(6357):262–5.
53. Willer JC, Sheng-Shu L, Bertagna X, Girard F. Pituitary beta-endorphin not involved in pain control in some pathophysiological conditions. *Lancet* (1984) 2(8397):295–6.
54. Estivariz FE, Iturriza F, McLean C, Hope J, Lowry PJ. Stimulation of adrenal mitogenesis by N-terminal proopiocortin peptides. *Nature* (1982) 297(5865):419–22.
55. Bicknell AB. N-terminal POMC peptides and adrenal growth. *J Mol Endocrinol* (2016) 56(4):T39–48. doi:10.1530/JME-15-0269
56. Fassnacht M, Hahner S, Hansen IA, Kreutzberger T, Zink M, Adermann K, et al. N-terminal proopiomelanocortin acts as a mitogen in adrenocortical tumor cells and decreases adrenal steroidogenesis. *J Clin Endocrinol Metab* (2003) 88(5):2171–9. doi:10.1210/jc.2002-021318
57. Pecori Giraldi F, Ambrogio AG. Pseudo-Cushing – a clinical challenge? *Front Horm Res* (2016) 46:1–14. doi:10.1159/000443859

11

Mouse Models Recapitulating Human Adrenocortical Tumors: What is Lacking?

*Felicia Leccia[1], Marie Batisse-Lignier[1,2], Isabelle Sahut-Barnola[1], Pierre Val[1], A-Marie Lefrançois-Martinez[1] and Antoine Martinez[1]**

[1] UMR6293, GReD, INSERM U1103, CNRS, Clermont Université, Clermont-Ferrand, France, [2] Endocrinology, Diabetology and Metabolic Diseases Department, Centre Hospitalier Universitaire, School of Medicine, Clermont-Ferrand, France

***Correspondence:**
Antoine Martinez
antoine.martinez@univ-bpclermont.fr

Adrenal cortex tumors are divided into benign forms, such as primary hyperplasias and adrenocortical adenomas (ACAs), and malignant forms or adrenocortical carcinomas (ACCs). Primary hyperplasias are rare causes of adrenocorticotropin hormone-independent hypercortisolism. ACAs are the most common type of adrenal gland tumors and they are rarely "functional," i.e., producing steroids. When functional, adenomas result in endocrine disorders, such as Cushing's syndrome (hypercortisolism) or Conn's syndrome (hyperaldosteronism). By contrast, ACCs are extremely rare but highly aggressive tumors that may also lead to hypersecreting syndromes. Genetic analyses of patients with sporadic or familial forms of adrenocortical tumors (ACTs) led to the identification of potentially causative genes, most of them being involved in protein kinase A (PKA), Wnt/β-catenin, and P53 signaling pathways. Development of mouse models is a crucial step to firmly establish the functional significance of candidate genes, to dissect mechanisms leading to tumors and endocrine disorders, and *in fine* to provide *in vivo* tools for therapeutic screens. In this article, we will provide an overview on the existing mouse models (xenografted and genetically engineered) of ACTs by focusing on the role of PKA and Wnt/β-catenin pathways in this context. We will discuss the advantages and limitations of models that have been developed heretofore and we will point out necessary improvements in the development of next generation mouse models of adrenal diseases.

Keywords: adrenal, tumor, mouse models, PKA, WNT

INTRODUCTION

Adrenocortical tumors (ACTs) are classified as benign adrenocortical adenomas (ACAs) and malignant adrenocortical carcinomas (ACCs). Most ACTs are benign, unilateral, and non-secreting adenomas, often discovered incidentally during abdominal imaging for reasons unrelated with adrenal gland (adrenal "incidentalomas"). Although less frequently, ACAs may be secreting tumors associated

---

Abbreviations: ACA, adrenocortical adenoma; ACC, adrenocortical carcinoma; ACT, adrenocortical tumor; ACTH, adrenocorticotropin hormone; APA, aldosterone-producing adenoma; CPA, cortisol-producing adenoma; CS, Cushing's syndrome; GIP, gastric inhibitor polypeptide; GPCR, G-protein-coupled receptors; LH/hCG, luteinizing hormone/choriogonaotropin; PA, primary aldosteronism; PBMAH, primary bilateral macronodular adrenal hyperplasia; PKA, protein kinase A; PPNAD, primary pigmented nodular adrenal hyperplasia; SF-1, steroidogenic factor 1.

with endocrine hyperfunction that leads to several symptoms and significant morbidity. Indeed, clinical manifestations of secreting ACAs differ depending on their secretion profile. Cortisol-producing adenomas (CPAs) lead to Cushing's syndrome (CS). Notably, hypercortisolism associated with unilateral ACAs is the most common form of adrenocorticotropin hormone (ACTH)-independent CS (1, 2). Aldosterone-producing adenomas (APAs) lead to primary aldosteronism (PA). APAs, together with bilateral hyperplasia, comprise 95% of all PA cases (3).

Although bilateral forms of ACTs are less frequent, several adrenal pathological conditions converge in the group of diseases termed adrenocortical hyperplasia, characterized by bilateral adrenal enlargement. Primary bilateral macronodular adrenal hyperplasia (PBMAH) is the most common and is a rare cause of CS. The report of familial forms and the bilateral nature suggest a genetic origin for PBMAH (4). Unlike PBMAH, primary pigmented nodular adrenal hyperplasia (PPNAD) is rarer but it may cause overt Cushing (5).

Contrary to ACAs, ACCs are extremely rare, with an annual incidence of 0.5–2 cases per million. However, they are highly aggressive tumors associated with poor prognosis and often diagnosed at an advanced stage (6, 7). They can occur at any age but the incidence in children is particularly high in southern Brazil due to the high prevalence of a specific TP53 mutation (8). Besides tumor growth and metastasis, clinical manifestations of ACCs are often the result of steroid hypersecretion caused by endocrine dysfunction, reminiscent of adrenal adenomas.

Over the last 5 years, genetic analyses of patients with sporadic or familial forms of ACTs has resulted in identification of alterations in a new set of genes, most of them being involved in cAMP/protein kinase A (PKA) and Wnt/β-catenin signaling pathways (9–11) (**Figures 1** and **2**). The major difference in the prevalence of ACA and ACC in patients suggests that adenomas are not precursors of malignant neoplasms. Moreover, the malignant transformation of a benign and non-functional adrenal tumor is very rare (12–14). Notably, the risk that an adrenal incidentaloma progresses to a malignant tumor has recently been estimated as almost zero by the *European Society of Endocrinology* (ESE). Consequently, European recommendations for the clinical management of patients with non-functional ACAs have been reconsidered and modified to avoid unnecessary procedures (European Congress of Endocrinology, May 2016, Munich, Germany – Symposium 5: ESE clinical guidelines: Management of adrenal incidentaloma: http://www.ece2016.org/scientific-programme/). By contrast, secreting ACAs are surgically removed, which prevents evaluation of a possible benign to malignant continuum in functional adenomas. In fact, the hypothesis that ACC could develop in a multistep process from normal adrenal to adenoma followed by malignant transformation relied on one case report in which a carcinoma emerged in the center of a surrounding benign ACT (15). However, some genome-wide approaches performed on independent cohorts to analyze genomic changes and gene regulation in ACTs suggests that cancers could result from pangenomic cumulative changes occurring in a multistep tumor progression (16–18). Although it is important to predict to what extent a benign lesion can be considered as the precursor of malignancy, analysis of patients' data may not be sufficient to provide a definitive conclusion.

The use of small animals for modeling tumors in a controlled experimental manner is a valuable strategy to explore the functional significance of mutations, to dissect mechanisms underlying both adrenocortical tumorigenesis and endocrine disorders, and to provide *in vivo* tools to screen for novel therapeutic approaches. To date, several genetically modified and xenografted mouse models have been developed to investigate the involvement of specific pathways and the heterogeneous nature of ACTs, respectively. Although models established until now have shed light on important aspects of adrenocortical diseases, many of them failed to fully mimic tumors found in human adrenals (**Table 1**). Hence, there is a strong need to develop relevant mouse models to shed light on mechanisms involved in the initiation and progression of adrenal tumors. In this article, we provide an overview of the existing mouse models (xenografted and genetically engineered) of ACTs relevant to human ACTs, including adrenal hyperplasia. We will discuss limitations of models that have been developed heretofore and we will point out necessary improvements in the development of next-generation mouse models of adrenal diseases. Notably, these models should allow, on the one hand, to firmly establish the role of newly identified genes in adrenocortical tumorigenesis and, on the other hand, to explore the interplay between pathways shown to be associated with ACTs (e.g., cAMP/PKA and Wnt/β-catenin).

BENIGN ADRENOCORTICAL TUMORS AND ASSOCIATED HYPERSECRETION SYNDROMES

Primary Bilateral Macronodular Adrenal Hyperplasia

Primary bilateral macronodular adrenal hyperplasia is a rare cause of CS, accounting for <2% of all endogenous CS cases (33, 34). PBMAH is characterized by the presence of adrenocortical nodules larger than 10 mm and it is often diagnosed in patients between 40 and 60 years of age, with clinical signs of cortisol excess and suppressed levels of plasma ACTH. PBMAH was first described by Kirschner and colleagues (35) and it was named ACTH-independent macronodular adrenal hyperplasia (AIMAH). However, it has been recently found that cortisol production in PBMAH is not truly ACTH independent, since a population of adrenocortical cells in the hyperplastic tissue can produce ACTH that in turn stimulates cortisol secretion through autocrine and paracrine mechanisms (36). Hence, the term "ACTH independent" is not entirely appropriate for this disorder. Although in the majority of cases, PBMAH appears to be sporadic, several cases of familial clustering have been reported in the last years (37–39). However, the true prevalence of the familial vs. sporadic form is unknown, as systematic familial screening has not been conducted.

Aberrant Hormone Receptors in PBMAH and Related Mouse Models

The mechanism by which cortisol production is stimulated in PBMAH, despite suppressed plasma ACTH, was previously

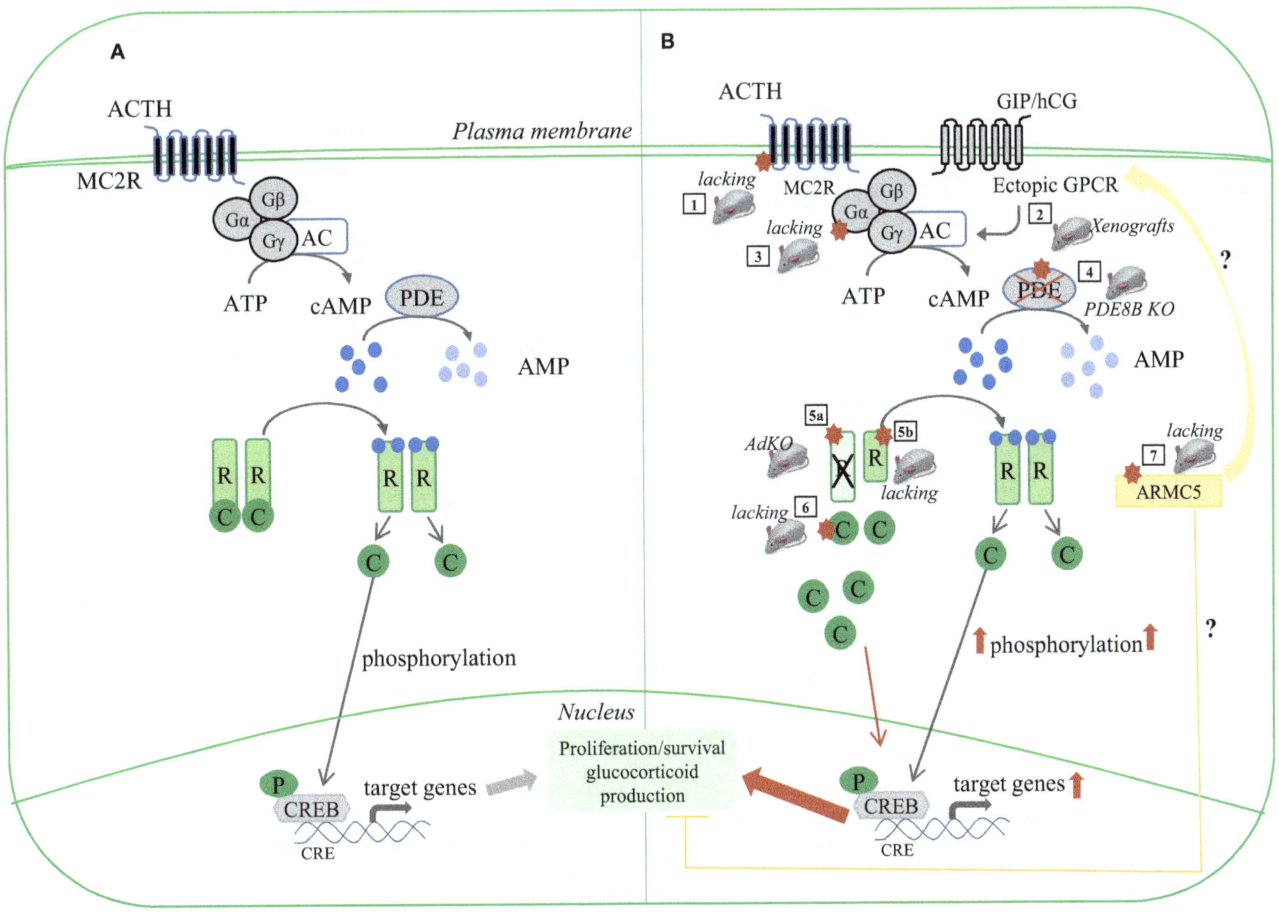

FIGURE 1 | PKA signaling pathway in adrenal tumorigenesis and related mouse models. (A) Under normal conditions, ACTH binds to MC2R, a G-protein-coupled receptor (GPCR) that activates adenylate cyclase (AC) *via* Gsα, thus increasing intracellular levels of cAMP. Upon binding of cAMP to regulatory subunits (R) of PKA, the complex dissociates releasing the catalytic subunits (C) which in turn phosphorylate (among others) the cAMP-responsive element-binding protein (CREB). Once phosphorylated, CREB transcription factor regulates the expression of steroidogenic and proliferative genes. In absence of ACTH, the pathway is repressed through the activity of several phosphodiesterases (PDE) that inactivate cAMP. **(B)** Molecular alterations of several components of cAMP/PKA signaling pathway cause adrenal hyperplasias and tumors. (1) Activating mutations of *MC2R* found in PBMAH patients lead to higher activation of the pathway. No mouse model is actually available for *Mcr2* activating mutations. (2) Hormones other than ACTH (GIP/hCG/LH), through ectopic expression of several GPCRs, may induce ACTH-independent hypercortisolism in PBMAH patients. Xenograft mouse models nicely recapitulate this pathologic context. (3) Activating mutations in *GNAS* gene, encoding for the subunit α of the stimulatory G protein, causes higher activation of the pathway. These mutations are the cause of adrenal hyperplasia associated with Cushing's syndrome in Mc-Cune Albright syndrome, whereas somatic mutations have been found in cortisol-producing adenomas. No mouse model is actually available for *Gnas*-activating mutations. (4) Inactivating mutations in PDE genes lead to an accumulation of cAMP, thus causing the persistent activation of the pathway in absence of ACTH and they have been associated with PBMAH and hypercortisolism. Whole-body *PDE8B* knockout mice developed mild hyperplasia. (5a) Most inactivating mutations in the *PRKAR1A* gene, encoding the 1α regulatory subunit (R1α) of the PKA, lead to aberrant transcripts and to the absence of the protein, resulting in constitutive activation of PKA. Adrenocortical-specific *Prkar1a* knockout (AdKO) mice develop a PPNAD-like syndrome with adrenal hyperplasia and ACTH-independent hypercorticosteronism. (5b) Some *PRKAR1A* gene mutations lead to expressed mutated (truncated) R1α proteins that also cause increased PKA activation. These mutations are associated with a more severe phenotype for reasons still not understood to date. No mouse model is available for expressed mutated R1α proteins. (6) Mutations in the *PRKACA* gene encoding for the catalytic subunit α (Cα) of the PKA alter its interaction with regulatory subunits leading to constitutive activation of PKA-Cα and increased steroidogenesis. These mutations have been identified in many patients with cortisol-producing adenomas. No mouse model is actually available for *Prkaca* activating mutations. (7) Inactivating germline and somatic mutations in the armadillo repeat-containing 5 (*ARMC5*) gene have been identified in ~50% of patients with PBMAH. The function and the mechanisms by which ARMC5 contributes to the pathogenesis of PBMAH are unknown. *In vitro* studies suggest a role in steroidogenesis and apoptosis processes and a possible interplay with the PKA pathway, which is supported by the association of *ARMC5* mutations with particular expression profile of GPCRs. No loss of function mouse model is actually available for *Armc5*.

unknown and was referred to as being "autonomous." Several groups have then shed light on the pathogenesis of hypercortisolism in PBMAH. They reported that in most patients with PBMAH and in some adenomas, cortisol secretion is regulated by hormones other than ACTH, through the aberrant expression of several G-protein-coupled receptors (GPCRs) that are normally absent (ectopic) or expressed at lower levels in the adrenal cortex (40–42). The GPCRs for gastric inhibitory polypeptide (GIP), catecholamines, vasopressin, serotonin, and luteinizing hormone/human chorionic gonadotropin (LH/hCG) have been

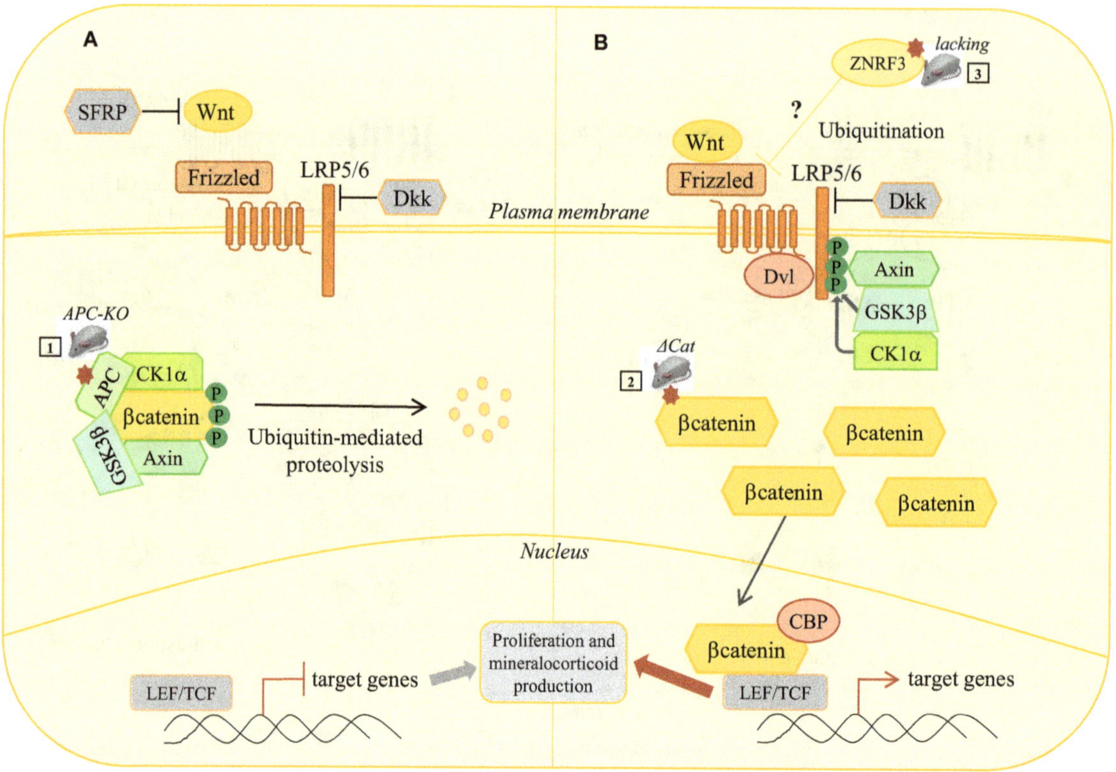

FIGURE 2 | WNT/β-catenin signaling pathway in adrenal tumorigenesis. (A) In the absence of Wnt ligands, b-catenin is phosphorylated by a complex composed of GSK3b, CK1, APC, and AXIN. This phosphorylation targets b-catenin to proteosomal degradation, thus preventing its nuclear translocation. In this context, the T cell-specific factors (Tcf)/lymphoid enhancer-binding factor (Lef) represses target genes expression through association with transcriptional inhibitors. Secreted frizzled related proteins (SFRP) can inhibit extracellular Wnt signaling. **(B)** When WNT signaling is active, binding of Wnt ligands to their receptor complex (Frizzled/LRP5/6) induces the recruitment of Disheveled (Dsv) to the cytoplasmic domain of Frizzled and the phosphorylation of the cytoplasmic tail of LRP5/6 by CK1 and GSK3b. This induces delocalization of Axin to LRP5/6 and sequestration of the degradation complex. b-catenin degradation is, thus, reduced and it accumulates. Accumulated b-catenin enters the nucleus, binds to LEF/TCF transcription factors, and activates transcription of target genes. Mutations in several members of WNT/β-catenin signaling pathway have been identified in adrenal hyperplasias, adenomas, and carcinomas. Several mouse models have been developed to induce constitutive β-catenin activation either through adrenal cortex specific loss of *Apc* (1) or the expression of a protein resistant to phosphorylation and ubiquitin-dependent degradation (2). Loss of ZNRF3, a potential Wnt signaling inhibitor, has been identified as the major genetic alteration in adrenal carcinoma. Mouse model with adrenal specific inactivation of *Znrf3* is required to assess its causal involvement in ACC.

shown to be involved in adrenal CS development (42). GIP-dependent CS has been reported in patients with PBMAH and with unilateral adenomas (33, 43, 44). In these patients, plasma cortisol levels were increased following meals, despite ACTH suppression, and paralleled postprandial elevation of GIP plasma concentrations. Hypercortisolism associated with aberrant LH/hCG receptors was first identified in a woman with transient CS during sequential pregnancies and persistent CS after menopause (45). Since then, several cases of PBMAH with aberrant LHR have been reported, alone or in association with GIPR (45, 46). The molecular mechanisms responsible for aberrant expression of these receptors are unknown as no genetic mutations have been found in the coding or regulatory regions of receptor genes. Furthermore, whether expression of these receptors is a primary or a secondary event in the pathogenesis of PBMAH is still a matter of debate. Several lines of evidence support the hypothesis that it is a causative factor. First, aberrant receptors are almost universally present in PBMAH and at early stages (47). Second, the same aberrant receptors were found in all members of some affected families (37, 48), although this was not found in a known Brazilian family (39). Further data supporting a triggering role of ectopic receptors in PBMAH came from xenotransplantation mouse models. Indeed, to investigate the role of ectopic GIPR and LHR expression in the development of PBMAH, Mazzuco and colleagues used an *in vivo* model of cell transplantation and tissue reconstruction. Primary bovine adrenocortical cells were genetically engineered to express GIPR or LHR (retrovirus-mediated enforced expression) and transplanted under the kidney capsule of adrenalectomized immunodeficient mice (49, 50). Transplantation of GIPR- or LHR-expressing cells induced the formation of hyperplasic and hypertrophic adrenocortical tissues. The growth advantage provided by aberrant receptors expression at least relied on increased proliferation rates of transplants but the downstream mechanisms supporting proliferation were not explored. These models nicely recapitulated the context of human PBMAH with GPCR-dependent CS. Indeed, LHR-dependent CS is not exclusively observed during pregnancies or after menopause (41). Likewise, in the LHR xenotransplanted

TABLE 1 | Current mouse models of adrenocortical tumors and their limitations.

Model	Gene	Promoter/driver	Adrenocortical phenotype	Limitation	Reference
$Men1^{\pm}$	*Men1*	Whole-body KO	Hyperplasia, adenoma, carcinoma (lack of tumor grade definition)	Multiple tumors	(19, 20)
$Prkar1a^{2\Delta/+}$	*Prkar1a*	*EIIA-Cre*	No adrenal phenotype	No adrenal phenotype	(21)
tTA/X2AS	*Prkar1a*	Tet-Off system	Hyperplasia maintaining of X-zone	Technical limitations, reproducibility	(22)
AdKO	*Prkar1a*	*0.5 Akr1b7-Cre*	Expansion of X-like zone with *zona fasciculata* features, autonomous corticosterone secretion	Late phenotype	(23)
$Pde8b^{-/-}$	*Pde8b*	Whole-body KO	Mild hyperplasia	No adrenal-specific ablation	(24)
ΔCat	*Ctnnb1*	*0.5 Akr1b7-Cre*	Hyperplasia, adenoma and ectopic *zona glomerulosa*, hyperaldosteronism	Rare carcinomas	(25)
APC-KO	*Apc*	*$Sf1\text{-}Cre^{low}$*	Hyperplasia progressed to microscopic and macroscopic adenomas	Progression to carcinoma was never observed	(26)
APC KO-$H19^{\Delta DMD}$	*Apc Igf2/H19 ICR*	*$Sf1\text{-}Cre^{low}$*	Hyperplasia and adenomas, more severe phenotype than APC-KO mice	One carcinoma	(26)
PEPCK-IGF	*Igf2*	*Pepck-Igf2*	Hyperplasia	No adrenocortical tumors	(27)
ΔCat; AdIgf2	*Ctnnb1 Igf2*	*0.5 Akr1b7-Cre* *0.5 Akr1b7-Igf2* *4.5 Scc-Igf2*	Hyperplasia, adenoma, slight increased proliferation compared to ΔCat mice	Moderate effect on tumor progression	(28)
$Acd^{acd/acd}$; $p53^{\pm}$	*Acd, Tp53*		Increased development of ACC compared to $Acd^{acd/acd}$	Multiple tumors	(29)
Inhα/TAg	*SV40 (large T antigen)*	*6kb inhibinα-TAg*	Malignant ACTs developing upon gonadectomy	Unrelated to human pathology	(30)
AdTAg	*SV40 (large T antigen)*	*0.5 Akr1b7-TAg*	Rapidly evolving tumors		(31)
YAC TR	*NR5A1*	YAC transgene	Hyperplasia and tumors	Tumors with gonadal phenotype	(32)

MEN1, multiple endocrine neoplasia type 1; Prkar1a, Protein kinase cAMP-dependent regulatory subunit type I alpha; Akr1b7, aldo-keto reductase family 1, member b7; Pde8b, phosphodiesterase 8b; Ctnnb1, catenin (cadherin-associated protein), beta 1; APC, adenomatous polyposis coli; KO, knockout; ICR, imprinting control region; PEPCK, phosphoenolpyruvate carboxykinase; IGF2, insulin-like growth factor 2; Acd, adrenocortical dysplasia; TP53, tumor protein P53; TAg, tumor antigen; SV40, simian virus 40; YAC, yeast artificial chromosome; Nr5a1, nuclear receptor subfamily; tTA/X2AS, transgenic mouse carrying an antisense transgene for Prkar1a exon 2 (X2AS) under the control of a tetracycline responsive promoter; ΔCat, $Catnb^{lox(ex3)}$ line x 0.5AkR1b7-Cre.

model, the hyperplastic tissue formed in the absence of supra-physiological levels of plasma LH. This shows a direct role of aberrant LHR expression in the pathogenesis of PBMAH with LH-responsive CS, even though the molecular mechanisms leading to ectopic expression of GPCRs in adrenocortical cells are still unknown.

Xenotransplantation models developed by Mazzuco et al. are not easy to manage for long-term follow-up or for assessment of therapeutic strategies, because immunodeficient mice with CS have short life expectancy. However, this elegant approach combining genetic engineering and cell transplantation of bovine adrenal cells in mice may be a useful tool to test the cooperation of multiple genetic alterations in the tumorigenic process (51) or when genetic alterations may be not relevant in mouse (e.g., *KCNJ5* gene, see Aldosterone-Producing Adenomas: WNT Pathway, KCNJ5, and Lack of Mouse Models).

Familial Forms of PBMAH, Genetic Alterations, and Related Mouse Models

Reports of rare familial forms and the bilateral nature of these tumors support a genetic origin of PBMAH. Many genes are associated with the development of PBMAH, including genes causing hereditary familial tumor syndromes, such as *APC* (52, 53), *MEN1* (54), and *FH* (55). Moreover, several reports pointed out genes involved in the cAMP/PKA signaling pathway, such as *PDE8B* and *PDE11A* (56, 57), *MC2R* (58), *GNAS* (59), and *PRKACA* (9) (**Figure 1**). Mutations in members of cAMP/PKA pathway are predicted to over-activate the pathway but they have been observed in a limited number of patients (**Figure 1**).

Germline inactivating mutations of the *MEN1* gene cause a complex genetic syndrome named multiple endocrine neoplasia type 1 (MEN1) characterized by endocrine and non-endocrine tumors (60). PBMAH occurs in ~21% of MEN1 patients (54). Two whole-body *Men1* KO mouse models have been reported. They nicely recapitulate the spectrum of tumors of MEN1 syndrome, including adrenocortical lesions. Specifically, whereas homozygous whole-body *Men1* KO is embryonic lethal (19, 20), heterozygous mice are viable and develop tumors similar to those found in the human disease, including adrenocortical hyperplasia that seems to progress from adenoma to carcinoma (20). Of note, characterization of the histological phenotype, allowing establishment of tumor grade, was not detailed in this paper. Therefore, the conclusion that a multi-step tumor progression process occurs in *Men1* adrenal tumors should be taken with caution (**Table 1**). Since *MEN1* has recently been identified as a significantly mutated gene in ACC (11), *Men1* KO mice could be useful to identify novel actors and mechanisms underlying the evolution of benign ACTs to malignancy.

Although the bilateral nature and the multifocal nodules suggest an important role of genetic factors in PBMAH, genetic defects summarized above account for only a few cases of this adrenal disease. More recently, inactivating germline and somatic mutations in the armadillo repeat-containing 5 (*ARMC5*) gene have been identified in ~50% of patients with apparently sporadic PBMAH and also in a large family with genetically transmitted PBMAH (10, 39, 61, 62). *ARMC5* is a tumor suppressor gene with the typical "two-hit" pattern of mutations: a first germline mutation and a second somatic one. The function and the mechanisms by which ARMC5 contributes to the pathogenesis of PBMAH are unknown. However, *in vitro* studies suggest a role in steroidogenesis and apoptosis processes (10). Indeed, *ARMC5* inactivation in cultured adrenocortical cells decreases the expression of *MC2R* and of various steroidogenic enzymes, both in basal conditions and after cAMP stimulation (10), suggesting that it may interfere with PKA pathway by impairing the stimulation of its target genes (**Figure 1**). Increased cell survival upon ARMC5 inactivation is proposed to trigger hyperplasia while subclinical CS could be the result of the major increase in adrenal mass that would compensate for decreased per-cell steroidogenic activity. Furthermore, *ARMC5* mutations seem to be associated with particular expression profile of GPCRs, i.e., beta-adrenergic and dopamine receptors (10). This observation supports the hypothesis of a link between ARMC5 and PKA signaling, as the abnormal expression of GPCRs leads to activation of PKA signaling, normally triggered by the ACTH receptor (MC2R) (**Figure 1**). Further *in vitro* studies and the development of knockout models are required to shed light on the ARMC5-dependent network that triggers development of PBMAH and CS. Notably, the combination of adrenal targeted GPCRs overexpression and *Armc5* knockout could provide information on a possible cooperation between ARMC5 and PKA signaling.

Primary Pigmented Nodular Adrenocortical Disease and Related Mouse Models

Primary pigmented nodular adrenocortical disease is a type of adrenal hyperplasia characterized by the presence of cortisol-secreting bilateral adrenal micronodules (<1 cm). PPNAD is the most common endocrine manifestation of Carney complex disease (CNC), an autosomal-dominant multiple neoplasia syndrome (63). More than 60% of CNC patients harbor mutations in the *PRKARIA* gene, encoding the regulatory subunit 1α (R1α) of PKA (64) (**Figure 1**). Specifically, inactivating heterozygous germline mutations are observed in about two-thirds of Carney Complex patients and loss of heterozygosity (LOH) has been reported, indicating that *PRKARIA* acts as a tumor suppressor gene (64). Interestingly, somatic inactivating mutations have also been found in ACTs (65). Several mouse models have been developed to target *Prkar1a* gene inactivation by different strategies (**Table 1**). Total *Prkar1a* KO mice had severe defects in mesoderm development and died at E9.5 (66). Mice heterozygous for a null allele of *Prkar1a* developed several tumors but had no adrenal phenotype (21). An antisense RNA approach was developed to achieve a more severe loss of R1α than in heterozygous KO mice (22). This allowed a 70% decrease in *Prkar1a*, causing several neoplastic manifestations, including mild adrenocortical hyperplasia. Interestingly, adrenocortical manifestations in the antisense RNA model included maintenance of the X-zone, a normally transient zone of fetal origin. To achieve bi-allelic inactivation without compromising mouse survival, we generated an *ad*renocortical-specific *Prkar1a* *k*nock*o*ut mouse model (AdKO) (23) by crossing *Prkar1a*-floxed strain with *Akr1b7*-Cre mice, thereby targeting specific genetic ablation in adrenocortical cells from E14.5 (67) (**Figures 1** and **3**; **Table 1**). These mice developed a PPNAD-like syndrome with ACTH-independent hyper-corticosteronism and adrenal hyperplasia, composed of hypertrophic cells emerging from the innermost cortex. Endocrine overactivity was associated with unbuffered PKA catalytic activity, which resulted in overexpression of steroidogenic genes. Interestingly, fetal-like hyperplasia centrifugally expanded with aging at the expense of the normal adult cortex, which underwent progressive atrophy. This mouse model confirmed the important role of PKA pathway in adrenal hyperplasia and shed light on possible mechanisms responsible for PPNAD. The most likely mechanism to explain the defective zonal differentiation and cell renewal in AdKO mice is an impaired capacity of adult progenitor cells of the outer cortex to undergo centripetal differentiation and increased survival of cells in the inner cortex that would then cumulate both fetal-like and fasciculata cell features. We further showed that PKA-dependent induction of mTOR signaling was one of the mechanisms participating in the resistance to apoptosis, leading to both hyperplasia and cell hypertrophy, typical of PPNAD (68, 69). Altogether, these observations suggest that PPNAD should be considered as a developmental disease.

To further elucidate the molecular mechanisms by which PKA pathway contributes to the initiation and/or development of adrenal disorders, it is essential to provide deeper insight of its interplay with other signaling pathways (**Figure 3**). Interestingly, WNT pathway activation has been involved in both PBMAH and PPNAD (70, 71) (**Figure 2**). Furthermore, as we will discuss in next sections, WNT pathway is also associated with ACA and ACC. A possible interplay between WNT/β-catenin and cAMP/PKA pathways in the pathogenesis of adrenal hyperplasia and tumors would be an important point to further investigate with mouse models (**Figure 3**).

Cortisol-Producing Adenomas: PKA Pathway, PRKACA Mutations, and Lack of Mouse Models

As discussed above (Sections "Familial Forms of PBMAH, Genetic Alterations, and Related Mouse Models" and "Primary Pigmented Nodular Adrenocortical Disease and Related Mouse Models"), a number of genetic defects in the cAMP/PKA pathway have been associated with adrenal hyperplasia and related to cortisol hypersecretion (**Figure 1**). Somatic mutations of *GNAS* (72–74) and *PRKAR1A* (75) have also been found in CPAs (**Figure 1**). However, these mutations only accounted for a small subset of CPAs, which represent a relevant cause of CS. Recently, Beuschlein and collaborators identified a hotpsot mutation (L205R) in the *PRKACA* gene, encoding the catalytic subunit α (Cα) of PKA, in

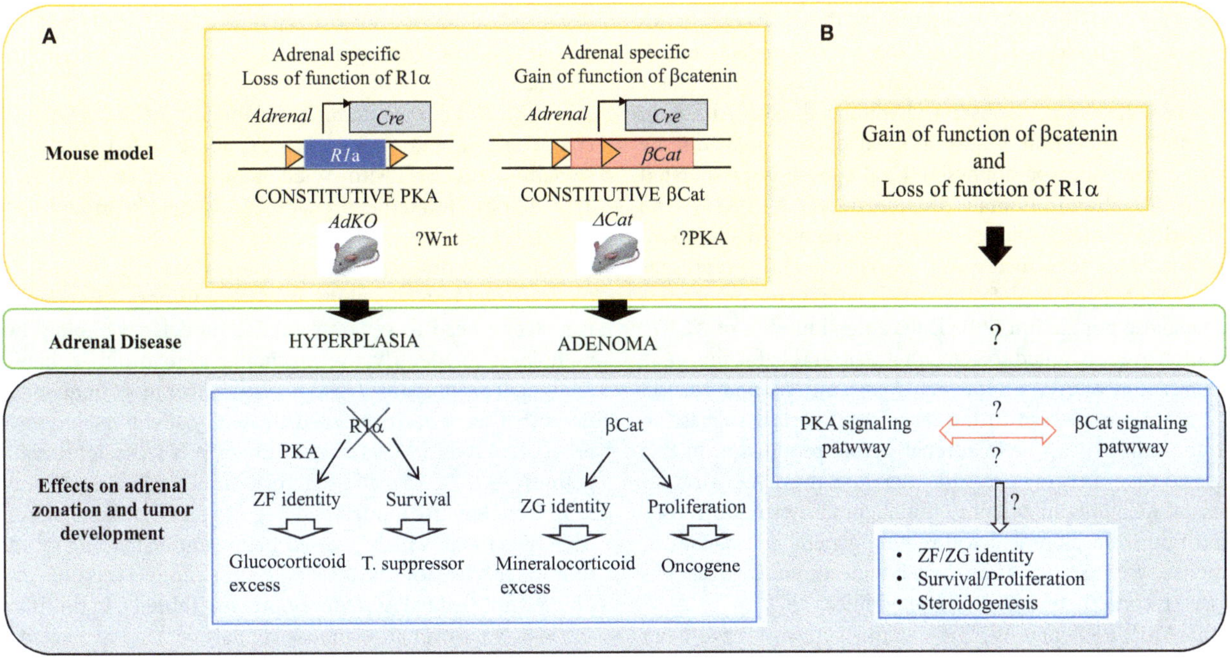

FIGURE 3 | Interplay between the WNT/β-catenin and the cAMP/PKA pathways in the pathogenesis of adrenal hyperplasias and tumors. (A) Two mouse models recapitulating some of the most frequent alterations found in adrenal tumors in patients. AdKO mice developed cortical hyperplasia as a result of constitutive PKA activation due to gene inactivation of R1a regulatory subunit of PKA. The increased PKA signaling also favored *zona fasciculata* cell identity and glucocorticoid excess. ΔCat mice developed cortical adenoma as a result of constitutive b-catenin due to deletion of exon 3 in the gene encoding the b-catenin (*Ctnnb1)* leading to protein stabilization. Increased b-catenin activation also induced ectopic differentiation of *zona glomerulosa* and aldosterone excess. **(B)** Our models demonstrated that *Prkar1a* is a tumor suppressor and *Ctnnb1* is an adrenal oncogene but secondary genetic alterations are required for malignant progression. A possible interplay between the WNT/β-catenin and the cAMP/PKA pathways in the adrenal cortex zonation and tumorigenesis is an important point to further investigate. The question can be genetically addressed by using compound transgenic mice based on previous available models and carrying both β-catenin and PKA constitutive activation.

more than one-third of patients with CPA (9). Four other groups subsequently reported the same mutation (72–74, 76). The *PRKACA* L205R mutation results in constitutive PKA activation (9, 74), which is a very likely cause of ACT formation (**Figure 1**). Supporting this hypothesis, patients with somatic mutations had adenomas, whereas patients with germline duplications had bilateral hyperplasias. Hence, *PRKACA* mutations, together with the previously identified *GNAS* and *PRKAR1A* inactivating mutations, strongly support a crucial role of cAMP/PKA pathway in the tumorigenesis of CPAs. The development of knock-in mouse models bearing *PRKACA* activating L205R mutation is required to evaluate its driver potential and to provide new insights into the mechanisms underlying PKA-dependent tumorigenesis in the context of cortisol-producing ACAs. In addition, adding extra copies of *Prkaca* in mouse, by additive transgenesis or targeted transgenesis at the *Rosa26* locus, would provide an opportunity to explore the pathogenic, maybe oncogenic, potential of PKA signaling. Such complementary mouse models would help understanding if gain-of-function mutations and gain of copy number alterations result in distinct adrenal lesions. Activating mutations in *CTNNB1*, the gene encoding β-catenin, have also been identified in CPAs (77). Interestingly, the recently identified *PRKACA* mutations were shown to be mutually exclusive with *CTNNB1* mutations (72–74, 76). Therefore, a possible interplay between WNT/β-catenin and cAMP/PKA pathways in CPAs remains to be investigated. Once again, mouse models should be invaluable tools to address this question *in vivo* (**Figure 3**).

Aldosterone-Producing Adenomas: WNT Pathway, KCNJ5, and Lack of Mouse Models

In recent years, high throughput next-generation sequencing technologies have allowed major advances in the knowledge of the genetic bases of APAs. By comparing the APA exome to the germline exome, recurrent somatic mutations have been identified in genes coding for ion channels and transporters regulating the cell membrane potential. Specifically, mutated genes encoding ion channels include *KCNJ5*, which encodes the G-protein activated potassium channel GIRK4, and is mutated in about 26–40% of APAs (78, 79) and *CACNA1D* and *CACNA1H* genes encoding for voltage-dependent calcium channels (80, 81). Genes encoding regulators of the cell membrane potential include two ATPases, *ATP1A1* and *ATP2B3* (82). All these mutations ultimately lead to increased intracellular calcium and abnormal activation of calcium–calmodulin-dependent kinase (Ca^{2+}–CAMK) signaling, which plays a central role in aldosterone production. Before identification of these novel APA-associated genes, several mouse models of potassium channels inactivation (*KCNK3/KCNK9* inactivation models) allowed understanding the effects of calcium homeostasis disruption and of some important aspects of PA (83–85). However, none of these models recapitulated hyperplasia and/or tumor development observed in human disease. Although one cannot exclude that mouse adrenal context may not be relevant to reproduce pathophysiological conditions associated with APA formation in humans, this suggests that in APAs, the tumorigenic potential could rely on a yet unidentified alteration. Among the newly identified genes, *KCNJ5* mutations represent the most frequent genetic defects in APAs, with higher prevalence in the Japanese population (79). Thus, animal models of *KCNJ5* inactivation are warranted to confirm a central role for this gene in the initiation of APAs. However, *Kcnj5* mRNA and KCNJ5 protein are not expressed in the rat adrenal cortex, suggesting that it does not play a role in adrenal steroid production in this species and very likely in mice (86). Therefore, the demonstration that loss of *KCNJ5* is sufficient to initiate both hyperaldosteronism and tumor development will require genetic approaches in non-mouse systems, such as primary bovine adrenocortical cells and tissue reconstruction in xenografted mice.

Both cAMP/PKA and WNT/β-catenin pathways have been involved in the development of CPAs. Similarly, WNT/β-catenin pathway plays an important role in APA development, in addition to calcium signaling. Indeed, by generating a mouse model with constitutive β-catenin activation in the adrenal gland (ΔCat model), we found that these mice developed progressive dysplasia and hyperplasia, ectopic differentiation of *zona glomerulosa* (ZG), and increased aldosterone production (**Table 1**). The ΔCat model will be further discussed in the ACC section. In a subsequent paper, Berthon and colleagues reported that WNT/β-catenin pathway was aberrantly activated in 70% of a series of 47 patients, which was the most frequent alteration reported in APAs (87). Furthermore, a recent study has reported *CTNNB1* mutations in 5.1% of a cohort of 198 APAs (88). These mutations were associated with stabilized β-catenin, suggesting activation of WNT pathway (**Figure 2**). Because of the higher frequency of WNT/β-catenin activation than of *CTNNB1* mutations, it is essential to expand our knowledge of the other causes of aberrant WNT/β-catenin activation, by investigating other members of the pathway or possible crosstalks with other pathways. Interestingly, decreased expression of the WNT inhibitor *SRFP2* was shown to contribute to deregulation of WNT/β-catenin pathway in the adrenal (87) (**Figure 2**).

ADRENOCORTICAL CARCINOMAS: THE LACK OF MOUSE MODELS

Adrenocortical carcinomas are extremely rare, with an annual incidence of 0.5–2 cases per million in adults. However, they are highly aggressive tumors associated with poor prognosis and often diagnosed at an advanced stage for which available treatments are rarely curative. The overall 5-year survival rates range from 10 to 40% (6, 7). ACCs can occur at any age, but the incidence in children is particularly high in southern Brazil due to the high prevalence of a specific germline mutation (p.R337H) of the *TP53* tumor suppressor gene (8). Pediatric and adult ACCs differ in genetics and many other ways (89, 90), as will be further discussed in Section "Pediatric ACCs: TP53, SF1, and Related Mouse Models." Although most ACCs arise sporadically, an increased incidence of ACCs has been reported in some genetic syndromes, such as familial adenomatous polyposis (FAP), characterized by mutations in *APC* and elevated Wnt/β-catenin signaling, and Beckwith–Wiedemann syndrome (BWS), characterized by elevated expression of insulin-like growth factor-2 (*IGF2*) (91, 92).

The developmental context of the disease is crucial for the treatment and management of adrenal tumors. Therefore, there is a strong need to generate mouse models resembling human pathology, to identify the mechanisms involved in benign to malignant progression. Up to now, the three most frequent alterations that have been reported in ACC patients include overexpression of IGF2 (93, 94), activation of WNT/β-catenin signaling pathway (11, 77, 95), and inactivation of TP53/RB pathway (96, 97). Several mouse models of deregulation of these pathways have been generated, which allowed better understanding of adrenal tumorigenesis. However, none of these models was able to recapitulate full-fledged ACC development (**Table 1**). In the following sections, we summarize mouse models of ACC generated up to now, and focus on what is still lacking for a better understanding of adrenal tumor initiation and progression.

Mouse Models of WNT/β-Catenin and IGF2 Signaling Activation Are Insufficient to Trigger ACC Formation

The WNT/β-catenin pathway is essential for embryonic development and cell renewal in adult adrenal cortex where β-catenin is expressed and active in ZG (98) (**Figure 3**). Several tumor profiling studies have reported mutations in β-catenin gene (*CTNNB1*) in both ACAs and ACCs (77, 99, 100), suggesting that β-catenin activating mutations could be involved in adrenal tumor initiation and progression to malignancy. To assess this hypothesis, we have generated a mouse model of constitutive β-catenin activation in the adrenal cortex (ΔCat mice) (25) (**Figures 2** and **3**; **Table 1**). ΔCat mice were generated by mating mice harboring a floxed allele of β-catenin [$Catnb^{lox(ex3)}$] (101) with mice expressing the Cre recombinase in steroidogenic cells of the adrenal cortex, through the *Akr1b7* promoter region (67). Cre-mediated excision of the third exon of *Ctnnb1* gene prevents β-catenin phosphorylation and ubiquitin-dependent degradation, which induces accumulation of the protein and constitutive activation of its target genes. ΔCat mice showed adrenal hyperplasia and ectopic differentiation of ZG. However, aggressive tumor formation was only observed in a subset of 17-month-old animals. Our model demonstrated that *Ctnnb1* was an adrenal oncogene but it also suggested that secondary genetic alterations were required for malignant progression. Through a different approach, Hammer and colleagues obtained similar results by generating mice with adrenal cortex specific loss of *Apc* (APC KO mice) (26), a component of the multi-protein destruction complex of β-catenin, to target WNT pathway activation (**Figure 2**). As ΔCat mice, APC KO mice displayed hyperplasia. Furthermore, hyperplasia progressed to microscopic and macroscopic adenomas as early as

15 weeks of age, but progression to carcinoma was never observed (**Table 1**). Results from our two groups suggest that constitutive activation of β-catenin initiates benign tumor development but is not sufficient to trigger malignant evolution.

Insulin-like growth factor-2 is a growth factor involved in the control of cell proliferation and inhibition of apoptosis and it was hypothesized to interact with the Wnt/β-catenin pathway. In sporadic adrenal tumors, IGF2 is overexpressed in 80–90% of ACCs but not in ACAs (93, 94). Several transgenic mouse models have been generated to explore the role of IGF2 in adrenal tumorigenesis (**Table 1**). Mice with overexpression of IGF2 under the control of phosphoenolpyruvate carboxykinase (*PEPCK*) promoter showed four- to sixfold elevation of serum IGF2 levels and mild adrenocortical hyperplasia but did not develop ACTs (27), suggesting that IGF2 overexpression was not involved in initiation of adrenal tumorigenesis. We have generated transgenic mice with *ad*renal cortex specific overexpression of *IGF2* (AdIgf2 mice) (28) (**Table 1**). These mice had up to sevenfold higher basal levels of IGF2 (up to 87-fold higher with ACTH stimulation), but again they did not show tumor formation despite a mild increase in cortical cell proliferation. These results indicated that IGF2 alone could stimulate adrenal cortex proliferation but it was not able to induce oncogenic transformation. The mitogenic effect of IGF2 overexpression suggests a role in tumor maintenance rather than initiation, which would rather be triggered by other actors, such as WNT pathway. This two-step model is supported by the fact that IGF2 overexpression is found only in ACCs, whereas mutations in β-catenin are reported in both ACAs and ACCs. To test the hypothesis of cooperation between IGF2 and WNT pathways, we generated a mouse model presenting both genetic alterations, by mating ΔCat mice with IGF2 overexpressing mice (28) (**Table 1**). Our analysis of this model clearly showed that IGF2 overexpression in the context of constitutive WNT/β-catenin pathway activation only had a moderate effect on tumor progression. In another approach, Hammer and collaborators generated a mouse model with both loss of *APC*, to achieve WNT activation, and loss of imprinting at the *Igf2/H19* region, to achieve elevated *IGF2* expression (26) (**Table 1**). These mice displayed adrenocortical hyperplasia, microscopic and macroscopic adenomas, and cancer formation. Although the phenotype was more severe than that observed in mice presenting loss of APC alone, only one cancer formation was observed. Taken together, these results have clearly shown that genetic alterations in WNT pathway and IGF2 overexpression are not sufficient to trigger malignant adrenocortical tumorigenesis. Interestingly, we recently reported that expression of enhancer of zeste 2 (EZH2), a histone methyl transferase of the polycomb repressive complex 2 (PRC2), positively correlated with malignancy and poor prognosis in three different cohorts of patients with ACTs (102). In this study, we provided evidence that in the H295R human adrenal cancer cell line, EZH2 down-regulation or pharmacological inhibition significantly decreased cell proliferation and aggressive behavior and induced apoptosis. Interestingly, EZH2 overexpression was shown to be the result of P53/RB/E2F pathway deregulation in good agreement with ACC omic studies. Although this remains to be demonstrated in a relevant animal model, these data suggest that EZH2 could be involved in malignant progression. Mouse models with various ability to express Ezh2 (loss- and gain-of-function) are, thus, required to decipher the molecular mechanisms involved in EZH2-mediated malignant progression, i.e., transcription repression through PRC2 recruitment or activation (103) and to identify the actors that cooperate with WNT pathway in this process. Altogether, these mouse models indicate that malignant tumors may arise from typical adenomas even if this progression only affects a small proportion of benign tumors and requires additional alterations, such as EZH2 overexpression. One challenge of these studies is the evaluation of tumor staging in mouse models. Until now, mouse tumors have been evaluated with the same criteria as human tumors, i.e., essentially Weiss's scoring. However, the transposability of these histologic criteria is unclear and the only undoubtful proof of malignant progression is metastatic dissemination, which was not observed in any of the models discussed above. Irrespective of this issue, inheritable tumors in mouse genetic models provide an invaluable tool to follow tumor initiation and progression. Whole genomic analyses in such models would provide a unique opportunity to demonstrate or invalidate the existence of a normal adrenal adenoma–carcinoma continuum in adrenocortical tumorigenesis.

Pediatric ACCs: TP53, SF1, and Related Mouse Models

In addition to overexpression of IGF2 and activation of WNT pathway, the third most frequent genetic alteration in ACCs is inactivation of TP53/RB pathway. Germline mutations in the *p53* tumor suppressor gene are associated with the development of Li–Fraumeni syndrome (LFS), an autosomal-dominant cancer syndrome resulting in multiple malignancies, including ACCs (104, 105). The rate of germline TP53 mutations in ACCs is age-dependent, ranging from up to 80% in pediatric ACCs (97) to 3–7% in adults (96). A 10-fold increased incidence of ACCs is observed in Southern Brazil due to a germline mutation within the oligomerization domain of *p53* (p.R337H). This germline mutation was first identified in 98% of children with ACCs (106). The p.R337H mutation was also present in 78% of children with sporadic ACTs in another series and in 13% of adult patients with ACCs (107). In adult ACTs, *TP53* mutations are mostly somatic and were considered to represent a later step in tumorigenesis (108, 109). Several mouse models of p53 dysfunction have been generated, including targeted mutations, replicating proteins identified in humans with LFS (110, 111). These mice developed a large spectrum of tumors but not ACCs. Mouse models of adrenal-specific *TP53* loss have not been generated to date, despite the high prevalence of *TP53* mutations in ACCs. However, the adrenocortical dysplasia (*Acd*) mouse model (112), carrying an inactivating mutation in *Tpp/Acd*, which normally functions to protect telomerase, was used to explore the consequences of *TP53* loss during adrenal tumorigenesis (**Table 1**). Interestingly, ablation of *p53* (obtained by mating *Acd* mice with *p53* null mice) rescued a number of characteristics of the *Acd* phenotype, including adrenal hypoplasia. This indicates that hypoplasia in *Acd* mice results from p53-mediated senescence. Moreover, the loss of *p53* in *Acd* mice leads to development of

ACC, suggesting that p53-mediated escape from senescence may contribute to adrenocortical carcinogenesis (29). Another approach to explore the consequences of p53 ablation during adrenal tumorigenesis consists in adrenal targeting of the Simian Virus 40 (SV40) large T antigen (TAg), a potent oncogene acting in part by inactivating p53 [reviewed in (113)]. TAg expressed under the control of several promoters has been used to induce ACTs in transgenic mice. In the *inhibin-α* (*inha*) promoter-TAg mouse, ACCs are induced by gonadectomy (30) (**Table 1**). This mouse model will not be discussed in details here as mouse models of gonadectomy-induced ACTs are beyond the scope of this review, being unrelated to the context of human adrenal tumors. In order to better recapitulate the context of human adrenal tumor development, we have generated a model in which TAg is expressed under the control of the adrenal cortex specific *Akr1b7* promoter (31) (**Table 1**). In this AdTAg model 2 of 3 surviving founder mice developed adrenal tumors that were used to generate cell lines for further *in vitro* analysis (114). As exome sequencing and SNP array recently confirmed that p53/RB is one of the most frequently altered pathways in ACCs (11), future mouse models are needed to further explore the role of TP53 in adrenal tumor formation and progression. Considering the well-characterized antagonism of large TAg toward p53 and Rb tumor suppressors, one would predict that the AdTAg model could provide one of the most relevant and simple models to explore adrenal tumorigenic processes.

Transcriptional profiling has demonstrated distinct signatures of adult and pediatric ACCs with the pediatric tumor transcriptome displaying similarities to that of fetal adrenal tissue (115). Moreover, pediatric and adult ACCs differ in several clinical, pathological, and molecular aspects [reviewed in (90)], suggesting that they may represent genetically distinct entities. In addition to *TP53*, the genetic locus containing steroidogenic factor 1 gene (*SF-1*) is commonly amplified and overexpressed in pediatric ACCs (116, 117). SF-1 is a nuclear receptor transcription factor that plays an important role in the regulation of steroidogenic genes, in development and function of the adrenal cortex, and in male sexual differentiation (118, 119). In contrast to children, the frequency of amplification and overexpression in adult patients is very low (120), but it is associated with poor outcome (121). A transgenic mouse model, harboring multiple copies of a yeast artificial chromosome, including the *SF-1* genetic locus, termed YACTR mice, has been generated (32) (**Table 1**). Although these mice developed adrenocortical hyperplasia that further progressed to adrenal tumors in a dose-dependent manner, the morphology of adrenal tumors differed from human ACTs and displayed a gonadal phenotype that was reminiscent of ACTs occurring in gonadectomized mice. These tumors are thought to arise from pluripotent adreno-gonadal precursor cells lying beneath the outer adrenal connective capsule, which have the potential to differentiate into cells of gonadal phenotype (122). Similarly, in YACTR mice, high levels of *SF-1* may trigger proliferation of pluripotent cells and the development of adrenal tumors with a gonadal phenotype. Despite the differences in tumor phenotypes in human and mice, SF-1 appears to play an important role in adrenal tumorigenesis in both species. Recently, it has been proposed that SF-1 overexpression induces alterations of redox mechanisms, which may contribute to adrenal tumorigenesis. Indeed, inactivation of SF1 target gene *Vnn1*, encoding the Vanin-1 protein involved in the response to oxidative stress, was found to antagonize the development of adrenocortical neoplasia in *SF-1* transgenic mice (123).

Novel Identified Genes in ACCs: Interplays with WNT Pathway and Need for In Vivo Studies

Recent OMIC studies confirmed that the most frequent genetic alterations in ACCs affect the tumor suppressor gene *TP53* and the oncogene *CTNNB1* (each being altered in ~16% of ACCs) (11, 124). In addition to pointing out alterations in already known drivers (*CTNNB1* and *TP53*), these studies identified new genes not previously reported in ACCs. Among these new genes, *ZNRF3* was found to be the most frequently altered (21% of ACCs). *ZNRF3* encodes a protein with E3 ubiquitin ligase activity, supposed to act as a negative regulator of the WNT/β-catenin pathway (125) (**Figure 2**). ACCs with alterations in *ZNRF3* locus showed activation of β-catenin target genes, but this activation was weaker than in tumors with *CTNNB1* mutations (11). Interestingly, *ZNRF3* and *CTNNB1* alterations were mutually exclusive. Further functional studies and novel mouse models are needed to further explore the role of *ZNRF3* in ACCs. Recurrent mutations have also been found in several known cell cycle regulators, including *CDKN2A*, *CDK4*, *RB1*, and *CCNE1*, confirming the notion that release from p53-sensitive checkpoints is a critical step in the process of adrenal tumorigenesis, a notion that previously emerged from analysis of p53 ablation in *Acd* mice.

Recently, mutations have also been found in *PRKAR1A* (126), a gene mutated in PPNAD (as discussed in Section "Primary Pigmented Nodular Adrenocortical Disease and Related Mouse Models") and much more rarely in ACAs (as discussed in Section "Cortisol-Producing Adenomas: PKA Pathway, PRKACA Mutations, and Lack of Mouse Models"). These recent reports of *PRKAR1A* mutations expand the role of PKA signaling in ACC. If any functional interplay exists between the WNT/β-catenin and the cAMP/PKA pathways in the pathophysiology of adrenal cortex, this is an important point that remains to be clarified *in vivo* (**Figure 3**). As reviewed in Drelon's study (127) data from the literature are in favor of such an interplay. This could influence normal adrenal cortex renewal/zonation as well as the pathophysiology of human adrenal tumors. However, whether these pathways cooperate or antagonize each other remains to be determined. This question could be genetically addressed by generating compound transgenic mice based on already available models carrying β-catenin and PKA constitutive activation (**Figure 3**) (23, 25).

FUTURE DIRECTIONS

The understanding of mechanisms of adrenal tumor progression is crucial for the management and treatment of the disease. Indeed, almost half of ACC patients present with metastatic disease and although mitotane alone or in combination with chemotherapy can improve patients' survival, there is no efficient treatment for advanced disease. There is, thus, a strong need to generate mouse models resembling human pathology to identify actors involved in adrenal carcinogenesis. Especially, mouse models testing the role of newly identified genes in pediatric and adult ACCs are warranted. Moreover, as recent OMIC approaches confirmed that p53/RB is one of the most frequently altered pathways in ACCs (11), the AdTAg mouse model, previously used to generate cell lines for *in vitro* analyses (114), now becomes a relevant model for the study of ACCs.

The study of molecular mechanisms underlying malignant tumor progression represents a crucial step to develop novel specific drugs. The next step is to test their efficacy through *in vitro* and *in vivo* experiments. The only available "*in vivo*" model is the ACC xenograft obtained by subcutaneous injection of the H295R cell line in nude mice (128). Although this model has been extensively used to evaluate new and established drugs, it is important to take its limitations into account. These include deregulated antitumoral response resulting from immunodeficiency and abnormal or deficient microenvironment associated with subcutaneous injection of cells. Therefore, the AdTAg mouse model could be a useful experimental platform to assess *in vivo* the role of newly identified candidates potentially involved in malignant progression, such as EZH2 (102), using genetic or pharmacological approaches. Considering pediatric adrenal cancers, knock-in mouse models reproducing *TP53* p.R337H mutation found in Brazilian families will be a major advance in our understanding of the pathogenesis of these destructive tumors. There is, thus, a strong need for novel mouse models for preclinical studies.

Finally, high throughput next-generation sequencing technologies have allowed major advances in the knowledge of the genetic bases of ACAs. Among the newly identified genes, *ARMC5*, *KCNJ5*, and *PRKACA* mutations represent the most frequent genetic defects in PBMAH, APAs, and CPAs, respectively (10, 39, 61, 62, 72–74, 79). Mouse models are required to confirm the driving potential of these genes in the initiation and/or progression of ACAs. In conclusion, we expect that the progress in gene editing methods and the recent identification of new recurrently mutated genes, will soon allow the development of novel mouse models capable of faithfully reproducing human adrenal diseases, overcoming the limitations of current models. These models will be useful, on the one hand, to investigate the mechanisms underlying malignant progression of adrenal tumors and, on the other hand, to develop novel therapeutic approaches.

AUTHOR CONTRIBUTIONS

FL and AM wrote the manuscript. All authors edited the manuscript.

FUNDING

We acknowledge the Université Blaise Pascal, Université d'Auvergne, Centre National de la Recherche Scientifique, Institut National de la Santé et de la Recherche Médicale, Agence National de la Recherche (grant ANR-14-CE12-0007), Fondation ARC pour la Recherche sur le Cancer (PJA 20141201894), and La Fondation de France, which supported our lab activity.

REFERENCES

1. Stratakis CA. Cushing syndrome caused by adrenocortical tumors and hyperplasias (corticotropin-independent Cushing syndrome). *Endocr Dev* (2008) 13:117–32. doi:10.1159/000134829
2. Calebiro D, Di Dalmazi G, Bathon K, Ronchi CL, Beuschlein F. cAMP signaling in cortisol-producing adrenal adenoma. *Eur J Endocrinol* (2015) 173:M99–106. doi:10.1530/EJE-15-0353
3. Fagugli RM, Taglioni C. Changes in the perceived epidemiology of primary hyperaldosteronism. *Int J Hypertens* (2011) 2011:162804. doi:10.4061/2011/162804
4. Hsiao H-P, Kirschner LS, Bourdeau I, Keil MF, Boikos SA, Verma S, et al. Clinical and genetic heterogeneity, overlap with other tumor syndromes, and atypical glucocorticoid hormone secretion in adrenocorticotropin-independent macronodular adrenal hyperplasia compared with other adrenocortical tumors. *J Clin Endocrinol Metab* (2009) 94:2930–7. doi:10.1210/jc.2009-0516
5. Bertherat J, Horvath A, Groussin L, Grabar S, Boikos S, Cazabat L, et al. Mutations in regulatory subunit type 1A of cyclic adenosine 5'-monophosphate-dependent protein kinase (PRKAR1A): phenotype analysis in 353 patients and 80 different genotypes. *J Clin Endocrinol Metab* (2009) 94:2085–91. doi:10.1210/jc.2008-2333
6. Wajchenberg BL, Albergaria Pereira MA, Medonca BB, Latronico AC, Campos Carneiro P, Alves VA, et al. Adrenocortical carcinoma: clinical and laboratory observations. *Cancer* (2000) 88:711–36. doi:10.1002/(SICI)1097-0142(20000215)88:4<711::AID-CNCR1>3.0.CO;2-W
7. Else T, Kim AC, Sabolch A, Raymond VM, Kandathil A, Caoili EM, et al. Adrenocortical carcinoma. *Endocr Rev* (2014) 35:282–326. doi:10.1210/er.2013-1029
8. Custódio G, Komechen H, Figueiredo FRO, Fachin ND, Pianovski MAD, Figueiredo BC. Molecular epidemiology of adrenocortical tumors in southern Brazil. *Mol Cell Endocrinol* (2012) 351:44–51. doi:10.1016/j.mce.2011.10.019
9. Beuschlein F, Fassnacht M, Assié G, Calebiro D, Stratakis CA, Osswald A, et al. Constitutive activation of PKA catalytic subunit in adrenal Cushing's syndrome. *N Engl J Med* (2014) 370:1019–28. doi:10.1056/NEJMoa1310359
10. Assié G, Libé R, Espiard S, Rizk-Rabin M, Guimier A, Luscap W, et al. ARMC5 mutations in macronodular adrenal hyperplasia with Cushing's syndrome. *N Engl J Med* (2013) 369:2105–14. doi:10.1056/NEJMoa1304603
11. Assié G, Letouzé E, Fassnacht M, Jouinot A, Luscap W, Barreau O, et al. Integrated genomic characterization of adrenocortical carcinoma. *Nat Genet* (2014) 46:607–12. doi:10.1038/ng.2953
12. Barzon L, Sonino N, Fallo F, Palu G, Boscaro M. Prevalence and natural history of adrenal incidentalomas. *Eur J Endocrinol* (2003) 149:273–85. doi:10.1530/eje.0.1490273
13. Cawood TJ, Hunt PJ, O'Shea D, Cole D, Soule S. Recommended evaluation of adrenal incidentalomas is costly, has high false-positive rates and confers a risk of fatal cancer that is similar to the risk of the adrenal lesion becoming malignant; time for a rethink? *Eur J Endocrinol* (2009) 161:513–27. doi:10.1530/EJE-09-0234
14. Kastelan D, Kraljevic I, Dusek T, Knezevic N, Solak M, Gardijan B, et al. The clinical course of patients with adrenal incidentaloma: is it time to reconsider the current recommendations? *Eur J Endocrinol* (2015) 173:275–82. doi:10.1530/EJE-15-0199
15. Bernard M-H, Sidhu S, Berger N, Peix J-L, Marsh DJ, Robinson BG, et al. A case report in favor of a multistep adrenocortical tumorigenesis. *J Clin Endocrinol Metab* (2003) 88:998–1001. doi:10.1210/jc.2002-021117

16. Ronchi CL, Sbiera S, Leich E, Henzel K, Rosenwald A, Allolio B, et al. Single nucleotide polymorphism array profiling of adrenocortical tumors – evidence for an adenoma carcinoma sequence? *PLoS One* (2013) 8:e73959. doi:10.1371/journal.pone.0073959
17. Gara SK, Wang Y, Patel D, Liu-Chittenden Y, Jain M, Boufraqech M, et al. Integrated genome-wide analysis of genomic changes and gene regulation in human adrenocortical tissue samples. *Nucleic Acids Res* (2015) 43:9327–39. doi:10.1093/nar/gkv908
18. Barreau O, de Reynies A, Wilmot-Roussel H, Guillaud-Bataille M, Auzan C, Rene-Corail F, et al. Clinical and pathophysiological implications of chromosomal alterations in adrenocortical tumors: an integrated genomic approach. *J Clin Endocrinol Metab* (2012) 97:E301–11. doi:10.1210/jc.2011-1588
19. Bertolino P, Radovanovic I, Casse H, Aguzzi A, Wang Z-Q, Zhang C-X. Genetic ablation of the tumor suppressor menin causes lethality at mid-gestation with defects in multiple organs. *Mech Dev* (2003) 120:549–60. doi:10.1016/S0925-4773(03)00039-X
20. Crabtree JS, Scacheri PC, Ward JM, Garrett-Beal L, Emmert-Buck MR, Edgemon KA, et al. A mouse model of multiple endocrine neoplasia, type 1, develops multiple endocrine tumors. *Proc Natl Acad Sci U S A* (2001) 98:1118–23. doi:10.1073/pnas.98.3.1118
21. Kirschner LS, Kusewitt DF, Matyakhina L, Towns WH, Carney JA, Westphal H, et al. A mouse model for the Carney complex tumor syndrome develops neoplasia in cyclic AMP-responsive tissues. *Cancer Res* (2005) 65:4506–14. doi:10.1158/0008-5472.CAN-05-0580
22. Griffin KJ, Kirschner LS, Matyakhina L, Stergiopoulos SG, Robinson-White A, Lenherr SM, et al. A transgenic mouse bearing an antisense construct of regulatory subunit type 1A of protein kinase A develops endocrine and other tumours: comparison with Carney complex and other PRKAR1A induced lesions. *J Med Genet* (2004) 41:923–31. doi:10.1136/jmg.2004.028043
23. Sahut-Barnola I, de Joussineau C, Val P, Lambert-Langlais S, Damon C, Lefrançois-Martinez A-M, et al. Cushing's syndrome and fetal features resurgence in adrenal cortex-specific Prkar1a knockout mice. *PLoS Genet* (2010) 6:e1000980. doi:10.1371/journal.pgen.1000980
24. Tsai L-CL, Shimizu-Albergine M, Beavo JA. The high-affinity cAMP-specific phosphodiesterase 8B controls steroidogenesis in the mouse adrenal gland. *Mol Pharmacol* (2011) 79:639–48. doi:10.1124/mol.110.069104
25. Berthon A, Sahut-Barnola I, Lambert-Langlais S, de Joussineau C, Damon-Soubeyrand C, Louiset E, et al. Constitutive beta-catenin activation induces adrenal hyperplasia and promotes adrenal cancer development. *Hum Mol Genet* (2010) 19:1561–76. doi:10.1093/hmg/ddq029
26. Heaton JH, Wood MA, Kim AC, Lima LO, Barlaskar FM, Almeida MQ, et al. Progression to adrenocortical tumorigenesis in mice and humans through insulin-like growth factor 2 and β-catenin. *Am J Pathol* (2012) 181:1017–33. doi:10.1016/j.ajpath.2012.05.026
27. Weber MM, Fottner C, Schmidt P, Brodowski KM, Gittner K, Lahm H, et al. Postnatal overexpression of insulin-like growth factor II in transgenic mice is associated with adrenocortical hyperplasia and enhanced steroidogenesis. *Endocrinology* (1999) 140:1537–43. doi:10.1210/endo.140.4.6660
28. Drelon C, Berthon A, Ragazzon B, Tissier F, Bandiera R, Sahut-Barnola I, et al. Analysis of the role of Igf2 in adrenal tumour development in transgenic mouse models. *PLoS One* (2012) 7:e44171. doi:10.1371/journal.pone.0044171
29. Else T, Trovato A, Kim AC, Wu Y, Ferguson DO, Kuick RD, et al. Genetic p53 deficiency partially rescues the adrenocortical dysplasia phenotype at the expense of increased tumorigenesis. *Cancer Cell* (2009) 15:465–76. doi:10.1016/j.ccr.2009.04.011
30. Kananen K, Markkula M, Mikola M, Rainio EM, McNeilly A, Huhtaniemi I. Gonadectomy permits adrenocortical tumorigenesis in mice transgenic for the mouse inhibin alpha-subunit promoter/simian virus 40 T-antigen fusion gene: evidence for negative autoregulation of the inhibin alpha-subunit gene. *Mol Endocrinol* (1996) 10:1667–77. doi:10.1210/mend.10.12.8961275
31. Sahut-Barnola I, Lefrancois-Martinez AM, Jean C, Veyssiere G, Martinez A. Adrenal tumorigenesis targeted by the corticotropin-regulated promoter of the aldo-keto reductase AKR1B7 gene in transgenic mice. *Endocr Res* (2000) 26:885–98. doi:10.3109/07435800009048613
32. Doghman M, Karpova T, Rodrigues GA, Arhatte M, De Moura J, Cavalli LR, et al. Increased steroidogenic factor-1 dosage triggers adrenocortical cell proliferation and cancer. *Mol Endocrinol* (2007) 21:2968–87. doi:10.1210/me.2007-0120
33. Lacroix A. ACTH-independent macronodular adrenal hyperplasia. *Best Pract Res Clin Endocrinol Metab* (2009) 23:245–59. doi:10.1016/j.beem.2008.10.011
34. Stratakis CA, Boikos SA. Genetics of adrenal tumors associated with Cushing's syndrome: a new classification for bilateral adrenocortical hyperplasias. *Nat Clin Pract Endocrinol Metab* (2007) 3:748–57. doi:10.1038/ncpendmet0648
35. Kirschner MA, Powell RD, Lipsett MB. Cushing's syndrome: nodular cortical hyperplasia of adrenal glands with clinical and pathological features suggesting adrenocortical tumor. *J Clin Endocrinol Metab* (1964) 24:947–55. doi:10.1210/jcem-24-10-947
36. Louiset E, Duparc C, Young J, Renouf S, Tetsi Nomigni M, Boutelet I, et al. Intraadrenal corticotropin in bilateral macronodular adrenal hyperplasia. *N Engl J Med* (2013) 369:2115–25. doi:10.1056/NEJMoa1215245
37. Vezzosi D, Cartier D, Régnier C, Otal P, Bennet A, Parmentier F, et al. Familial adrenocorticotropin-independent macronodular adrenal hyperplasia with aberrant serotonin and vasopressin adrenal receptors. *Eur J Endocrinol* (2007) 156:21–31. doi:10.1530/eje.1.02324
38. Watson TD, Patel SJ, Nardi PM. Case 121: familial adrenocorticotropin-independent macronodular adrenal hyperplasia causing Cushing syndrome. *Radiology* (2007) 244:923–6. doi:10.1148/radiol.2443041507
39. Alencar GA, Lerario AM, Nishi MY, Mariani BM, Almeida MQ, Tremblay J, et al. ARMC5 mutations are a frequent cause of primary macronodular adrenal Hyperplasia. *J Clin Endocrinol Metab* (2014) 99:E1501–9. doi:10.1210/jc.2013-4237
40. Lacroix A, Ndiaye N, Tremblay J, Hamet P. Ectopic and abnormal hormone receptors in adrenal Cushing's syndrome. *Endocr Rev* (2001) 22:75–110. doi:10.1210/edrv.22.1.0420
41. Bourdeau I, D'Amour P, Hamet P, Boutin JM, Lacroix A. Aberrant membrane hormone receptors in incidentally discovered bilateral macronodular adrenal hyperplasia with subclinical Cushing's syndrome. *J Clin Endocrinol Metab* (2001) 86:5534–40. doi:10.1210/jcem.86.11.8062
42. Lacroix A, Baldacchino V, Bourdeau I, Hamet P, Tremblay J. Cushing's syndrome variants secondary to aberrant hormone receptors. *Trends Endocrinol Metab* (2004) 15:375–82. doi:10.1016/j.tem.2004.08.007
43. Reznik Y, Allali-Zerah V, Chayvialle JA, Leroyer R, Leymarie P, Travert G, et al. Food-dependent Cushing's syndrome mediated by aberrant adrenal sensitivity to gastric inhibitory polypeptide. *N Engl J Med* (1992) 327:981–6. doi:10.1056/NEJM199210013271403
44. Groussin L, Perlemoine K, Contesse V, Lefebvre H, Tabarin A, Thieblot P, et al. The ectopic expression of the gastric inhibitory polypeptide receptor is frequent in adrenocorticotropin-independent bilateral macronodular adrenal hyperplasia, but rare in unilateral tumors. *J Clin Endocrinol Metab* (2002) 87:1980–5. doi:10.1210/jcem.87.5.8458
45. Lacroix A, Hamet P, Boutin JM. Leuprolide acetate therapy in luteinizing hormone – dependent Cushing's syndrome. *N Engl J Med* (1999) 341:1577–81. doi:10.1056/NEJM199911183412104
46. Goodarzi MO, Dawson DW, Li X, Lei Z, Shintaku P, Rao CV, et al. Virilization in bilateral macronodular adrenal hyperplasia controlled by luteinizing hormone. *J Clin Endocrinol Metab* (2003) 88:73–7. doi:10.1210/jc.2002-021292
47. Bertherat J, Contesse V, Louiset E, Barrande G, Duparc C, Groussin L, et al. In vivo and in vitro screening for illegitimate receptors in adrenocorticotropin-independent macronodular adrenal hyperplasia causing Cushing's syndrome: identification of two cases of gonadotropin/gastric inhibitory polypeptide-dependent hypercortisolism. *J Clin Endocrinol Metab* (2005) 90:1302–10. doi:10.1210/jc.2004-1256
48. Lee S, Hwang R, Lee J, Rhee Y, Kim DJ, Chung U-I, et al. Ectopic expression of vasopressin V1b and V2 receptors in the adrenal glands of familial ACTH-independent macronodular adrenal hyperplasia. *Clin Endocrinol (Oxf)* (2005) 63:625–30. doi:10.1111/j.1365-2265.2005.02387.x
49. Mazzuco TL, Chabre O, Sturm N, Feige J-J, Thomas M. Ectopic expression of the gastric inhibitory polypeptide receptor gene is a sufficient genetic event to induce benign adrenocortical tumor in a xenotransplantation model. *Endocrinology* (2006) 147:782–90. doi:10.1210/en.2005-0921
50. Mazzuco TL, Chabre O, Feige J-J, Thomas M. Aberrant expression of human luteinizing hormone receptor by adrenocortical cells is sufficient to provoke both hyperplasia and Cushing's syndrome features. *J Clin Endocrinol Metab* (2006) 91:196–203. doi:10.1210/jc.2005-1975

51. Herbet M, Salomon A, Feige J-J, Thomas M. Acquisition order of Ras and p53 gene alterations defines distinct adrenocortical tumor phenotypes. *PLoS Genet* (2012) 8:e1002700. doi:10.1371/journal.pgen.1002700
52. Groen EJ, Roos A, Muntinghe FL, Enting RH, de Vries J, Kleibeuker JH, et al. Extra-intestinal manifestations of familial adenomatous polyposis. *Ann Surg Oncol* (2008) 15:2439–50. doi:10.1245/s10434-008-9981-3
53. Berthon A, Martinez A, Bertherat J, Val P. Wnt/β-catenin signalling in adrenal physiology and tumour development. *Mol Cell Endocrinol* (2012) 351:87–95. doi:10.1016/j.mce.2011.09.009
54. Gatta-Cherifi B, Chabre O, Murat A, Niccoli P, Cardot-Bauters C, Rohmer V, et al. Adrenal involvement in MEN1. Analysis of 715 cases from the Groupe d'etude des Tumeurs Endocrines database. *Eur J Endocrinol* (2012) 166:269–79. doi:10.1530/EJE-11-0679
55. Shuch B, Ricketts CJ, Vocke CD, Valera VA, Chen CC, Gautam R, et al. Adrenal nodular hyperplasia in hereditary leiomyomatosis and renal cell cancer. *J Urol* (2013) 189:430–5. doi:10.1016/j.juro.2012.07.139
56. Rothenbuhler A, Horvath A, Libé R, Faucz FR, Fratticci A, Raffin Sanson ML, et al. Identification of novel genetic variants in phosphodiesterase 8B (PDE8B), a cAMP-specific phosphodiesterase highly expressed in the adrenal cortex, in a cohort of patients with adrenal tumours. *Clin Endocrinol (Oxf)* (2012) 77:195–9. doi:10.1111/j.1365-2265.2012.04366.x
57. Vezzosi D, Libe R, Baudry C, Rizk-Rabin M, Horvath A, Levy I, et al. Phosphodiesterase 11A (PDE11A) gene defects in patients with acth-independent macronodular adrenal hyperplasia (AIMAH): functional variants may contribute to genetic susceptibility of bilateral adrenal tumors. *J Clin Endocrinol Metab* (2012) 97:E2063–9. doi:10.1210/jc.2012-2275
58. Swords FM, Noon LA, King PJ, Clark AJL. Constitutive activation of the human ACTH receptor resulting from a synergistic interaction between two naturally occurring missense mutations in the MC2R gene. *Mol Cell Endocrinol* (2004) 213:149–54. doi:10.1016/j.mce.2003.10.052
59. Salpea P, Stratakis CA. Carney complex and McCune Albright syndrome: an overview of clinical manifestations and human molecular genetics. *Mol Cell Endocrinol* (2014) 386:85–91. doi:10.1016/j.mce.2013.08.022
60. Agarwal R, Szalkiewicz ERH, Warner RRP, Roayaie S, Hechtman JF, Zhu H, et al. Multiple endocrine neoplasia type 1 associated with a new mutation in the menin gene and a midgut neuroendocrine tumor. *Pancreas* (2014) 43:145–6. doi:10.1097/MPA.0b013e31829f9d3d
61. Faucz FR, Zilbermint M, Lodish MB, Szarek E, Trivellin G, Sinaii N, et al. Macronodular adrenal hyperplasia due to mutations in an armadillo repeat containing 5 (ARMC5) gene: a clinical and genetic investigation. *J Clin Endocrinol Metab* (2014) 99:E1113–9. doi:10.1210/jc.2013-4280
62. Gagliardi L, Schreiber AW, Hahn CN, Feng J, Cranston T, Boon H, et al. ARMC5 mutations are common in familial bilateral macronodular adrenal hyperplasia. *J Clin Endocrinol Metab* (2014) 99:E1784–92. doi:10.1210/jc.2014-1265
63. Stratakis CA, Kirschner LS, Carney JA. Clinical and molecular features of the Carney complex: diagnostic criteria and recommendations for patient evaluation. *J Clin Endocrinol Metab* (2001) 86:4041–6. doi:10.1210/jcem.86.9.7903
64. Kirschner LS, Carney JA, Pack SD, Taymans SE, Giatzakis C, Cho YS, et al. Mutations of the gene encoding the protein kinase A type I-alpha regulatory subunit in patients with the Carney complex. *Nat Genet* (2000) 26:89–92. doi:10.1038/79238
65. Espiard S, Ragazzon B, Bertherat J. Protein kinase A alterations in adrenocortical tumors. *Horm Metab Res* (2014) 46:869–75. doi:10.1055/s-0034-1385908
66. Amieux PS, Howe DG, Knickerbocker H, Lee DC, Su T, Laszlo GS, et al. Increased basal cAMP-dependent protein kinase activity inhibits the formation of mesoderm-derived structures in the developing mouse embryo. *J Biol Chem* (2002) 277:27294–304. doi:10.1074/jbc.M200302200
67. Lambert-Langlais S, Val P, Guyot S, Ragazzon B, Sahut-Barnola I, De Haze A, et al. A transgenic mouse line with specific Cre recombinase expression in the adrenal cortex. *Mol Cell Endocrinol* (2009) 300:197–204. doi:10.1016/j.mce.2008.10.045
68. de Joussineau C, Sahut-Barnola I, Levy I, Saloustros E, Val P, Stratakis CA, et al. The cAMP pathway and the control of adrenocortical development and growth. *Mol Cell Endocrinol* (2012) 351:28–36. doi:10.1016/j.mce.2011.10.006
69. de Joussineau C, Sahut-Barnola I, Tissier F, Dumontet T, Drelon C, Batisse-Lignier M, et al. mTOR pathway is activated by PKA in adrenocortical cells and participates in vivo to apoptosis resistance in primary pigmented nodular adrenocortical disease (PPNAD). *Hum Mol Genet* (2014) 23:5418–28. doi:10.1093/hmg/ddu265
70. Bourdeau I. Clinical and molecular genetic studies of bilateral adrenal hyperplasias. *Endocr Res* (2004) 30:575–83. doi:10.1081/ERC-200043735
71. Horvath A, Mathyakina L, Vong Q, Baxendale V, Pang ALY, Chan W-Y, et al. Serial analysis of gene expression in adrenocortical hyperplasia caused by a germline PRKAR1A mutation. *J Clin Endocrinol Metab* (2006) 91:584–96. doi:10.1210/jc.2005-1301
72. Cao Y, He M, Gao Z, Peng Y, Li Y, Li L, et al. Activating hotspot L205R mutation in PRKACA and adrenal Cushing's syndrome. *Science* (2014) 344:913–7. doi:10.1126/science.1249480
73. Goh G, Scholl UI, Healy JM, Choi M, Prasad ML, Nelson-Williams C, et al. Recurrent activating mutation in PRKACA in cortisol-producing adrenal tumors. *Nat Genet* (2014) 46:613–7. doi:10.1038/ng.2956
74. Sato Y, Maekawa S, Ishii R, Sanada M, Morikawa T, Shiraishi Y, et al. Recurrent somatic mutations underlie corticotropin-independent Cushing's syndrome. *Science* (2014) 344:917–20. doi:10.1126/science.1252328
75. Bertherat J, Groussin L, Sandrini F, Matyakhina L, Bei T, Stergiopoulos S, et al. Molecular and functional analysis of PRKAR1A and its locus (17q22-24) in sporadic adrenocortical tumors: 17q losses, somatic mutations, and protein kinase A expression and activity. *Cancer Res* (2003) 63(17):5308–19.
76. Di Dalmazi G, Kisker C, Calebiro D, Mannelli M, Canu L, Arnaldi G, et al. Novel somatic mutations in the catalytic subunit of the protein kinase A as a cause of adrenal Cushing's syndrome: a European multicentric study. *J Clin Endocrinol Metab* (2014) 99:E2093–100. doi:10.1210/jc.2014-2152
77. Tissier F, Cavard C, Groussin L, Perlemoine K, Fumey G, Hagneré A-M, et al. Mutations of beta-catenin in adrenocortical tumors: activation of the Wnt signaling pathway is a frequent event in both benign and malignant adrenocortical tumors. *Cancer Res* (2005) 65:7622–7. doi:10.1158/0008-5472.CAN-05-0593
78. Choi M, Scholl UI, Yue P, Björklund P, Zhao B, Nelson-Williams C, et al. K+ channel mutations in adrenal aldosterone-producing adenomas and hereditary hypertension. *Science* (2011) 331:768–72. doi:10.1126/science.1198785
79. Zennaro M-C, Boulkroun S, Fernandes-Rosa F. An update on novel mechanisms of primary aldosteronism. *J Endocrinol* (2015) 224:R63–77. doi:10.1530/JOE-14-0597
80. Azizan EAB, Poulsen H, Tuluc P, Zhou J, Clausen MV, Lieb A, et al. Somatic mutations in ATP1A1 and CACNA1D underlie a common subtype of adrenal hypertension. *Nat Genet* (2013) 45:1055–60. doi:10.1038/ng.2716
81. Scholl UI, Stölting G, Nelson-Williams C, Vichot AA, Choi M, Loring E, et al. Recurrent gain of function mutation in calcium channel CACNA1H causes early-onset hypertension with primary aldosteronism. *Elife* (2015) 4:e06315. doi:10.7554/eLife.06315
82. Beuschlein F, Boulkroun S, Osswald A, Wieland T, Nielsen HN, Lichtenauer UD, et al. Somatic mutations in ATP1A1 and ATP2B3 lead to aldosterone-producing adenomas and secondary hypertension. *Nat Genet* (2013) 45:e1–2. doi:10.1038/ng.2550
83. Aller MI, Veale EL, Linden A-M, Sandu C, Schwaninger M, Evans LJ, et al. Modifying the subunit composition of TASK channels alters the modulation of a leak conductance in cerebellar granule neurons. *J Neurosci* (2005) 25:11455–67. doi:10.1523/JNEUROSCI.3153-05.2005
84. Heitzmann D, Derand R, Jungbauer S, Bandulik S, Sterner C, Schweda F, et al. Invalidation of TASK1 potassium channels disrupts adrenal gland zonation and mineralocorticoid homeostasis. *EMBO J* (2008) 27:179–87. doi:10.1038/sj.emboj.7601934
85. Guyon A, Tardy MP, Rovère C, Nahon J-L, Barhanin J, Lesage F. Glucose inhibition persists in hypothalamic neurons lacking tandem-pore K+ channels. *J Neurosci* (2009) 29:2528–33. doi:10.1523/JNEUROSCI.5764-08.2009
86. Chen AX, Nishimoto K, Nanba K, Rainey WE. Potassium channels related to primary aldosteronism: expression similarities and differences between human and rat adrenals. *Mol Cell Endocrinol* (2015) 417:141–8. doi:10.1016/j.mce.2015.09.011
87. Berthon A, Drelon C, Ragazzon B, Boulkroun S, Tissier F, Amar L, et al. WNT/β-catenin signalling is activated in aldosterone-producing adenomas and controls aldosterone production. *Hum Mol Genet* (2014) 23:889–905. doi:10.1093/hmg/ddt484

88. Åkerström T, Maharjan R, Sven Willenberg H, Cupisti K, Ip J, Moser A, et al. Activating mutations in CTNNB1 in aldosterone producing adenomas. *Sci Rep* (2016) 6:19546. doi:10.1038/srep19546
89. Almeida MQ, Latronico AC. The molecular pathogenesis of childhood adrenocortical tumors. *Horm Metab Res* (2007) 39:461–6. doi:10.1055/s-2007-981476
90. Faria AM, Almeida MQ. Differences in the molecular mechanisms of adrenocortical tumorigenesis between children and adults. *Mol Cell Endocrinol* (2012) 351:52–7. doi:10.1016/j.mce.2011.09.040
91. Gaujoux S, Pinson S, Gimenez-Roqueplo A-P, Amar L, Ragazzon B, Launay P, et al. Inactivation of the APC gene is constant in adrenocortical tumors from patients with familial adenomatous polyposis but not frequent in sporadic adrenocortical cancers. *Clin Cancer Res* (2010) 16:5133–41. doi:10.1158/1078-0432.CCR-10-1497
92. Else T. Association of adrenocortical carcinoma with familial cancer susceptibility syndromes. *Mol Cell Endocrinol* (2012) 351:66–70. doi:10.1016/j.mce.2011.12.008
93. Giordano TJ, Kuick R, Else T, Gauger PG, Vinco M, Bauersfeld J, et al. Molecular classification and prognostication of adrenocortical tumors by transcriptome profiling. *Clin Cancer Res* (2009) 15:668–76. doi:10.1158/1078-0432.CCR-08-1067
94. Ribeiro TC, Latronico AC. Insulin-like growth factor system on adrenocortical tumorigenesis. *Mol Cell Endocrinol* (2012) 351:96–100. doi:10.1016/j.mce.2011.09.042
95. Giordano TJ, Thomas DG, Kuick R, Lizyness M, Misek DE, Smith AL, et al. Distinct transcriptional profiles of adrenocortical tumors uncovered by DNA microarray analysis. *Am J Pathol* (2003) 162:521–31. doi:10.1016/S0002-9440(10)63846-1
96. Raymond VM, Else T, Everett JN, Long JM, Gruber SB, Hammer GD. Prevalence of germline TP53 mutations in a prospective series of unselected patients with adrenocortical carcinoma. *J Clin Endocrinol Metab* (2013) 98:E119–25. doi:10.1210/jc.2012-2198
97. Wasserman JD, Novokmet A, Eichler-Jonsson C, Ribeiro RC, Rodriguez-Galindo C, Zambetti GP, et al. Prevalence and functional consequence of TP53 mutations in pediatric adrenocortical carcinoma: a children's oncology group study. *J Clin Oncol* (2015) 33:602–9. doi:10.1200/JCO.2013.52.6863
98. Kim AC, Reuter AL, Zubair M, Else T, Serecky K, Bingham NC, et al. Targeted disruption of beta-catenin in Sf1-expressing cells impairs development and maintenance of the adrenal cortex. *Development* (2008) 135:2593–602. doi:10.1242/dev.021493
99. Tadjine M, Lampron A, Ouadi L, Bourdeau I. Frequent mutations of beta-catenin gene in sporadic secreting adrenocortical adenomas. *Clin Endocrinol (Oxf)* (2008) 68:264–70. doi:10.1111/j.1365-2265.2007.03033.x
100. Gaujoux S, Grabar S, Fassnacht M, Ragazzon B, Launay P, Libé R, et al. β-catenin activation is associated with specific clinical and pathologic characteristics and a poor outcome in adrenocortical carcinoma. *Clin Cancer Res* (2011) 17:328–36. doi:10.1158/1078-0432.CCR-10-2006
101. Harada N, Tamai Y, Ishikawa T, Sauer B, Takaku K, Oshima M, et al. Intestinal polyposis in mice with a dominant stable mutation of the beta-catenin gene. *EMBO J* (1999) 18:5931–42. doi:10.1093/emboj/18.21.5931
102. Drelon C, Berthon A, Mathieu M, Ragazzon B, Kuick R, Batisse-Lignier M, et al. EZH2 is overexpressed in adrenocortical carcinoma and is associated with disease progression. *Hum Mol Genet* (2016). doi:10.1093/hmg/ddw136
103. Deb G, Thakur VS, Gupta S. Multifaceted role of EZH2 in breast and prostate tumorigenesis: epigenetics and beyond. *Epigenetics* (2013) 8:464–76. doi:10.4161/epi.24532
104. Li FP, Fraumeni JF, Mulvihill JJ, Blattner WA, Dreyfus MG, Tucker MA, et al. A cancer family syndrome in twenty-four kindreds. *Cancer Res* (1988) 48:5358–62.
105. Malkin D, Li FP, Strong LC, Fraumeni JF, Nelson CE, Kim DH, et al. Germ line p53 mutations in a familial syndrome of breast cancer, sarcomas, and other neoplasms. *Science* (1990) 250:1233–8. doi:10.1126/science.1978757
106. Ribeiro RC, Sandrini F, Figueiredo B, Zambetti GP, Michalkiewicz E, Lafferty AR, et al. An inherited p53 mutation that contributes in a tissue-specific manner to pediatric adrenal cortical carcinoma. *Proc Natl Acad Sci U S A* (2001) 98:9330–5. doi:10.1073/pnas.161479898
107. Latronico AC, Pinto EM, Domenice S, Fragoso MC, Martin RM, Zerbini MC, et al. An inherited mutation outside the highly conserved DNA-binding domain of the p53 tumor suppressor protein in children and adults with sporadic adrenocortical tumors. *J Clin Endocrinol Metab* (2001) 86:4970–3. doi:10.1210/jcem.86.10.7957
108. Gicquel C, Bertagna X, Gaston V, Coste J, Louvel A, Baudin E, et al. Molecular markers and long-term recurrences in a large cohort of patients with sporadic adrenocortical tumors. *Cancer Res* (2001) 61(18):6762–7.
109. Ragazzon B, Libé R, Gaujoux S, Assié G, Fratticci A, Launay P, et al. Transcriptome analysis reveals that p53 and {beta}-catenin alterations occur in a group of aggressive adrenocortical cancers. *Cancer Res* (2010) 70(18):8276–81. doi:10.1158/0008-5472.CAN-10-2014
110. Lang GA, Iwakuma T, Suh Y-A, Liu G, Rao VA, Parant JM, et al. Gain of function of a p53 hot spot mutation in a mouse model of Li-Fraumeni syndrome. *Cell* (2004) 119:861–72. doi:10.1016/j.cell.2004.11.006
111. Olive KP, Tuveson DA, Ruhe ZC, Yin B, Willis NA, Bronson RT, et al. Mutant p53 gain of function in two mouse models of Li-Fraumeni syndrome. *Cell* (2004) 119:847–60. doi:10.1016/j.cell.2004.11.004
112. Keegan CE, Hutz JE, Else T, Adamska M, Shah SP, Kent AE, et al. Urogenital and caudal dysgenesis in adrenocortical dysplasia (acd) mice is caused by a splicing mutation in a novel telomeric regulator. *Hum Mol Genet* (2005) 14:113–23. doi:10.1093/hmg/ddi011
113. Colvin EK, Weir C, Ikin RJ, Hudson AL. SV40 TAg mouse models of cancer. *Semin Cell Dev Biol* (2014) 27:61–73. doi:10.1016/j.semcdb.2014.02.004
114. Ragazzon B, Lefrançois-Martinez A-M, Val P, Sahut-Barnola I, Tournaire C, Chambon C, et al. Adrenocorticotropin-dependent changes in SF-1/DAX-1 ratio influence steroidogenic genes expression in a novel model of glucocorticoid-producing adrenocortical cell lines derived from targeted tumorigenesis. *Endocrinology* (2006) 147:1805–18. doi:10.1210/en.2005-1279
115. West AN, Neale GA, Pounds S, Figueredo BC, Rodriguez Galindo C, Pianovski MAD, et al. Gene expression profiling of childhood adrenocortical tumors. *Cancer Res* (2007) 67:600–8. doi:10.1158/0008-5472.CAN-06-3767
116. Figueiredo BC, Cavalli LR, Pianovski MAD, Lalli E, Sandrini R, Ribeiro RC, et al. Amplification of the steroidogenic factor 1 gene in childhood adrenocortical tumors. *J Clin Endocrinol Metab* (2005) 90:615–9. doi:10.1210/jc.2004-0942
117. Pinto EM, Chen X, Easton J, Finkelstein D, Liu Z, Pounds S, et al. Genomic landscape of paediatric adrenocortical tumours. *Nat Commun* (2015) 6:6302. doi:10.1038/ncomms7302
118. Parker KL, Schimmer BP. Steroidogenic factor 1: a key determinant of endocrine development and function. *Endocr Rev* (1997) 18:361–77. doi:10.1210/edrv.18.3.0301
119. Val P, Lefrancois-Martinez A-M, Veyssiere G, Martinez A. SF-1 a key player in the development and differentiation of steroidogenic tissues. *Nucl Recept* (2003) 1:8. doi:10.1186/1478-1336-1-8
120. Almeida MQ, Soares IC, Ribeiro TC, Fragoso MCBV, Marins LV, Wakamatsu A, et al. Steroidogenic factor 1 overexpression and gene amplification are more frequent in adrenocortical tumors from children than from adults. *J Clin Endocrinol Metab* (2010) 95:1458–62. doi:10.1210/jc.2009-2040
121. Sbiera S, Schmull S, Assie G, Voelker H-U, Kraus L, Beyer M, et al. High diagnostic and prognostic value of steroidogenic factor-1 expression in adrenal tumors. *J Clin Endocrinol Metab* (2010) 95:E161–71. doi:10.1210/jc.2010-0653
122. Bielinska M, Genova E, Boime I, Parviainen H, Kiiveri S, Leppäluoto J, et al. Gonadotropin-induced adrenocortical neoplasia in NU/J nude mice. *Endocrinology* (2005) 146:3975–84. doi:10.1210/en.2004-1643
123. Latre de Late P, El Wakil A, Jarjat M, de Krijger RR, Heckert LL, Naquet P, et al. Vanin-1 inactivation antagonizes the development of adrenocortical neoplasia in Sf-1 transgenic mice. *Endocrinology* (2014) 155:2349–54. doi:10.1210/en.2014-1088
124. Juhlin CC, Stenman A, Haglund F, Clark VE, Brown TC, Baranoski J, et al. Whole-exome sequencing defines the mutational landscape of pheochromocytoma and identifies KMT2D as a recurrently mutated gene. *Genes Chromosomes Cancer* (2015) 54:542–54. doi:10.1002/gcc.22267

125. Hao H-X, Xie Y, Zhang Y, Charlat O, Oster E, Avello M, et al. ZNRF3 promotes Wnt receptor turnover in an R-spondin-sensitive manner. *Nature* (2012) 485:195–200. doi:10.1038/nature11019
126. Zheng S, Cherniack AD, Dewal N, Moffitt RA, Danilova L, Murray BA, et al. Comprehensive pan-genomic characterization of adrenocortical carcinoma. *Cancer Cell* (2016) 29:723–36. doi:10.1016/j.ccell.2016.04.002
127. Drelon C, Berthon A, Mathieu M, Martinez A, Val P. Adrenal cortex tissue homeostasis and zonation: a WNT perspective. *Mol Cell Endocrinol* (2015) 408:156–64. doi:10.1016/j.mce.2014.12.014
128. Logie A, Boudou P, Boccon-Gibod L, Baudin E, Vassal G, Schlumberger M, et al. Establishment and characterization of a human adrenocortical carcinoma xenograft model. *Endocrinology* (2000) 141:3165–71. doi:10.1210/endo.141.9.7668

12

Thirty-Eight-Year Follow-Up of Two Sibling Lipoid Congenital Adrenal Hyperplasia Patients Due to Homozygous Steroidogenic Acute Regulatory (STARD1) Protein Mutation: Molecular Structure and Modeling of the STARD1 L275P Mutation

*Khalil Khoury[1], Elie Barbar[2], Youssef Ainmelk[3], Annie Ouellet[3], Pierre Lavigne[2] and Jean-Guy LeHoux[2]**

[1] Department of Pediatrics, Faculty of Medicine, University of Sherbrooke, Sherbrooke, QC, Canada, [2] Department of Biochemistry, Faculty of Medicine, University of Sherbrooke, Sherbrooke, QC, Canada, [3] Department of Obstetrics and Gynecology, Faculty of Medicine, University of Sherbrooke, Sherbrooke, QC, Canada

***Correspondence:**
Jean-Guy LeHoux
jean-guy.lehoux@usherbrooke.ca

Objective: Review the impact of StAR (STARD1) mutations on steroidogenesis and fertility in LCAH patients. Examine the endocrine mechanisms underlying the pathology of the disorder and the appropriate therapy for promoting fertility and pregnancies.

Design: Published data in the literature and a detailed 38-year follow-up of two sibling LCAH patients. Molecular structure and modeling of the STARD1 L275P mutation.

Setting: University hospital.

Patients: Patient A (46,XY female phenotype) and patient B (46,XX female) with LCAH bearing the L275P mutation in STARD1.

Interventions: Since early-age diagnosis, both patients underwent corticoid replacement therapy. Patient A received estrogen therapy at pubertal age. Clomiphene therapy was given to Patient B to induce ovulation. Pregnancies were protected with progesterone administration.

Main Outcome Measures: Clinical and molecular assessment of adrenal and gonadal functions.

Results: Both patients have classic manifestations of corticosteroid deficiency observed in LCAH. Time of onset and severity were different. Patient A developed into a female phenotype due to early and severe damage of Leydig cells. Patient B started a progressive pubertal development, menarche and regular non-ovulatory cycle. She was able to have successful pregnancies.

Conclusions: Understanding the molecular structure and function of STARD1 in all steroidogenic tissues is the key for comprehending the heterogeneous clinical manifestations of LCAH, and the development of an appropriate strategy for the induction of ovulation and protecting pregnancies in this disease.

Keywords: LCAH, spontaneous puberty, fertility, pregnancy, steroidogenic acute regulatory protein (StAR, STARD1), cholesterol, molecular structure, therapy

INTRODUCTION

Classical lipoid congenital adrenal hyperplasia (LCAH), which was originally described by Prader and Siebenmann (1957) is a severe form of congenital adrenal hyperplasia inherited as an autosomal recessive disease. Patients bearing this disorder show an impaired production of glucocorticoids, mineralocorticoids, and sex steroids. Their basal levels of adrenocorticotropin (ACTH) and plasma renin activity (PRA) are high with no steroidal response to ACTH, or human chorionic gonadotropin (hCG) treatment. Signs of adrenal insufficiency and hyperpigmentation occur in phenotypic female infants regardless of the karyotype (Bose et al., 1996).

In LCAH, the destruction in early fetal life of Leydig cells of 46,XY subjects, by the toxic effect of stored cholesterol and derivatives, eliminates testosterone biosynthesis and normal virilization. In such cases, external genitalia are female with blind vaginal pouch and absence of cervix, uterus, and fallopian tubes due to undamaged Sertoli cells producing the Müllerian inhibitory hormone. Occasionally reported development of Wolffian ducts testifies for the presence of testosterone synthesis early in fetal life (Ogata et al., 1989). When adequately treated, 46,XX subjects may undergo spontaneous puberty, feminization and even cyclic vaginal bleeding (Matsuo et al., 1994; Bose et al., 1997; Fujieda et al., 1997). Despite the presence of sufficient amounts of estrogens to produce secondary sexual development and endometrial growth, progesterone levels remain undetectable, indicating that the periodic vaginal bleeding is of a non-ovulatory nature (Fujieda et al., 1997). Thus, affected individuals are all phenotypically female with a severe salt-wasting crisis and hyperpigmentation and may die shortly after birth unless treated with steroid-replacement therapy (Hauffa et al., 1985). Non-classical LCAH has also been reported: Affected individuals present with a phenotype of late onset adrenal insufficiency with only mild or minimally disordered sexual development (Baker et al., 2006; Sahakitrungruang et al., 2010).

Because mitochondria from affected adrenal and gonads fail to transform cholesterol to pregnenolone, it has been postulated for many years that LCAH disease was due to a defect in the cholesterol side chain cleavage enzyme complex cytochrome P450 (P450scc) (Degenhart et al., 1972; Koizumi et al., 1977; Matteson et al., 1986) which is the first step in steroidogenesis: The conversion of cholesterol to pregnenolone. In searching for such defect, Lin et al. (1991), Sakai et al. (1994) and Fukami et al. (1995) found no mutations in the *CYP11A1* gene of affected individuals. However, mutations in CYP11A gene were subsequently reported resulting in indistinguishable clinical and hormonal phenotypes when compared to LCAH cases (Tajima et al., 2001; Katsumata et al., 2002; Hiort et al., 2005). In addition, these patients do not have the massive adrenal hyperplasia that characterizes LCAH (Miller, 2016).

With the discovery of STARD1 (STeroidogenic Acute Regulatory) protein (Clark et al., 1994), the leading cause of LCAH was then attributed to mutations in that protein (Lin et al., 1995; Bose et al., 1996). STARD1 is produced in the cytoplasm and mediates the biosynthesis of steroid hormones by controlling the transfer of cholesterol from the outer mitochondrial membrane (OMM) to the inner mitochondrial membrane (IMM) where P450scc is located (Farkash et al., 1986; Geuze et al., 1987). Moreover, numerous mutations disrupting STARD1 activity were found in the carboxyl-terminal of the protein (Lin et al., 1995; Bose et al., 1996; Bhangoo et al., 2005, 2006) suggesting that this is a biologically important domain. Another crucial domain for STARD1 is the cholesterol binding pocket which contains a putative salt bridge between Glu^{169} and Arg^{188} (Mathieu et al., 2002a). Other clinical STARD1 mutations are found at the binding site, in particular Glu^{169} and Met^{225}, and they lead to LCAH (Miller, 1997).

In the absence of STARD1, steroidogenesis proceeds, for a temporary period, at about 14% of the STARD1 induced level (Lin et al., 1995; Tee et al., 1995; Bose et al., 1996; Miller, 1997; Khoury et al., 2006a). The pathogenesis of the different manifestations of LCAH involves STARD1-dependent and STARD1-independent steps of steroidogenesis (Bose et al., 1996; Miller, 1997). The STARD1-dependent phase would be the loss of the protein activity leading to a decrease of more than 80% of adrenal and gonad steroidogenesis. The STARD1-independent stage is characterized by a destruction of the steroidogenic capacity due to the accumulation of cholesterol, cholesterol esters and oxidation products. This engorges the cells and damages its cytoarchitecture through both physical displacement and biochemical actions.

Abbreviations: StAR, steroidogenic acute regulatory protein (STARD1); LCAH, lipoid congenital adrenal hyperplasia; P450scc, cytochrome P450 side chain cleavage; Testo, testosterone; Andro, androstenedione; DHEA, dehydroepiandrosterone; Prog, progesterone; E_2, 17β-estradiol; LH, luteinizing hormone; FSH, follicular stimulating hormone; 17 OH-Prog, 17 hydroxy-progesterone; 17 OH-Preg, 17 hydroxy-pregnenolone; ACTH, adrenocorticotropin; hCG, human chorionic gonadotropin; PRA, plasma renin activity; PCR, polymerase chain reaction; PMSG, post-menopausal stimulating gonadotropin; IVF; *in vitro* fertilization; PPROM, premature preterm rupture of membranes.

We have previously communicated the cases of LCAH in two children (46,XX and 46,XY) of a French Canadian family due to a homozygous L275P STARD1 mutation (Khoury et al., 2004). Furthermore, ovulation and pregnancies in the 46,XX patient were possible with Clomiphene stimulation and progesterone administration during the first trimester (Khoury et al., 2006b, 2009). Here, we review data collected over a three-decade follow-up of these patients focusing on their clinical evolution, gonadal function, puberty and fertility. Finally, the STARD1 mechanism of action and the impact of the clinical mutants on the protein's structure/activity will be addressed. An informed consent form was signed by all participants for blood sampling and analysis, and studies were approved by the institutional *"Comité d'éthique de la recherche en santé chez l'humain du CHUS"*.

PATIENT A (46,XY KARYOTYPE)

Patient A was born in summer 1977 after 41 weeks of normal gestation, weighing 3960 g and measuring 53 cm (Khoury et al., 2004). External genitalia were described as normal female phenotype with bilateral inguinal hernia. This was surgically repaired at the age of 5 weeks with no complications. Both gonads observed during surgery were pushed into the abdomen. At the age of 11 months, the patient suffered from gastroenteritis, hyperthermia, and dehydration. Blood pressure was 100/50, heart rate 120/min, and respiratory rate 24–28/min. Blood glucose was 3.8 mmol/L, sodium 121 mmol/L, chloride 93 mmol/L, potassium 5.4 mmol/L, and serum bicarbonate was 7 mmol/L. Intravenous fluid and glucose were administered to correct this situation. Four days after the cessation of the intravenous therapy, electrolytes disturbance and metabolic acidosis relapsed (sodium 126 mmol/L, chloride 103 mmol/L, potassium 6.3 mmol/L, sodium bicarbonate 14 mmol/L, and blood glucose 4.6 mmol/L). Intravenous rehydration was restarted. Physical examination was normal except for generalized and moderate hyperpigmentation, hypertrichosis on arms and on the lower part of her back. The external genitalia corresponded to those of a normal female with normal clitoris and vaginal orifice. There were no palpable gonads in the inguinal region and the scar of the previous surgical procedure appeared normal.

Adrenal Function

At the age of 11 months, serum cortisol was 640 nmol/L at 8 h 00 and 361 nmol/L at 16 h 00 (N = 165–635 nmol/L); serum aldosterone was respectively 641 and 319 pmol/L (N = 168–2570 pmol/L) and plasma renin activity was 11.9 ng/ml/s at 16 h (N < 4.17 ng/ml/s), and urine pregnanetriol 0.0 μmol/d (N = 0.06–0.6). Further investigations showed that serum cortisol, aldosterone as well as urinary pregnanetriol did not respond to intramuscular ACTH stimulation for 3 days (**Table 1**). Substitution therapy with mineralocorticoid (fludrocortisone acetate) and glucorticoid (cortisone acetate) was then started. Four months later, we decided to stop cortisone acetate to obtain more data on her glucocorticoid secretion.

For the following 20 months, the child was growing well (50 percentile for height and weight) and has no specific symptoms. From 35 to 41 months of age, the patient was admitted to the hospital for 3 episodes of hypoglycemia and acidosis during infectious illnesses. Blood glucose was 1.4–4.0 mmol/L, electrolytes were normal with high renin activity and elevated urinary sodium. Basal steroid hormones (while receiving fludrocortisone acetate 0.025 mg every 12 h) revealed low cortisolemia* 69 and 8.28 nmol/L at 8 and 16 h respectively, normal aldosterone** 737 and 208 pmol/L, 17 OH-progesterone 0.15 nmol/L (N = 0.1–2.7), DHEA 0.69 nmol/L (N = 0.38–2.52), DHEA-S 0.54 μmol/L (N = 0.13–0.54) testosterone 0.1 nmol/L (N = 0.07–0.9), and ACTH 33 pmol/L (N = 2–11). ACTH stimulation test was repeated at that time (intramuscular injections of ACTH-Gel 25 IU/m^2 every 12 h × 5 days) under replacement therapy with fludrocortisone acetate 0.025 mg every 12 h and Dexamethasone 0.25 mg every 8 h. The higher values of blood cortisol and aldosterone obtained during this stimulation was 19.3 and 263 pmol/L respectively, urinary free cortisol*** was < 5.5 nmol/day and pregnanetriol**** 0.11 μmol/day at that moment. The result of previously ordered blood karyotype revealed the suspected 46,XY. Then clinical, biochemical and genetic studies confirmed the suspected diagnosis of what was believed at that time as 20,22 desmolase deficiency. Substitution therapy with fludrocortisone acetate and hydrocortisone continues, doses were regularly adjusted according to clinical symptoms, blood glucose and electrolytes as well as serum level of ACTH and PRA in addition to observations of growth and bone maturation.

Normal basal values from 2–5 years:

* Cortisol 166–525 nmol/L (mean Δ after ACTH stimulation 400 nmol/L)

** Aldosterone 83–971 pmol/L (mean Δ after ACTH stimulation 500 pmol/L)

*** Urinary free cortisol 8.28–24.8 nmol/d

**** Urinary pregnanetriol < 1.5 μmol/d

Radiological Investigations

At the moment of her first admission, at 11 months of age, the IV pyelography was normal. Several pelvic and abdominal echographies were performed from the age of 3 6/12 to 13 years. These showed no uterus, no visible gonads and no adrenal hypertrophy, the bone age was always significantly delayed (growth curve not shown).

Gonadal Function

FSH, LH and different androgens were measured at regular intervals from the age of ~3 years until the patient was 13 year old (**Table 2**). As can be seen, the levels of serum androstenedione, dehydroepiandrosterone, total and free testosterone were low to not detectable. hCG stimulation test (intramuscular injections 4000 IU/day for 5 days) was performed at the age of 13 years (while the patient was receiving fludrocortisone acetate and Dexamethasone). As shown in **Table 2**, hCG stimulation did not increase circulating levels of 17 OH-pregnenolone, 17 OH-progesterone, DHEA, androstenedione, and total and free testosterone.

TABLE 1 | Patient A.

Dates	Serum cortisol nmol/L (165–635)	Serum aldosterone pmol/L (168–2520)	Plasma renin ng/L/s (<4.17)	Urine pregnanetriol μmol/day (0.06–0.6)
Day 2	966	670	19.46	0
Day 1	634	621	22.2	<0.03
Day 0	739	474	11.95	<0.03
Day 3	811	244	15.29	<0.03
Day 4	497	357	13.34	<0.09

ACTH stimulation test: Injection of ACTH-Gel 25 IU/m² /q 12 h/3 days During this test, the patient received NaCl 70 meq/d, the serum sodium was 120–131 mmol/L, potassium 6.0–6.9 mmol/L and urinary sodium 51–64 mmol/L, at 8 and 16 h respectively. Age of patient A, 11 months.

TABLE 2 | Patient A.

Hormones age	FSH IU/L	LH IU/L	17 OH-Preg nmol/L	17 OH-Prog nmol/L	DHEA nmol/L	Andro nmol/L	Testo (total) nmol/L	Testo (free) nmol/L
~3 years	–	–	–	0.15	0.69	–	0.1	–
~4 years	–	–	–	–	< 0.35	< 0.3	< 0.35	–
5 10/12 years	3.9	< 2.7	–	–	1.73	< 0.3	< 0.35	–
6 7/12 years	13.8	< 5	–	–	2.08	< 0.7	< 0.35	–
7 6/12 years	8.6	< 5	–	–	–	–	< 0.35	–
8 years	23	< 5	–	–	–	–	< 0.35	-
8 9/12 years	11.8	5.1	–	–	–	–	< 0.35	< 0.6
10 4/12 years	11.6	< 2	–	–	–	–	< 0.35	< 2
12 6/12 years	4.6	< 0.5	–	–	< 1.7	< 0.3	< 0.7	< 3
hCG (IM) 4000 IU/dX5 days D 0	33.2	1.8	< 0.16	< 0.3	< 1.5	< 0.3	< 0.7	< 1.0
D 3	–	–	< 0.16	< 0.3	< 1.5	< 0.3	< 0.7	–
D 4	–	–	< 0.16	< 0.3	< 1.5	< 0.3	< 0.7	–
D 6	–	–	< 0.16	< 0.3	< 1.5	< 0.3	< 0.7	< 2.1

T, total; F, free; D, day; –, not available. Normal values are indicated for different ages:
FSH: Prepubertal 0.26–3 IU/L, puberty Tanner II, III 0.6–10.9 IU/L.
LH: Prepubertal 0.02–0.3 IU/L, puberty Tanner II, III 0.2–5.0 IU/L.
17-OH pregnenolone: Puberty Tanner II, III 0.6–10.9 nmol/L.
17-OH progesterone: Prepubertal 0.09–2.7 nmol/L, puberty Tanner II, III 0.3–3.9 nmol/L.
DHEA: 2–5 years 0.38–2.52 nmol/L, 6–10 years 0.9–5.3 nmol/L, puberty Tanner II, III 0.87–10.5 nmol/L.
Androstenedione: 1–10 years 0.18–1.78 nmol/L, puberty Tanner II, III 0.6–2.87 nmol/L.
Testosterone (total): 3–10 years 0.07–0.66 nmol/L, puberty Tanner II, III 0.63–11.2 nmol/L.
Testosterone (free): Prepubertal 0.52–2.0 pmol/L, adult male 180–971 pmol/L.
Gonadal function of Patient A measured at different interval from age 3 to 13 years old.

Gonadal Histology

A laparotomy was performed at the age of 13 5/12 years: The left gonad (3 × 1.5 × 1 cm) was removed. The exploration of the right side was negative and showed no Müllerian or Wolffian structures. The histology of the removed gonad is illustrated in **Figure 1**. Worth noticing is the atrophy and hyalinization of the seminiferous tubules, the presence of some germinal cells without spermatogonia, the presence of some Sertoli cells and the important engorgement of Leydig cells with fat.

Growth

The patient's growth velocity decreased regularly from the age of 10 years until she was 14 year old. Bone age was always significantly delayed (curve not shown). The thyroid function and growth hormone secretions were normal. Progressive ethinyl estradiol therapy was started at the age of 14 leading to a gradual pubertal development (good breast development, moderate pubic hair) and an increase of the growth rate. Final adult height was in the normal mid-parental range.

PATIENT B (46,XX KARYOTYPE)

Patient B was born in spring 1979 (Koizumi et al., 1977; Khoury et al., 2004). She had skin hyperpigmentation since the age of 1.5 months. At 4.5 months, she was hospitalized for fever, anorexia, fatigue and weight loss, and was treated with antibiotics (pharyngitis) for 10 days. Furthermore, she suffered from somnolence, vomiting and dehydration with hyponatremia and hyperkalemia (Khoury et al., 2009).

Adrenal Function

The endocrine investigations revealed a low/normal serum cortisol 174 nmol/L (N = 77–635), low/normal aldosterone 138.7 pmol/L (N = 166–1970) and renin activity 3.3 ng/L/s

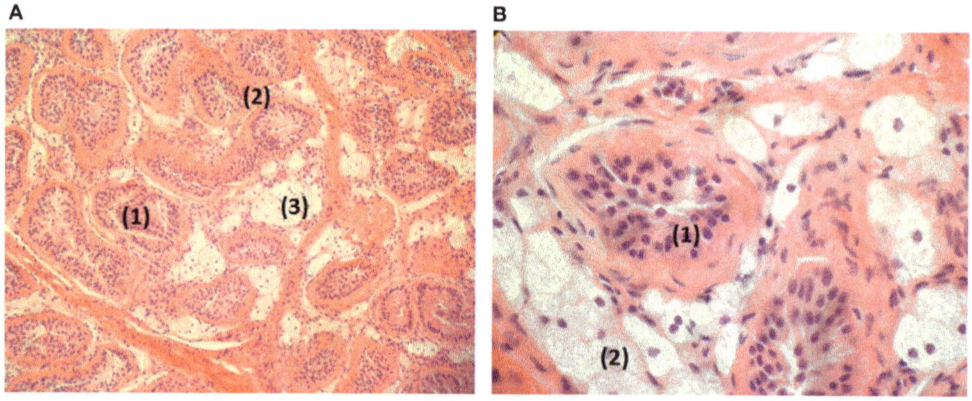

FIGURE 1 | Histology of the removed gonad. (A) Testis in low magnification: atrophic seminiferous tubules (1). Hyaline thickening of the basal membranes (2). Hyperplasia and clarification of the Leydig cells (3). **(B)** Testis in higher magnification: atrophic seminiferous tubules (1) containing Sertoli cells in the absence of spermatogonia. Lipid overload of the Leydig cells (2).

TABLE 3 | Patient B.

Time	Serum cortisol nmol/L (166–525)	Serum aldosterone pmol/L (139–1498)	Plasma renin ng/L/s (<2.8)
Day 1	18.2	136	0.88
Day 0	5.52	161	6.47
Day 2	8.28	136	3.27
Day 4	13.8	180	5.36

ACTH stimulation test: Injection of ACTH-Gel 25 IU/m^2/12 h/3 days. Age of Patient B, 21 months. Normal values are in parentheses.

($N < 4.17$). The urinary pregnanetriol was 0.59 μmol/day ($N = 0.06$–0.6). The ACTH stimulation (IM injections of ACTH-Gel 25 IU/m^2 q 12 h. × 3 days) resulted of very small increases in cortisol (220 nmol/L) and aldosterone (277.4 pmol/L). She was growing well with no specific symptoms while treated only with fludrocortisone acetate 0.025 mg bid, up to the age of 15 months. From that age to 21 months she suffered 3 episodes of hypoglycemia during a varicella illness and otitis media. Her serum cortisol level was 8.28 nmol/L ($N = 166$–690), serum aldosterone and plasma renin activity were 141.3 pmol/L ($N = 139$–1498) and 0.67 ng/L/s ($N < 2.8$) respectively. Then Dexamethasone 0.25 mg p.o. every 8 h was added to fludrocortisone acetate before to undergo her second ACTH stimulation test. Results illustrated in **Table 3** indicate a very low basal cortisol and incapacity of the zona fasciculata-reticularis to respond to ACTH stimulation; the same table shows low level of aldosterone with no response of the zona glomerulosa to ACTH stimulation. Consequently, the doses of glucocorticoids (Dexamethasone changed for hydrocortisone) and fludrocortisone acetate, were adjusted regularly during all the next years, according to her clinical evolution, blood glucose and electrolytes, as well as plasma ACTH and renin activity.

Gonadal Function

The patient's serum levels* of FSH and LH were normal up to puberty. Serum levels of 17 OH-Prog, DHEA, androstenedione, and testosterone were very low. Plasma ACTH varied from 43–4.6 pmol/L during that period. She started thelarche and pubarche at the age of 11 7/12 and 12 years, respectively. The hypophyso-gonadal function was previously summarized (Khoury et al., 2009). A spontaneous normal menarche started at the age of 14 2/12 years. The menstruations were regular with no dysmenorrhea. The basal temperature registered between 21 and 24 years indicated a monophasic non-ovulatory curve. Shortly after a Clomiphene stimulation, circulating 17β-estradiol level increased from 703 to 1428 pmol/L and progesterone level increased from 3.4 to 9.4 nmol/L (Khoury et al., 2004).

*Normal prepubertal values: FSH 1.0–4.2 IU/L, LH 0.02–0.18 IU/L, 17-OH progesterone 0.09–2.72 nmol/L, DHEA 0.4–6.6 nmol/L, androstenedione 0.28–1.75 nmol/L, testosterone 0.07–0.35 nmol/L.

Radiological Investigations

An abdominal and pelvic echography was performed at the age of 2 5/12 years. It revealed a normal uterus and ovaries. Adrenal glands have no particular aspect. This examination was repeated at 11 1/12 years and 12 3/12 years and showed a prepubertal uterus and normal ovaries with small follicles. A small delay of bone age was noted at different ages.

Growth

Regular growth was observed. Peak height velocity began around the age of 13 years. Final adult height was in the normal mid-parental range.

Fertility Studies and Childbirth

Clomiphene stimulation, to increase gonadal activities and induce ovulation, was started at the age of 25 years. First pregnancy occurred at the age of 25 4/12 years, unfortunately interrupted by spontaneous abortion 6 weeks later (Khoury et al., 2009). A second pregnancy (quadruple) was initiated later on with Clomiphene stimulation, and was protected with progesterone supplementation at the 17th day of the cycle. One fetus was naturally lost at 7 weeks of gestation and one feticide was done 1 ½ weeks later, so progesterone was continued up to the 25th week of gestation. In October 2005, two normal boys were born prematurely. This first child delivery was previously communicated in an international meeting in 2006 (Khoury et al., 2006b). At 28 years old, a third pregnancy initiated with Clomiphene stimulation, and progesterone was taken from the 17th day of the cycle up to the 17th week of gestation. After 36 weeks of normal gestation, a female child was born in October 2008 (Khoury et al., 2009).

Molecular Biology Studies

Genomic DNA was extracted from the gonadal tissue of patient-A. The seven exons of the STARD1 gene were PCR-amplified using primers and conditions previously described (Bose et al., 1996) and PCR products were sequenced. A mutation was found in exon 7 which was located at the amino acid residue 275, a leucine being substituted by a proline. Genomic DNA was subsequently extracted from the blood leukocytes of the two patients, their two parents and a normal individual. The exon 7 was analyzed for each individual. For the mutation L275P, the control was +/+, the two parents were +/−, and the two children were −/− (**Figure 2**).

COS-1 cells were used to determine STARD1 activity and quantification. **Figure 3A** shows results obtained by western blotting analysis, and **Figure 3B** shows that the L275P mutant activity was 87% impaired compared to wild type (Khoury et al., 2004).

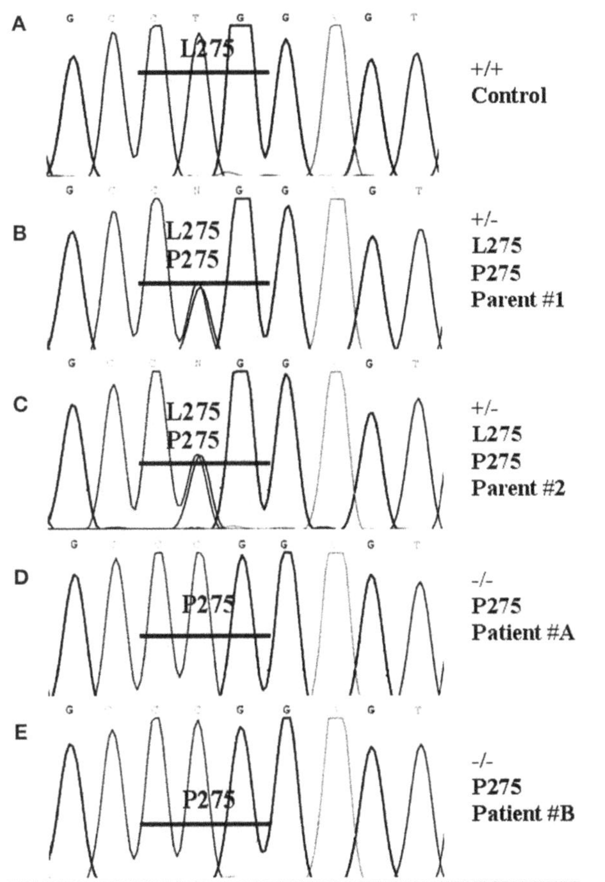

FIGURE 2 | DNA sequencing. Genomic DNA was extracted from the blood of two patients, their two parents and a normal individual as control **(A)** using the Invitrogen DNAzol BD reagent. The seven exons of the STARD1 gene were PCR and sequenced. A mutation was found in exon 7. For exon 7 oligonucleotides used for PCR were (5′ to 3′) ATGAGCGTGTGTACCAGTGACG, (5′ to 3′) CCTGGCAGCCTGTTTGTGATAG; the annealing temperature was $60^{\circ}C$ and the reaction processed for 30 cycles. The PCR products were sequenced. The mutation found in exon 7 was located at the amino acid residue 275, a leucine being substituted by a proline. The two parents **(B,C)** were +/−, and the two children **(D,E)** were −/−.

MECHANISM OF CHOLESTEROL TRANSFER BY STARD1

In order to better explain how clinical mutations affect steroidogenesis, we will discuss the mechanism of action of STARD1 at the molecular level. STARD1 delivers cholesterol from the outer to the inner membrane of mitochondria is poorly understood. STARD1 may act as a sterol transfer protein and enhance sterol desorption from the outer to the inner side of mitochondria (Kallen et al., 1998; Petrescu et al., 2001). In this model STARD1 is directed to the mitochondria via its N-terminus recognition sequence and then, utilizing C-terminal sequences, produces as yet unidentified alterations in the OMM that results in the transfer of cholesterol to the inner side. It is established that STARD1 acts on the OMM and that its level of activity is proportionate to the time it remains at that site (Arakane et al., 1998; Bose et al., 2002).

MLN64, a protein involved in cholesterol transfer in malignant breast cancer, has a significant homology to the C-terminal region of STARD1 and can promote cholesterol transfer (Watari et al., 1997). The C-terminus of STARD1 contains the StAR-Related Lipid Transfer (START) domain which is conserved across a large family of proteins including MLN64 and STARD1 (Ponting and Aravind, 1999; Stocco, 2000; Tsujishita and Hurley, 2000). START domain in MLN64 is homologous to the START domain of the STARD1 protein. Both, functionally similar, are able to bind cholesterol in a 1:1 ratio (Tsujishita and Hurley, 2000; Petrescu et al., 2001). It was first proposed that STARD1 acts as a cholesterol shuttle for transferring cholesterol to the IMM via a hydrophobic tunnel revealed by the crystal structure of MLN64-START (Tsujishita and Hurley, 2000), but the exact mechanism by which STARD1 releases cholesterol to the IMM is unknown (Stocco, 2001). According to computer homology models based on MLN64 structure, STARD1 does not contain a tunnel, but a hydrophobic pocket that can accommodate one molecule of cholesterol (Mathieu et al., 2002a,b; Baker et al., 2005; Yaworsky et al., 2005; Murcia et al., 2006; Lavigne et al., 2010; Thorsell et al., 2011; Létourneau et al., 2014, 2015); the STARD1 crystal structure corroborates this hydrophobic pocket. Several mutations that result in LCAH were mapped onto the MLN64-START structure, in positions residing within the hydrophobic tunnel; these mutations would destabilize the tunnel. In parallel, the residues Glu^{169}, Met^{225}, and Leu^{275} are part of STARD1's sterol binding pocket and the hydrophobic environment provided by α-helices 2, 3, and 4 (**Figure 4**). Two regions of STARD1 appear important

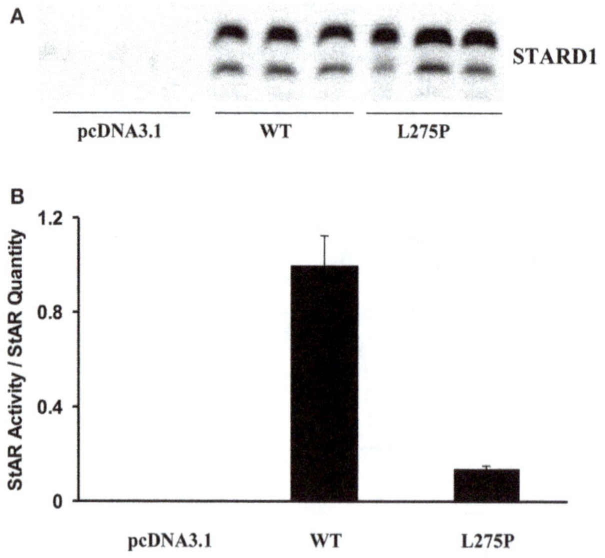

FIGURE 3 | STARD1 activity and quantification. COS-1 cells were cotransfected with the F2 construct (Harikrishna et al., 1993) (500 ng) and 200 ng pcDNA3.1 harboring the wild type (WT) human STARD1 cDNA. (WT STARD1-pcDNA3.1) or the mutant L275P STARD1-pcDNA3.1 and 300 ng of pcDNA3.1. Cells were incubated for 24 h. **(A)** 20 μg of whole cell homogenate were analyzed by immunoblotting. The membranes were exposed to anti-STARD1 antibody, followed by a horseradish peroxidase-conjugated anti-rabbit secondary antibody (Fleury et al., 2004). Immunoreactive proteins were visualized with ECL Plus (Amersham Biosciences, U.K. Ltd., Little Chalfont, Buckinghamshire, England) on a Storm 860 laser scanner instrument (Molecular Dynamics, Sunnyvale, CA) and the band intensity was quantified using ImageQuant software. **(B)** Pregnenolone from cell media was analyzed by radioimmunoassay (Fleury et al., 2004). Results are expressed as STARD1 activity/STARD1 quantity after background subtraction.

for the binding of cholesterol and its release during its transfer to the IMM. A cholesterol gating region containing the C-terminal α-helix 4 and a cholesterol binding region buried inside the STARD1 molecule (Roostaee et al., 2008). More specifically, the importance of STARD1's C-terminal region in cholesterol transfer is confirmed by many observations; deletion of 28 amino acids from the C-terminal results in a complete loss of steroids production (Arakane et al., 1996; Wang et al., 1998). This C-terminal deletion corroborates with the truncated STARD1 mutant Q258X and lead to LCAH (Miller, 1997).

In vitro experiments have highlighted the role of α-helix 4 as a gate for cholesterol binding (Baker et al., 2005; Roostaee et al., 2008). The helix would be in thermodynamic equilibrium between a partially-unfolded (open) and folded (closed) states (Mathieu et al., 2002a). Upon cholesterol binding, the equilibrium is shifted to the more stable closed state (Baker et al., 2005; Roostaee et al., 2008; Barbar et al., 2009a), until the subsequent release of the ligand by other mechanisms, such as interactions with other mitochondrial proteins, to trigger the transfer of cholesterol from the outer to the inner mitochondrial membrane (Liu et al., 2006; Bose et al., 2008a).

The hypothesis is that the STARD1 C-terminal α-helix 4 movement is a key factor for STARD1-mediated cholesterol transfer inside mitochondria (Mathieu et al., 2002a,b; LeHoux et al., 2003). For instance, biochemical and structural studies of the L275P mutation at the α-helix 4 led to a dramatic reduction in cholesterol binding that correlated with a decrease in the steroidogenic activity of STARD1 (Roostaee et al., 2008).

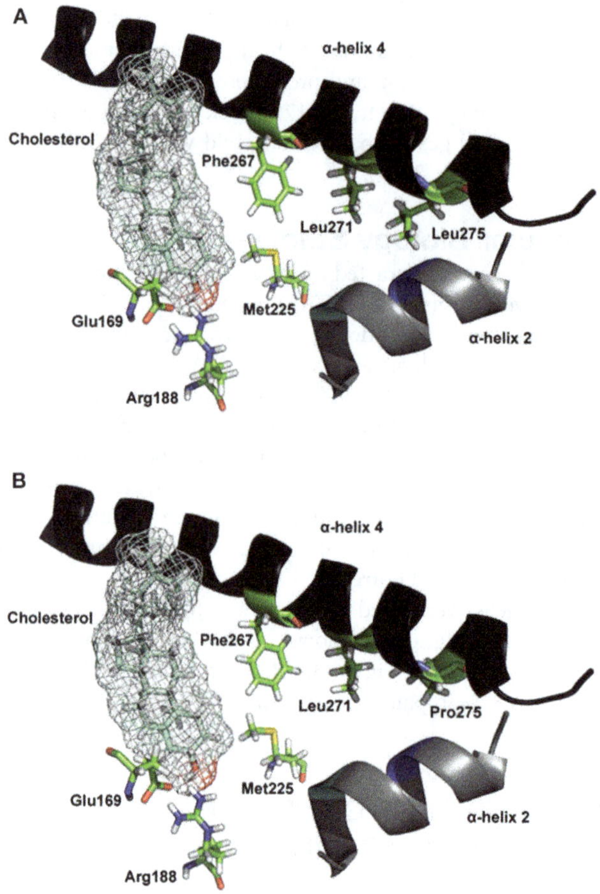

FIGURE 4 | Molecular model of STARD1 L275P mutation. (A) The essential elements of the wild-type STARD1 are shown. The salt bridge formed by Glu^{169}/Arg^{188} putatively interacts with the β-OH of cholesterol, while the α-helix 4 is in a closed state. The line of hydrophobic residues $Phe^{267}/Leu^{271}/Leu^{275}$ interacting with α-helix 2, Met^{225} and other hydrophobic residues (not shown for image simplicity) help stabilize the STARD1 /cholesterol complex. **(B)** The long hydrophobic side chain for Leu^{275} is absent in the clinical mutation L275P, thereby creates a void in the hydrophobic environment necessary for stabilizing holo- STARD1, leading to a reduction in cholesterol binding and steroidogenic activity (Roostaee et al., 2008). Initial coordinates for the molecular modeling of STARD1 were retrieved from the Protein Databank (code 1IMG). Site-directed mutagenesis and energy minimization were done *in silico* using the molecular modeling software SYBYL 8.0 (Tripos Inc, St. Louis, MO). All the rendering was done using PYMOL (DeLano, W. L. The PyMOL Molecular Graphics System, 2002, DeLano Scientific, Palo Alto, CA).

Several amino acids are in contact with the sterol binding pocket. **Figure 4A** shows Leu^{275} and other residues forming a hydrophobic core near the end of the C-terminal α-helix 4, and **Figure 4B** shows the model for the mutation Leu^{275} to proline. Any alterations in these residues, forming a line of hydrophobic residues, would affect the binding and the steroidogenic activity of STARD1. In the case of the L275P mutation, it yielded a 13%

pregnenolone production in isolated mitochondria (Roostaee et al., 2008); such a level of steroidogenesis is in agreement with previous studies (Bose et al., 1996; Khoury et al., 2004).

The far-UV CD spectra of STARD1 WT has a 32.5% α-helical content, which is close to the 40% maximum helical content calculated for the three-dimensional model. The L271N and L275P mutants showed a reduced α-helical content of 28.8 and 29.4% respectively compared with STARD1 WT. As discussed above, these mutants were expected to lead to the weakening of the hydrophobic interface and hence to a reduction in the amount of α-helical content and stable tertiary structure (Roostaee et al., 2008). Also, short molecular dynamics simulations have indicated that the L275P mutation confers a higher flexibility to STARD1's α-helix 4 (Barbar et al., 2009b), which suggests a more open state of the helix, thereby reducing its gating capacity, which is related to the decrease in cholesterol binding and the steroidogenic activity previously studied (Bose et al., 1998; Roostaee et al., 2008).

Interestingly, another clinical leucine to proline mutation (L260P) at the α-helix 4 has been found in Swiss LCAH patients and exhibited a similar *in vitro* steroidogenic activity as the L275P mutant (Flück et al., 2005). Hence, one would expect that the L260P mutant might structurally behave in a similar fashion as L275P, by affecting the α-helix 4 gating mechanism.

FUNCTIONAL ACTIVITIES

Functional activities determined in transfected COS-1 cells revealed differences between different mutants. On the two LCAH patients reported in the study of Lin et al. (1995), the Q258X STARD1 mutant had a functional activity of 17% and the R193X mutant had 14%. Bose et al. reported that the L275P mutant converted 10% more cholesterol to pregnenolone than the vector control (Bose et al., 1996). In 19 Japanese patients, Nakae et al. reported 8 different mutations and in functional studies only the M225T mutation was found to have a partial activity of 44% (Nakae et al., 1997). All other mutants had activities not greater than that of the vector plasmid. STARD1-independent pregnenolone production in the three above mentioned studies was about 14%. Nakae et al. reported on a patient with Q258X, M225T (heterozygous compound) mutations who had a cliteromegaly at the time of diagnosis and moderate elevation of serum testosterone in response to hCG stimulation (Nakae et al., 1997). This patient had the onset of symptoms of adrenocortical insufficiency at the age of 10 months. These authors suggested that late onset of LCAH results from mutations that do not completely inactivate STARD1. The Canadian patient cited by Bose et al. (1996) had the heterozygous compound mutation A218V, L275P, and 46,XY karyotype; her manifestations of corticosteroid deficiency were noted at the age of 2 months.

STARD1 INDEPENDENCE

STARD1 is mainly expressed under acute tropic hormone stimulation. In the absence of STARD1, several elements may account for the basal level of steroid hormone production. For example, MLN64 may be able to enhance the basal low level of steroidogenesis since it is present in human granulosa and theca cells as well as in the fetal adrenal cortex (Watari et al., 1997). Other proteins with a START domain (like STARD4 and D6) might contribute to the basal steroidogenic activity (Soccio et al., 2002; Bose et al., 2008b), but their precise distribution in steroidogenic tissues and role are yet to be clarified. The synthesis or uptake of hydroxysterols might also contribute to the STARD1-independent steroidogenesis; for example, soluble 22R-OH and 25 OH-cholesterol can diffuse to the inner mitochondrial membrane without the participation of STARD1 and be used as substrate for pregnenolone formation (Lin et al., 1995; Roostaee et al., 2008).

LCAH AND STARD1 MUTATION IN CANADA

In this review, we report the first detailed study of LCAH due to homozygous STARD1 mutation in Canada and, to our knowledge, the first successful pregnancy in a 46,XX female with this disease. Since the discovery of STARD1 in 1994 (Clark et al., 1994), many important works contributed to increase our understanding on the role played by this protein in the steroidogenesis and the physiology of LCAH. We have identified a homozygous recessive mutation on the STARD1 gene of our two patients and the heterozygous mutation in their mother and father. This mutation resulted in the substitution of a leucine by a proline (L275P) in the STARD1 protein (Khoury et al., 2004), which did not conserve more than 13% of its steroidogenesis activity compared to wild type STARD1, as analyzed in COS-1 cells. This is in agreement with Bose et al. (1996) who reported that the mutated L275P STARD1, found in another Canadian, converted 10% more cholesterol to pregnenolone than the control vector. The Canadian patient cited by Bose et al. (1996) had the heterozygous compound mutation A218V, L275P, and 46,XY karyotype; her manifestations of corticosteroid deficiency were noted at the age of 2 months. We did not have the opportunity to obtain a genetic history for this patient; we know however (personal communication from Dr. Rose Girgis, Edmonton, Canada) that the parents are from French Canadian origin who lived in the province of Quebec before moving to the west. It is unknown if any parental connection exists between these two families who share the allele L275P. Although the number of patients bearing the L275P mutation is too small to be conclusive, it might indicate a possible founder effect for this disease in Canada (Bose et al., 1996).

CLINICAL MANIFESTATION AND EFFICIENCY OF CHOLESTEROL TRANSFER SYSTEM

The two patients, A and B, described in this study had a normal health before their first admission to the hospital for severe manifestations of mineralocorticoid deficiency and hyperpigmentation at the age of 11 and 4 1/2 months respectively. Some residual secretion of aldosterone was present and basal blood cortisol was in the low normal level, but without any significant response to ACTH stimulation up to the age of 3 years for patient A and only 15 months for her sister. Consequently, patient A seemed to have less severe corticosteroid deficiency than patient B and both patients have less severe mineralocorticoid and glucocorticoid deficiencies than reported in similar cases (Bose et al., 1996).

To date, at least 97 patients with LCAH and more than 35 different mutations have been reported in the STARD1 gene (Bhangoo et al., 2005, 2006; Papadimitriou et al., 2006; Abdulhadi-Atwan et al., 2007). Two distinct genetic clusters were initially reported: More than 70% of Japanese alleles and all Korean alleles carry the Q258X mutation; a second genetic cluster is found among Palestinian Arabs, most of whom carry the R182L mutation. Many publications underline that some correlations exist between the severity of STARD1 mutation and the age of onset of a clinical salt-wasting crisis, hypoglycemia and gonadal function (Bose et al., 1996; Miller, 1997; Bhangoo et al., 2005, 2006). Patients with the mutation Q258X or R182L are generally symptomatic by the age of 1 day to some weeks. Three unrelated patients of Swiss ancestry, L260P mutant, had their onset of symptoms at the age 2.5–5.5 months (Flück et al., 2005). Furthermore, as reported by Chen et al. (2005) patients from eastern Saudi Arabia who carry the R182H mutation, very close to the Palestinian mutation R182L, had a milder disease starting at the age of 1–14 months, and 4 out of 7 of them had the onset of their symptoms from 7–14 months of age; functional study in this group showed a complete loss of STARD1 activity. One patient from Qatar, with R182H mutation, had the onset of clinical symptoms and laboratory evidence of salt loss at the age of 3 weeks (Achermann et al., 2001); the *in vitro* STARD1 activity of this patient was not determined. The patients reported by Chen et al. (2005) as well as our two patients raise the question about the different clinical manifestations and time of onset with the same genetic mutations, in the same ethnic group or family members and the same geographic region. There is, clearly, a limited sensitivity of the different functional assays for determination of STARD1 activity which may explain the poor correlation frequently observed between the clinical findings and the results of *in vitro* studies. There is also a wide spectrum of heterogeneity in the clinical manifestations and biochemistry, as well as, the time of onset of different symptoms in LCAH. However, in our case, since the assays for Patients A and B are relatively standardized, the sensitivity is the same.

Interestingly, both patients carry the same mutation, yet the clinical manifestation of LCAH was delayed between them. The physiological conditions are different from one pregnancy to another and the demand for different steroids is variable during fetal development. Indeed, during pregnancy, conditions such as nutrition, hydration/dehydration, disease and other stress, may have an influence on steroidogenesis. In addition, the circumstances of delivery and the neonatal environment may have different patterns of tropic hormone stimulation which may modulate the extent of acute steroidogenic demands.

The STARD1 -dependent and STARD1 -independent steroidogenesis seem to be good descriptive models to explain the chronology of events in non-placental steroidogenic tissues. It is not clear however what determines the length of time an infant with LCAH can survive before experiencing a salt-wasting crisis (Hauffa et al., 1985; Fujieda et al., 2003; Bhangoo et al., 2006). We still need more information concerning the function or loss of function of the mutated STARD1 and what determines the longevity and efficiency of the STARD1 -independent system. It is clear, however, that early appeal and continuous stimulation of steroidogenesis in the gonads (by the hormones hCG, FSH, LH) and the adrenals (by ACTH and the renin-angiotensin system) are the starting point initiating the failure of both systems. In this study, our two patients, Patient A, 46,XY and Patient B, 46,XX, members of the same family with the same homozygous (L275P) mutation, have different severity of the disease and different time of onset of corticosteroid deficiency. Clinical manifestations and hormonal data prove the severe deficiency of testosterone secretion in Patient A, the milder ovary dysfunction in Patient B and the presence of some residual corticosteroid secretion and progressive post natal adrenal failure for both.

GONADAL FUNCTION IN LCAH AND 46,XY GENOTYPE

Patient A in this study is a 46,XY genotype with female external genitalia and blind vaginal pouch. **Figure 1** shows lipid accumulation in Leydig cells typical of LCAH. The absence of androgen secretion, basal and after hCG stimulation, as well as the absence of Wolffian structures testify on the early and severe deficiency of testosterone secretion necessary for differential sexual development and virilization. In fact, during the early weeks of embryonic development, the fetus is exposed to acute hCG stimulation which may lead to lipid accumulation in the cell due to the lack of STARD1 activity, thereby destroying Leydig cells. This is clearly contrasting with the relatively moderate severity of mineralocorticoid and glucocorticoid deficiency of this patient. Generally, all 46,XY reported patients had a profound impairment of testosterone synthesis (Bose et al., 1996), however Wolffian duct derivatives are sometimes well developed as reported by Nakae et al. (1997) on patient 7 (Q258X, M225T) who had a cliteromegaly and moderate secretion of testosterone in response to hCG stimulation.

This seems to be concordant with the hypothesis of the earlier mentioned STARD1-dependent steroidogenesis deficiency and STARD1-independent impairment of steroidogenesis due to Leydig cells destruction following lipid accumulation caused by an early and continuous stimulation (placental hCG, fetal pituitary LH). Such patients should be raised as females (Bose et al., 1996) and should undergo orchidectomy due to the risk of *in situ* testicular carcinoma development (Korsch et al., 1999).

GONADAL FUNCTION IN LCAH AND 46,XX GENOTYPE

Spontaneous Puberty

Patient B in this study is a unique case. While she had an earlier and more severe corticosteroid deficiency than her sibling, her ovarian function was less disturbed than what was observed in other similar cases (Bose et al., 1996). By the end of 1990, at the age of 11 7/12 years, she started a progressive pubertal development; her ovarian response to hCG stimulation was normal and she had menarche at the age of 14 2/12 years (Khoury et al., 2004). This was unexpected for LCAH in 1993. Our observations are in agreement with Matsuo's report in 1994 (Matsuo et al., 1994) that 5/5 46,XX patients with LCAH aged more than 13 years expressed a spontaneous development of secondary sex characters and vaginal bleeding at the time of puberty, their estrogen level ranging from 22–85 pg/ml. Bose et al. (1997) described in 1997 the first genetic analysis in a 46,XX female homozygous for STARD1 shift mutation 261ΔT and spontaneous feminization. Three other cases were reported by Fujieda et al. (1997, 2003)who found that the ovaries of such patients were enlarged in the post pubertal stage with many cysts occupying the entire volume of the ovary and with hypertrophied ovarian stroma. This phenomenon was not observed on repeated echographies in our Patient B. The heterogeneity in the pubertal development of 46,XX female patients with STARD1 mutation was also described by Nakae et al. (1997) who reported on 6/10 46,XX patients who experienced spontaneous pubertal changes, irregular menstruations, anovulatory cycles and in some a polycystic aspect of ovaries. All these reports show that the difference in the extent of impairment of the testis and ovaries is dramatic in LCAH. However, although initially unexpected, even the most severely affected 46,XX female patients undergo spontaneous feminization, breast development and cyclical vaginal bleeding at the usual age of puberty (Matsuo et al., 1994; Bose et al., 1997; Nakae et al., 1997).

The fetal ovary cells are quiescent and in affected 46,XX patients these–cells should remain undamaged since they should not accumulate cholesterol esters until they first undergo gonadotropin stimulation. This would explain why these cells retain steroidogenic capacity and hence at the time of puberty can make estrogens, albeit, in subnormal amounts, resulting in high gonadotropin secretion. However, only the cells in the individually recruited follicles undergo stimulation, and hence only these cells accumulate cholesterol esters and lose steroidogenic capacity. Regular monthly cycles are possible, because a large number of follicles remain relatively undamaged before recruitment. Such monthly cycles, which may persist for years, are probably anovulatory and can produce a large quantity of ovarian cysts.

STARD1 EXPRESSION IN THE OVARIES

The study of Sandhoff and McLean (1996) shows that in rat ovaries STARD1 mRNA expression is controlled by tropic hormones PMSG (post-menopausal stimulating gonadotropin) and hCG. hCG increases the steady-state level of STARD1 mRNA in the ovary during follicular and luteal development. The rise in STARD1 expression paralleled the rise in serum progesterone levels, consistent with STARD1's presumed role in the regulation of steroidogenesis. Furthermore. STARD1 gene expression in primary cultures of porcine granulosa cells is stimulated above control levels by FSH, 8-bromo-cAMP and IGF-1 respectively. FSH and IGF-1 interact synergistically to induce amplification of STARD1 mRNA and protein expression in serum-free monolayer culture of immature swine granulosa cells (Balasubramanian et al., 1997). During follicular development in the rat ovary, Ronen-Fuhrmann et al. (1998) have examined the time-dependent expression of STARD1 mRNA and protein in PMSG/hCG-treated immature rats. They found that in the early phase, before the administration of tropic hormones, granulosa cells did not express STARD1. The first peak of STARD1expression was generated by PMSG administration. The expression was restricted to the ovarian secondary interstitial tissue as well as to a fewer scattered theca interna cells producing androgens which can synergistically potentiate FSH-induced actions in granulosa cells, and P450 aromatase for estrogen production in granulosa cells of Graafian follicles. This also seems to initiate the transition of follicles from the small antral stage to the preovulatory stage. After hCG administration, both the granulosa (until now devoid of STARD1) and the theca-interstitial cell types joined in synchronized production of STARD1. At this phase of follicular development, usually perceived as the onset of the luteinization process, high STARD1mRNA levels resumed in the all-ovarian interstitium and high levels of STARD1were also expressed in the granulosa cells; however, in the later cell type, STARD1 expression was strictly confined to periovulatory follicles.

INDUCTION OF OVULATION

The measurement of blood FSH, LH, E2, and other hormones, at different ages in patient B, argues for a normal function of the hypothalamus-pituitary axis with a progressive increase of 17β-estradiol secretion to induce progressive pubertal feminization and regular menstruations. This was probably due to an efficient mechanism of STARD1 -independent steroidogenesis still undamaged by the toxic accumulation of cholesterol and its derivatives, during the short life of stimulated follicles. However, data showed that she failed to demonstrate the spontaneous estrogen surge of the end of follicular phase, necessary for the secretion of ovulatory peak of LH, ovulation and consequently the normal increase of progesterone and basal temperature during the next theoretical luteal phase. The menstrual cycles of this patient were anovulatory for many years before consulting for infertility problems. Interestingly, during her early pubertal development, a hCG stimulation test resulted in a small increase in androstenedione and substantial enhancement of 17β-estradiol secretion (Khoury et al., 2009).

The mechanism of this response is subject to speculation, but more importantly it indicates that the steroidogenic systems retained some capacity to respond to tropic hormones. Thus, during the follow-up in the fertility clinic, we proposed to observe the function of the hypothalamus-hypophyso-ovarian axis during a Clomiphene stimulation test. This was done at the age of 25 years. Endocrine data shows that pituitary gonadotrophins, induced by Clomiphene stimulation, enhanced the steroidogenesis process in the granulosa cells, in the same manner as was observed with the hCG stimulation test, 13 years earlier. Furthermore, the high levels of progesterone and 17β-estradiol observed during the second half of her menstrual cycle is a clear confirmation of a process of ovulation and luteinization (Khoury et al., 2006b, 2009). According to Ronen-Fuhrmann et al. (1998) this is due, in the normal rat, to the high STARD1 expression induced by tropic hormones in all ovarian interstitium and the granulosa cells of periovulatory follicles. In our patient, this may indicate that hCG stimulation or increased secretion of pituitary FSH and LH induced by Clomiphene, as well as the ovulatory peak of LH, may have a role of further activation of the STARD1-independent system (Watari et al., 1997). It is also plausible to think that the amplification of the mutated STARD1 expression by those tropic hormones may contribute, via its partial steroidogenic activity, to the production of estrogen surge necessary for the ovulatory peak of LH and ovulation.

STARD1, CORPUS LUTEUM, AND PREGNANCY

Pregnancy is the ultimate proof of the induction of ovulation. In our patient this was produced by Clomiphene stimulation. We believe that any other protocols of ovulation induction by gonadotrophins will also have a good chance of success. Our patient had a first pregnancy at the age of 25 4/12 years. However, a spontaneous abortion occurred 6 weeks later. The human corpus luteum derived from the ovulated follicle is an active producer of progesterone, an essential hormone for establishing and sustaining early pregnancy (Carr, 1992). Placental progesterone becomes sufficient to maintain pregnancy only after about 6 weeks of gestation, the so-called "luteoplacental shift." Consequently, human maternal ovariectomy in the first 6 weeks will cause spontaneous abortion, but maternal ovariectomy thereafter will not (Csapo et al., 1973; Csapo and Pulkkinen, 1978). The critical step in luteal progesterone secretion is the movement of cholesterol from the OMM to the IMM (Devoto et al., 2002). Examination of corpora lutea of different luteal phases revealed that the basal expression of STARD1 transcript and protein was greatest in early and mid-luteal phase to decline in the late-luteal phase. Furthermore, under hCG stimulation, the expression of the major 1.6 kb STARD1 mRNA transcript is rapidly enhanced. The rise in STARD1 expression paralleled an increase in progesterone levels (Chung et al., 1998; Devoto et al., 2001). In human corpus luteum, the theca-lutein cells and granulosa-lutein cells exhibited marked heterogeneity in STARD1 protein concentration, with theca-lutein cells expressing greater levels of STARD1 than granulosa-lutein cells, irrespective of the stage of the luteal phase (Devoto et al., 2001; Christenson and Devoto, 2003). Human chorionic gonadotropin treatment during the late-luteal phase causes a pronounced increase in both theca-and granulosa-lutein cell STARD1 gene expression. In some species, including human, PGF2α is believed to be the physiological agent responsible for causing corpus luteum regression at the end of a non-fertile cycle. This luteolytic compound has been shown to cause a pronounced decline in STARD1 gene expression, altering cholesterol transport to the mitochondria, inhibiting progesterone production and leading to substantial stores of lipids (Devoto et al., 2001; Christenson and Devoto, 2003). The distribution of STARD1 inside theca and granulosa-lutein cells of human corpus luteum was assessed by electron microscopy (Sierralta et al., 2005). Greater levels of STARD1 immunolabeling was found in the cells from early- and mid- than in the late-luteal phase of corpus luteum, and lower levels in cells from women treated with GnRH antagonist in the mid-luteal phase. There is also a substantial amount of mature STARD1 protein (30 kDa) in the cytoplasm of luteal cells (Sierralta et al., 2005). The presence of STARD1 in the cytoplasm was also reported in rat adrenal homogenates (LeHoux et al., 1999). The administration of GnRH antagonist during mid-luteal phase causes a dramatic reduction in STARD1 immunolabeling in both the cytosol and mitochondria of theca and granulosa-lutein cells of mid-luteal corpus luteum suggesting that, the levels of STARD1 protein in both cell compartments are LH dependent. Also, the presence of MLN64 in the supernatant of human corpus luteum extract throughout the luteal phase (Watari et al., 1997; Kishida et al., 2004) supports the idea that in cells with high steroidogenic activities, proteins with a START domain, other than STARD1, might participate in the intracellular trafficking of cholesterol or other lipids.

We conclude that the early spontaneous abortion at the first pregnancy was due to a dysfunction of this mutated STARD1 inside the theca and granulosa cells of the corpus luteum. The STARD1-dependent steroidogenesis was highly solicited during the early and middle phase of the corpus luteum development by an acute and important stimulation of hCG. The incapacity of the mutated STARD1 to transport the high quantity of cholesterol to the IMM will result in an accumulation of cholesterol, cholesterol esters, and oxidative products in the steroidogenic cells of the corpus luteum. This leads to the destruction of both the STARD1-dependent and STARD1-independent systems, in agreement with the two-hit theory concerning STARD1mutations in steroidogenic tissues. Moreover, this explains the failure of the corpus luteum to produce the progesterone necessary for preparing and stabilizing the endometrium, and protecting the embryo during the early first trimester (Christenson and Devoto, 2003; Sierralta et al., 2005). Substitution therapy with progesterone was then indicated. It was recommended to start progesterone at the 17th day of the cycle and to continue this treatment, during the first trimester, if pregnancy was confirmed later. This technique was successful since a second pregnancy occurred. Progesterone treatment was initially recommended throughout the pregnancy hoping to optimize uterine quiescence and prevent premature delivery in her multiple gestations (Meis, 2005); but for some reason, it was stopped at 25 weeks. Delivery of two normal boys occurred at 30 weeks of gestation. The same treatment was used for a third pregnancy, however progesterone administered up to the 17th week was deemed sufficient to support a single gestation. This led to the delivery of a normal girl at 36 weeks of gestation (October 2008).

In 2008, Sertedaki et al. reported a female LCAH patient bearing a 11-bp deletion in exon 6 of her STARD1 gene (Sertedaki et al., 2009). She did have "cysts in the ovaries" and the LH/FSH ratio was very high. After many unsuccessful attempts to conceive, she entered a program of IVF. Follicle development and growth was easily obtained by the administration of recombinant FSH and recombinant LH and follicle maturation was initiated by hCG administration before oocyte retrieval. After IVF and implantation, vaginal administration of progesterone was conducted to support pregnancy up to the 11th week. A female baby was born by cesarean section in 2007 with no perinatal complications. The used protocol was a classic strategy for IVF. Furthermore, it is fully concordant with our strategy for induction of ovulation and protecting pregnancy in LCAH during the first trimester of gestation. In our case, we used Clomiphene for ovulation induction and only 400–600 mg/d of progesterone (Prometrium) (oral and/or vaginal) was given (Smitz et al., 1992; Progesterone supplementation, 2008).

PREGNANCIES OBSERVATIONS

Ovulation induction with Clomiphene citrate is associated, in 6–8 % of cases, with multiple pregnancies, mainly twins (Messinis, 2005). During her last two pregnancies, the patient B developed high blood pressure. Because it first started during pregnancy and it returned to normal after delivery, we classified it as gestational hypertension. She never met preeclampsia criteria. The onset of high blood pressure was earlier in the second pregnancy (16 + 6 weeks GA) than in the third one (34 weeks GA), perhaps because of the twin pregnancy status which represents a risk factor (Creasy et al., 2004).

We do not know exactly the cause of the two preterm deliveries preceded by premature preterm rupture of membranes (PPROM). Although high dosages and regular daily oral steroid administration during pregnancy has been associated with preterm delivery and PPROM (Laskin et al., 1997), this was

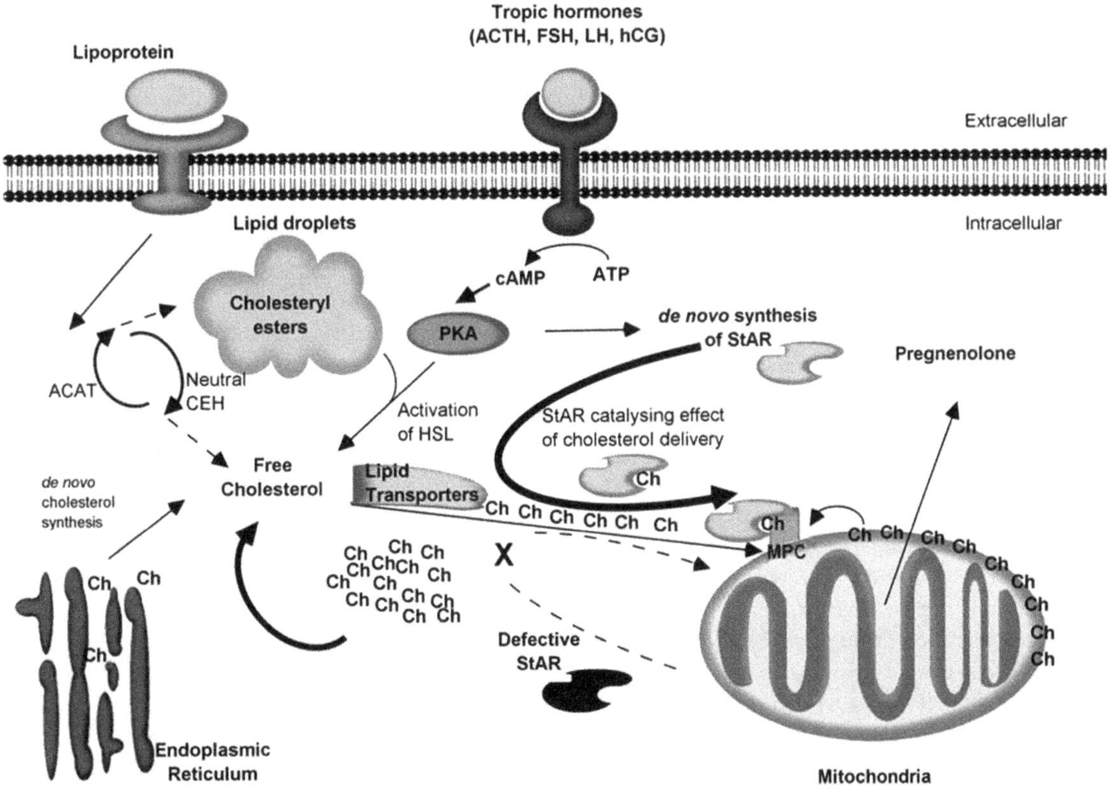

FIGURE 5 | Cellular model of steroidogenesis and LCAH. Low and high density lipoproteins (LDL and HDL) are captured by receptors on the cell membrane. Initial metabolism of LDL lipids occurs in the lysosome where cholesteryl esters are hydrolyzed by acidic cholesteryl ester hydrolases (acidic CEH). The resulting free cholesterol (Ch) is re-esterified by the cytosolic acyl-CoA:cholesterol acyltransferase (ACAT) and stored in lipid droplets. Cholesterol can also be synthesized *de novo* in the endoplasmic reticulum. In the resting cell, cholesterol is constantly hydrolyzed/re-esterified by neutral CEH and ACAT. With the help of lipid transporters, free cholesterol can be conveyed at the OMM. Then cholesterol present at the OMM can be transferred to the IMM for conversion to pregnenolone without STARD1. This *low capacity* system may explain the basal level of hormone production (10–13%) for homeostasis. Following an acute event (stress, dehydration, puberty, etc.), tropic hormones stimulate steroidogenic cells and activate PKA, which in turn leads to three actions: The activation of the hormone-sensitive lipase (HSL) which releases cholesterol from lipid droplets, the *de novo* synthesis of STARD1, and the formation of a multiprotein complex (MPC) somehow involved in the transfer of cholesterol to the IMM (Liu et al., 2006; Bose et al., 2008a). Then STARD1 may act as a *high capacity* system by catalyzing the delivery of cholesterol to the OMM and the MPC complex for its transfer to P450scc in response to the acute demand for steroid hormones. In the case of LCAH, the STARD1 high capacity system is impaired cannot support the substantial throughput of cholesterol, and the latter accumulates in the cytosol; lipid droplets become engorged with cholesterol. As lipid droplets accumulate, the cell becomes less functional and LCAH is onset.

probably not the case for our patient who received physiological doses of hydrocortisone and fludrocortisone acetate during her pregnancies. Furthermore, in this case, we not believe that there is an association between preterm delivery from PPROM and cessation of progesterone, since the patient did not complain of premature contraction or significant uterine activity before the delivery. Also, stimulation with oxytocine has been necessary for delivery. Finally, even if infection is a main causative agent in PPROM, she didn't have any criteria associated with that.

CONCLUSION

We have described clinical data collected over 38 years of follow-up on two French-Canadian patients with 46,XY and 46,XX karyotype and presenting the classical clinical manifestations of LCAH due to a homozygous STARD1 mutation (L275P).

The two patients presented the classic picture of LCAH. Mineralocorticoids and glucocorticoids deficiencies are less severe in Patient A than Patient B. Both patients have had less severe manifestations of corticosteroid deficiency and a later onset of clinical symptoms than the vast majority of patients suffering from STARD1 mutations described in the literature. Patient A (46,XY) portrayed clinical and biochemical signs of early and severe deficiency of testosterone secretion. Testosterone is necessary for differential sexual development and virilization in the early weeks of fetal life during the period of high stimulation by hCG.

Patient B, 46,XX karyotype, is probably one of the first patients with LCAH in which spontaneous pubertal development was observed. She had menarche and spontaneous regular non-ovulatory menstruations for many years before consulting the fertility clinic. hCG and Clomiphene stimulation tests proved the possibility of increasing estrogen secretion by an acute stimulation of the ovarian theca interstitia and the granulosa cells. Clomiphene stimulation restored the surge of 17β-estradiol and LH secretion of the mid-cycle to induce ovulation and open the door for pregnancy. Our understanding of the physiological role of STARD1 during the different phases of the corpus luteum was essential to explain the miscarriage at 6 weeks of the first pregnancy, and then to develop a preventive therapy by progesterone administration during the first trimester of the following pregnancies. We were able to describe and present the first case of pregnancy in the patient with LCAH. It was a very long way from a fatal disease to a normal healthy life and restoration of the reproductive function in a female with the L275P mutation of STARD1.

The clinical and biochemical data of our two patients are concordant with the STARD1-dependent and STARD1 -independent mechanisms of steroidogenesis. However, the non-STARD1 steroidogenesis system is, in our opinion, the basal physiologic system of steroid synthesis producing normal adrenal and gonadic steroids during the normal physiological circumstances. Furthermore, the STARD1 -dependent steroidogenesis system seems to be a key rate-limiting mediator in the acute regulation of steroidogenesis by tropic hormones. It is acting during the acute need for more production of steroids during physiologic periods of normal development (as sexual differentiation and virilization in the early fetal life of the male), surgical or infection stress, normal surge of estrogen production in the mid-cycle necessary for ovulation, or the high production of progesterone during the first trimester of pregnancy. The incapacity of the mutated STARD1 to assume this high speed function, during stress situations and tropic hormone stimulation, leads to the accumulation of high levels of cholesterol, cholesterol esters and oxidative products in the cell. Early appeal and continuous stimulation of steroidogenesis in the gonads (by the hormones hCG, FSH, LH) and the adrenal (by ACTH and renin-angiotensin system) are the starting points initiating the failure of both systems of steroid production.

Figure 5 shows an up to date model of steroidogenesis and LCAH. Despite all the progress made during the last 20 years in the physiology of the transfer of cholesterol to the IMM (Liu et al., 2006; Bose et al., 2008a; Miller, 2016), we still need to understand the detailed interplay between STARD1 and its delivery of cholesterol to a multiprotein complex (MPC) (Liu et al., 2006; Bose et al., 2008a) somehow involved in the transfer of cholesterol to the IMM.

Finally, we wish to point the reader to our recent progress on the dynamics and mechanism of ligand binding and release of the START domain of STARD6 (Létourneau et al., 2016).

AUTHOR CONTRIBUTIONS

KK was in charge of patients. EB and PL contributed to figures. JGL, EB, and KK contributed to the writing of this article. YA and AO did the clinical follow-ups of the pregnancies.

ACKNOWLEDGMENTS

This work was supported by grant MT-10983 from the Canadian Institutes of Health Research. We thank Dr. W. L. Miller for the gift of F2 construct. We also thank Dr. Mélanie Arbor-Levert for her assistance with the clinical follow-ups of the pregnancies as well as Dr. Nadia, Ekindi Ndongo for her comments concerning histology results.

REFERENCES

1. Abdulhadi-Atwan, M., Jean, A., Chung, W. K., Meir, K., Ben Neriah, Z., Stratigopoulos, G., et al. (2007). Role of a founder c.201_202delCT mutation and new phenotypic features of congenital lipoid adrenal hyperplasia in Palestinians. *J. Clin. Endocrinol. Metab.* 92, 4000–4008. doi: 10.1210/jc.200 7-1306
2. Achermann, J. C., Meeks, J. J., Jeffs, B., Das, U., Clayton, P. E., Brook, C. G., et al. (2001). Molecular and structural analysis of two novel StAR mutations in patients with lipoid congenital adrenal hyperplasia. *Mol. Genet. Metab.* 73, 354–357. doi: 10.1006/mgme.2001.3202
3. Arakane, F., Kallen, C. B., Watari, H., Foster, J. A., Sepuri, N. B., Pain, D., et al. (1998). The mechanism of action of steroidogenic acute regulatory protein (StAR). StAR acts on the outside of mitochondria to stimulate

steroidogenesis. *J. Biol. Chem.* 273, 16339–16345. doi: 10.1074/jbc.273.26.16339

4. Arakane, F., Sugawara, T., Nishino, H., Liu, Z., Holt, J. A., Pain, D., et al. (1996). Steroidogenic acute regulatory protein (StAR) retains activity in the absence of its mitochondrial import sequence: implications for the mechanism of StAR action. *Proc. Natl. Acad. Sci. U.S.A.* 93, 13731–13736. doi: 10.1073/pnas.93.24.13731
5. Baker, B. Y., Lin, L., Kim, C. J., Raza, J., Smith, C. P., Miller, W. L., et al. (2006). Nonclassic congenital lipoid adrenal hyperplasia: a new disorder of the steroidogenic acute regulatory protein with very late presentation and normal male genitalia. *J. Clin. Endocrinol. Metab.* 91, 4781–4785. doi: 10.1210/jc.2006- 1565
6. Baker, B. Y., Yaworsky, D. C., and Miller, W. L. (2005). A pH-dependent molten globule transition is required for activity of the steroidogenic acute regulatory protein, StAR. *Biol. Chem.* 280, 41753–41760. doi: 10.1074/jbc.M510241200
7. Balasubramanian, K., Lavoie, H. A., Garmey, J. C., Stocco, D. M., and Veldhuis, J. D. (1997). Regulation of porcine granulosa cell steroidogenic acute regulatory protein (StAR) by insulin-like growth factor I: synergism with follicle- stimulating hormone or protein kinase A agonist. *Endocrinology* 138, 433–439.
8. Barbar, É., Lavigne, P., and LeHoux, J.-G. (2009b). Validation of the mechanism of cholesterol binding by StAR using short molecular dynamics simulations. *J. Steroid Biochem. Mol. Biol.* 113, 92–97. doi: 10.1016/j.jsbmb.2008.11.008
9. Barbar, É., LeHoux, J.-G., and Lavigne, P. (2009a). Toward the NMR structure of StAR. *Mol. Cell Endocrinol.* 300, 89–93. doi: 10.1016/j.mce.2008.12.007
10. Bhangoo, A., Anhalt, H., Ten, S, and King, S. R. (2006). Phenotypic variations in lipoid congenital adrenal hyperplasia. *Pediatr. Endocrinol. Rev.* 3, 258–271. Bhangoo, A., Gu, W. X., Pavlakis, S., Anhalt, H., Heier, L., Ten, S., et al.
11. (2005). Phenotypic features associated with mutations in steroidogenic acute regulatory protein. *J. Clin. Endocrinol. Metab.* 90, 6303–6309. doi: 10.1210/jc.2005-0434
12. Bose, H. S., Baldwin, M. A., and Miller, W. L. (1998). Incorrect folding of steroidogenic acute regulatory protein (StAR) in congenital lipoid adrenal hyperplasia. *Biochemistry* 37, 9768–9775.
13. Bose, H. S., Lingappa, V. R., and Miller, W. L. (2002). Rapid regulation of steroidogenesis by mitochondrial protein import. *Nature* 417, 87–91. doi: 10.1038/417087a
14. Bose, H. S., Pescovitz, O. H., and Miller, W. L. (1997). Spontaneous feminization in a 46,XX female patient with congenital lipoid adrenal hyperplasia due to a homozygous frameshift mutation in the steroidogenic acute regulatory protein. *J. Clin. Endocrinol. Metab.* 82, 1511–1515. doi: 10.1210/jc.82.5.1511
15. Bose, H. S., Sugawara, T., Strauss, J. F. III., and Miller, W. L. (1996). The pathophysiology and genetics of congenital lipoid adrenal hyperplasia. International Congenital Lipoid Adrenal Hyperplasia Consortium. *N. Engl. J. Med.* 335, 1870–1878. doi: 10.1056/nejm199612193352503
16. Bose, H. S., Whittal, R. M., Ran, Y., Bose, M., Baker, B. Y., and Miller, W. L. (2008b). StAR-like activity and molten globule behavior of StARD6, a male germ-line protein. *Biochemistry* 47, 2277–2288. doi: 10.1021/bi701966a
17. Bose, M., Whittal, R. M., Miller, W. L., and Bose, H. S. (2008a). Steroidogenic activity of StAR requires contact with mitochondrial VDAC1 and phosphate carrier protein. *J. Biol. Chem.* 283, 8837–8845. doi: 10.1074/jbc.M7092 21200
18. Carr, B. R. (1992). "Disorders of the ovary and female productive tract," in *Williams Textbook of Endocrinology*, eds J. D. Wilson and D. W. Foster (Philadelphia: WB *Saunders*), 733–98.
19. Chen, X., Baker, B. Y., Abduljabbar, M. A., and Miller, W. L. (2005). A genetic isolate of congenital lipoid adrenal hyperplasia with atypical clinical findings. *J. Clin. Endocrinol. Metab.* 90, 835–840. doi: 10.1210/jc.2004-1323
20. Christenson, L. K., and Devoto, L. (2003). Cholesterol transport and steroidogenesis by the corpus luteum. *Reprod. Biol. Endocrinol.* 1:90. doi: 10.1186/1477-7827-1-90
21. Chung, P. H., Sandhoff, T. W., and McLean, M. P. (1998). Hormone and prostaglandin F2 alpha regulation of messenger ribonucleic acid encoding steroidogenic acute regulatory protein in human corpora lutea. *Endocrine* 8, 153–160.
22. Clark, B. J., Wells, J., King, S. R., and Stocco, D. M. (1994). The purification, cloning, and expression of a novel luteinizing hormone-induced mitochondrial protein in MA-10 mouse Leydig tumor cells. Characterization of the steroidogenic acute regulatory protein (StAR). *J. Biol. Chem.* 269, 28314–28322.
23. Creasy, R. K., Resnik, R., Iams, J., Lockwood, C., and Moore, T. (2004). *Maternal- Fetal Medicine, Principles and Practice.* 5th Edn., Philadelphia: W. B. Saunders.
24. Csapo, A. I., and Pulkkinen, M. (1978). Indispensability of the human corpus luteum in the maintenance of early pregnancy. Luteectomy evidence. *Obstet. Gynecol. Surv.* 33, 69–81. doi: 10.1097/00006254-197802000-00001
25. Csapo, A. I., Pulkkinen, M. O., and Wiest, W. G. (1973). Effects of luteectomy and progesterone replacement therapy in early pregnant patients. *Am. J. Obstet. Gynecol.* 115, 759–765. doi: 10.1016/0002-9378(73)90517-6
26. Degenhart, H. J., Visser, H. K., Boon, H., and O'Doherty, N. J. (1972). Evidence for deficient 20α -cholesterol-hydroxylase activity in adrenal tissue of a patient with lipoid adrenal hyperplasia. *Acta Endocrinol.* 71, 512–518.
27. Devoto, L., Kohen, P., Gonzalez, R. R., Castro, O., Retamales, I., Vega, M., et al. (2001). Expression of steroidogenic acute regulatory protein in the human corpus luteum throughout the luteal phase. *J. Clin. Endocrinol. Metab.* 86, 5633–5639. doi: 10.1210/jcem.86.11.7982
28. Devoto, L., Kohen, P., Vega, M., Castro, O., González, R. R., Retamales, I., et al. (2002). Control of human luteal steroidogenesis. *Mol. Cell. Endocrinol.* 186, 137–141. doi: 10.1016/S0303-7207(01)00654-2
29. Farkash, Y., Timberg, R., and Orly, J. (1986). Preparation of antiserum to rat cytochrome P-450 cholesterol side chain cleavage, and its use for ultrastructural localization of the immunoreactive enzyme by protein A-gold technique. *Endocrinology* 118, 1353–1365.
30. Fleury, A., Mathieu, A. P., Ducharme, L., Hales, D. B., and LeHoux, J. G. (2004). Phosphorylation and function of the hamster adrenal steroidogenic acute regulatory protein (StAR). *J. Steroid Biochem. Mol. Biol.* 91, 259–271. doi: 10.1016/j.jsbmb.2004.04.010
31. Flück, C. E., Maret, A., Mallet, D., Portrat-Doyen, S., Achermann, J. C., Leheup, B., et al. (2005). A novel mutation L260P of the steroidogenic acute regulatory protein gene in three unrelated patients of Swiss ancestry with congenital lipoid adrenal hyperplasia. *J. Clin. Endocrinol. Metab.* 90, 5304–5308. doi: 10.1210/jc.2005-0874
32. Fujieda, K., Okuhara, K., Abe, S., Tajima, T., Mukai, T., and Nakae, J. (2003). Molecular pathogenesis of lipoid adrenal hyperplasia and adrenal hypoplasia congenita. *J. Steroid Biochem. Mol. Biol.* 85, 483–489. doi: 10.1016/S0960-0760(03)00232-2
33. Fujieda, K., Tajima, T., Nakae, J., Sageshima, S., Tachibana, K., Suwa, S., et al. (1997). Spontaneous puberty in 46,XX subjects with congenital lipoid adrenal hyperplasia. Ovarian steroidogenesis is spared to some extent despite inactivating mutations in the steroidogenic acute regulatory protein (StAR) gene. *J. Clin. Invest.* 99, 1265–1271. doi: 10.1172/JCI119284
34. Fukami, M., Sato, S., Ogata, T., and Matsuo, N. (1995). Lack of Mutations in P450scc Gene (CYP11A) in Six Japanese Patients with Congenital Lipoid Adrenal Hyperplasia. *Clin. Pediatr. Endocrinol.* 4, 39–46. doi: 10.1297/cpe.4.39
35. Geuze, H. J., Slot, J. W., Yanagibashi, K., McCracken, J. A., Schwartz, A. L., and Hall, P. F. (1987). Immunogold cytochemistry of cytochromes P-450 in porcine adrenal cortex. Two enzymes (side-chain cleavage and 11 beta-hydroxylase) are co-localized in the same mitochondria. *Histochemistry* 86, 551–557.
36. Harikrishna, J. A., Black, S. M., Szklarz, G. D., and Miller, W. L. (1993).
37. Construction and function of fusion enzymes of the human cytochrome P450scc system. *DNA Cell Biol.* 12, 371–379. doi: 10.1089/dna.1993.12.371
38. Hauffa, B. P., Miller, W. L., Grumbach, M. M., Conte, F. A., and Kaplan, S. L. (1985). Congenital adrenal hyperplasia due to deficient cholesterol side-chain cleavage activity (20, 22-desmolase) in a patient treated for 18 years. *Clin. Endocrinol.* 23, 481–493. doi: 10.1111/j.1365-2265.1985.tb01107.x
39. Hiort, O., Holterhus, P. M., Werner, R., Marschke, C., Hoppe, U., Partsch, C. J., et al. (2005). Homozygous disruption of P450 side-chain cleavage (CYP11A1) is associated with prematurity, complete 46,XY sex reversal, and severe adrenal failure. *J. Clin. Endocrinol. Metab.* 90, 538–541. doi: 10.1210/jc.2004-1059
40. Kallen, C. B., Billheimer, J. T., Summers, S. A., Stayrook, S. E., Lewis, M., and Strauss, J. F. III. (1998). Steroidogenic acute regulatory protein (StAR) is a sterol transfer protein. *J. Biol. Chem.* 273, 26285–26288. doi: 10.1074/jbc.273.41.26285

41. Katsumata, N., Ohtake, M., Hojo, T., Ogawa, E., Hara, T., Sato, N., et al. (2002). Compound heterozygous mutations in the cholesterol side-chain cleavage enzyme gene (CYP11A) cause congenital adrenal insufficiency in humans. *J. Clin. Endocrinol. Metab.* 87, 3808–3813. doi: 10.1210/jcem.87.8.8763
42. Khoury, K., Ainmelk, Y., Ouellet, A., and LeHoux, J. G. (2006a). "A spontaneous pubertal development and a first case of pregnancy in a patient with Lipoid congenital adrenal hyperplasia (CAH) due to homozygous StAR protein mutation," in *Scientific Program and Abstracts of the XIIth Adrenal Cortex and Vth Molecular Steroidogenesis Conference.* (Boston, MA).
43. Khoury, K., Ainmelk, Y., Ouellet, A., and Lehoux, J. G. (2006b). A spontaneous pubertal development and a first case of pregnancy in a patient with lipoid congenital adrenal hyperplasia (CAH) due to homozygous StAR protein mutation [Abstract]. *Gynecol. Endocrinol.* 22(Suppl. 1), 226. 12th World Congress of Gynecological Endocrinology.
44. Khoury, K., Barbar, E., Ainmelk, Y., Ouellet, A., and Lehoux, J. G. (2009). Gonadal Function, First Cases of Pregnancy and Child Delivery in a Woman with LCAH. *J. Clin. Endocrinol. Metab.* 94, 1333–1337. doi: 10.1210/jc.2008-1694
45. Khoury, K., Ducharme, L., and LeHoux, J. G. (2004). Family of two patients with congenital lipoid adrenal hyperplasia due to StAR mutation. *Endocr. Res.* 30, 925–929. doi: 10.1081/ERC-200044151
46. Kishida, T., Kostetskii, I., Zhang, Z., Martinez, F., Liu, P., Walkley, S. U., et al. (2004). Targeted mutation of the MLN64 START domain causes only modest alterations in cellular sterol metabolism. *J. Biol. Chem.* 279, 19276–19285. doi: 10.1074/jbc.M400717200
47. Koizumi, S., Kyoya, S., Miyawaki, T. M., Kidani, H., and Funabashi, T. (1977). Cholesterol side-chain cleavage enzyme activity and cytochrome P-450 content in adrenal mitochondria of a patient with congenital lipoid adrenal hyperplasia (Prader disease). *Clin. Chim. Acta* 77, 301–306. doi: 10.1016/0009- 8981(77)90233-9
48. Korsch, E., Peter, M., Hiort, O., Sippell, W. G., Ure, B. M., Hauffa, B. P., et al. (1999). Gonadal histology with testicular carcinoma *in situ* in a 15-year- old 46,XY female patient with a premature termination in the steroidogenic acute regulatory protein causing congenital lipoid adrenal hyperplasia. *J. Clin. Endocrinol. Metab.* 84, 1628–1632. doi: 10.1210/jcem.84.5.5694
49. Laskin, C. A., Bombardier, C., Hannah, M. E., Mandel, F. P., Ritchie, J. W., Farewell, V., et al. (1997). Prednisone and aspirin in women with autoantibodies and unexplained recurrent fetal loss. *N. Engl. J. Med.* 337, 148–153. doi: 10.1056/NEJM199707173370302
50. Lavigne, P., Najmanivich, R., and Lehoux, J. G. (2010). Mammalian StAR-related lipid transfer (START) domains with specificity for cholesterol: structural conservation and mechanism of reversible binding. *Subcell. Biochem.* 51, 425–437. doi: 10.1007/978-90-481-8622-8_15
51. LeHoux, J. G., Hales, D. B., Fleury, A., Briere, N., Martel, D., and Ducharme, L. (1999). The *in vivo* effects of adrenocorticotropin and sodium restriction on the formation of the different species of steroidogenic acute regulatory protein in rat adrenal. *Endocrinology* 140, 5154–5164.
52. LeHoux, J. G., Mathieu, A., Lavigne, P., and Fleury, A. (2003). Adrenocorticotropin regulation of steroidogenic acute regulatory protein. *Microsc. Res. Tech.* 61, 288–299. doi: 10.1002/jemt.10338
53. Létourneau, D., Bédard, M., Cabana, J., Lefebvre, A., LeHoux, J. G., and Lavigne, P. (2016). STARD6 on steroids: solution structure, multiple timescale backbone dynamics and ligand binding mechanism. *Sci. Rep.* 6:28486. doi: 10.1038/srep28486
54. Létourneau, D., Lavigne, P., Lefebvre, A., and LeHoux, J.-G. (2014). "START domain protein structure and ligand specificity," in *Cholesterol Transporters of the START Domain Protein Family in Health and Disease,* eds B. J. Clark and D. M. Stocco (New York, NY: Springer), 49–72.
55. Létourneau, D., Lefebvre, A., Lavigne, P., and LeHoux, J. G. (2015). The binding site specificity of STARD4 subfamily: breaking the cholesterol paradigm. *Mol. Cell Endocrinol.* 408, 53–61. doi: 10.1016/j.mce.2014.12.016
56. Lin, D., Gitelman, S. E., Saenger, P., and Miller, W. L. (1991). Normal genes for the cholesterol side chain cleavage enzyme, P450scc, in congenital lipoid adrenal hyperplasia. *J. Clin. Invest.* 88:1955–1962. doi: 10.1172/JCI115520
57. Lin, D., Sugawara, T., Strauss, J. F. III., Clark, B. J., Stocco, D. M., Saenger, P., et al. (1995). Role of steroidogenic acute regulatory protein in adrenal and gonadal steroidogenesis. *Science* 267, 1828–1831.
58. Liu, J., Rone, M. B., and Papadopoulos, V. (2006). Protein-protein interactions mediate mitochondrial cholesterol transport and steroid biosynthesis. *J. Biol. Chem.* 281, 38879–38893.
59. Mathieu, A. P., Fleury, A., Ducharme, L., Lavigne, P., and LeHoux, J. G. (2002a). Insights into steroidogenic acute regulatory protein (StAR)-dependent cholesterol transfer in mitochondria: evidence from molecular modeling and structure-based thermodynamics supporting the existence of partially unfolded states of StAR. *J. Mol. Endocrinol.* 29, 327–345. doi: 10.1677/jme.0.02 90327
60. Mathieu, A. P., Lavigne, P., and LeHoux, J. G. (2002b). Molecular modeling and structure-based thermodynamic analysis of the StAR protein. *Endocr. Res.* 28, 419–423.
61. Matsuo, N., Tsuzaki, S., Anzo, M., Ogata, T., and Sato, S. (1994). The phenotypic definition of congenital Lipoid adrenal hyperplasia: analysis of the 67 Japanese patients. *Horm. Res.* 41(Suppl.), 106.
62. Matteson, K. J., Chung, B. C., Urdea, M. S., and Miller, W. L. (1986). Study of cholesterol side-chain cleavage (20,22 desmolase) deficiency causing congenital lipoid adrenal hyperplasia using bovine-sequence P450scc oligodeoxyribonucleotide probes. *Endocrinology* 118, 1296–1305. doi: 10.1210/endo-118-4-1296
63. Meis, P. J. (2005). 17 hydroxyprogesterone for the prevention of preterm delivery. *Obstet. Gynecol.* 105, 1128–1135. doi: 10.1097/01.AOG.0000160432.95395.8f
64. Messinis, I. E. (2005). Ovulation induction: a mini review. *Hum. Reprod.* 20, 2688–2697. doi: 10.1093/humrep/dei128
65. Miller, W. L. (1997). Congenital lipoid adrenal hyperplasia: the human gene knockout for the steroidogenic acute regulatory protein. *J. Mol. Endocrinol.* 19, 227–240. doi: 10.1677/jme.0.0190227
66. Miller, W. L. (2016). Disorders in the initial steps of steroid hormone synthesis.
67. *J. Steroid Biochem. Mol. Biol.* doi: 10.1016/j.jsbmb.2016.03.009. [Epub ahead of print].
68. Murcia, M., Faráldo-Gómez, J. D., Maxfield, F. R., and Roux, B. (2006). Modeling the structure of the StART domains of MLN64 and StAR proteins in complex with cholesterol. *J. Lipid Res.* 47, 2614–2630. doi: 10.1194/jlr.M600232-JLR200
69. Nakae, J., Tajima, T., Sugawara, T., Arakane, F., Hanaki, K., Hotsubo, T., et al. (1997). Analysis of the steroidogenic acute regulatory protein (StAR) gene in Japanese patients with congenital lipoid adrenal hyperplasia. *Hum. Mol. Genet.* 6, 571–576. doi: 10.1093/hmg/6.4.571
70. Ogata, T., Matsuo, N., Saito, M., and Prader, A. (1989). The testicular lesion and sexual differentiation in congenital lipoid adrenal hyperplasia. *Helv. Paediatr. Acta* 43, 531–538.
71. Papadimitriou, A., Fountzoula, I., Nicolaidou, P., and Tzortzatou, G. (2006). Ovarian insufficiency in congenital lipoid adrenal hyperplasia begins in infancy. *J. Pediatr. Endocrinol. Metab.* 19, 271–274. doi: 10.1515/JPEM.2006.19.3.271
72. Petrescu, A. D., Gallegos, A. M., Okamura, Y., Strauss, J. F. III., and Schroeder, F. (2001). Steroidogenic acute regulatory protein binds cholesterol and modulates mitochondrial membrane sterol domain dynamics. *J. Biol. Chem.* 276, 36970–36982. doi: 10.1074/jbc.M101939200
73. Ponting, C. P., and Aravind, L. (1999). START: a lipid-binding domain in StAR, HD-ZIP and signalling proteins. *Trends Biochem. Sci.* 24:130–132. doi: 10.1016/S0968-0004(99)01362-6
74. Prader, A., and Siebenmann, R. E. (1957). Nebenniereninsuffizienz bei kongenitaler Lipoidhyperplasie der Nibennieren. *Helv. Paediatr. Acta* 12, 569–595.
75. Progesterone supplementation (2008). Progesterone supplementation during the luteal phase and in early pregnancy in the treatment of infertility: an educational bulletin. *Fertil. Steril.* 90, S150–S153. doi: 10.1016/j.fertnstert.2008.02.012
76. Ronen-Fuhrmann, T., Timberg, R., King, S. R., Hales, K. H., Hales, D. B., Stocco, D. M., et al. (1998). Spatio-temporal expression patterns of steroidogenic acute regulatory protein (StAR) during follicular development in the rat ovary. *Endocrinology* 139, 303–315. doi: 10.1210/en.139.1.303
77. Roostaee, A., Barbar, E., Lavigne, P., and LeHoux, J. G. (2008). The mechanism of specific binding of free cholesterol by the Steroidogenic Acute Regulatory Protein: Evidence for a role of the C-terminal helix in the gating of the binding site. *Biosci. Rep.* 29, 89–101. doi: 10.1042/BSR20080111
78. Sahakitrungruang, T., Soccio, R. E., Lang-Muritano, M., Walker, J. M., Achermann, J. C., and Miller, W. L. (2010). Clinical, genetic, and functional

characterization of four patients carrying partial loss-of-function mutations in the steroidogenic acute regulatory protein (StAR). *J. Clin. Endocrinol. Metab.* 95:3352–3359. doi: 10.1210/jc.2010-0437

79. Sakai, Y., Yanase, T., Okabe, Y., Hara, T., Waterman, M. R., Takayanagi, R., et al. (1994). No mutation in cytochrome P450 side chain cleavage in a patient with congenital lipoid adrenal hyperplasia. *J. Clin. Endocrinol. Metab.* 79, 1198–1201. doi: 10.1210/jcem.79.4.7962293
80. Sandhoff, T. W., and McLean, M. P. (1996). Hormonal regulation of steroidogenic acute regulatory (StAR) protein messenger ribonucleic acid expression in the rat ovary. *Endocrine* 4, 259–267.
81. Sertedaki, A., Pantos, K., Vrettou, C., Kokkali, G., Christofidou, C., Kanavakis, E., et al. (2009). Conception and pregnancy outcome in a patient with 11-bp deletion of the steroidogenic acute regulatory protein gene. *Fertil. Steril.* 91, 934.e15–934.e18. doi: 10.1016/j.fertnstert.2008.07.1770
82. Sierralta, W. D., Kohen, P., Castro, O., Muñoz, A., Strauss, J. F. III., and Devoto, L. (2005). Ultrastructural and biochemical evidence for the presence of mature steroidogenic acute regulatory protein (StAR) in the cytoplasm of human luteal cells. *Mol. Cell. Endocrinol.* 242, 103–110. doi: 10.1016/j.mce.2005.08.003
83. Smitz, J., Erard, P., Camus, M., Devroey, P., Tournaye, H., Wisanto, A., et al. (1992). Pituitary gonadotrophin secretory capacity during the luteal phase in superovulation using GnRH-agonists and HMG in a desensitization or flare-up protocol. *Hum. Reprod.* 7, 1225–1229.
84. Soccio, R. E., Adams, R. M., Romanowski, M. J., Sehayek, E., Burley, S. K., and Breslow, J. L. (2002). The cholesterol-regulated StarD4 gene encodes a StAR-related lipid transfer protein with two closely related homologues, StarD5 and StarD6. *Proc. Natl. Acad. Sci. U.S.A.* 99, 6943–6948. doi: 10.1073/pnas.052143799
85. Stocco, D. M. (2000). StARTing to understand cholesterol transfer. *Nat. Struct. Biol.* 7, 445–447. doi: 10.1038/75834
86. Stocco, D. M. (2001). Tracking the role of a star in the sky of the new millennium. *Mol. Endocrinol.* 15, 1245–1254. doi: 10.1210/mend.15.8.0697
87. Tajima, T., Fujieda, K., Kouda, N., Nakae, J., and Miller, W. L. (2001). Heterozygous mutation in the cholesterol side chain cleavage enzyme (p450scc) gene in a patient with 46,XY sex reversal and adrenal insufficiency. *J. Clin. Endocrinol. Metab.* 86:3820–3825. doi: 10.1210/jcem.86.8.7748
88. Tee, M. K., Lin, D., Sugawara, T., Holt, J. A., Guiguen, Y., Buckingham, B., et al. (1995). T->A transversion 11 bp from a splice acceptor site in the human gene for steroidogenic acute regulatory protein causes congenital lipoid adrenal hyperplasia. *Hum. Mol. Genet.* 4, 2299–2305. doi: 10.1093/hmg/4.12.2299
89. Thorsell, A. G., Lee, W. H., Persson, C., Siponen, M. I., Nilsson, M., Busam, R. D., et al. (2011). Comparative structural analysis of lipid binding START domains. *PLoS ONE* 6:e19521. doi: 10.1371/journal.pone.0019521
90. Tsujishita, Y., and Hurley, J. H. (2000). Structure and lipid transport mechanism of a StAR-related domain. *Nat. Struct. Biol.* 7, 408–414. doi: 10.1038/ 75192
91. Wang, X., Liu, Z., Eimerl, S., Timberg, R., Weiss, A. M., Orly, J., et al. (1998). Effect of truncated forms of the steroidogenic acute regulatory protein on intramitochondrial cholesterol transfer. *Endocrinology* 139, 3903–3912.
92. Watari, H., Arakane, F., Moog-Lutz, C., Kallen, C. B., Tomasetto, C., Gerton, G. L., et al. (1997). MLN64 contains a domain with homology to the steroidogenic acute regulatory protein (StAR) that stimulates steroidogenesis. *Proc. Natl. Acad. Sci. U.S.A.* 94, 8462–8467. doi: 10.1073/pnas.94.16.8462
93. Yaworsky, D. C., Baker, B. Y., Bose, H. S., Best, K. B., Jensen, L. B., Bell, J. D., et al. (2005). pH-dependent Interactions of the carboxyl-terminal helix of steroidogenic acute regulatory protein with synthetic membranes. *J. Biol. Chem.* 280, 2045–2054. doi: 10.1074/jbc.M410937200

13

ACTH Action on Messenger RNA Stability Mechanisms

*Agnès Desroches-Castan[1,2,3], Jean-Jacques Feige[1,2,3] and Nadia Cherradi[1,2,3]**

[1] Institut National de la Santé et de la Recherche Médicale, INSERM U1036, Grenoble, France, [2] Commissariat à l'Energie Atomique et aux Energies Alternatives, Institut de Biosciences et Biotechnologies de Grenoble, Laboratoire Biologie du Cancer et de l'Infection, Grenoble, France, [3] Université Grenoble Alpes, Unité Mixte de Recherche-S1036, Grenoble, France

***Correspondence:** Nadia Cherradi nadia.cherradi@cea.fr*

The regulation of mRNA stability has emerged as a critical control step in dynamic gene expression. This process occurs in response to modifications of the cellular environment, including hormonal variations, and regulates the expression of subsets of proteins whose levels need to be rapidly adjusted. Modulation of messenger RNA stability is usually mediated by stabilizing or destabilizing RNA-binding proteins (RNA-BP) that bind to the 3′-untranslated region regulatory motifs, such as AU-rich elements (AREs). Destabilizing ARE-binding proteins enhance the decay of their target transcripts by recruiting the mRNA decay machineries. Failure of such mechanisms, in particular mis-expression of RNA-BP, has been linked to several human diseases. In the adrenal cortex, the expression and activity of mRNA stability regulatory proteins are still understudied. However, ACTH- or cAMP-elicited changes in the expression/phosphorylation status of the major mRNA-destabilizing protein TIS11b/BRF1 or in the subcellular localization of the stabilizing protein Human antigen R have been reported. They suggest that this level of regulation of gene expression is also important in endocrinology.

Keywords: ACTH, AU-rich elements, RNA-binding proteins, TIS11b/BRF1, HuR, tristetraprolin, mRNA stability

INTRODUCTION

Transcriptional regulation of the cellular responses to hormones has been the primary focus of many endocrinological research studies during the past decades. Although the transcriptional mechanisms that regulate the production of specific mRNAs are undoubtedly important, it has become increasingly evident that processes regulating the stability of mRNAs also represent critical steps in the control of dynamic gene expression. In particular, acute changes in gene expression are now recognized to be controlled by RNA-binding proteins (RNA-BP) and microRNAs through their binding to target transcripts and their positive or negative regulation of mRNA turnover. Because the ability to respond to rapid changes in ACTH levels is essential for maintaining steroid hormone homeostasis, posttranscriptional mechanisms are expected to be involved in ACTH action. The pleiotropic effects exerted by ACTH on adrenocortical cell functions are regulated through a multiplicity of mechanisms. Through binding to its adenylate-cyclase-coupled receptor MC2R, ACTH stimulates the release of cAMP and the activation of the cAMP-dependent protein kinase A (PKA), which in turn phosphorylates and regulates a number of specific substrates including the steroidogenic acute regulatory protein (StAR) (1) and the cAMP response element-binding protein (CREB) (2). ACTH also strongly regulates the transcription of a number of genes involved in the

---

Abbreviations: TIS11b, TPA-inducible sequence 11b; BRF1, butyrate response factor 1; ZFP36, zinc finger protein; TTP, tristetraprolin; CCR4, carbon catabolite repressor protein 4; CNOT1, CCR4-NOT transcription complex subunit 1; Dcp1a, decapping enzyme 1a.

steroidogenic response including those encoding several steroidogenic enzymes (3), components of the extracellular matrix (4) and many others. Another less characterized level of regulation through which ACTH exerts its actions is the control of mRNA stability through the activity of specific proteins that bind the 3′-untranslated region (3′-UTR) of target mRNAs. We were first to observe that the increase in vascular endothelial growth factor-A (VEGF-A) mRNA induced by ACTH in primary adrenocortical fasciculata cells did not result from increased transcription (5) but from stabilization of its mRNA (6). Here, we will present the proteins that mediate the regulation of short-lived mRNA stability/degradation and focus on those which are regulated by ACTH in adrenocortical cells.

mRNA STABILITY MECHANISMS: AN INTERPLAY BETWEEN *CIS*-ACTING ELEMENTS AND *TRANS*-ACTING FACTORS

The steady-state level of any mRNA in an eukaryotic cell results from the balance between its synthesis through gene transcription and its degradation through the mRNA decay machinery. Regulation of mRNA stability implies both *cis* elements mainly located in the 3′-UTR of mRNAs and *trans*-acting factors. These latter factors comprise a number of RNA-BP that specifically bind distinct *cis* elements, form multimolecular scaffolds that favor or prevent the subsequent recruitment of the mRNA deadenylation and mRNA degradation machineries (**Figure 1A**) (7). Eukaryotic mRNAs are protected at both extremities by a 7-methyl guanosine cap at their 5′-end that confers resistance to 5′ to 3′ exonucleases and by a poly(A)-tail recruiting the poly(A)-binding protein (PABP) at their 3′-end that confers resistance to 3′ to 5′ exonuclease attack by the exosome complex (8). The most frequently distributed and best-studied *cis* elements are the AU-rich elements (AREs) that are often arranged in mRNA 3′-UTRs as repeated AUUUA pentameric sequences that eventually overlap (9). More than 6,000 human ARE-containing mRNAs have been listed in the last upgrade of the ARED 3.0 database (http://brp.kfshrc.edu.sa/ARED/) (10). Many of them have a short half-life, rendering this regulatory process highly effective to rapidly turn down a cellular function.

AREs BINDING PROTEINS

Among the more than 20 ARE-binding proteins (ARE-BP) identified so far, some are destabilizing the target mRNA by recruiting deadenylases and exonucleases and some are stabilizing them by protecting them from these degradation enzymes. The competition between both types of proteins for a given ARE will ultimately determine the fate of the target mRNA. The best characterized stabilizing ARE-BP is human antigen R (HuR), which is a member of the ELAV (homologs of the *Drosophila* proteins *embryonic lethal abnormal vision*) family (11). HuR is ubiquitously expressed and is predominantly localized in the nucleus of non-stimulated cells where it forms messenger ribonucleoprotein complexes that are assembled during splicing of primary transcripts, prior to transport of mature mRNAs to the cytoplasm (12). Upon cell activation by various stimuli, HuR undergoes CRM1-dependent nuclear-cytoplasmic shuttling, directed by localization signals (13). Binding of HuR to ARE may play important roles in controlling the processing, splicing, and polyadenylation of the nuclear transcript, together with the nuclear export and stabilization/translation in the cytoplasm. The exact mechanism by which HuR stabilizes target mRNAs is still unclear, but HuR has been reported in many cell types to prevent the degradation of target mRNAs by competing with destabilizing proteins and thereby preventing their recruitment of the exosome machinery (6, 14). A larger number of destabilizing proteins has been described. Among them, the tristetraprolin (TTP) family, which comprises three distinct members in mammals (TTP/TIS11/ZFP36, TIS11b/BRF1/ZFP36-L1, and TIS11d/BRF2/ZFP36-L2) is one of the best characterized. Although they all bind to similar synthetic sequences *in vitro*, members of the TTP family present specific sites of action and preferential targets *in vivo*, as demonstrated by the distinct phenotypes of the mice that have been genetically invalidated for each of these genes. In TTP-KO mice, the TNFα mRNA is significantly stabilized in macrophages, resulting in a fatal postnatal inflammatory syndrome (15). Deletion of TIS11b/BRF1 gene in mice results in embryonic lethality due to abnormal placentation and major vascular defects (16, 17). This is mainly caused by the failure of TIS11b to repress the expression of VEGF at the end of the developmental angiogenic process. The complete invalidation of the TIS11d gene causes postnatal lethality due to defective definitive hematopoiesis (18). Structural studies have shown that the tandem zing finger repeats of TTP family proteins bind to the 5′-UUAUUUA(U/A)(U/A)-3′ recognition motif while the C-terminal and N-terminal domains of the proteins participate in the recruitment of the mRNA deadenylation and mRNA degradation enzymes (19, 20). Other destabilizing ARE-BP include KH-splicing regulatory protein (KSRP) and the AU-rich RNA-binding factor 1 (AUF1/HnRNP D).

ACTH ACTION ON mRNA DECAY MECHANISMS: FROM TRANSCRIPTION TO PHOSPHORYLATION OF ARE-BP

TIS11b, also named BRF1 or ZFP36-L1, was identified in the adrenal cortex through a differential display RT-PCR analysis of ACTH-stimulated versus non-stimulated adrenocortical cells (21). HuR and alternatively spliced isoforms of AUF1/hnRNPD are also expressed in adrenal cells (6, 22). Recently, it was established that ACTH induced *zfp36-L1* gene transcription in bovine adrenocortical cells (BAC) through phosphorylation of CREB transcription factor and CREB-mediated activation of TIS11b promoter (23). A highly conserved cAMP response element (CRE) was found at -402 to -394 relative to the transcription start site (TSS) of human *zfp36-L1* gene. TIS11b mRNA is also rapidly stimulated by 8-bromo-cAMP in murine adrenocortical Y-1 cells or Leydig MA-10 cells (22), suggesting that the protein is a key regulator of endocrine tissue biology. Interestingly, no classical CRE was identified within the −2,000 bp upstream of the TSS of the two other family members TTP and TIS11d. In agreement

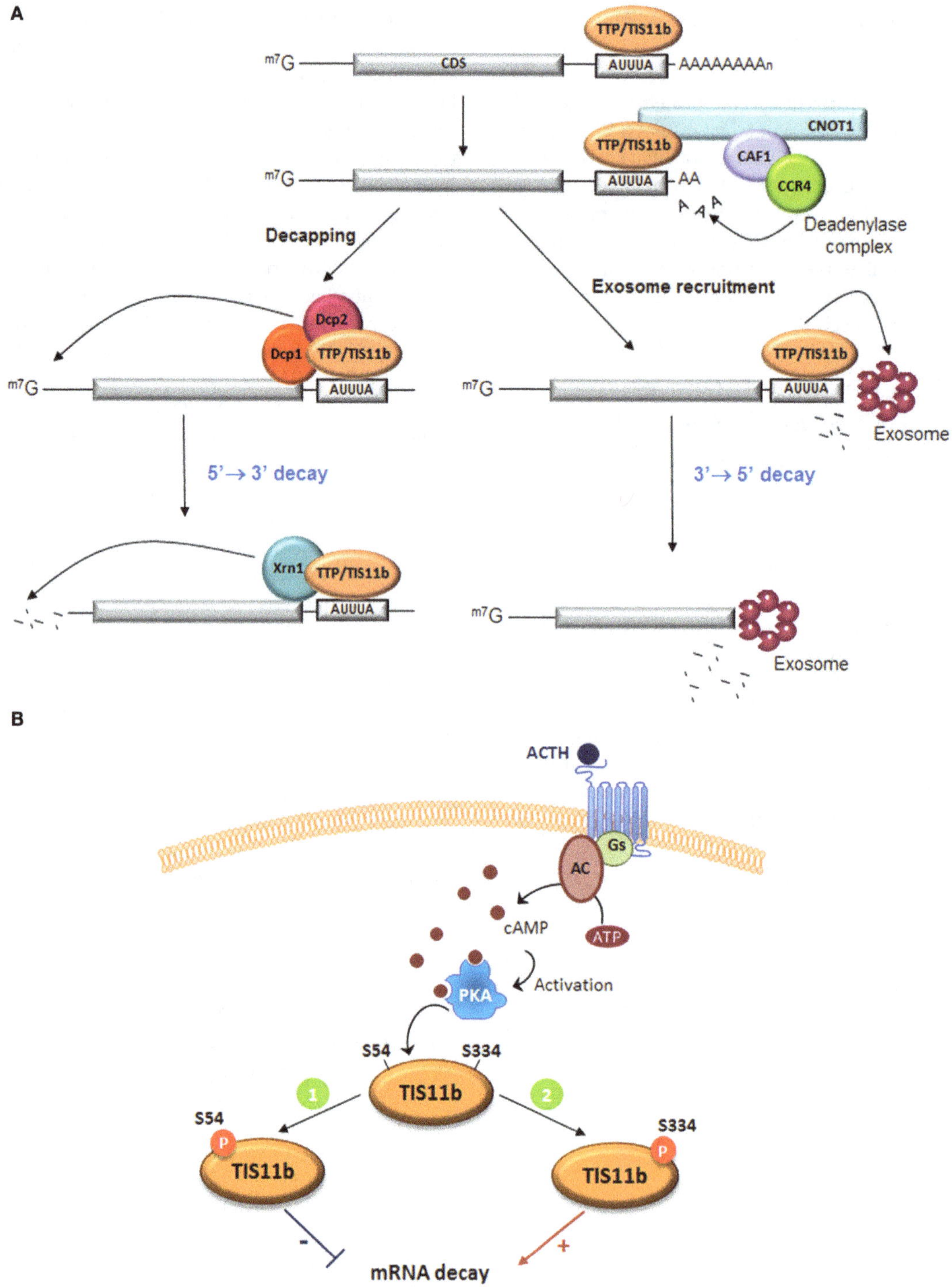

FIGURE 1 | Function of tristetraprolin (TTP) and TIS11b in ARE-mediated mRNA decay. (A) TTP and TIS11b bind to AU-rich elements in the 3′-UTR of target mRNAs and recruit the deadenylase complex directly (CCR4–CAF–NOT1 complex) to trigger mRNA deadenylation. Deadenylated transcripts are degraded through TTP- or TIS11b-mediated recruitment of the exosome, a multiprotein complex that promotes the 3′ to 5′ mRNA decay. Alternatively, deadenylation can be followed by mRNA decapping by the decapping enzymes Dcp1/Dcp2 and the 5′ to 3′ mRNA degradation by the Xrn1 exonuclease. CDS, coding sequence. **(B)** Two putative protein kinase A (PKA) phosphorylation sites, S54 and S334, were identified in TIS11b protein sequence with important roles in protein activity and stability. ACTH stimulation increases intracellular cAMP levels through the action of the G protein Gs and the adenylyl cyclase. This leads to activation of PKA (1). Phosphorylation of TIS11b at S54 by PKA inhibits protein activity. TIS11b-phospho-S54 is sequestered in the cytoplasm due to enhanced interaction with 14-3-3 proteins. This mechanism would promote vascular endothelial growth factor (VEGF) mRNA induction (2). To turn down VEGF production, phosphorylation of TIS11b at S334 by PKA increases protein stability and activity. Dephosphorylation of both serines presumably by the phosphatase PP2A leads to degradation of TIS11b *via* the proteasome.

with this observation, TTP or TIS11d mRNA levels were not changed upon ACTH challenge, pointing at a specific induction of TIS11b by the hormone in the adrenal cortex (23).

Two major target transcripts of TIS11b have been identified in the adrenal cortex. The first one is the message encoding the angiogenic cytokine VEGF (24). Knowing that VEGF mRNA was rapidly but transiently induced by ACTH in fasciculata cells through a transcription-independent mechanism, the contribution of TIS11b and HuR to this transient induction was investigated. Using HuR- and TIS11b-specific siRNAs, it was established that (i) ACTH induced nucleo-cytoplasmic translocation of HuR to trigger VEGF mRNA stabilization in the cytoplasm and (ii) TIS11b, which is induced later by ACTH, participates in the downregulation of VEGF mRNA levels. A short 75-bp long sequence in VEGF mRNA 3′-UTR was shown to bind TIS11b through two adjacent UUAUUUAAU and AUUUA motifs. The second identified target of TIS11b in endocrine cells is the StAR mRNA whose PKA-stimulated transcription paralleled TIS11b induction (22). *StAR* mediates intramitochondrial cholesterol transport in most steroidogenic tissues in response to hormonal changes (1). Cyclic AMP stimulates two major StAR transcripts of 3.5 and 1.6 kb, which arise from differential use of polyadenylation signals and therefore differ only in their 3′-UTR (lengths 0.7 and 2.8 kb, respectively). In mouse MA-10 and Y-1 cells, 8-bromo-cAMP stimulates StAR 3.5-kb mRNA as the predominant form. In BAC, similar long and short forms appear equally (21), whereas in human adrenocortical carcinoma cells H295R, di-butyryl-cAMP selectively stimulates the short form of StAR mRNA (25). Following translation, the 3.5-kb StAR message is preferentially degraded after removal of the stimulus through the action of TIS11b binding to UAUUUAUU repeats in the extended 3′-UTR. This attenuation process provides a rapid mechanism to inactivate StAR when hormonal stimulation ceases.

ARE-binding proteins are also distal targets of several signaling pathways. TTP and TIS11b are phosphorylated by a variety of protein kinases. However, the impact of these phosphorylations on their mRNA-destabilizing activity is still a matter of debate, with some studies indicating that phosphorylations of TTP decrease its affinity for ARE-rich mRNAs (26) and other studies reporting that phosphorylations by ERK, p38 MAP-Kinase/MK2, or JNK kinase do not impact this affinity (27). Similarly, phosphorylation of TIS11b by PKB/Akt or MK2 at conserved serine residues did not affect its ability to bind AREs but nevertheless inhibited its ability to promote ARE-mRNA degradation (28, 29). The current accepted model suggests that protein-kinase activation leads to phosphorylation of TTP or TIS11b, favors their sequestration by 14.3.3 proteins, and thereby reduces their mRNA-destabilizing action. Upon signal extinction, dephosphorylation of TTP and TIS11b occurs probably *via* protein phosphatase PP2A and allows the recruitment of the mRNA decay ribonucleases. A new ACTH-regulated phosphorylation site recently identified in TIS11b seems, however, to mediate a different biological response. ACTH-mediated activation of PKA was reported to induce the phosphorylation of TIS11b on two serine residues, S54 and S334 (23) (**Figure 1B**). Analysis of phospho-dead (S54A, S334A) and phospho-mimick (S54D, S334D) TIS11b mutants revealed that S54 regulates the binding of TIS11b to 14.3.3 protein but that S334 does not play a significant role in this interaction. In contrast, the C-terminal S334 phospho-site appears to be involved in the interaction with the CCR4–NOT1 deadenylation complex. TIS11b S334D phospho-mimick mutants presented a reduced association with CNOT1, a core subunit of the CCR4–NOT deadenylase complex, but however displayed an enhanced interaction with the decapping enzyme Dcp1a. Unexpectedly, this interaction was associated with an increased mRNA-destabilizing activity of TIS11b S334D as compared to the dephospho-form of TIS11b (23). These observations suggest that combinatorial phosphorylations of TIS11b on specific residues do not systematically abrogate their mRNA-destabilizing capability but rather fine-tune their interactions with the mRNA decay machineries.

EXPRESSION OF TTP FAMILY MEMBERS IN ADRENOCORTICAL TUMORS

Overexpression of ARE-containing transcripts encoding factors promoting growth, inflammation, angiogenesis, and invasion has been observed in carcinogenesis (30). These aberrant expressions results from dysfunctional ARE-mediated posttranscriptional control, which seems to be mainly due to deregulations in ARE-binding proteins rather than to ARE mutations. Downregulation of TTP expression has been found in a variety of human malignancies including breast, colon, prostate, and lung cancers (31–33). The loss of TTP expression seems to be an early event during tumorigenesis. Nevertheless, apart from single-nucleotide polymorphisms associated with decreased translation efficiency, the mechanisms leading to TTP suppression in cancer remain obscure. Analysis of the mRNA expression levels of TTP family members (TTP, TIS11b, and TIS11d) and HuR in human adrenocortical tumors revealed that TTP mRNA was dramatically decreased in adrenocortical adenoma (ACA) and adrenocortical carcinomas (ACC) as compared to normal adrenal cortex (NAC) (**Figure 2**). By contrast, TIS11b mRNA is highly expressed in ACC as compared to ACA and NAC while the expression of the third member of the family TIS11d was similar in all the tissues examined. No significant difference in HuR expression was found between normal cortex and adrenocortical tumors. Remarkably, the expression patterns of TTP and TIS11b are symmetrically opposite in normal adrenal cortex and malignant tumors. The relevance of these variations to human physiology and the pathology of adrenocortical cancer remains to be determined. In addition, these results will require validation by measurement of TTP and TIS11b protein levels.

CLOSING REMARKS AND PERSPECTIVES

Transcriptional regulation has been considered the primary control point of protein production in eukaryotic cells. However, there is growing evidence of pivotal posttranscriptional regulation for many genes, including those involved in differentiated functions of the adrenal cortex such as the *StAR* gene. This has prompted extensive investigations to elucidate the mechanisms controlling RNA processing, mRNA nuclear export and localization, mRNA stability, and turnover, in addition to translational

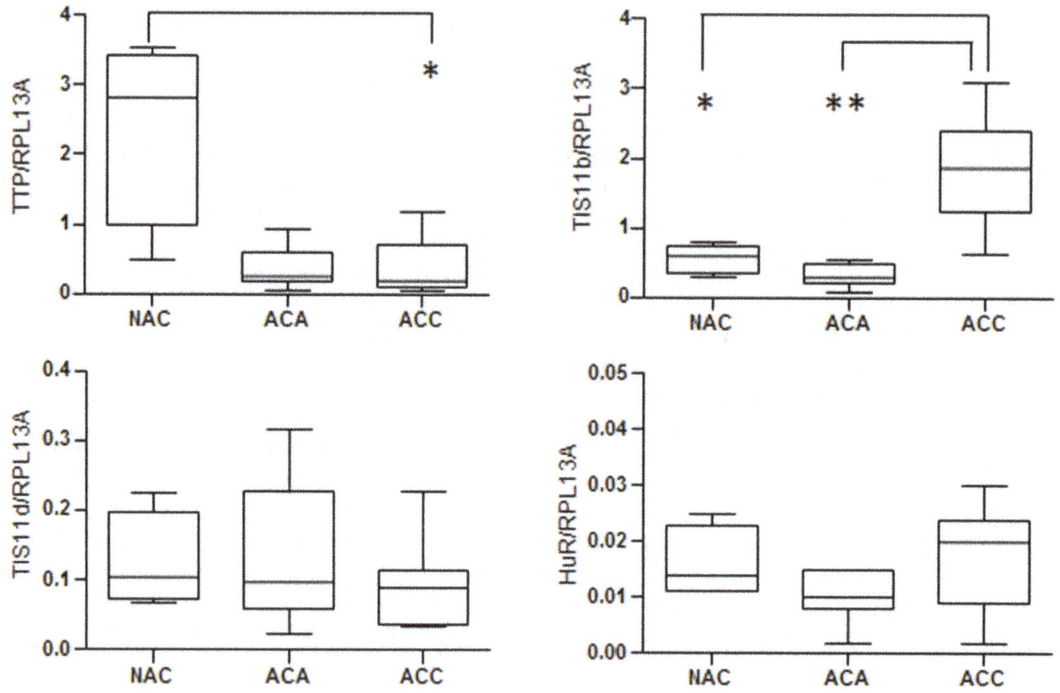

FIGURE 2 | Expression of mRNA stability regulators in human adrenocortical tumors. Relative expression of mRNA stability factors in adrenocortical tumor samples from the French COMETE (COrtico et MEdullosurrénales, Tumeurs Endocrines) Network. TTP family members (TTP, TIS11b, and TIS11d) and HuR were quantified by reverse transcription-quantitative PCR in 4 normal adrenal cortex, 11 cortisol-producing adrenocortical adenomas, and 15 adrenocortical carcinomas. RPL13A was used as housekeeping gene for normalization. The graphs show median with interquartile range. All data were analyzed using the GraphPad Prism Software and were considered as statistically different when $p < 0.05$ (*) and $p < 0.01$ (**).

rates and posttranslational events. The regulation of mRNA stability has emerged as a critical control step in determining the cellular mRNA level, which is regulated through specific RNA sequence elements–protein interactions. In this context, study of the hormonal control of mRNA stability regulatory proteins and their activity in adrenal cortex function is just beginning. Considering that acute ACTH treatment affects a large number of transcripts, it seems very likely that mRNA stability regulations might play an important role in these transient gene expressions. These mechanisms are expected to also operate in response to other cAMP-mobilizing hormones in their respective target organs. For example, parathyroid hormone has been shown to decrease sodium/hydrogen exchanger 3 mRNA stability through the action of the destabilizing protein KSRP in kidney epithelial cells (34). Importantly, few mRNA stability regulatory factors have been identified so far that appear to control a large pool of target mRNAs. This suggests that a slight alteration in the control mechanism may generate large-scale effects that could contribute to the development of complex disorders, including adrenal diseases. Efforts in studying mRNA stability regulators in adrenal cortex and their hormonal regulations should be made in order to better understand their potential contribution to adrenocortical pathologies and possibly discover potential biomarkers and therapeutic targets.

AUTHOR CONTRIBUTIONS

All authors listed have contributed to the work.

FUNDING

This work was funded through institutional support from INSERM, University Grenoble-Alpes and Commissariat à l'Energie Atomique et aux Energies Alternatives, and through grant support from the Fondation pour la Recherche Médicale and the Fondation ARC pour la Recherche sur le Cancer.

REFERENCES

1. Stocco DM. StAR protein and the regulation of steroid hormone biosynthesis. *Annu Rev Physiol* (2001) 63:193–213. doi:10.1146/annurev.physiol.63.1.193
2. Lefrancois-Martinez AM, Blondet-Trichard A, Binart N, Val P, Chambon C, Sahut-Barnola I, et al. Transcriptional control of adrenal steroidogenesis: novel connection between Janus kinase (JAK) 2 protein and protein kinase A (PKA) through stabilization of cAMP response element-binding protein (CREB) transcription factor. *J Biol Chem* (2011) 286:32976–85. doi:10.1074/jbc.M111.218016
3. Sewer MB, Waterman MR. Insights into the transcriptional regulation of steroidogenic enzymes and StAR. *Rev Endocr Metab Disord* (2001) 2:269–74. doi:10.1023/A:1011516532335

4. Feige JJ, Keramidas M, Chambaz EM. Hormonally regulated components of the adrenocortical cell environment and the control of adrenal cortex homeostasis. *Horm Metab Res* (1998) 30:421–5. doi:10.1055/s-2007-978908
5. Gaillard I, Keramidas M, Liakos P, Vilgrain I, Feige JJ, Vittet D. ACTH-regulated expression of vascular endothelial growth factor in the adult bovine adrenal cortex: a possible role in the maintenance of the micro-vasculature. *J Cell Physiol* (2000) 185:226–34. doi:10.1002/1097-4652(200011)185:2<226::AID-JCP7>3.0.CO;2-E
6. Cherradi N, Lejczak C, Desroches-Castan A, Feige JJ. Antagonistic functions of tetradecanoyl phorbol acetate-inducible-sequence 11b and HuR in the hormonal regulation of vascular endothelial growth factor messenger ribonucleic acid stability by adrenocorticotropin. *Mol Endocrinol* (2006) 20:916–30. doi:10.1210/me.2005-0121
7. Stoecklin G, Muhlemann O. RNA decay mechanisms: specificity through diversity. *Biochim Biophys Acta* (2013) 1829:487–90. doi:10.1016/j.bbagrm.2013.04.002
8. Planel S, Rataj F, Feige JJ, Cherradi N. Posttranscriptional regulation of angiogenesis through AU-rich mRNA degradation: potential application in cancer therapy. In: Feige JJ, Pagès G, Soncin F, editors. *Molecular Mechanisms of Angiogenesis from Ontogenesis to Oncogenesis*. France: Springer-Verlag (2014). p. 353–72.
9. Hitti E, Khabar KS. Sequence variations affecting AU-rich element function and disease. *Front Biosci (Landmark Ed)* (2012) 17:1846–60. doi:10.2741/4023
10. Bakheet T, Williams BR, Khabar KS. ARED 3.0: the large and diverse AU-rich transcriptome. *Nucleic Acids Res* (2006) 34:D111–4. doi:10.1093/nar/gkj052
11. Simone LE, Keene JD. Mechanisms coordinating ELAV/Hu mRNA regulons. *Curr Opin Genet Dev* (2013) 23:35–43. doi:10.1016/j.gde.2012.12.006
12. Matsumoto K, Wassarman KM, Wolffe AP. Nuclear history of a pre-mRNA determines the translational activity of cytoplasmic mRNA. *EMBO J* (1998) 17:2107–21. doi:10.1093/emboj/17.7.2107
13. Fan XC, Steitz JA. HNS, a nuclear-cytoplasmic shuttling sequence in HuR. *Proc Natl Acad Sci U S A* (1998) 95:15293–8. doi:10.1073/pnas.95.26.15293
14. Linker K, Pautz A, Fechir M, Hubrich T, Greeve J, Kleinert H. Involvement of KSRP in the post-transcriptional regulation of human iNOS expression-complex interplay of KSRP with TTP and HuR. *Nucleic Acids Res* (2005) 33:4813–27. doi:10.1093/nar/gki797
15. Taylor GA, Carballo E, Lee DM, Lai WS, Thompson MJ, Patel DD, et al. A pathogenetic role for TNF alpha in the syndrome of cachexia, arthritis, and autoimmunity resulting from tristetraprolin (TTP) deficiency. *Immunity* (1996) 4:445–54. doi:10.1016/S1074-7613(00)80411-2
16. Stumpo DJ, Byrd NA, Phillips RS, Ghosh S, Maronpot RR, Castranio T, et al. Chorioallantoic fusion defects and embryonic lethality resulting from disruption of Zfp36L1, a gene encoding a CCCH tandem zinc finger protein of the Tristetraprolin family. *Mol Cell Biol* (2004) 24:6445–55. doi:10.1128/MCB.24.14.6445-6455.2004
17. Bell SE, Sanchez MJ, Spasic-Boskovic O, Santalucia T, Gambardella L, Burton GJ, et al. The RNA binding protein Zfp36l1 is required for normal vascularisation and post-transcriptionally regulates VEGF expression. *Dev Dyn* (2006) 235:3144–55. doi:10.1002/dvdy.20949
18. Stumpo DJ, Broxmeyer HE, Ward T, Cooper S, Hangoc G, Chung YJ, et al. Targeted disruption of Zfp36l2, encoding a CCCH tandem zinc finger RNA-binding protein, results in defective hematopoiesis. *Blood* (2009) 114:2401–10. doi:10.1182/blood-2009-04-214619
19. Hudson BP, Martinez-Yamout MA, Dyson HJ, Wright PE. Recognition of the mRNA AU-rich element by the zinc finger domain of TIS11d. *Nat Struct Mol Biol* (2004) 11:257–64. doi:10.1038/nsmb738
20. Lykke-Andersen J, Wagner E. Recruitment and activation of mRNA decay enzymes by two ARE-mediated decay activation domains in the proteins TTP and BRF-1. *Genes Dev* (2005) 19:351–61. doi:10.1101/gad.1282305
21. Chinn AM, Ciais D, Bailly S, Chambaz E, LaMarre J, Feige JJ. Identification of two novel ACTH-responsive genes encoding manganese-dependent superoxide dismutase (SOD2) and the zinc finger protein TIS11b [tetradecanoyl phorbol acetate (TPA)-inducible sequence 11b]. *Mol Endocrinol* (2002) 16:1417–27. doi:10.1210/mend.16.6.0844
22. Duan H, Cherradi N, Feige JJ, Jefcoate C. cAMP-dependent posttranscriptional regulation of steroidogenic acute regulatory (STAR) protein by the zinc finger protein ZFP36L1/TIS11b. *Mol Endocrinol* (2009) 23:497–509. doi:10.1210/me.2008-0296
23. Rataj F, Planel S, Desroches-Castan A, Le Douce J, Lamribet K, Denis J, et al. The cAMP pathway regulates mRNA decay through phosphorylation of the RNA-binding protein TIS11b/BRF1. *Mol Biol Cell* (2016) 27:3841–54. doi:10.1091/mbc.E16-06-0379
24. Ciais D, Cherradi N, Bailly S, Grenier E, Berra E, Pouyssegur J, et al. Destabilization of vascular endothelial growth factor mRNA by the zinc-finger protein TIS11b. *Oncogene* (2004) 23:8673–80. doi:10.1038/sj.onc.1207939
25. Clark BJ, Combs R. Angiotensin II and cyclic adenosine 3′,5′-monophosphate induce human steroidogenic acute regulatory protein transcription through a common steroidogenic factor-1 element. *Endocrinology* (1999) 140:4390–8. doi:10.1210/en.140.10.4390
26. Hitti E, Iakovleva T, Brook M, Deppenmeier S, Gruber AD, Radzioch D, et al. Mitogen-activated protein kinase-activated protein kinase 2 regulates tumor necrosis factor mRNA stability and translation mainly by altering tristetraprolin expression, stability, and binding to adenine/uridine-rich element. *Mol Cell Biol* (2006) 26:2399–407. doi:10.1128/MCB.26.6.2399-2407.2006
27. Chrestensen CA, Schroeder MJ, Shabanowitz J, Hunt DF, Pelo JW, Worthington MT, et al. MAPKAP kinase 2 phosphorylates tristetraprolin on in vivo sites including Ser178, a site required for 14-3-3 binding. *J Biol Chem* (2004) 279:10176–84. doi:10.1074/jbc.M310486200
28. Maitra S, Chou CF, Luber CA, Lee KY, Mann M, Chen CY. The AU-rich element mRNA decay-promoting activity of BRF1 is regulated by mitogen-activated protein kinase-activated protein kinase 2. *RNA* (2008) 14:950–9. doi:10.1261/rna.983708
29. Schmidlin M, Lu M, Leuenberger SA, Stoecklin G, Mallaun M, Gross B, et al. The ARE-dependent mRNA-destabilizing activity of BRF1 is regulated by protein kinase B. *EMBO J* (2004) 23:4760–9. doi:10.1038/sj.emboj.7600477
30. Benjamin D, Moroni C. mRNA stability and cancer: an emerging link? *Expert Opin Biol Ther* (2007) 7:1515–29. doi:10.1517/14712598.7.10.1515
31. Brennan SE, Kuwano Y, Alkharouf N, Blackshear PJ, Gorospe M, Wilson GM. The mRNA-destabilizing protein tristetraprolin is suppressed in many cancers, altering tumorigenic phenotypes and patient prognosis. *Cancer Res* (2009) 69:5168–76. doi:10.1158/0008-5472.CAN-08-4238
32. Griseri P, Bourcier C, Hieblot C, Essafi-Benkhadir K, Chamorey E, Touriol C, et al. A synonymous polymorphism of the Tristetraprolin (TTP) gene, an AU-rich mRNA-binding protein, affects translation efficiency and response to Herceptin treatment in breast cancer patients. *Hum Mol Genet* (2011) 20:4556–68. doi:10.1093/hmg/ddr390
33. Al-Souhibani N, Al-Ahmadi W, Hesketh JE, Blackshear PJ, Khabar KS. The RNA-binding zinc-finger protein tristetraprolin regulates AU-rich mRNAs involved in breast cancer-related processes. *Oncogene* (2010) 29:4205–15. doi:10.1038/onc.2010.168
34. Murray RD, Merchant ML, Hardin E, Clark B, Khundmiri SJ, Lederer ED. Identification of an RNA-binding protein that is phosphorylated by PTH and potentially mediates PTH-induced destabilization of Npt2a mRNA. *Am J Physiol Cell Physiol* (2016) 310:C205–15. doi:10.1152/ajpcell.00192.2015

14

The Potential of ACTH in the Genesis of Primary Aldosteronism

*John W. Funder**

Hudson Institute of Medical Research and Monash University, Clayton, VIC, Australia

***Correspondence:**
John W. Funder
john.funder@hudson.org.au

Aldosterone is a homeostatic hormone, rising in volume depletion, sodium deficiency, and potassium loading, in response to angiotensin11 and elevation of plasma potassium. Pathophysiologically, in primary aldosteronism (PA) aldosterone levels are inappropriate for the patient's sodium and potassium status, and thus outside the normal feedback loop. ACTH is equivalent with A11 and [K^+] in elevating aldosterone: its effects differ from those of the other secretagogues in four ways. First, it is not sustained; second, it raises aldosterone and cortisol secretion with equal potency; third, it is outside the normal feedback loops, reflecting the epithelial action of aldosterone; and finally its possible role in driving inappropriate aldosterone secretion (aka PA) is not widely recognized. Thirty years ago, it was shown that on a fixed sodium intake of 175 meq/day 36 of 100 unselected hypertensives, in whom PA has been excluded on contemporary criteria, had 24 h urinary aldosterone levels above the upper limit of normotensive controls. More recently, the dexamethasone enhanced fludrocortisone suppression test (FDST) showed 29% of unselected hypertensives to have plasma aldosterone concentrations above the upper limit of normotensive controls. In subjects negative for PA on the FDST, 27% were extremely hyper-responsive to ultra-low dose ACTH infusion; the remaining 73% showed minimal aldosterone elevation, as did normotensive controls: all three groups had negligible cortisol responses. On treadmill testing, no differences were found between groups in (minimally altered) ACTH and cortisol levels: hyper-responders to ultra-low ACTH, however, showed a major elevation in PAC. The implications of these studies, when validated, are substantial for PA, in that approximately half of hypertensive patients appear to show inappropriate aldosterone levels for their sodium status. The physiological role(s) of ACTH as an acute aldosterone secretagogue, and the mechanisms whereby its continuous secretion is curtailed, remain to be established.

Keywords: aldosterone, ACTH, cardiovascular, cortisol, circadian rhythm

BACKGROUND

For many years, most studies on aldosterone have focused on its action on renal salt and water transport, undeniably its major homeostatic role. More recently, following the RALES trial of the effects of spironolactone in progressive cardiac failure (1), a range of extraepithelial effects, primarily cardiovascular, has been shown in animal studies (2–4). The doses of aldosterone (or DOCA) used, and the extent of salt loading, make extrapolation to physiology difficult, and to human pathophysiology doubly difficult. That said, PA clearly has a higher cardiovascular risk profile than age-, sex-, and blood pressure-matched essential hypertension (EH) (5, 6): whether this is a primary effect of aldosterone on the heart and/or blood vessels, or secondary to the increased total body sodium, is yet to be established (7).

The secretory response to what are commonly regarded as its principal regulators (angiotensin II, plasma potassium concentration) is prolonged as long as the stimulus persists. In contrast, ACTH elevates aldosterone acutely but transiently. At least two features of this response are unclear. The first is the organ(s) and processes targeted by the acute elevation; the second the mechanism(s) whereby this acute response is curtailed. Given that the circadian rhythm of aldosterone secretion clearly precedes that of cortisol, both steroids may have roles as "Zeitgebers," effecting diurnal changes in their respective physiologic target tissues. In addition to its circadian variation, however, ACTH is elevated by stress, physical, or psychological. Whereas stress responses to elevated cortisol have been widely studied, those in response to elevated aldosterone appear to have escaped attention. It may be that they form part of the classical "fight or flight" response, by acutely (non-genomically) activating mineralocorticoid receptors (MR) in the vasculature, a physiologic aldosterone target tissue expressing the specificity-conferring enzyme 11β-hydroxysteroid dehydrogenase type 2 (11β-HSD2) (8). A similar rapid vasoconstrictor response follows the acute aldosterone elevation upon orthostasis.

What curtails the elevation of aldosterone secretion despite continued high ACTH levels is currently unclear. One attractive possibility is that it reflects a genomic effect of maintained high levels of glucocorticoid secretion. Heterozygous glucocorticoid receptor (GR) (±) null mice show persistently elevated levels of both corticosterone and aldosterone levels, consistent with elevated levels of ACTH and impaired glucocorticoid negative feedback on aldosterone secretion (9). To date, there appear to be no reports on levels of aldosterone in patients with hypercortisolism due to GR abnormalities leading to increased ACTH levels. There are, of course, additional/other mechanisms whereby the acute elevation of aldosterone in response to ACTH might be curtailed.

Finally, it is accepted that under normal circumstances, ACTH acts with equivalent potency as a secretagogue for cortisol and aldosterone. Recently, as will be discussed in detail below, there is evidence that aldosterone secretion appears supersensitive to very low dose ACTH at levels which do not elevate cortisol secretion (10).

PRIMARY ALDOSTERONISM

The first description of the role of ACTH came over 50 years ago, with the description by Sutherland et al. of a patient with "hypertension, increased aldosterone secretion and low plasma renin activity relieved by dexamethasone" (11). This constellation, variously termed glucocorticoid-suppressive hyperaldosteronism (GSH) or glucocorticoid-remediable aldosteronism (GRA) is now termed familial hyperaldosteronism Type-1, and its genesis demonstrated in an early paper from the Lifton laboratory (12). This heritable condition reflects a crossover event during ancestral meiosis, wherein a chimeric gene with the 5′ end of CYP11 B1 (11β hydroxylase) and the 3′ end of CYP11 B2 (aldosterone synthase) are fused. This results in a sequence, which is expressed throughout the zona fasciculata, producing high levels of aldosterone in response to normal levels of ACTH, rather than the normally much lower levels from aldosterone producing cell clusters (13) in the zona glomerulosa. Suppression of ACTH secretion by dexamethasone lowers aldosterone levels and replaces (more or less) the secretion of endogenous glucocorticoid.

Arguably, the first of the studies directly addressing the potential role of ACTH in PA was by Kem et al. (14). Seven PA patients [three ideopathic adrenal hyperplasia (IAH) and four aldosterone producing adenoma (APA)] were studied, with the conclusion that "these data indicate that ACTH frequently is the dominant stimulus of the episodic secretion of aldosterone in patients with either adrenal adenomas or hyperplasia." Couple this with a report 4 years later by Helber et al. (15) entitled "Evidence for a subgroup of essential hypertensives with non-suppressible excretion of aldosterone during sodium loading." The effect of sodium loading (175 μg/day for 6 days) on 24 h urinary aldosterone (UA) was determined in three groups – 56 healthy controls, 100 patients with EH, and 16 patients with PA (12 APA, 4 IAH). In healthy controls, the upper limit of UA was <6 μg/day; all the PA patients were unsuppressed (IAH 8–20, APA 23–64 μg/day); 64 of the EH patients suppressed UA to levels in the normal range; but 36 did not, with values above 6 and up to 16 μg/day. Non-suppressing EH patients showed a mean UA value of 10 ± 3 (SD) μg/day; those who suppressed a mean of 2.7 ± 1.4 (SD). Plasma [K^+] in the 36 non-suppressors was 3.81 ± 0.44 meq/L and in the 64 EH suppressors was 4.26 ± 0.37 meq/L ($p < 0.001$). Finally, in response to 4 weeks on 200 mg/day spironolactone, blood pressure fell by 22 mmHg in non-suppressors, 21 mmHg in the PA patients, and 9 mmHg in the 64 EH patients who suppressed. The authors conclude, "We believe, therefore, that our patient groups with inadequate high aldosterone suppression during Na^+ loading may reflect qualitatively a similar pathogenetic defect in mineralocorticoid secretion as "hyperplasia patients" with hypermineralocorticoidism."

These data, based on 24 h urinary rather than spot plasma aldosterone, remained unremarked for more than three decades. By the use of variously stringent cut-offs in both the screening test for aldosterone [the aldosterone to renin ratio (ARR)] followed by confirmatory testing, PA is currently gazetted to affect 5–13% of referred hypertensives. Add the 16 confirmed PA to the 36 non-suppressors found by Helber et al. in patients referred to the University of Cologne, and the figure stands at 45%, which would currently be regarded as totally out of court, given the understandable focus on the most florid expression of PA, sometimes dubbed "low hanging fruit."

Where this at face value improbable figure starts to make sense is the incorporation of ACTH status into confirmatory/exclusion testing. Currently, any one of half a dozen procedures are used around the world, of which the fludrocortisone-saline suppression test (FST) is sometimes regarded as the "gold standard" – 4 days of fludrocortisone, sodium, potassium supplementation, and often (but not always) hospitalization. In a series of papers from the Piaditis group in Athens (10, 16–19), the potentially confounding effect of ACTH on values obtained in the FST has been addressed in two ways. First is the inclusion of 2 mg dexamethasone at midnight on the last day of testing [fludrocortisone suppression test (FDST)], with initial results that were arresting, in both a group of control normotensives with normal adrenals on imaging, and a second group of essentially unselected hypertensives (16).

On the FDST, the 97.5% upper limit of normal for plasma aldosterone concentration (PAC) was found to be 74 pmol/L, and for ARR 32 pmol/mL, in the 72 normotensive controls. Among the 180 hypertensives, 56 (31%) showed upright PAC values above 74 pmol/L, combined with an ARR >32 pmol/mU on day 5, evidence for a much higher percentage of unselected hypertensives having inappropriate aldosterone secretion, i.e., PA. In prior studies from the same group, the classical saline infusion test (SIT) was compared with a post-dexamethasone SIT; the latter showed a similar (24%) prevalence of PA, more than double the 11% found on the commonly used SIT (17). More recently, much larger groups of controls ($n = 100$) and hypertensives (327) have been studied, with results essentially identical to the initial study, and a prevalence of PA of 29% (18). A recent overview by Piaditis and colleagues (19) compares these latter figures for prevalence with those from other centers absent dexamethasone loading, which range from 1 to 18%.

There are a number of factors that may conspire toward explaining the difference with and without dexamethasone. The first is the reliance on plasma cortisol as a surrogate for ACTH: just as their circadian secretion appears different, the responses to stress (see below) may differ. Second is the single make-or-break value for PAC, close to the nadir of circadian levels, on which both screening (ARR, PAC above some arbitrary cut-off) depend. It is just possible that Helber et al. got it right, and that UA integrates secretion over 24 h, which may be more pathophysiologically relevant. Finally, it may be that in the historically nephrocentric universe of stimuli to aldosterone secretion angiotensin II reigns supreme, plasma [K^+] admitted almost as an afterthought, and a continuous role of ACTH almost entirely neglected. We may have to extend the sentence quoted earlier from Kem et al. "These data indicate that ACTH frequently is the dominant stimulus of the episodic secretion of aldosterone in patients with either adrenal adenomas or hyperplasia" (14) from the pathophysiological to the realm of physiology, in control normotensives [to halve the 97.5% cut-off in the FST (6 meq/L) to 3 meq/L in the FDST], and (incidentally) in only ~70% of essential hypertensives.

There would also appear to be another dimension in which ACTH may be a probable actor in inappropriate hypersecretion of aldosterone. The data also come from the Athens group, and address patients with EH who previously tested negative for PA by the FDST. In this study (10), 113 of such hypertensives and 61 normotensive controls underwent an ultra-low dose ACTH-stimulation test, followed by a treadmill test. On the basis of the cut-off values for aldosterone (47 ng/dL) and ARR (2.7 ng/dL/μU/mL) at 15- or 30-min post ACTH (97.5% percentile value in controls), 30/113 (27%) of hypertensives recorded values for both PAC and ARR above the cut-off (HYPER group), and 83/113 (73%) did not (EH: ESHT group). Mean values for aldosterone post-ACTH were identical in the control and ESHT groups, and approximately threefold higher at both 15 and 30 min in the HYPER group; cortisol levels post-ACTH were the same in all three groups.

The authors then extended their studies from testing the adrenal responses to ultra-low ACTH to real life (more or less), with all participants undergoing a treadmill stress test to 80% of age-adjusted maximal cardiac pulse, 24 h after the ultra-low ACTH test in each project. When the results of both tests were aggregated and analysed, the 30 patients in the HYPER group showed a twofold to threefold greater elevation over baseline compared with controls or ESHT: no group showed an elevation in plasma cortisol at peak or recovery.

These studies are prismatic, but not perfect. In addition to issues canvassed in the accompanying editorial (20), other questions might be raised. Variances for all groups in terms of response to ultra-low ACTH are extraordinarily low, even when expressed as they are at SEM; this is much less the case for aldosterone responses to treadmill testing, but those for the other two groups remain tight. In contrast, the variances in terms of cortisol response are enormous. The FDST test was done on days 4–7, after ultra-low ACTH on day 2 and the treadmill on day 3. While this may have been convenient, it presumably excluded an unspecified number of subjects who had undergone the two previous tests. There would thus appear to be a corpus of data on such subjects, in addition to the 113 hypertensives who "failed" the FDST. From this perspective, these patients may have been of more interest than the adventitious KCNJ5 data.

These questions said and done, the data from these studies (10, 16–19) taken together argue powerfully that we need to reconsider our currently accepted values for the prevalence of inappropriate aldosterone secretion (aka PA). The current figures of 1–18% of hypertension – on the basis of strict or relaxed cut-offs, referred or general practice patients – are testimony to diagnostic frailty rather than variation in patient populations: what the first three of the Athens studies have shown is a potential confounder in unrecognized roles for ACTH in testing. The implication of the three studies (16–18) is that ~ 30% of unselected hypertensives have autonomous aldosterone secretion independent of the classic secretagogues, a much higher figure than is currently acknowledged.

The ultra-low ACTH/treadmill studies open a quite distinct scenario, that of heightened zona glomerulosa sensitivity to everyday stresses, accounting for a similar fraction of hypertensive subjects. Just as the driver of PA is unclear in the majority of PA diagnosed post-FDST, so it is for the genesis of the adrenal sensitivity. What needs to be done is to validate the generalizability of past findings, not by slavishly repeating the present protocols, given the difficulty in persuading control subjects to undergo imaging and FDST, but by doing a comparison of the seated saline suppression test (SSST) with and without 2 mg dexamethasone at midnight on the day before (FSSST). In preliminary studies, Michael Stowasser's laboratory has shown excellent comparability between the SSST and the FST (21). Subjects negative on the FSSST might then be enrolled in an ultra-low dose ACTH study, including if possible a 24 h urine to measure integrated aldosterone secretion, in addition to values obtained during the test.

If, as I anticipate, this series of findings from Athens can be generalized, we need to recognize that PA affects not ~ 10%

of hypertensives but over half. Currently, major interest and considerate resources are devoted to seeking, for example, additional somatic mutations possibly involved in oversecretion of aldosterone from APA: it may be much less fun grinding through clinical studies, but the outcome for hypertensive patients is likely to be far greater. If over half of hypertensive patients have PA, and fewer than 1% are even screened let alone diagnosed and treated in any jurisdiction, the case for inclusion of low dose MR antagonist in first line antihypertensive therapy would appear to be incontrovertible.

AUTHOR CONTRIBUTIONS

The author confirms being the sole contributor of this work and approved it for publication.

FUNDING

This work is supported by the Victorian Government's Operational Infrastructure Support Program and is a local Australian program. This funding does not fully influence this work.

REFERENCES

1. Pitt B, Zannad F, Remme WJ, Cody R, Castaigne A, Perez A, et al. The effect of spironolactone on morbidity and mortality in patients with severe heart failure. Randomized Aldactone Evaluation Study Investigation. *N Engl J Med* (1999) **341**:709–17. doi:10.1056/NEJM199909023411001
2. Brilla CG, Weber KT. Mineralocorticoid excess, dietary sodium, and myocardial fibrosis. *J Lab Clin Med* (1992) **120**:893–901.
3. Young MJ, Funder JW. The renin-angiotensin-aldosterone system in experimental mineralocorticoid-salt induced cardiac fibrosis. *Am J Physiol* (1996) **271**:E883–8.
4. Young MJ, Funder JW. Eplerenone, but not steroid withdrawal, reverses cardiac fibrosis in DOC/salt rats. *Endocrinology* (2004) **145**:3153–7. doi:10.1210/en.2004-0005
5. Milliez P, Girerd X, Plouin P-F, Blacher J, Safar ME, Mourad J-J. Evidence for an increased rate of cardiovascular events in patients with primary aldosteronism. *J Am Coll Cardiol* (2005) **45**:1243–8. doi:10.1016/j.jacc.2005.01.015
6. Savard S, Amar L, Plovin PF, Steichen O. Cardiovascular complications associated with primary aldosteronism: a controlled cross-proportional study. *Hypertension* (2013) **62**:331–6. doi:10.1161/HYPERTENSIONAHA.113.01060
7. Funder JW. Primary aldosteronism and salt. *Pflugers Arch* (2015) **467**:587–94. doi:10.1007/s00424-014-1658-0
8. Funder JW, Pearce PT, Smith R, Campbell J. Vascular type I aldosterone binding sites are physiological mineralocorticoid receptors. *Endocrinology* (1989) **125**:2224–6. doi:10.1210/endo-125-4-2224
9. Michailidou Z, Carter RN, Marshall E, Sutherland HG, Brownstein DG, Owen E, et al. Glucocorticoid receptor haploinsufficiency causes hypertension and attenuates hypothalamic-pituitary-adrenal axis and blood pressure adaptions to high-fat diet. *FASEB J* (2008) **22**:3896–907. doi:10.1096/fj.08-111914
10. Markou A, Sertedak A, Kaltsas G, Androulakis I, Marakaki C, Pappa T, et al. Stress-induced aldosterone hypersecretion in a substantial subset of patients with essential hypertension. *J Clin Endocrinol Metab* (2015) **100**(8):2857–64. doi:10.1210/jc.2015-1268
11. Sutherland DJ, Ruse JL, Laidlaw JC. Hypertension, increased aldosterone secretion and low plasma renin activity relieved by dexamethasone. *Can Med Assoc J* (1966) **95**:1109–19.
12. Lifton RP, Dluhy RG, Powers M, Rich GM, Cook S, Ulick S, et al. A chimeric 11 beta-hydroxylase/aldosterone synthase gene causes glucocorticoid-remediable aldosteronism and human hypertension. *Nature* (1992) **355**:262–5. doi:10.1038/355262a0
13. Nishimoto K, Tomlins SA, Luick R, Cani AK, Giordano TJ, Hoveson DH, et al. Aldosterone-stimulating somatic gene mutations are common in normal adrenal glands. *Proc Natl Acad Sci USA* (2015) **112**:E4591–9. doi:10.1073/pnas.1505529112
14. Kem DC, Weinberger MH, Gomez-Sanchez C, Higgins JR, Kramer NJ. The role of ACTH in the episodic release of aldosterone in patients with idiopathic adrenal hyperplasia, hypertension, and hyperaldosteronism. *J Lab Clin Med* (1976) **88**:261–70.
15. Helber A, Wambach G, Hummerich W, Bonner G, Meurer KA, Kaufmann W. Evidence for a subgroup of essential hypertensives with non-suppressible excretion of aldosterone during sodium loading. *Klin Wochenschr* (1980) **58**:439–47. doi:10.1007/BF01476798
16. Gouli A, Kaltsas G, Tzonou A, Markou A, Androulakis II, Ragkou D, et al. High prevalence of autonomous aldosterone secretion among patients with essential hypertension. *Eur J Clin Invest* (2011) **41**:1227–36. doi:10.1111/j.1365-2362.2011.02531.x
17. Piaditis GP, Kaltsas GA, Androulakis II, Gouli A, Makras P, Papadogias D, et al. High prevalence of autonomous cortisol and aldosterone secretion from adrenal adenomas. *Clin Endocrinol* (2009) **71**:772–8. doi:10.1111/j.1365-2265-2009.03551.x
18. Papanastasiou L, Markou A, Pappa T, Gouli A, Tsounas P, Fountoulakis S, et al. Primary aldosteronism in hypertensive patients: clinical implications and target therapy. *Eur J Clin Invest* (2014) **44**:697–706. doi:10.1111/eci.12286
19. Piaditis G, Markou A, Papanastasiou L, Androulakis II, Kaltsas G. Progress in aldosteronism. A review of the prevalence of primary aldosteronism in re-hypertension and hypertension. *Eur J Endocrinol* (2015) **172**:R191–203. doi:10.1530/EJE-14-0537
20. Funder JW. Commentary: primary aldosteronism: seismic shifts. *J Clin Endocrinol Metab* (2015) **100**:2853–5. doi:10.1210/jc.2015-2800
21. Ahmed AH, Cowley D, Wolley M, Gordon RD, Xu S, Taylor PJ, et al. Seated saline suppression testing for the diagnosis of primary aldosteronism: a preliminary study. *J Clin Endocrinol Metab* (2014) **99**:2745–53. doi:10.1210/jc.2014-1153

15

Role of EPAC in cAMP-Mediated Actions in Adrenocortical Cells

Aurélia E. Lewis[1]*, *Reidun Aesoy*[2] *and Marit Bakke*[2]

[1] *Department of Molecular Biology, University of Bergen, Bergen, Norway,* [2] *Department of Biomedicine, University of Bergen, Bergen, Norway*

***Correspondence:**
Aurélia E. Lewis
aurelia.lewis@uib.no

Adrenocorticotropic hormone regulates adrenal steroidogenesis mainly via the intracellular signaling molecule cAMP. The effects of cAMP are principally relayed by activating protein kinase A (PKA) and the more recently discovered exchange proteins directly activated by cAMP 1 and 2 (EPAC1 and EPAC2). While the intracellular roles of PKA have been extensively studied in steroidogenic tissues, those of EPACs are only emerging. EPAC1 and EPAC2 are encoded by the genes *RAPGEF3* and *RAPGEF4*, respectively. Whereas EPAC1 is ubiquitously expressed, the expression of EPAC2 is more restricted, and typically found in endocrine tissues. Alternative promoter usage of *RAPGEF4* gives rise to three different isoforms of EPAC2 that vary in their N-termini (EPAC2A, EPAC2B, and EPAC2C) and that exhibit distinct expression patterns. EPAC2A is expressed in the brain and pancreas, EPAC2B in steroidogenic cells of the adrenal gland and testis, and EPAC2C has until now only been found in the liver. In this review, we discuss current knowledge on EPAC expression and function with focus on the known roles of EPAC in adrenal gland physiology.

Keywords: ACTH, steroidogenesis, cyclic AMP, EPAC, HPA axis, adrenal glands, adrenal cortex hormones

INTRODUCTION

In response to stress, the hypothalamic–pituitary–adrenal (HPA) axis is activated. Parvocellular neurons, located in the paraventricular nucleus of the hypothalamus release corticotrophin-releasing factor (CRF), which is transported to the anterior pituitary where it stimulates the corticotropes by binding to type I CRF receptors (1). In response to CRF, these cells release the prohormone pro-opiomelanocortin (POMC) (2). Through posttranscriptional modifications, the inert POMC is converted to biologically active peptides, including adrenocorticotropic hormone (ACTH) (3). ACTH enters the systemic circulation, binds to specific receptors located on the surface of adrenocortical cells, and stimulates the production of adrenocorticosteroid hormones, including cortisol, aldosterone, and adrenal androgens (4). Steroid hormones are produced from the same precursor, cholesterol, by a set of cytochrome P450 steroid hydroxylases (CYP11A1, CYP11B1 and CYP11B2, CYP17 and CYP21) and the steroid dehydrogenase 3βHSD (5). The enzymes are differentially expressed in the three zones of the adrenal cortex (zona glomerulosa, zona fasciculata, and zona reticularis) giving rise to zone-specific hormone production. In humans, the primary source of cholesterol for steroid hormone production is low density lipoprotein (LDL), which is imported via the LDL receptor (LDLR) from the blood stream. Once cholesterol enters the cell, hormone-sensitive lipase (HSL) converts it to free cholesterol substrate (6). Free cholesterol is then delivered to the inner mitochondrial membrane by the actions of steroidogenic acute regulatory protein (StAR) and cholesterol-binding proteins. CYP11A1 (or P450 cholesterol side chain cleavage) catalyses the first and rate-limiting enzymatic step in the biosynthesis of all steroid hormones, the conversion of cholesterol to pregnenolone (7, 8). Pregnenolone can be further converted into different hormone intermediates in the endoplasmic reticulum and the final production of cortisol and aldosterone occurs in mitochondria within the zona fasciculata and zona glomerulosa, respectively (5).

In the adrenal cortex, ACTH coordinates the biosynthesis of steroid hormones via the second messenger cAMP. In response to ACTH binding to its receptor, conformational changes induce the release of G-proteins, which then activate membrane bound adenylyl cyclases (ACs). Upon activation, ACs generates cAMP from ATP (**Figure 1A**). cAMP relays ACTH-mediated functions via the activation of the serine–threonine kinase cAMP-dependent protein kinase A (PKA) or the exchange proteins directly activated by cAMP (EPAC1 and 2 also named cAMP-regulated guanine nucleotide exchange factors (cAMP-GEFs) I and II). Following cAMP activation, PKA and EPAC transmit signals differently. PKA phosphorylates numerous substrates, while EPACs act as guanine exchange factors (GEFs) catalyzing the conversion of the small GTPases Rap1 and Rap2 from an inactive (GDP-bound) to active form [guanine triphosphate (GTP)-bound] (9, 10). While cAMP signaling by PKA in steroidogenic cells has been intensely investigated, the roles of EPAC are only beginning to emerge. This review summarizes our current knowledge of EPAC2 in tissues of the hypothalamus–pituitary–adrenal axis.

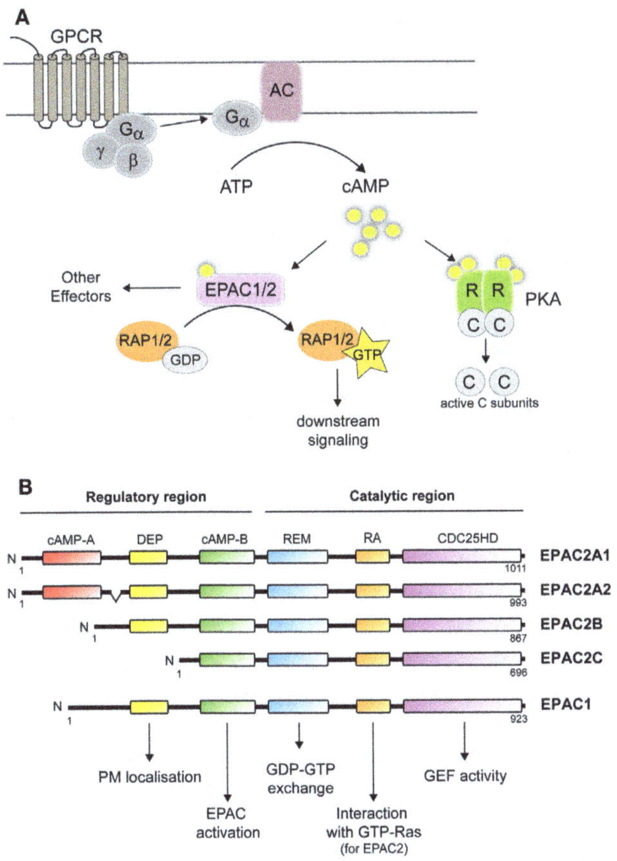

FIGURE 1 | cAMP-mediated signaling and EPAC1 and 2 isoforms. (A) cAMP signaling: following ligand binding of G-protein-coupled receptor, the membrane bound adenylate cyclase (AC) is activated, and generate cAMP from ATP. cAMP subsequently activates PKA and/or EPAC1/2. Binding of cAMP to PKA causes the release of the catalytic subunits, which phosphorylate a variety of targets. Binding of cAMP to EPAC leads to guanosine diphosphate (GDP) to guanine triphosphate (GTP) exchange on Rap1 or Rap2. **(B)** Domain structure illustration of EPAC1 and EPAC2 isoforms consisting of: cAMP-binding domains A and B, disheveled, Egl-10, pleckstrin (DEP) domain, Ras-exchange motif (REM), Ras association (RA) domain, and CDC25-homology domain (HD). The protein structure of EPAC2A2 is shown in accordance to EPAC2A1. Functional roles of each domain are also indicated. PM, plasma membrane; GEF, guanine nucleotide exchange factor activity.

STRUCTURE AND FUNCTION OF EPAC ISOFORMS

The identification of EPACs was reported in 1998 by two separate groups using different approaches. EPAC1 was discovered by de Rooij and colleagues in a database search for proteins containing cAMP-binding domains with the ultimate goal to explain the PKA-independent cAMP-induced activation of Rap1 (9). The same year, Kawasaki et al. identified both EPAC1 and EPAC2 in a screen for brain-specific genes with cAMP-binding motifs (11). In recent years, it has become evident that the EPAC proteins play essential roles in many biological processes, in some where EPAC and PKA collaborate to achieve a common biological response and in some where the two cAMP effectors have separate functions [reviewed in Ref. (12–14)].

Expression of EPAC Isoforms

The EPAC proteins are encoded by two different genes: *RAPGEF3* (EPAC1) and *RAPGEF4* (EPAC2), which both give rise to multiple transcripts. Three transcripts are produced from *RAPGEF3*, but only variant 1, encoding EPAC1, has been studied (13). EPAC1 is relatively ubiquitously expressed (9, 11). Specific parts of the brain, thyroid gland, proximal tubules of the kidney, ovary, and skeletal muscle express the highest levels of EPAC1, but lower levels of EPAC1 have been found in virtually all tissues examined, as well as in hematopoietic cells (15). Studies on murine tissues suggest that EPAC1, as well as EPAC2, mRNA expression is also regulated at different stages of development in embryos and after birth (16).

At the transcript level, four different isoforms arise from *RAPGEF4*, termed EPAC2A1, EPAC2A2, EPAC2B, and EPAC2C (**Figure 1B**) (17–20). The EPAC2A2 transcript might be specifically expressed in the brain (20), but the existence of a corresponding protein is yet to be demonstrated. Thus, potential biological roles for this isoform remain unknown. By contrast, the three other mRNAs are known to give rise to the proteins EPAC2A, EPAC2B, and EPAC2C. EPAC2A was the initial EPAC2 isoform identified (11), and is expressed predominantly in brain (with high levels in the cerebral cortex, hippocampus, habenula, cerebellum, and hypothalamus), pituitary, and endocrine pancreas (11, 17, 20). The EPAC2B isoform was identified by the group of Dr. Seino during their efforts in developing an EPAC2 knockout model (19). While confirming deletion of EPAC2A, they discovered the presence of a shorter transcript in the adrenal gland that lacked the N-terminal cAMP-binding domain [(19); **Figure 1B**]. Until now, EPAC2B expression has only been demonstrated in the adrenal gland (19–21), in the Leydig cell-derived cell line MA10 (21) and in endocrine pancreas (20). The physiological roles of EPAC2B appear to diverge from those of EPAC2A since EPAC2B is not able to substitute for EPAC2A in cellular assays monitoring insulin secretion (19). The shortest EPAC2 isoform, EPAC2C, was also identified by the group of Dr. Seino (17, 18) and has so far only been found in the liver, presumably solely in hepatocytes (18, 20). The strict tissue-specific expression of the different EPAC2 isoforms is controlled, at least in part, by DNA methylation. Detailed analyses of the EPAC2 gene have led to the identification of alternative promoters for the different isoforms (18, 20) and bisulfite sequencing demonstrated that the methylation status of the different promoters nearly perfectly mimics their activity and the expression pattern of the corresponding isoform (20).

Structure and Activation of EPAC Proteins

EPACs are multidomain proteins consisting of two main parts, i.e., an N-terminal regulatory region and a C-terminal catalytic region (**Figure 1B**). The regulatory region is built up by a cAMP-binding domain and a disheveled, Egl-10, pleckstrin (DEP) domain. EPAC2A contains two cAMP-binding domains, cAMP-A and cAMP-B, while EPAC1 has only one such domain. The domain structure of EPAC2B is similar to EPAC1 and lacks the first cAMP-A binding domain, while EPAC2C lacks both the cAMP-A and DEP domains (18, 19). The N-terminal cAMP-A domain in EPAC2A binds cAMP with low affinity and is not believed to be important for cAMP-induced activation (10). Instead, this domain appears to be important for the localization of EPAC2A near the plasma membrane (19). The DEP domain, by its ability to interact with phosphatidic acid, is also important in targeting EPAC to the plasma membrane upon activation by cAMP (22). The catalytic region consists of a CDC25 homology domain (CDC25HD) that catalyzes Rap1 activation, a Ras-exchange motif (REM) domain, and a Ras association (RA) domain (23). The regulatory regions of EPAC1 and EPAC2 function as inhibitors of the C-terminal GEF domain in the absence of cAMP. Binding of cAMP induces a conformational change that opens the catalytic CDC25HD domain from auto-inhibitory restraints and thereby permits GTP loading of Rap (10, 24–26). Both EPAC1 and EPAC2 contain potential RA domains, but only EPAC2 has been shown to interact with Ras-GTP, which contributes in recruiting EPAC2 to the plasma membrane. The enrichment of EPAC2 on the membrane through Ras binding is crucial for EPAC2-mediated Rap1 activation (27, 28). In addition to the plasma membrane, other subcellular localizations have been observed, such as the perinuclear region, nuclear membranes, and mitochondria for EPAC1 [reviewed in Ref. (29)] and the Golgi apparatus and the nucleus for EPAC2B (21).

Physiological Roles of EPAC

EPACs regulate a multitude of cAMP-mediated cellular processes in many different tissues [extensively reviewed in Ref. (23)], including the formation of cell–cell adhesion (24, 30–33), cell proliferation (34, 35), differentiation (36, 37), cell survival (38), ion channels regulation (39–41), and Ca^{2+}-mediated signaling (23, 42, 43). The development of EPAC knockout mice models has led to a better insight into the biological functions of these proteins. In spite of the involvement of EPAC in multiple cellular pathways, mice lacking EPAC1, EPAC2, or both EPAC1 and EPAC2 do not show gross developmental or reproductive abnormalities. However recent studies have revealed that EPAC1−/− and EPAC2−/− mice display various phenotypes in response to stress or other challenges. For example, mice lacking EPAC1 or EPAC2 exhibit impaired glucose tolerance and dysfunctional insulin secretion after glucose challenge when compared with their wild-type littermates (44–46). Double knockout mice of both EPACs in the forebrain showed defects in long-term potentiation, spatial learning, and social interactions (47), whereas knocking out only EPAC2 is sufficient to induce social interactions impairment (48). Loss of EPAC2 also causes defects in memory retrieval in a fear condition paradigm (49). Interestingly, single nucleotide polymorphisms within the gene encoding EPAC2 have been linked to autism. Screening of 48 autistic individuals for mutations in the RAPGEF4 gene showed that four rare missense mutations may be a cause of autism (50). In spine synapses, these mutations alter the protein function of EPAC2 by affecting its Rap-GEF activity, the synaptic protein distribution and spine morphology (51). Activation of EPAC2 results in shrinkage of dendritic spine size as well as increased motility and turnover of the spines, thereby contributing to the plasticity of brain circuits (51, 52). Mice lacking EPAC1 or EPAC2 also present with phenotypes in the heart. Deletion of EPAC1 causes a mild decrease in basal cardiac functions, but more interestingly protects mice hearts from various stressors, such as arrhythmogenic stress (53). However, partly in contrast to this study, deletion of EPAC1 was reported to have no effect in cardiac function (54). Instead, loss of EPAC2 was shown to protect against β-adrenergic receptor-dependent arrhythmia (54). Most of the biological functions aforementioned have been attributed retrospectively to EPAC1 and EPAC2A due to their expression pattern. The roles of EPAC2B and EPAC2C, which were discovered later, are overall less studied. The potential roles of EPAC2B are discussed in chapter 2. In the liver, EPAC2C has been shown to suppress apoptosis and iNOS expression and activity in hepatocytes (55). EPAC2C may also control bile acid-stimulated canalicular formation in the liver (56).

EPAC IN THE HPA AXIS

EPAC2A is expressed in the hypothalamus and pituitary gland and EPAC2B in the adrenal gland. cAMP is known to be an essential regulator at all levels in the HPA axis (57) and, here, we review how EPAC2 is emerging to contribute to cAMP-mediated actions.

EPAC in the Hypothalamus and the Pituitary

In response to various stress factors, the expression of CRF is stimulated in the PVN of the hypothalamus. CRF synthesis is dependent in part upon the neuropeptide pituitary adenylate cyclase-activating polypeptide (PACAP) and a subsequent elevation of cAMP (57, 58). So far, only PKA-dependent signaling has been reported to relay the stimulatory effect of cAMP on CRF expression. PKA inhibition was indeed shown to prevent binding of cAMP response element (CRE)-binding protein (CREB) on the CRF gene promoter and to inhibit transcriptional activation (59). EPAC has not been studied in PACAP-mediated actions in the PVN. However, EPAC was shown to mediate the effects of PACAP on long-term depression of synaptic transmission in the hippocampus through Rap in murine hippocampal slices (60), and in mice deleted for both Epac1 and Epac2 (47). These studies may, therefore, suggest a potential contribution of EPAC in PACAP-responsive PVN. In the suprachiasmatic nuclei of the hypothalamus, EPAC has been associated with leptin signaling (61) and the regulation of factors involved in setting circadian rhythms in Ref. (62). In noradrenergic neurons isolated from locus coeruleus (LC) in culture, EPAC, but not PKA, was shown to be involved in mediating the actions of cAMP (63). Thus, upon CRF binding to type-1 CRF receptor, LC neurons differentiate into norepinephrine-producing neurons via the activation of cAMP–EPAC–ERK/MAPK pathway, by potentiating brain-derived neurotrophic factor-stimulated synaptic plasticity via tyrosine kinase B signaling (63). Since LC neurons innervate PVN neurons, EPAC may, hence, indirectly stimulate the secretion of CRF from the hypothalamus [reviewed in Ref. (64)].

EPAC2A is also the dominant isoform expressed in the pituitary (19), but we still have very limited information about the potential roles of EPAC2 in this gland. Experiments in AtT20 pituitary cells demonstrated that EPAC, presumably EPAC2A, acts as a mediator of CRF_1-induced signaling in corticotropes (65) and in HEK-293 overexpressing CRH-R2β cells (66). Upon activation of the CRH receptor, EPAC2A is involved in cAMP-mediated induction of ERK signaling (65), a pathway previously reported to induce POMC transcription in a PKA-independent manner (67). In addition, CRF receptor activation via Gq is known to signal to phospholipase Cε (PLCε) and, hence, inositol (1,4,5) triphosphate (IP3) to induce calcium stores mobilization that contributes to ACTH secretion (1, 2, 68). Considering that the activation of PLCε by EPAC–Rap2 has been reported to activate Ca^{2+} release and the secretion of hormones in different tissues (23), EPAC may also contribute to the secretion of ACTH in corticotropes.

EPAC in Adrenal Physiology

Role of EPAC versus PKA in Steroidogenesis

In the adrenal cortex, PKA is undoubtedly the major mediator by which cAMP regulates steroidogenesis (69–71). Once PKA is activated, both an acute and a chronic response occur, which contribute to increased steroid hormone synthesis. During the acute response, PKA phosphorylates HSL, which converts cholesterol esters to free cholesterol. This rapid response also involves an increase in StAR, which facilitates the movement of cholesterol to the inner mitochondrial membrane where the rate-limiting enzyme CYP11A1 resides (72). The chronic response corresponds to the transcriptional activation of all the other steroidogenic enzymes (73, 74). In a study by Schimmer et al., using microarray technology to investigate the effects of ACTH in mouse adrenal Y1 cells, the involvement of PKA was shown to account for up to 60% of the effects of ACTH on transcription, while only 6% could be assigned to PKC (70). This study clearly validated the dominant role of PKA in steroidogenesis, but left about 34% of the ACTH effects to be independent of PKA and PKC. In addition, another study had pointed to the importance of cAMP signaling, mediated independently of PKA, for aldosterone production in the adrenal zona glomerulosa (75). These findings suggest a role for EPAC in the regulation of adrenal function. The specific expression of the EPAC2B isoform in steroidogenic cells (19, 21) also points to roles for EPAC-dependent signaling in these cells. We, therefore, systematically assessed the involvement of PKA versus EPAC in steroidogenesis using cell permeable cAMP analogs specific for PKA and EPAC1/2 (N6-benzoyl-cAMP and 8-p-chlorophenylthio-2-O-methyl-cAMP) in adrenocortical cell lines (21). Our study demonstrated that PKA, and not EPAC2B, is the essential cAMP-induced regulator of factors involved in steroid hormone production (such as StAR, CYP11A1, and CYP17) as well as for the biosynthesis of cortisol and aldosterone. The role of EPAC2 was also studied in bovine zona fasciculata, expressing high levels of EPAC2 mRNA (76), using the same EPAC-specific cAMP analog (77). Although this analog induced cortisol biosynthesis, a non-hydrolyzable EPAC activator had no effect. The study concluded that metabolites of the hydrolyzable EPAC-specific analog induced the increase in cortisol observed in a cAMP-independent manner. Although seemingly opposite results were obtained with the same EPAC activating compound, these two studies indicate that EPAC is not important for cortisol production. cAMP rapidly induces the transcription factor nerve growth factor-induced clone B (NGFI-B), a regulator of several steroid hydroxylase genes (78–80). In adrenocortical cells in culture, we also found that NGFI-B-induction by cAMP is mediated by PKA and not by EPAC (21). Current investigations on HPA axis regulation in mouse knockout models will provide insights into the potential roles for EPAC1/2 in this neuroendocrine system.

EPAC2B Contributes to Cytoskeletal Remodeling in the Adrenal Cortex

In adrenocortical cells in culture, cAMP characteristically induces changes in cell shape and a concomitant reorganization of F-actin microfilaments [reviewed in Ref. (81)]. Furthermore, cytoskeletal reorganization has been shown to contribute to steroidogenic hormone production by allowing the correct positioning of lipid droplets, the ER and mitochondria where cholesterol and its metabolites are transported and metabolized (82–84). While using PKA- and EPAC-specific agonists to study their effect on steroidogenesis in adrenocortical cell lines, we observed that the activation of both cAMP effectors contributed to cell rounding and the reorganization of F-actin fibers (21). Considering that PKA activation contributes to the regulation and expression of many enzymes necessary for steroidogenesis, the additional effect mediated by PKA on F-actin remodeling would, hence, correlate well with enzymatic outputs. By contrast, the effects of EPAC on F-actin remodeling are not correlated to steroidogenesis and may, therefore, contribute to other aspects of adrenal physiology. In line with this, we also found that activation of EPAC2B induced a marked decrease in migration (21). This finding implies that EPAC2B plays a role in cell motility and this suggests wider implications, such as adrenal cancer cell invasion. Although EPAC2 has so far not been implicated in cancer development, several studies have demonstrated roles, albeit contradictory, for EPAC1 in cell migration and metastasis (85). The molecular mechanisms implicated include, at least, an increase of Ca^{2+} release mediated by PLC-IP3 promoting actin remodelling and cell migration of melanoma cells (86) as well as integrin activation important for cell migration and metastasis of pancreatic cancer cells (87). EPAC2B may, hence, act in the same way as EPAC1 in the adrenal gland.

CONCLUSION

Since the discovery of EPACs in 1998, our understanding of cAMP-induced signaling and its roles in physiological processes has changed dramatically. Important initial *in vitro* studies on EPAC paved the way for current phenotypic analyses of genetic mouse models lacking EPAC in single or double knockouts. Based on these gene knockout models an important picture has emerged, namely that although deletion of EPAC does not cause gross defects in mice kept at standard protected conditions in the animal facility, exposure to stressful situations provoke significant phenotypes. EPAC2 is expressed along the HPA axis, and it is interesting to note that whereas the hypothalamus and pituitary specifically express EPAC2A, the adrenal cortex expresses solely the EPAC2B isoform. While EPAC has been shown to mediate potential roles in the hypothalamus, putative functions in the PVN are yet to be determined. At the hypophyseal level, EPAC2A has been implicated in the regulation of POMC expression, and in the adrenal cortex, EPAC2B affects the migration of adrenocortical cells in culture. The generation of spatial and temporal conditional gene knockout models is now required to pinpoint the specific roles of the different EPAC isoforms during development and adult life. Moreover, the ongoing efforts to develop isoform-specific agonists and antagonists hold great promise for insights into isoform-specific functions. Such compounds will also be important potential new drugs to treat diseases in which EPAC plays a role. Several studies do indeed suggest that EPACs are promising drug targets (88), giving hope that small molecules targeting EPACs will serve as useful treatments in the future.

AUTHOR CONTRIBUTIONS

AEL, RA, and MB wrote parts of the manuscript. AL coordinated editing.

REFERENCES

1. Hauger RL, Risbrough V, Oakley RH, Olivares-Reyes JA, Dautzenberg FM. Role of CRF receptor signaling in stress vulnerability, anxiety, and depression. *Ann N Y Acad Sci* (2009) 1179:120–43. doi:10.1111/j.1749-6632.2009.05011.x
2. Stojilkovic SS, Tabak J, Bertram R. Ion channels and signaling in the pituitary gland. *Endocr Rev* (2010) 31:845–915. doi:10.1210/er.2010-0005
3. Smith AI, Funder JW. Proopiomelanocortin processing in the pituitary, central nervous system, and peripheral tissues. *Endocr Rev* (1988) 9:159–79. doi:10.1210/edrv-9-1-159
4. Gallo-Payet N. Adrenal and extra-adrenal functions of ACTH. *J Mol Endocrinol* (2016). doi:10.1530/JME-15-0257
5. Payne AH, Hales DB. Overview of steroidogenic enzymes in the pathway from cholesterol to active steroid hormones. *Endocr Rev* (2004) 25:947–70. doi:10.1210/er.2003-0030
6. Kraemer FB, Shen WJ. Hormone-sensitive lipase: control of intracellular tri-(di-)acylglycerol and cholesteryl ester hydrolysis. *J Lipid Res* (2002) 43:1585–94. doi:10.1194/jlr.R200009-JLR200
7. Ishimura K, Fujita H. Light and electron microscopic immunohistochemistry of the localization of adrenal steroidogenic enzymes. *Microsc Res Tech* (1997) 36:445–53. doi:10.1002/(SICI)1097-0029(19970315)36:6<445::AID-JEMT2>3.0.CO;2-H
8. Miller WL, Bose HS. Early steps in steroidogenesis: intracellular cholesterol trafficking. *J Lipid Res* (2011) 52:2111–35. doi:10.1194/jlr.R016675
9. de Rooij J, Zwartkruis FJ, Verheijen MH, Cool RH, Nijman SM, Wittinghofer A, et al. Epac is a Rap1 guanine-nucleotide-exchange factor directly activated by cyclic AMP. *Nature* (1998) 396:474–7. doi:10.1038/24884
10. de Rooij J, Rehmann H, van Triest M, Cool RH, Wittinghofer A, Bos JL. Mechanism of regulation of the Epac family of cAMP-dependent RapGEFs. *J Biol Chem* (2000) 275:20829–36. doi:10.1074/jbc.M001113200
11. Kawasaki H, Springett GM, Mochizuki N, Toki S, Nakaya M, Matsuda M, et al. A family of cAMP-binding proteins that directly activate Rap1. *Science* (1998) 282:2275–9. doi:10.1126/science.282.5397.2275
12. Almahariq M, Mei FC, Cheng X. Cyclic AMP sensor EPAC proteins and energy homeostasis. *Trends Endocrinol Metab* (2014) 25:60–71. doi:10.1016/j.tem.2013.10.004
13. Banerjee U, Cheng X. Exchange protein directly activated by cAMP encoded by the mammalian rapgef3 gene: structure, function and therapeutics. *Gene* (2015) 570:157–67. doi:10.1016/j.gene.2015.06.063
14. Sugawara K, Shibasaki T, Takahashi H, Seino S. Structure and functional roles of Epac2 (Rapgef4). *Gene* (2016) 575:577–83. doi:10.1016/j.gene.2015.09.029
15. Tiwari S, Felekkis K, Moon EY, Flies A, Sherr DH, Lerner A. Among circulating hematopoietic cells, B-CLL uniquely expresses functional EPAC1, but EPAC1-mediated Rap1 activation does not account for PDE4 inhibitor-induced apoptosis. *Blood* (2004) 103:2661–7. doi:10.1182/blood-2003-06-2154
16. Ulucan C, Wang X, Baljinnyam E, Bai Y, Okumura S, Sato M, et al. Developmental changes in gene expression of Epac and its upregulation in myocardial hypertrophy. *Am J Physiol Heart Circ Physiol* (2007) 293:H1662–72. doi:10.1152/ajpheart.00159.2007
17. Ozaki N, Shibasaki T, Kashima Y, Miki T, Takahashi K, Ueno H, et al. cAMP-GEFII is a direct target of cAMP in regulated exocytosis. *Nat Cell Biol* (2000) 2:805–11. doi:10.1038/35041046
18. Ueno H, Shibasaki T, Iwanaga T, Takahashi K, Yokoyama Y, Liu LM, et al. Characterization of the gene EPAC2: structure, chromosomal localization, tissue expression, and identification of the liver-specific isoform. *Genomics* (2001) 78:91–8. doi:10.1006/geno.2001.6641
19. Niimura M, Miki T, Shibasaki T, Fujimoto W, Iwanaga T, Seino S. Critical role of the N-terminal cyclic AMP-binding domain of Epac2 in its subcellular localization and function. *J Cell Physiol* (2009) 219:652–8. doi:10.1002/jcp.21709
20. Hoivik EA, Witsoe SL, Bergheim IR, Xu Y, Jakobsson I, Tengholm A, et al. DNA methylation of alternative promoters directs tissue specific expression of Epac2 isoforms. *PLoS One* (2013) 8:e67925. doi:10.1371/journal.pone.0067925
21. Aumo L, Rusten M, Mellgren G, Bakke M, Lewis AE. Functional roles of protein kinase A (PKA) and exchange protein directly activated by 3',5'-cyclic adenosine 5'-monophosphate (cAMP) 2 (EPAC2) in cAMP-mediated actions in adrenocortical cells. *Endocrinology* (2010) 151:2151–61. doi:10.1210/en.2009-1139
22. Consonni SV, Gloerich M, Spanjaard E, Bos JL. cAMP regulates DEP domain-mediated binding of the guanine nucleotide exchange factor Epac1

to phosphatidic acid at the plasma membrane. *Proc Natl Acad Sci U S A* (2012) 109:3814–9. doi:10.1073/pnas.1117599109

23. Schmidt M, Dekker FJ, Maarsingh H. Exchange protein directly activated by cAMP (epac): a multidomain cAMP mediator in the regulation of diverse biological functions. *Pharmacol Rev* (2013) 65:670–709. doi:10.1124/pr.110.003707
24. Rehmann H, Prakash B, Wolf E, Rueppel A, De Rooij J, Bos JL, et al. Structure and regulation of the cAMP-binding domains of Epac2. *Nat Struct Biol* (2003) 10:26–32. doi:10.1038/nsb878
25. Rehmann H, Arias-Palomo E, Hadders MA, Schwede F, Llorca O, Bos JL. Structure of Epac2 in complex with a cyclic AMP analogue and RAP1B. *Nature* (2008) 455:124–7. doi:10.1038/nature07187
26. Rehmann H, Das J, Knipscheer P, Wittinghofer A, Bos JL. Structure of the cyclic-AMP-responsive exchange factor Epac2 in its auto-inhibited state. *Nature* (2006) 439:625–8. doi:10.1038/nature04468
27. Li Y, Asuri S, Rebhun JF, Castro AF, Paranavitana NC, Quilliam LA. The RAP1 guanine nucleotide exchange factor Epac2 couples cyclic AMP and Ras signals at the plasma membrane. *J Biol Chem* (2006) 281:2506–14. doi:10.1074/jbc.M508165200
28. Liu C, Takahashi M, Li Y, Song S, Dillon TJ, Shinde U, et al. Ras is required for the cyclic AMP-dependent activation of Rap1 via Epac2. *Mol Cell Biol* (2008) 28:7109–25. doi:10.1128/MCB.01060-08
29. Grandoch M, Roscioni SS, Schmidt M. The role of Epac proteins, novel cAMP mediators, in the regulation of immune, lung and neuronal function. *Br J Pharmacol* (2010) 159:265–84. doi:10.1111/j.1476-5381.2009.00458.x
30. Rangarajan S, Enserink JM, Kuiperij HB, de Rooij J, Price LS, Schwede F, et al. Cyclic AMP induces integrin-mediated cell adhesion through Epac and Rap1 upon stimulation of the beta 2-adrenergic receptor. *J Cell Biol* (2003) 160:487–93. doi:10.1083/jcb.200209105
31. Bos JL. Epac: a new cAMP target and new avenues in cAMP research. *Nat Rev Mol Cell Biol* (2003) 4:733–8. doi:10.1038/nrm1197
32. Fukuhara S, Sakurai A, Sano H, Yamagishi A, Somekawa S, Takakura N, et al. Cyclic AMP potentiates vascular endothelial cadherin-mediated cell-cell contact to enhance endothelial barrier function through an Epac-Rap1 signaling pathway. *Mol Cell Biol* (2005) 25:136–46. doi:10.1128/MCB.25.1.136-146.2005
33. Lorenowicz MJ, Fernandez-Borja M, Kooistra MR, Bos JL, Hordijk PL. PKA and Epac1 regulate endothelial integrity and migration through parallel and independent pathways. *Eur J Cell Biol* (2008) 87:779–92. doi:10.1016/j.ejcb.2008.05.004
34. Aivatiadou E, Ripolone M, Brunetti F, Berruti G. cAMP-Epac2-mediated activation of Rap1 in developing male germ cells: RA-RhoGAP as a possible direct down-stream effector. *Mol Reprod Dev* (2009) 76:407–16. doi:10.1002/mrd.20963
35. Hochbaum D, Hong K, Barila G, Ribeiro-Neto F, Altschuler DL. Epac, in synergy with cAMP-dependent protein kinase (PKA), is required for cAMP-mediated mitogenesis. *J Biol Chem* (2008) 283:4464–8. doi:10.1074/jbc.C700171200
36. Bryn T, Mahic M, Enserink JM, Schwede F, Aandahl EM, Tasken K. The cyclic AMP-Epac1-Rap1 pathway is dissociated from regulation of effector functions in monocytes but acquires immunoregulatory function in mature macrophages. *J Immunol* (2006) 176:7361–70. doi:10.4049/jimmunol.176.12.7361
37. Petersen RK, Madsen L, Pedersen LM, Hallenborg P, Hagland H, Viste K, et al. Cyclic AMP (cAMP)-mediated stimulation of adipocyte differentiation requires the synergistic action of Epac- and cAMP-dependent protein kinase-dependent processes. *Mol Cell Biol* (2008) 28:3804–16. doi:10.1128/MCB.00709-07
38. Cullen K, McCool J, Anwer MS, Webster CR. Activation of cAMP-guanine exchange factor (cAMP-GEF) confers protein kinase A independent protection from hepatocyte apoptosis. *Am J Physiol Gastrointest Liver Physiol* (2004) 2:G334–43. doi:10.1152/ajpgi.00517.2003
39. Honegger KJ, Capuano P, Winter C, Bacic D, Stange G, Wagner CA, et al. Regulation of sodium-proton exchanger isoform 3 (NHE3) by PKA and exchange protein directly activated by cAMP (EPAC). *Proc Natl Acad Sci U S A* (2006) 103:803–8. doi:10.1073/pnas.0503562103
40. Tengholm A. Cyclic AMP dynamics in the pancreatic beta-cell. *Ups J Med Sci* (2012) 117:355–69. doi:10.3109/03009734.2012.724732
41. Zhang CL, Katoh M, Shibasaki T, Minami K, Sunaga Y, Takahashi H, et al. The cAMP sensor Epac2 is a direct target of antidiabetic sulfonylurea drugs. *Science* (2009) 325:607–10. doi:10.1126/science.1172256
42. Kang G, Chepurny OG, Malester B, Rindler MJ, Rehmann H, Bos JL, et al. cAMP sensor Epac as a determinant of ATP-sensitive potassium channel activity in human pancreatic beta cells and rat INS-1 cells. *J Physiol* (2006) 573:595–609. doi:10.1113/jphysiol.2006.107391
43. Morel E, Marcantoni A, Gastineau M, Birkedal R, Rochais F, Garnier A, et al. cAMP-binding protein Epac induces cardiomyocyte hypertrophy. *Circ Res* (2005) 97:1296–304. doi:10.1161/01.RES.0000194325.31359.86
44. Shibasaki T, Takahashi H, Miki T, Sunaga Y, Matsumura K, Yamanaka M, et al. Essential role of Epac2/Rap1 signaling in regulation of insulin granule dynamics by cAMP. *Proc Natl Acad Sci U S A* (2007) 104:19333–8. doi:10.1073/pnas.0707054104
45. Kai AK, Lam AK, Chen Y, Tai AC, Zhang X, Lai AK, et al. Exchange protein activated by cAMP 1 (Epac1)-deficient mice develop beta-cell dysfunction and metabolic syndrome. *FASEB J* (2013) 27:4122–35. doi:10.1096/fj.13-230433
46. Song WJ, Mondal P, Li Y, Lee SE, Hussain MA. Pancreatic beta-cell response to increased metabolic demand and to pharmacologic secretagogues requires EPAC2A. *Diabetes* (2013) 62:2796–807. doi:10.2337/db12-1394
47. Yang Y, Shu X, Liu D, Shang Y, Wu Y, Pei L, et al. Impairs learning and social interactions via aberrant regulation of miR-124 and Zif268 translation. *Neuron* (2012) 73:774–88. doi:10.1016/j.neuron.2012.02.003
48. Srivastava DP, Jones KA, Woolfrey KM, Burgdorf J, Russell TA, Kalmbach A, et al. Social, communication, and cortical structural impairments in Epac2-deficient mice. *J Neurosci* (2012) 32:11864–11878.
49. Ostroveanu A, van der Zee EA, Eisel UL, Schmidt M, Nijholt IM. Exchange protein activated by cyclic AMP 2 (Epac2) plays a specific and time-limited role in memory retrieval. *Hippocampus* (2010) 20:1018–26. doi:10.1002/hipo.20700
50. Bacchelli E, Blasi F, Biondolillo M, Lamb JA, Bonora E, Barnby G, et al. Screening of nine candidate genes for autism on chromosome 2q reveals rare nonsynonymous variants in the cAMP-GEFII gene. *Mol Psychiatry* (2003) 8:916–24. doi:10.1038/sj.mp.4001340
51. Woolfrey KM, Srivastava DP, Photowala H, Yamashita M, Barbolina MV, Cahill ME, et al. Epac2 induces synapse remodeling and depression and its disease-associated forms alter spines. *Nat Neurosci* (2009) 12:1275–84. doi:10.1038/nn.2386
52. Penzes P, Woolfrey KM, Srivastava DP. Epac2-mediated dendritic spine remodeling: implications for disease. *Mol Cell Neurosci* (2011) 46:368–80. doi:10.1016/j.mcn.2010.11.008
53. Okumura S, Fujita T, Cai W, Jin M, Namekata I, Mototani Y, et al. Epac1-dependent phospholamban phosphorylation mediates the cardiac response to stresses. *J Clin Invest* (2014) 124:2785–801. doi:10.1172/JCI64784
54. Pereira L, Cheng H, Lao DH, Na L, van Oort RJ, Brown JH, et al. Epac2 mediates cardiac beta1-adrenergic-dependent sarcoplasmic reticulum Ca2+ leak and arrhythmia. *Circulation* (2013) 127:913–22. doi:10.1161/CIRCULATIONAHA.12.148619
55. Zhang B, Nweze I, Lakshmanan J, Harbrecht BG. Activation of a cyclic amp-guanine exchange factor in hepatocytes decreases nitric oxide synthase expression. *Shock* (2013) 39:70–6. doi:10.1097/SHK.0b013e3182760530
56. Fu D, Wakabayashi Y, Lippincott-Schwartz J, Arias IM. Bile acid stimulates hepatocyte polarization through a cAMP-Epac-MEK-LKB1-AMPK pathway. *Proc Natl Acad Sci U S A* (2011) 108:1403–8. doi:10.1073/pnas.1018376108
57. Kageyama K, Tamasawa N, Suda T. Signal transduction in the hypothalamic corticotropin-releasing factor system and its clinical implications. *Stress* (2011) 14:357–67. doi:10.3109/10253890.2010.536279
58. Kageyama K, Suda T. Regulatory mechanisms underlying corticotropin-releasing factor gene expression in the hypothalamus. *Endocr J* (2009) 56:335–44. doi:10.1507/endocrj.K09E-075
59. Agarwal A, Halvorson LM, Legradi G. Pituitary adenylate cyclase-activating polypeptide (PACAP) mimics neuroendocrine and behavioral manifestations of stress: evidence for PKA-mediated expression of the corticotropin-releasing hormone (CRH) gene. *Brain Res Mol Brain Res* (2005) 138:45–57. doi:10.1016/j.molbrainres.2005.03.016
60. Ster J, de Bock F, Bertaso F, Abitbol K, Daniel H, Bockaert J, et al. Epac mediates PACAP-dependent long-term depression in the hippocampus. *J Physiol* (2009) 587:101–13. doi:10.1113/jphysiol.2008.157461
61. Fukuda M, Williams KW, Gautron L, Elmquist JK. Induction of leptin resistance by activation of cAMP-Epac signaling. *Cell Metab* (2011) 13:331–9. doi:10.1016/j.cmet.2011.01.016

62. O'Neill JS, Maywood ES, Chesham JE, Takahashi JS, Hastings MH. cAMP-dependent signaling as a core component of the mammalian circadian pacemaker. *Science* (2008) 320:949–53. doi:10.1126/science.1152506
63. Traver S, Marien M, Martin E, Hirsch EC, Michel PP. The phenotypic differentiation of locus ceruleus noradrenergic neurons mediated by brain-derived neurotrophic factor is enhanced by corticotropin releasing factor through the activation of a cAMP-dependent signaling pathway. *Mol Pharmacol* (2006) 70:30–40. doi:10.1124/mol.106.022715
64. Dunn AJ, Swiergiel AH. The role of corticotropin-releasing factor and noradrenaline in stress-related responses, and the inter-relationships between the two systems. *Eur J Pharmacol* (2008) 583:186–93. doi:10.1016/j.ejphar.2007.11.069
65. Van Kolen K, Dautzenberg FM, Verstraeten K, Royaux I, De Hoogt R, Gutknecht E, et al. Corticotropin releasing factor-induced ERK phosphorylation in AtT20 cells occurs via a cAMP-dependent mechanism requiring EPAC2. *Neuropharmacology* (2010) 58:135–44. doi:10.1016/j.neuropharm.2009.06.022
66. Markovic D, Punn A, Lehnert H, Grammatopoulos DK. Molecular determinants and feedback circuits regulating type 2 CRH receptor signal integration. *Biochim Biophys Acta* (2011) 1813:896–907. doi:10.1016/j.bbamcr.2011.02.005
67. Kovalovsky D, Refojo D, Liberman AC, Hochbaum D, Pereda MP, Coso OA, et al. Activation and induction of NUR77/NURR1 in corticotrophs by CRH/cAMP: involvement of calcium, protein kinase A, and MAPK pathways. *Mol Endocrinol* (2002) 16:1638–51. doi:10.1210/mend.16.7.0863
68. Gutknecht E, Van der Linden I, Van Kolen K, Verhoeven KF, Vauquelin G, Dautzenberg FM. Molecular mechanisms of corticotropin-releasing factor receptor-induced calcium signaling. *Mol Pharmacol* (2009) 75:648–57. doi:10.1124/mol.108.050427
69. Clark BJ, Ranganathan V, Combs R. Post-translational regulation of steroidogenic acute regulatory protein by cAMP-dependent protein kinase A. *Endocr Res* (2000) 26:681–9. doi:10.3109/07435800009048587
70. Schimmer BP, Cordova M, Cheng H, Tsao A, Goryachev AB, Schimmer AD, et al. Global profiles of gene expression induced by adrenocorticotropin in Y1 mouse adrenal cells. *Endocrinology* (2006) 147:2357–67. doi:10.1210/en.2005-1526
71. Aesoy R, Mellgren G, Morohashi K, Lund J. Activation of cAMP-dependent protein kinase increases the protein level of steroidogenic factor-1. *Endocrinology* (2002) 143:295–303. doi:10.1210/en.143.1.295
72. Stocco DM. The role of the StAR protein in steroidogenesis: challenges for the future. *J Endocrinol* (2000) 164:247–53. doi:10.1677/joe.0.1640247
73. Sewer MB, Waterman MR. ACTH modulation of transcription factors responsible for steroid hydroxylase gene expression in the adrenal cortex. *Microsc Res Tech* (2003) 61:300–7. doi:10.1002/jemt.10339
74. Sewer MB, Waterman MR. Adrenocorticotropin/cyclic adenosine 3',5'-monophosphate-mediated transcription of the human CYP17 gene in the adrenal cortex is dependent on phosphatase activity. *Endocrinology* (2002) 143:1769–77. doi:10.1210/endo.143.5.8820
75. Gambaryan S, Butt E, Tas P, Smolenski A, Allolio B, Walter U. Regulation of aldosterone production from zona glomerulosa cells by ANG II and cAMP: evidence for PKA-independent activation of CaMK by cAMP. *Am J Physiol Endocrinol Metab* (2006) 290:E423–33. doi:10.1152/ajpendo.00128.2005
76. Liu H, Enyeart JA, Enyeart JJ. ACTH inhibits bTREK-1 K+ channels through multiple cAMP-dependent signaling pathways. *J Gen Physiol* (2008) 132:279–94. doi:10.1085/jgp.200810003
77. Enyeart JA, Enyeart JJ. Metabolites of an Epac-selective cAMP analog induce cortisol synthesis by adrenocortical cells through a cAMP-independent pathway. *PLoS One* (2009) 4:e6088. doi:10.1371/journal.pone.0006088
78. Bassett MH, Suzuki T, Sasano H, De Vries CJ, Jimenez PT, Carr BR, et al. The orphan nuclear receptor NGFIB regulates transcription of 3beta-hydroxysteroid dehydrogenase. implications for the control of adrenal functional zonation. *J Biol Chem* (2004) 279:37622–30. doi:10.1074/jbc.M405431200
79. Wilson TE, Mouw AR, Weaver CA, Milbrandt J, Parker KL. The orphan nuclear receptor NGFI-B regulates expression of the gene encoding steroid 21-hydroxylase. *Mol Cell Biol* (1993) 13:861–8. doi:10.1128/MCB.13.2.861
80. Zhang P, Mellon SH. Multiple orphan nuclear receptors converge to regulate rat P450c17 gene transcription: novel mechanisms for orphan nuclear receptor action. *Mol Endocrinol* (1997) 11:891–904. doi:10.1210/mend.11.7.9940
81. Gallo-Payet N, Payet MD. Mechanism of action of ACTH: beyond cAMP. *Microsc Res Tech* (2003) 61:275–87. doi:10.1002/jemt.10337
82. Sewer MB, Li D. Regulation of steroid hormone biosynthesis by the cytoskeleton. *Lipids* (2008) 43:1109–15. doi:10.1007/s11745-008-3221-2
83. Sewer MB, Li D. Regulation of adrenocortical steroid hormone production by RhoA-diaphanous 1 signaling and the cytoskeleton. *Mol Cell Endocrinol* (2013) 371:79–86. doi:10.1016/j.mce.2012.11.014
84. Issop L, Rone MB, Papadopoulos V. Organelle plasticity and interactions in cholesterol transport and steroid biosynthesis. *Mol Cell Endocrinol* (2013) 371:34–46. doi:10.1016/j.mce.2012.12.003
85. Almahariq M, Mei FC, Cheng X. The pleiotropic role of exchange protein directly activated by cAMP 1 (EPAC1) in cancer: implications for therapeutic intervention. *Acta Biochim Biophys Sin (Shanghai)* (2016) 48:75–81. doi:10.1093/abbs/gmv115
86. Baljinnyam E, De Lorenzo MS, Xie LH, Iwatsubo M, Chen S, Goydos JS, et al. Exchange protein directly activated by cyclic AMP increases melanoma cell migration by a Ca2+-dependent mechanism. *Cancer Res* (2010) 70:5607–17. doi:10.1158/0008-5472.CAN-10-0056
87. Almahariq M, Chao C, Mei FC, Hellmich MR, Patrikeev I, Motamedi M, et al. Pharmacological inhibition and genetic knockdown of exchange protein directly activated by cAMP 1 reduce pancreatic cancer metastasis in vivo. *Mol Pharmacol* (2015) 87:142–9. doi:10.1124/mol.114.095158
88. Parnell E, Palmer TM, Yarwood SJ. The future of EPAC-targeted therapies: agonism versus antagonism. *Trends Pharmacol Sci* (2015) 36:203–14. doi:10.1016/j.tips.2015.02.003

16

T-Type Calcium Channel: A Privileged Gate for Calcium Entry and Control of Adrenal Steroidogenesis

Michel F. Rossier[1,2]*

[1] *Service of Clinical Chemistry and Toxicology, Hospital of Valais, Sion, Switzerland,* [2] *Department of Human Protein Science, Faculty of Medicine, University of Geneva, Geneva, Switzerland*

***Correspondence:**
Michel F. Rossier
michel.rossier@hopitalvs.ch

Intracellular calcium plays a crucial role in modulating a variety of functions such as muscle contraction, hormone secretion, gene expression, or cell growth. Calcium signaling has been however shown to be more complex than initially thought. Indeed, it is confined within cell microdomains, and different calcium channels are associated with different functions, as shown by various channelopathies. Sporadic mutations on voltage-operated L-type calcium channels in adrenal glomerulosa cells have been shown recently to be the second most prevalent genetic abnormalities present in human aldosterone-producing adenoma. The observed modification of the threshold of activation of the mutated channels not only provides an explanation for this gain of function but also reminds us on the importance of maintaining adequate electrophysiological characteristics to make channels able to exert specific cellular functions. Indeed, the contribution to steroid production of the various calcium channels expressed in adrenocortical cells is not equal, and the reason has been investigated for a long time. Given the very negative resting potential of these cells, and the small membrane depolarization induced by their physiological agonists, low threshold T-type calcium channels are particularly well suited for responding under these conditions and conveying calcium into the cell, at the right place for controlling steroidogenesis. In contrast, high threshold L-type channels are normally activated by much stronger cell depolarizations. The fact that dihydropyridine calcium antagonists, specific for L-type channels, are poorly efficient for reducing aldosterone secretion either *in vivo* or *in vitro*, strongly supports the view that these two types of channels differently affect steroid biosynthesis. Whether a similar analysis is transposable to fasciculata cells and cortisol secretion is one of the questions addressed in the present review. No similar mutations on L-type or T-type channels have been described yet to affect cortisol secretion or to be linked to the development of Cushing syndrome, but several evidences suggest that the function of T channels is also crucial in fasciculata cells. Putative molecular mechanisms and cellular structural organization making T channels a privileged entry for the "steroidogenic calcium" are also discussed.

Keywords: adrenal cortex, steroidogenesis, aldosterone, cortisol, ACTH, calcium signaling, electrophysiology, T-type calcium channels

---

Abbreviations: APA, aldosterone-producing adenoma; BK, broad conductance calcium-activated potassium channel; CPA, cortisol-producing adenoma; I_0, maximal current; I_{stst}, steady-state current; ISH, *in situ* hybridization; PA, primary aldosteronism; PMA, phorbol 12 myristate 13-acetate ester; SK, small conductance calcium-activated potassium channel; StAR, steroidogenic acute regulatory protein; ZF, zona fasciculata; ZG, zona glomerulosa.

INTRODUCTION

Voltage-operated calcium channels play a crucial role in signal transduction of many excitable and non-excitable cell types (1). While a rapid modulation of their activity by hormone-stimulated kinases and/or G proteins has been recognized for a long time (2, 3), a control of their expression levels in the cell has been also described (4).

Among these channels, low threshold-activated, T-type (for transient and tiny current) calcium channels appear distinct concerning their electrophysiological and molecular properties. Although their existence has been shown early by studies of their voltage-dependence, kinetics, and single channel conductance (5–7), their cloning and their molecular characterization has been delayed, in part because of a lack of specific pharmacological tools and because they share less structural homology with the rest of the voltage-operated calcium channels. Thus, in the light of their molecular structure (8, 9), T-type calcium channels have been proposed to play specific physiological roles within the cells, and it has been suggested that they could be involved, depending on the levels of their expression, in the development of several diseases, such as hypertension, cardiac failure, epilepsy, or cancer (4).

Electrophysiological Properties of T-Type Calcium Channels

An important and discriminating property of T channels is their ability to activate upon small depolarization of the membrane, allowing a surge of calcium entry into excitable cells at the beginning of an action potential (when the electrochemical gradient is highly favorable for cation entry), as well as in only slightly depolarized non-excitable cells, like isolated adrenal cortex steroidogenic cells. Their rapid, voltage-dependent inactivation and their slow deactivation (**Figure 1A**) make their gating characteristics distinct from those of other channels. This feature not only allows isolating specifically the corresponding currents thanks to defined voltage patch clamp protocols but also is responsible for the specific role played by these channels in the modulation of cardiac and neuronal cell excitability (10, 11). In cells devoid of action potential, such as isolated adrenal glomerulosa cells in culture, a sustained calcium entry within a permissive window of voltage is possible thanks to a significant overlap between the activation and inactivation potential ranges of the channel (12).

Indeed, voltage-operated calcium channels are classically characterized by their activation curve, reflecting the probability of channel opening at various membrane potentials (and, therefore, the proportion of channels activating at each voltage), and their steady-state inactivation curve, showing the proportion of channels remaining available (not inactivated) at different voltages (**Figure 1B**). These curves are produced experimentally by measuring currents under specific protocols, normalizing them and mathematically fitting data to Boltzmann's equation. Examination of these curves reveals, for each type of channel, the presence of a *permissive window of voltage*, in which activation and inactivation overlap. A *sustained* flux of calcium through the channels is theoretically possible in this window, where a significant proportion of channels are already activated but not yet completely inactivated. This window delimits the range of voltages over which a steady-state current can flow through the channels, and the relative amplitude of this current can be calculated as a function of voltage using Ohm's law (15). It is important to realize at this point that, because only a small fraction of channels is open at any time in this mode (upon slight membrane depolarization), the current amplitude is tiny as compared to the maximal current observed within the same cell when all channels open together during a putative action potential or upon a strong depolarization. However, because the channel activation is *sustained* for minutes (due to lack of complete inactivation), calcium accumulated within the cell during this period is huge in comparison to the amount entering during a single action potential that leads the cell to voltages less favorable for calcium influx.

Low threshold T-type calcium channels activate (and inactivate) at lower voltages than high-threshold L-type calcium channels, and, as a consequence, also present their permissive window at lower voltages. In fact, any channel modification (through phosphorylation, binding of G protein or genetic mutation) affecting its activation and/or inactivation curves will result in a marked change of the properties of the steady state current. Indeed, not only the position of the window will be shifted under these conditions but also the maximal amplitude of the steady-state current, which depends on both the extent of the overlap of the activation and inactivation curves and on the electrochemical gradient for calcium entry.

The resting potential of glomerulosa cells from different species has been measured to be between −86 and −73 mV (16–19), values that are at the left edge of the T channel window (see **Figure 1B**, right panel), but farther from that of L-type channel. Values reported for fasciculata cells are between −76 and −66 mV (16, 20, 21), showing that fasciculata cells are slightly depolarized (by 8–10 mV) as compared to glomerulosa cells under resting conditions. Moreover, depolarization of the cells by *physiological concentrations* of agonists like AngII, ACTH, or potassium (see below) has been determined to be maximally 10–20 mV (18–20, 22), which is sufficient for increasing the steady-state current through T channels by several folds. Increasing extracellular potassium, progressively from low to supra-physiological concentrations, has been shown to increase aldosterone secretion in parallel to the size of the predicted T-channel steady-state calcium current (12).

Whether adrenal cortical cells are naturally excitable (i.e., able to generate action potentials) has been debated. Indeed, when cell to cell contacts are preserved, several authors observed low frequency action potentials in both resting and stimulated glomerulosa and fasciculata cells. *Isolated* glomerulosa cells have been conventionally considered as non-excitable because their membrane potential rests close to the equilibrium potential for potassium (16) and remains negative to −60 mV upon stimulation with AngII or physiological concentrations of potassium. In contrast, some mouse zona glomerulosa cells *within adrenal slices* spontaneously generate membrane potential oscillations of low periodicity (0.44 Hz), as shown under whole cell current clamp conditions (17). Similar properties of rat, rabbit, and cat glomerulosa, and fasciculata cells had been previously reported

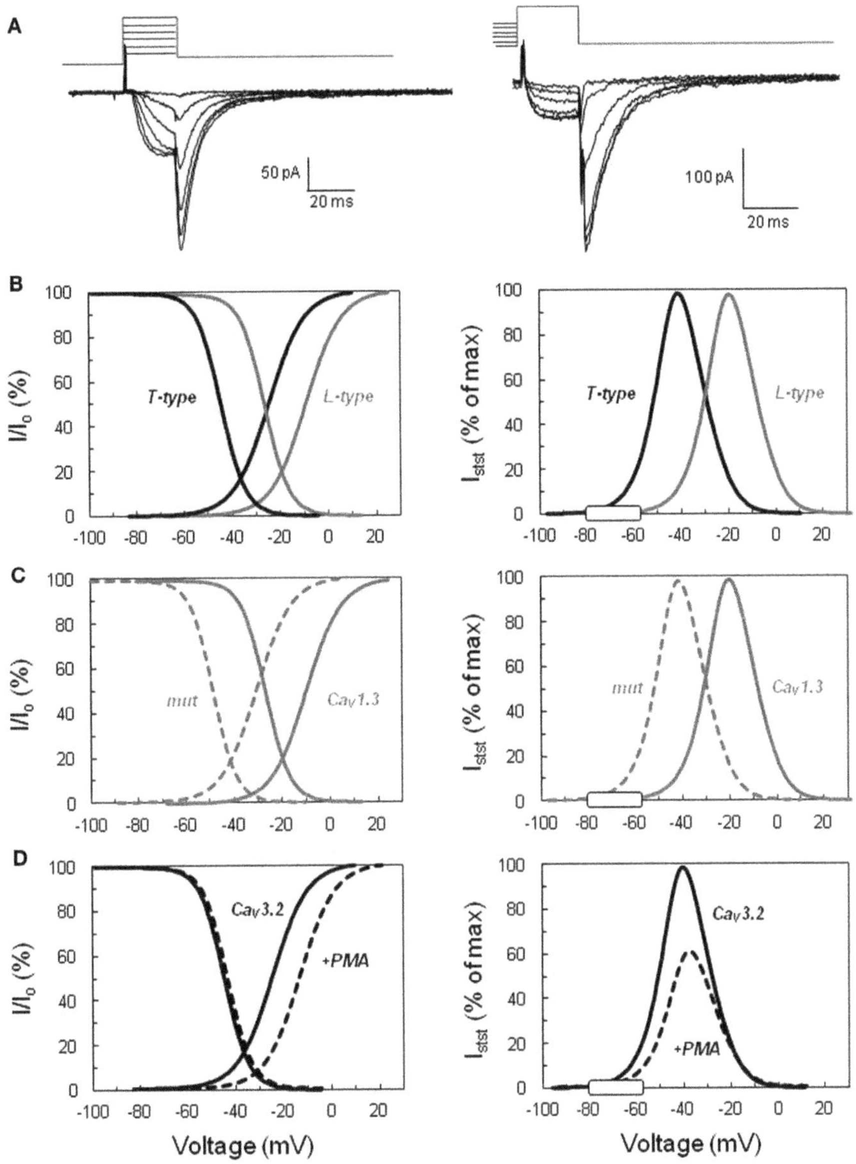

FIGURE 1 | Activation and inactivation of voltage-operated calcium channels and steady-state "window" currents. (A) Examples of slowly deactivating (T-type) Ba^{2+} currents recorded in the whole cell configuration of the patch clamp technique. Left. Voltage protocol for determining the activation curve: tail currents were evoked by repolarizing the cell to −65 mV after a short period (20 ms) of depolarization at various voltages (−45 to +5 mV for this selection of traces) from a holding potential of −90 mV. Right. Voltage protocol for determining the steady-state inactivation curve: tail currents were elicited in the same cell at −65 mV, but after steady-state inactivation of the channels for 10 s at various holding potentials (here from −80 to −30 mV) and 20 ms activation at +20 mV. Current amplitude upon cell repolarization was then determined by fitting tail currents to an exponential function (the time constant was approximately 7 ms). **(B)** Comparison of low (T-type) versus high (L-type) threshold voltage-operated calcium channels. Left panel shows normalized activation and inactivation curves determined for T-type channels using the same type of protocol as shown in panel A. Tail current amplitudes were plotted as a function of the test voltage, fitted to Boltzmann's equation, and normalized to the maximal current (I_0). Curves for L-type channels were similarly defined from L-current amplitudes determined with a different voltage protocol, including the inactivation of T currents. Right panel displays the calculated normalized steady-state current (I_{stst}) expected through T-type and L-type channels within their respective permissive window of voltage. The theoretical steady-state currents were obtained from the activation and inactivation curves according to Ohm's law and expressed as a percentage of the maximal current. The white rectangle on the voltage axis indicates the range of membrane potentials reached in naive glomerulosa cells and in cells stimulated with physiological concentrations of angiotensin II or extracellular potassium. **(C)** Effect of the Ile770Met mutation described in the CACNA1D L-type calcium channel (13) on the channel activation, inactivation, and steady-state current. Curves have been determined as in **(B)** for the wild-type channel (continuous line, Ca$_V$1.3) and for the mutant channel (dotted line, mut) and show the significant shift of the channel permissive window toward lower voltages. **(D)** Effect of PKC activation on CACNA1H T channel activation, inactivation, and steady-state current. Curves have been determined as in **(B)** for the naive channel (continuous line, Ca$_V$3.2) and for the channel in glomerulosa cells treated with the PKC activator phorbol 12 myristate 13-acetate ester (dotted line, +PMA) and show the significant reduction of the amplitude of the maximal steady-state current with the slight shift of the permissive window toward higher voltages. The graphs of this figure have been constructed based on data available in Ref. (14, 13).

(16, 18, 23). Electrical activity has generally to be induced in silent cells by depolarization with secretagogues (AngII, ACTH, or potassium) or by injecting depolarizing current in the current clamp mode (16, 18, 20), which is coherent with thresholds for triggering the action potential observed above −64 mV (17). Spontaneous or evoked voltage oscillations appear insensitive to inhibition by tetrodotoxin or nifedipine, but completely abolished by low nickel concentrations, suggesting that they are supported by calcium currents carried by low threshold T-type calcium channels ($Ca_V3.2$) (17, 20). Moreover, the frequency of the electrical oscillator is regulated positively by potassium and AngII (17), providing an additional way to these agonists for controlling steroid production.

Indeed, the presence of action potentials on top of the mechanism previously described as being responsible for the steady state calcium entry through T-type channels is expected to affect calcium signaling and therefore steroidogenesis. However, the exact role and influence of the spontaneous or evoked action potentials on steroid production (mostly measured experimentally from isolated cells, devoid of action potentials) have not been precisely and specifically quantified yet, probably given the strong relationship existing between this electrical activity and calcium entry. For example, it is not known whether a low but sustained entry of calcium is not more efficient for stimulating and maintaining steroid production than pulsatile peaks of high calcium with intermittent periods of channel inactivation.

Calcium Channel Mutations in Primary Aldosteronism

Aldosterone secretion from adrenal glomerulosa cells is under the control of AngII and extracellular potassium (24, 25), and indirectly regulates blood pressure through stimulation of renal sodium reabsorption. A dysregulation of aldosterone production may lead to systemic hypertension and hypokalemia (26). Adrenal aldosterone-producing adenomas (APA) constitutively produce aldosterone (27) and are a common cause of severe hypertension. About 5–10% of patients referred to hypertension clinics have APA (28, 29), which are typically benign and well circumscribed, and their removal cures or ameliorates hypertension. The principal genetic cause of APA development [present in 40% of these tumors (30)] has been attributed to recurrent mutations in the KCNJ5 potassium channel, affecting its ion selectivity filter and therefore responsible for a sustained depolarization of the glomerulosa cell with the subsequent activation of low voltage-operated calcium channels (31). Other mutations associated to the presence of APA were identified by whole exome sequencing. Somatic mutations affected two members of the P-type ATPase gene family, ATP1A1 (the α1 subunit of the Na/K-ATPase) and ATP2B3 (the plasma membrane calcium ATPase), highlighting again the importance of maintaining a strongly negative resting potential and a low cytosolic calcium concentration in adrenal glomerulosa cells for maintaining a low basal aldosterone production (32).

More recently, one additional gene, coding for a calcium channel, was identified with somatic and germline mutations present in other APA tumors without KCNJ5 mutation (13). CACNA1D encodes the α1 (pore-forming) subunit of $Ca_V1.3$, a high-threshold L-type calcium channel. CACNA1D mutations were identified in 9% of APA and represent the second most frequent cause of the disease (30). In contrast to patients with KCNJ5 mutations who are more frequently females, CACNA1D carriers are mostly males. Paradoxically, APA are generally composed of large cells with the morphological appearance of fasciculata cells (ZF-like cells) but still express markers of glomerulosa cells, including the enzymes required for aldosterone biosynthesis (33). While KCNJ5 mutations were associated with large ZF-like APA, CACNA1D mutations are present in small ZG-like APA, suggesting that the cellular composition influences the adenoma size (32, 34). Whether the resting potential of these cells, expected to be less negative in KCNJ5 mutant APAs (like in fasciculata cells) than in normal glomerulosa or in CACNA1D mutant cells, is involved in the determination of cell size and morphology remains to be demonstrated, which is probably a difficult task given the reported heterogeneity of the lesions.

Mutations identified in CACNA1D and associated with APA were affecting two conserved amino acids of the L-type $Ca_V1.3$ channel, Gly403 and Ile770, both located near the cytosolic end of S6 transmembrane segments in domains I and II (**Figure 2**), regions implicated in channel gating (13). To assess the effect of these mutations on channel function, wild type and mutant channels were expressed in HEK293T cells and their electrophysiological properties investigated with the patch clamp technique. Compared to wt channels, both mutants showed maximum current amplitude at less depolarized potentials, as well as a significant leftward shift (by 20 mV) of their activation and steady-state inactivation curves (**Figure 1C**). As a consequence, the permissive window of the channel is also shifted to more negative voltages, corresponding to membrane potentials reached upon physiological stimulations. In other words, these gain-of-function mutations of the channel, by shifting its threshold of activation, make the $Ca_V1.3$ channel "T-like."

Recently, using whole exome sequencing in subjects with unexplained primary aldosteronism (PA) diagnosed at a young age (<10 years), a new mutation has been identified that affect a T-type calcium channel (CACNA1H). Interestingly, the mutation (M1549V) is located within the S6 segment of domain III (**Figure 2**). Electrophysiology demonstrates that this variant causes a 10 times reduction of the rate of channel inactivation and a modest shift of the activation curve to more hyperpolarized potentials, two effects inferred to produce increased calcium influx and aldosterone hypersecretion (35).

Clearly, these observations highlight the importance of low threshold T-type calcium channels in the control of aldosterone biosynthesis, and they recently reactivated the general interest for a comprehensive understanding of the functional specificity of these channels in steroidogenesis. This review aims at recapitulating the arguments in favor of a privileged functional role for T channels in the control of steroid production, at comparing their involvement in aldosterone and cortisol secretion, and, finally, at discussing whether similar mutations on calcium channels, as observed in PA patients, are susceptible to occur in fasciculata cells and to be responsible of some forms of Cushing syndrome.

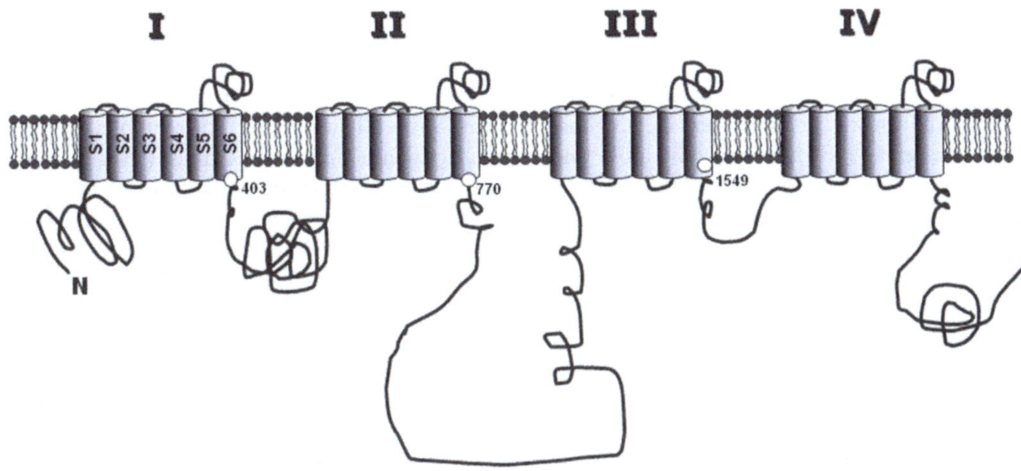

FIGURE 2 | Common structure of the alpha 1 subunit of voltage-operated calcium channels. The main, pore-forming α_1 subunits of the various voltage-operated calcium channels share a common general structure, with four homologous repeats (I–IV), each composed of six hydrophobic, putative membrane-spanning alpha helix domains (S1–S6). The three large loops connecting repeats together, as well as the N- and C-terminal extremities are located in the cytosol. The positions of Gly403 and Ile770 mutated in CACNA1D (13), and of Met1549 in CACNA1H (35), are indicated at the end of the S6 segments in repeats I, II, and III, respectively.

STRUCTURE, EXPRESSION, AND PROPERTIES OF T-TYPE CALCIUM CHANNELS IN ADRENAL CORTEX

Although most studies of low-threshold T-type calcium current expression have focused on the analysis of neuronal and cardiac tissues, the presence of similar currents has been demonstrated throughout the body in both excitable and non-excitable cells, including adrenal glomerulosa (36–44) and fasciculata cells (45–48) from various species.

Three different genes code for the various T channels that are all composed of a single, large α_1 subunit (49). According to the proposed nomenclature of voltage-gated calcium channels (50), α_1G, α_1H, and α_1I T channel isoforms have been renamed $Ca_V3.1$, 3.2, and 3.3, respectively (**Table 1**).

TABLE 1 | Nomenclature of T-type calcium channels.

Channel name	Protein isoform	Gene name
$Ca_V3.1$	α_1G	CACNA1G
$Ca_V3.2$	α_1H	CACNA1H
$Ca_V3.3$	α_1I	CACNA1I

The expression in *Xenopus* oocytes or HEK293 cells of each of the three cloned α_1 subunits coding for T channels generates typical low threshold transient currents with classical properties associated with T channels (51–54). Currents induced by $Ca_V3.1$ and $Ca_V3.2$ channels are nearly identical but can be easily distinguished by the higher sensitivity of $Ca_V3.2$ to inhibition by nickel (55).

As for high threshold calcium channels and sodium channels (56, 57), the α_1 subunits of T channels consist of four homologous repeats (I–IV), each being composed of six transmembrane segments (S1–S6), including a highly conserved pore loop (between S5 and S6) and a distinct voltage sensor (S4) (**Figure 2**). In contrast, more divergence between isoform sequences is found within the large intracellular loops, particularly that linking domains II and III, which also contains a site for alternative splicing in α_1G (58). Interestingly, this variable region of the channel is responsible for the interaction of several calcium channels with specific cell proteins [such as the ryanodine receptor binding to the skeletal muscle L-type channel (59), or syntaxin binding to the neuronal N-type channel (60)], and could therefore participate to the establishment of specific functions for each channel isoform within the cell (see below).

The T channel family presents only 28% sequence identity with other voltage-gated calcium channels, while L ($Ca_V1.x$) and non-L ($Ca_V2.x$) high threshold channel families share more than 50% of their sequence. Replacement of two out of the four glutamate residues generally present in each P (pore-forming) region of the channel by aspartate seems to be responsible for the specific ion selectivity and permeation of T channels (61). Like for other calcium channels, molecular diversity among T channels is increased by alternative splicing of the mRNA of each of the three isotypes, and the properties of some of the 24 putative $Ca_V3.1$ splice variants have been described by several groups (58, 62–64).

Physiological roles for T-type channels have been proposed in several tissues, including pacing of the heart (10), smooth muscle contraction (65), pain neurotransmission (5), fertilization (66), or adrenal steroid biosynthesis (38, 46). The tissue-selective expression of these channels and their isoforms has been determined at the molecular level by Northern blot analysis, *in situ* hybridization (ISH), RT-PCR, as well as by immunohistochemistry (IH) in human and other species. $Ca_V3.1$ has been shown to be expressed predominantly in brain as well as in heart, while $Ca_V3.2$ is mostly found in kidney and liver, but can be also observed in adrenal cortical cells.

The analysis of the expression pattern of the various T channel isoforms revealed that mRNA coding for each of the three α_1 subunits is detectable in the adrenal gland, although in varying quantities. The molecular identity of the channels has been determined more specifically in the adrenal cortex, showing that the predominant subtype expressed in both glomerulosa and fasciculata cells from various species is $Ca_V3.2$ (**Table 2**), a finding in agreement with the high sensitivity to nickel of the T currents recorded in these cells (67). In several studies, a stronger expression of the channel was reported to be present in glomerulosa cells as compare to fasciculata cells (35, 67, 68). Similarly, $Ca_V3.2$ has been found to be the main isoform expressed in the human adrenocortical cell line H295R (69), but $Ca_V3.1$ could be induced in the same cells by changing culture conditions (70).

Indeed, besides short-term modulation of T channels by hormones through the transduction mechanisms described below, a slower and more sustained regulation of channel activity results from the control of the expression of the α_1 subunit. Such a regulation of T channel expression has been observed during the development of various organs, suggesting that these channels could play important roles at specific stages of the fetal life. The density of T channels has been shown to be relatively elevated in H295R cells, a cell line derived from a human adrenocarcinoma, as compared to corresponding normal tissue. This is reminiscent of the many pathological situations where re-expression of fetal genes has been observed during the evolution of oncologic diseases. Interestingly, aldosterone, which is produced by H295R cells, has been shown to significantly increase the T current amplitude, as well as the α_1H transcript levels (69). Because T channels support steroidogenesis in various cells, including H295R cells, this autocrine action of aldosterone on channel expression represents a positive feedback loop that could help tumor cells to maintain differentiated functions like steroidogenesis.

Treatment of isolated rat (47) or bovine (71) fasciculata cells with ACTH for 3–6 days has been shown to induce the expression of CACNA1H mRNA and to markedly increase the amplitude of the T-type calcium currents, a response efficiently blocked by cycloheximide, an inhibitor of protein synthesis. ACTH treatment did not affect L-type current expression in these cells. Interestingly, the putative role of cAMP in this response to ACTH has been challenged by the use of distinct cellular messenger analogs and metabolites mimicking ACTH action without PKA activation (71, 73), and by the fact that ACTH-induced T current up-regulation was not affected by the PKA antagonist H89 (47).

Recently, the relative expression of four distinct calcium channels ($Ca_V1.2$, 1.3, 2.2, and 3.2) has been analyzed at the mRNA and protein levels in human normal adrenal cortex, as well as in aldosterone (APA) and in cortisol-producing adenoma (CPA). While RT-PCR results showed that $Ca_V3.2$ (CACNA1H) was the second most expressed channel in APA (after $Ca_V1.3$), $Ca_V3.2$ was clearly dominant in CPA (68), which is consistent with the prevalence of the T-current in fasciculata cell, as shown by electrophysiological recordings (45, 47). This also suggests a much stronger expression of T channels in CPA than in normal fasciculata cells. Moreover, in APA, only the T subunit $Ca_V3.2$ was positively correlated among patients with individual peripheral blood aldosterone levels (68). In CPA cases, however, this correlation was not observed with cortisol levels.

The electrophysiological properties of endogenous T-type calcium channels have been extensively investigated with the patch clamp technique in rat (19, 47, 74), bovine (15, 45, 74–76), and human (43, 72) glomerulosa and fasciculata cells (**Table 3**), and compared to those of recombinant $Ca_V3.2$ expressed in 293 cells (77). The threshold of current activation, the peak current voltage, and the half-maximal activation and steady-state inactivation ($V_{1/2}$) were all within the range of voltages expected for low threshold T-type calcium channels. In other studies, using slow ramp depolarization, T current activation threshold in rat or bovine glomerulosa cells was determined to be at around −70 mV and that for L-type current at −55 mV (14, 78).

Interestingly, in spite of the fact that the same channel isoform as in glomerulosa cells ($Ca_V3.2$) is apparently expressed in zona fasciculata (71, 72), what has been confirmed by the high sensitivity of the current to inhibition by nickel in these cells, all parameters appear slightly shifted toward more depolarized potentials in fasciculata cells. The reason for this difference is unknown and could be in part related to the selection of the reviewed literature.

The functional relevance of these observations, as previously mentioned, resides in the fact that, in the absence of action potentials and upon limited cell depolarization induced by low physiological concentrations of potassium or AngII, the membrane potential is expected to rapidly reach the region of the T channel permissive window, allowing calcium influx, but not that of L channels. As a consequence, T-type channels appear to be the main contributors to *sustained* calcium influx in response to AngII or physiological concentrations of potassium in glomerulosa cells, because the resting potential of these cells is highly negative, close to the potassium inversion potential (−80 mV), and the agonists do not depolarize the cell enough to reach the threshold of L-type channel activation (**Figure 1B**).

In contrast, it is probable that upon strong cell depolarization induced by supra-physiological concentrations of agonists, or

TABLE 2 | Adrenal cortex expression of T-type calcium channel isotypes.

Cell/tissue	Species	α_1G/CaV3.1	α_1H/CaV3.2
Adrenal zona glomerulosa	Bovine	–	Cloning/ISH (67)
Adrenal zona glomerulosa	Rat	–	ISH (67)
Adrenal zona fasciculata	Bovine		Northern blot (71)
Adrenal zona fasciculata	Human		Northern blot (72)
Adrenal cortex	Human		IH (35, 68)
H295R cells	Human	RT-PCR (70)	RT-PCR (69, 70)

TABLE 3 | Electrophysiological properties of T channels in adrenocortical cells.

	Glomerulosa	Fasciculata	Reference
Threshold of activation (mV)	−80 to −60	−70 to −50	(15, 19, 43, 45, 47, 74–76)
Peak current voltage (mV)	−40 to −30	−30 to −10	(19, 43, 45, 47, 72, 74–76)
Half-maximal activation $V_{1/2}$ (mV)	−47 to −23	−50 to −17	(15, 19, 45, 47, 72, 76)
Half-maximal inactivation $V_{1/2}$ (mV)	−74 to −50	−65 to −43	(15, 19, 45, 47, 72, 74, 76)

under particular conditions, T channels discharge altogether, generating pulses of action potentials able to secondly activate high threshold L-type channels (75). However, the relative contribution to steroidogenesis of calcium entering the cell trough L-type channels in this mode appears quite limited, given the poor efficiency of dihydropyridines or other specific L-type channel calcium antagonists for inhibiting aldosterone or cortisol secretion, *in vivo* or *in vitro* (see below).

PHARMACOLOGICAL DEMONSTRATION OF T-CHANNEL FUNCTION IN STEROIDOGENESIS

Adrenocortical T-type currents have been implicated early in the control of steroid biosynthesis (14, 38, 46, 79, 80), and this specific role for T channels has been extensively reviewed in the literature (12, 24, 81, 82). A direct demonstration of the crucial role played by these channels involved their inhibition by pharmacological agents. However, in spite of strong efforts to develop or isolate highly selective calcium antagonists during the last decades, only a few of the characterized pharmacological compounds appeared to preferentially affect T-type channels. Some of these drugs have been recently tested on heterologously expressed recombinant channels and sometimes display weak channel subtype selectivity. The reported potency (IC_{50}) of these compounds on the various T channel isoforms is indicated in **Table 4**.

Inorganic polyvalent cations were among the first chemicals used to block T-type currents and their efficacy varies depending on the tissue examined, reflecting different channel isoform expression patterns (96). For example, nickel revealed to be useful for discriminating between $Ca_V3.2$ (IC_{50} <15 μM) and $Ca_V3.1$ (IC_{50} >250 μM). In contrast, the relative efficacy of zinc to inhibit T currents in various neuronal tissues (97, 98) suggests that this cation could have a higher affinity for $Ca_V3.1$.

Mibefradil, a derivative of verapamil initially developed as a promising antihypertensive drug (99), and kurtoxin, a purified scorpion toxin (92), have been shown to preferentially inhibit T currents than high voltage-activated currents. Unfortunately, at the same concentrations, mibefradil also attenuates potassium currents (100), and kurtoxin interacts with sodium channels (92), therefore limiting their use for determining endogenous T channel function.

Dihydropyridines are widely used as antihypertensive drugs and are generally considered as specific L-type channel antagonists. However, some of these molecules also efficiently affect T channel activity. Indeed, while all these compounds inhibit L channels with similar potency (with IC_{50} around 0.1 μM), niguldipine and nicardipine are also efficient T channel antagonists, while nimodipine and nifedipine are much more useful for discriminating between L and T currents (101). As expected, dihydropyridine efficacy varies from one cell type to the other (96). Interestingly, while their binding affinity on L channels is clearly voltage-dependent, this dependence is much less pronounced in their interaction with T channels (102), suggesting that the selectivity of these drugs should also vary from one cell type to the other in part because of the difference in their resting potential.

Many other substances, such as succinimide derivatives, phenytoin, pimozide, flunarizine, zonisamide, barbiturates, some anesthetics, and benzodiazepines, employed in clinic essentially for treating neurological or psychiatric disorders, have been shown to also affect T channel activity in non-neuronal cells (96). However, it is noteworthy that none of the above mentioned pharmacological agents is absolutely selective for T-type channels and most of them also affect other types of ionic channels, particularly high threshold calcium channels, when employed at slightly higher concentrations.

The role of T channels in the control of steroidogenesis has been thoroughly investigated by comparing the effects of different classes of calcium antagonists. Aldosterone secretion by adrenal glomerulosa cells, either *in vivo*, or *in vitro* in response to AngII or potassium, is efficiently inhibited by several T channel blockers, like tetrandrine (103, 104), mibefradil (19, 105), zonisamide (14), peripheral-type benzodiazepines (106), nickel (104), efonidipine (107, 108), or nicardipine (109), but not by highly selective L channel antagonists (14, 79, 107, 108). The relative lack of effect *in vivo* of several dihydropyridine antihypertensive drugs on circulating aldosterone concentrations in human has been previously discussed (110). In a recent meta-analysis (111), T channel antagonists appeared more efficient than L channel blockers for reducing aldosterone secretion and improving renal function, but not for decreasing blood pressure.

TABLE 4 | Pharmacology of T-type calcium channel isotypes.

Agent (type/class)	$Ca_V3.1$	$Ca_V3.2$	$Ca_V3.3$	$Ca_V1.x$	Reference
			IC_{50} (μM)		
Nickel (inorganic ion)	250–470	**5.4–13.0**	180–216	>200	(53, 55, 83–86)
Mibefradil (antihypertensive)	**0.12–1.20**	1.0–1.4	1.5	>12	(51, 53, 84, 87–90)
Phenytoin (anticonvulsant)	75–140	8–192	?	>360	(83, 91)
Propofol (anesthetic)	20	27	?		(91)
Pentobarbital (barbiturate)	310	345	?	>600	(91)
Kurtoxin (scorpion toxin)	**0.015**	0.061	?	>10	(92)
Pimozide (neuroleptic)	0.035	0.054	0.030		(93)
Flunarizine (neuroleptic)	**0.53 (K_D)**	3.55 (K_D)	0.84 (K_D)		(93)
Anandamide (cannabinoid)	4.15	**0.33**	1.10		(94)
Amiloride (diuretics)		156–167			(53, 86)
Curcumin (condiment)		20			(95)
TTA-P2 (antinociceptive)		0.35		>3	(75)

Bold indicates the channel isoform with the highest sensitivity to the most discriminant drugs.

An extensive pharmacological characterization of both T-type and L-type channels appears particularly relevant in cases of APA, not only for defining the treatment of hyperaldosteronism but also for diagnostic purposes. Indeed, if the cause of the disease is linked to a mutation on the potassium channel (KCNJ5), leading to sustained cell depolarization and calcium influx through T-type channels, most dihydropyridines will be expected to be quite inefficient for preventing aldosterone hypersecretion. In contrast, if a mutation on the L-type channel subunit α1D (CACNA1D) is causal (see above), and the mutant channel retains the same sensitivity to this class of calcium antagonists as the wild-type channel, the drugs will probably reduce aldosterone secretion. This hypothesis has been recently supported by the observation that a patient identified as affected by a *de novo* germline CACNA1D mutation responded particularly well to treatment with the dihydropyridine amlodipine, which normalized blood pressure and resolved ventricular hypertrophy in this patient (13).

Adrenocorticotropic hormone-induced cortisol secretion from bovine adrenal fasciculata cells has been similarly shown to be inhibited by low nickel concentrations (45). A parallel inhibition of T-type currents in these cells with an IC_{50} of 20 μM strongly suggests that the $Ca_V3.2$ channel isoform is also mostly responsible for the steroidogenic response in fasciculata cells (45, 47). This was confirmed by the observation that mibefradil also inhibited both T-type calcium current and cortisol secretion induced by ACTH in bovine fasciculata cells with IC_{50}'s of 1.0 and 3.5 μM, respectively (76). Curcumin directly modulates the activity of several types of ion channels, including $Ca_V3.2$. In addition to a slight stimulatory effect on cortisol production from naive fasciculata cells, attributed to cell depolarization in response to potassium current inhibition, this compound has been shown to markedly reduce in parallel the large cortisol responses to both ACTH or AngII, and the $Ca_V3.2$ current (95). Similar results were obtained recently with the organic compound TT-P2, a recently developed potent and quite selective antagonist of T-type calcium channels (75).

The relative lack of selectivity of most of these calcium antagonists has been partially circumvented by combining the information collected with several unrelated compounds and comparing their individual action on both T currents and steroid production in a comprehensive way (112). Indeed, the degree of aldosterone inhibition by a large series of calcium antagonists has been shown to be strongly correlated to the extent of T current inhibition, but not to that of L current inhibition (see below).

MODULATION OF T-CHANNEL ACTIVITY BY HORMONES

The unique signaling function of T channels suggests that their activity must be rapidly modulated by various hormones and extracellular modulators. While such a control of channel activity has been extensively described for high voltage-activated calcium channels (113, 114), much less information is available concerning T channels.

Nevertheless, rapid changes of T channel activity, positive or negative, have been reported in response to various agonists in several tissues, including adrenal cortical cells (**Table 5**).

For example, the effect of angiotensin II (AngII) on several different calcium channels has been thoroughly reviewed (126). Basically, the hormone can affect the activity of voltage-operated calcium channels either indirectly, by inducing cell depolarization, or directly, by modifying the channel intrinsic electrophysiological properties.

Modulation of Channel Activity through Membrane Depolarization

A modulation by AngII of the glomerulosa cell membrane potential has been known for a long time (22). Indeed, application of AngII on isolated rat glomerulosa cells induces a biphasic response: a brief hyperpolarization phase followed by a sustained and reversible decrease of membrane conductance accompanied by a depolarization from the resting potential, estimated in these cells to be around −80 mV. This observation was confirmed by means of fluorescent probes for measuring membrane potential (127), or the patch clamp technique in the perforated patch configuration (19). As previously discussed, at low physiological concentrations, AngII did not evoke action potentials in naive glomerulosa cells, but only shifted the voltage by 10–20 mV. The hormone-induced cell depolarization observed in rat, bovine, and human glomerulosa cells was always due to the inhibition of potassium permeability (128), but some differences between species were seen in the characteristics of the potassium currents involved. Four distinct types

TABLE 5 | T-type calcium channel modulation by hormones in adrenal cortex.

Agonists	Tissue/cell type (species)	Effect	Cellular messenger	Reference
AngII	Adrenal glomerulosa (bovine)	+	Gi protein	(38, 42, 115)
AngII	Adrenal glomerulosa (bovine)	+	CaMKII	(116–118)
AngII	Adrenal glomerulosa (bovine)	−	PKC	(15, 119, 120)
ANP	Adrenal glomerulosa (bovine)	−	cGMP?	(40, 41, 121)
Dopamine	Adrenal glomerulosa (rat)	−	G prot (βγ)/PKA	(122, 123)
Serotonin	Adrenal glomerulosa (rat)	+	Gs/PKA	(124)
Endozepine	Adrenal (frog)	+	PKA	(125)
ACTH/AngII	Adrenal fasciculata (human)	+	n/a	(72)
ACTH/AngII	Adrenal fasciculata (bovine)	+	n/a	(46, 75)
ACTH/VIP	Adrenal fasciculata (rat)	+	n/a	(47)
Aldosterone	H295R (human)	+	Gene expression	(69)

of potassium channels were identified in rat and bovine glomerulosa cells (129), but AngII induced a substantial inhibition of only inward rectifier and delayed rectifier potassium channel activities in these species (130). This action was reversible and blocked by the AT1 receptor antagonist losartan (131, 132). In contrast, AngII has been shown to also inhibit a charybdotoxin-sensitive current in rat glomerulosa cells (133), suggesting that a large conductance calcium-activated (BK) potassium channel is also modulated by the hormone.

The modulation of potassium permeability by AngII has been also investigated in bovine glomerulosa cells by measuring the efflux of ^{86}Rb or ^{43}K (134–136). The authors found that after a transient activation that was sensitive to apamin, a blocker of calcium-sensitive (SK) potassium channels, the efflux was then inhibited in a concentration-dependent manner by AngII, and that changes in potassium conductance reflect changes in membrane potential. Thus, the transient hyperpolarization would be due to the activation of calcium-activated potassium channels responding to the transient elevation of cytosolic free calcium concentration ($[Ca^{2+}]_c$) occurring upon calcium release from intracellular stores, while other types of potassium channels, such as the delayed rectifier, are later inhibited in a sustained fashion and are responsible for the depolarization phase. The latter effect of AngII on the potassium permeability being mimicked by diacylglycerol, a role for PKC in this process has been suggested (137). The functional link between potassium conductance modulation and aldosterone secretion was also supported by the demonstration that AngII-induced steroidogenesis is markedly affected by potassium ionophores like valinomycin (138), or by various potassium channel antagonists (139) or agonists (140), and, more recently, by the demonstration of the role of the KCNJ5 channel in maintaining a very negative resting potential within these cells and therefore a low basal aldosterone production (31).

Similar results have been obtained with adrenal fasciculata cells. Indeed, in bovine cells, AngII induces a biphasic response corresponding to a transient hyperpolarization followed by a sustained depolarization (141). The hyperpolarization phase appears to be due to the activation of calcium-dependent potassium currents, but also to chloride currents, the resting potential of fasciculata cells being less negative than that of glomerulosa cells. The identity of the conductance responsible for the fasciculata cell depolarization upon AngII challenge is less clearly defined. A cholera toxin-sensitive potassium current has been proposed to maintain the resting potential of bovine fasciculata cells and to be reduced by AngII and ACTH (142). However other mechanisms have been also suggested, such as the activation of a non-selective cationic conductance, the capacitative calcium influx triggered by calcium release from the stores, or the stimulation of the electrogenic 3Na/1Ca exchanger by elevated $[Ca^{2+}]_c$.

It should be repeated here that the cell depolarization evoked by hormones like AngII or ACTH is sustained but very limited in amplitude. As previously discussed, the consequence therefore is a selective activation of low threshold T-type calcium channels, particularly in cells displaying a very negative resting potential. These particular conditions also explain the exquisite sensitivity of glomerulosa cells to small variations of extracellular potassium, within its physiological range of concentrations.

However, it is important to remember that isolating glomerulosa and fasciculata cells from the adrenal cortex could prevent the occurrence of spontaneous or evoked electrical activity. The presence of action potentials in these cells would allow bringing the membrane depolarization transiently up to voltage values corresponding to L-channel activation and T-channel inactivation and, therefore, the relative contribution of low and high voltage channels in the steroidogenic response to secretagogues could have been wrongly estimated in isolated cells devoid of AP. Nevertheless, because T channels are apparently involved in the triggering and the propagation of the putative action potentials required for L channel activation (17), their function remains crucial even in cells able to work in an "excitable mode."

Modulation of Channel Activity through Protein Modification

The modulation of calcium channels by G proteins has been recognized for a long time as one on the main mechanisms employed by hormones to control the influx of calcium into their target cells (3, 114, 143). In most cases, G proteins that interact with calcium channels are sensitive to pertussis toxin treatment. This toxin, which efficiently blocks the activation of both G_i and G_o proteins, therefore represents a valuable tool for determining the intracellular signaling pathway leading to channel modulation. Moreover, the interaction between the receptor, the G protein and the channel is generally considered to be restricted to a small area of the membrane because it can be observed in the excised patch configuration of the patch-clamp technique, in contrast to other mechanisms involving diffusible molecules acting on channels located at distance from the receptor. It is important to realize that, depending on the mechanism involved, a given receptor can influence calcium influx very locally or broadly within the cell, a distinction that can have physiological consequences depending on the structural and functional organization of the cell (see below).

The modulation of T-type channels by AngII in bovine adrenal glomerulosa cells has been the object of some controversy. Indeed, early observations suggest that, in these cells, AngII increases the amplitude of the slowly deactivating and rapidly inactivating calcium currents, linked to the T-type channel activity (38). Further studies revealed that AngII, in fact, induces a shift of the channel activation curve toward more negative potential values (making the channel more prone to opening upon limited cell depolarization), an effect requiring the presence of GTP in the patch pipette and mimicked by the addition of GTPγS (42). These results, as well as the fact that AngII action is prevented by pertussis toxin treatment or introduction of a monoclonal antibody generated against recombinant Gαi (115), are in favor of the involvement of a Gi protein in the activation of T channels. However, a direct interaction between the G protein and the channel is questioned by the observation that the hormone can increase the single channel opening probability in the cell attached configuration (42). Indeed, the latter observation strongly suggests that a rapidly diffusible second messenger is generated by AngII and responsible for the modulation of T channels. In fact the possibility that, in adrenal glomerulosa cells, AngII modulates T channel activity by more than one single mechanism has been raised by the following observation: although activation of CaMKII by the rise of intracellular calcium also shifts the activation curve of T channels to more negative potentials, as demonstrated with pharmacological inhibitors of the kinase (116), these inhibitors only minimally reduced AngII action (115).

In contrast, in another series of experiments, AngII has been shown to markedly *reduce* T channel activity in bovine glomerulosa cells through a PKC-mediated shift of the channel activation curve to more *positive* values (15). This inhibition of T channels was mimicked by PMA (**Figure 1D**) and correlated with the reduction of the potassium-induced aldosterone production observed in the presence of the same agent. The functional link between the T channel activity and aldosterone production evoked by extracellular potassium was further demonstrated by the observation that PMA did not affect either L-type channel activity (120) or steroidogenesis triggered with a calcium ionophores (14). This paradoxical inhibitory action of AngII is somehow balanced by the cell depolarization evoked by the hormone and can have some physiological relevance. Indeed, aldosterone production induced by extracellular potassium, which is highly dependent on the activity of T-type channels, is reduced in a PKC-dependent manner by AngII in rat glomerulosa cells, putatively to prevent overstimulation in the presence of both agonists (144).

The multiplicity of the mechanisms involved by a same hormone like AngII to modulate T currents, sometimes in opposite directions, could reflect the presence of various T channel isoforms within the cell under specific culture conditions. It would be therefore relevant to determine whether the expression of the various channel isoforms is changing during development or upon specific pathological states, in order to better predict the hormone action on calcium influx.

Several other physiological modulators of steroidogenesis and/or their intracellular messengers have been reported to affect T channel activity in adrenocortical cells (**Table 5**). Moreover, activation of ectopic receptors for serotonin or GIP, illegitimately expressed in human fasciculata cells, and causing Cushing syndrome through stimulation of cAMP in ACTH-independent macronodular adrenal hyperplasia, has been also reported to enhance T channel activity through a PKA-dependent mechanism (145).

Finally, it is noteworthy that channel modulation, being through phosphorylation or binding to G proteins, not only affects the electrophysiological properties of the channel but could also modify channel interaction with cellular proteins involved in the calcium signal transduction.

PUTATIVE MECHANISMS CONFERRING FUNCTIONAL SPECIFICITY TO T-CHANNELS IN STEROIDOGENESIS

As previously discussed, a close correlation has been observed in many instances between the production of aldosterone and the activity of T channels (but not L channels) upon modulation with potassium (12, 38), AngII (144), ANP (40), or several pharmacological agents affecting PKC (15, 144). Similarly, the steroidogenic response of glomerulosa cells to prolactin (103) or serotonin (124) has been shown to rely, at least partially, on the modulation of T channels, as well as the inhibition of aldosterone secretion by dopamine (122, 123, 146). The production of glucocorticoids by fasciculata cells was also dependent on T-type calcium channels when stimulated either by ACTH (46) or by an endozepine triakontetraneuropeptide (125).

Because a specific role in the modulation of steroid biosynthesis and secretion has been attributed to T-type channels in adrenal cortical cells, the challenge then consisted in understanding how their molecular and electrophysiological characteristics and how the structural organization of the cell confer a functional advantage to these channels.

In a few experiments, both T-type and L-type calcium currents have been simultaneously determined under various discriminating pharmacological conditions, and this concomitantly with measurement of cytosolic calcium fluctuations in the same single cell (14). Potassium-induced cytosolic calcium elevation and aldosterone production in response to the same agents were also determined in parallel. Steroidogenesis appeared systematically linked to T channel (but not to L channel) activity while cytosolic calcium fluctuations depended principally on L current amplitude (112). This finding suggests dissociation between the cytosolic calcium signaling evoked by extracellular potassium and the rate-limiting steps of aldosterone biosynthesis, known to occur within the mitochondria (147, 148). According to our working hypothesis, in order to exert their preferential stimulatory action on steroid biosynthesis, T channels have to fulfill at least two prerequisites: (a) maintain a sustained influx of calcium into the cell, and (b) direct a part of this calcium toward the mitochondria.

The first point is addressed by considering the particular electrophysiological properties of T channels. Indeed, how can transient (T-type) calcium currents, which inactivate within a fraction of a second in excitable cells, support activation of steroidogenesis in response to potassium for minutes or even hours? As previously discussed, upon slight depolarization of the cell, and in the absence of action potentials, a sustained entry of calcium within a permissive window of voltage is possible due to the significant overlap between the activation and inactivation potential ranges of the channel (12, 15, 40). This steady-state current is tiny and barely detectable with the conventional patch-clamp technique, but, because it is *sustained*, in the long run it allows a large amount of calcium to enter and accumulate within the cell, at least sufficiently for activating steroidogenesis. The resting potential of the rat and bovine glomerulosa cells has been estimated to be around −80 mV, a value close to the low voltage edge of this window. As a consequence, a small depolarization of the membrane, induced by a slight increase of extracellular potassium in the physiological range, may increase by several folds the steady-state influx of calcium through T channels (**Figure 1B**). While L-type channels also display a similar window of voltage, this is located at much more positive potentials, rarely reached under physiological conditions (19).

In addition to the establishment of a permissive window of voltage in which calcium can enter the cells near the resting potential, the specific function of T channels is probably also conferred by their localization within the cell membrane. Indeed, it should be noted here that, at supraphysiological cell depolarization, even in the absence of regenerative electrical activity, other types of calcium channels are simultaneously activated in the same cells, leading to an apparent redundancy of the calcium entry pathways. However, only a part of the functions attributed to T channels is actually shared by these other channels, which sometimes even exert opposite effects on steroidogenesis (79). This fact suggests that the cell is able to decipher the calcium signal specifically resulting from T channel activation. This is theoretically possible for two reasons: (1) the signal is confined due to the compartmentalization of calcium within the cell, and (2) there is a strict organization of the transduction mechanisms at the molecular level (149). In other words, the close environment of the channel (the proximity of specific calcium-binding protein and/or cellular organelles) dictates the function of calcium entering the cell at this precise location.

Mitochondria play a particular role in intracellular calcium homeostasis. Indeed, because of the very negative potential of their inner membrane (around −180 mV), and the presence of a specific calcium uniporter, they avidly take up calcium when its concentration rises in the cytosol. Mitochondrial calcium influx is rapidly balanced by an equivalent efflux of calcium out of the organelle, which is dependent on sodium exchange, but only up to a given cytosolic concentration called the "mitochondrial set-point" (147). Above this set-point, fluxes are no more balanced and calcium rapidly accumulates within the mitochondrial matrix. This allows the cytosolic calcium concentration to come back down to this critical set-point. This property of mitochondria makes them very efficient cytosolic buffers, able to attenuate large calcium transients within the cell. At the same time, the mitochondria are also a *target* for calcium, particularly in steroidogenic cells. Indeed, steroids are synthesized by successive oxidations of a common precursor, cholesterol. Some important enzymatic steps in this process require molecular oxygen and, for this reason, must occur within the mitochondria. The rate limiting step in steroid biosynthesis is indeed the intramitochondrial conversion of cholesterol to pregnenolone, which requires the transfer of the substrate from the cytosol across the double membrane into the organelle. This early step in steroidogenesis is controlled by cytosolic and mitochondrial calcium levels as shown by several independent experimental observations: (a) rising ambient calcium stimulates aldosterone production in permeabilized glomerulosa cells and this response is prevented by the addition of ruthenium red, a blocker of the mitochondrial calcium uniporter (148), (b) intracellular calcium stimulates both intramitochondrial cholesterol transfer (150) and the expression of the steroidogenic acute regulatory (StAR) protein (151), which is required for efficient cholesterol transport into the mitochondria, and (c) cytosolic calcium fluctuations evoked by AngII are relayed and amplified within the mitochondrial matrix (152).

Interestingly, when mitochondrial calcium fluctuations induced by AngII were recorded at the *single organelle* levels with a GFP-derived probe (153), all mitochondria of the same cell did not respond simultaneously to the hormone, but calcium hot spots appeared in different regions of the cell, at different time points, and in an apparent stochastic manner (112). This observation suggests that the mitochondrial calcium response does not result from calcium uptake upon diffusion of calcium across the entire cytosol, but more probably upon local calcium release from intracellular stores located in proximity of the organelles.

Because calcium stimulates early, rate limiting steps of steroidogenesis occurring within the mitochondria, and because calcium entering the cell through T channels is not detected within the cytosol of bovine adrenal glomerulosa cells (14), we have proposed that calcium is directly conveyed from the plasma membrane to the mitochondria *via* the lumen of the endoplasmic reticulum, which would act as a sort of "*intracellular calcium pipeline*" (112, 149) (**Figure 3**).

This functional model is structurally supported by the distribution of the reticulum endoplasmic and the mitochondria within glomerulosa cells (and other cell types), with the presence of many "quasi synaptic" physical contacts observed between these organelles, as shown by electron microscopy, as well as by a close apposition of the reticulum with the plasma membrane in many points at the cell periphery (**Figures 3A–C**). This model therefore predicts specific interactions between T channels embedded within the plasma membrane and some components of the reticulum (**Figure 3D**). This proposal has been supported by the observation that disrupting physically the interaction between the reticulum and the cell membrane impairs the transduction of calcium signal elicited by potassium to the mitochondria, and therefore steroidogenesis in H295R cells (154). It is noteworthy that this organization of calcium influx, involving the local transfer of calcium entering the cell directly into the endoplasmic reticulum, is somehow reminiscent of the early "capacitative" model proposed by Putney (155), before revisiting it for taking into account results obtained with thapsigargin (156, 157), and it is quite intriguing that the α_1H isoform of T channels, which is the most abundant in glomerulosa cells, has been proposed to mediate a capacitative calcium entry in non-excitable cancer cells (158).

The application of the pipeline model to the control of cortisol within fasciculata cells has not yet been specifically evaluated. The dichotomy between T-type and L-type channel functions is probably less obvious in these cells, where ACTH-induced steroid secretion is more efficiently inhibited by nifedipine and potentiated by Bay K8644, consistent with the involvement of L-type channels in the steroidogenic response (159, 160), in spite of the relatively low levels of expression of these channels reported in bovine fasciculata cells (45). However, species differences have been reported in term of dihydropyridine efficiency for reducing cortisol secretion (160). Clearly, additional investigations are still required for clarifying the functional relationship existing between calcium channels and limiting steps of cortisol biosynthesis, and therefore more specifically defining the role of each calcium channel.

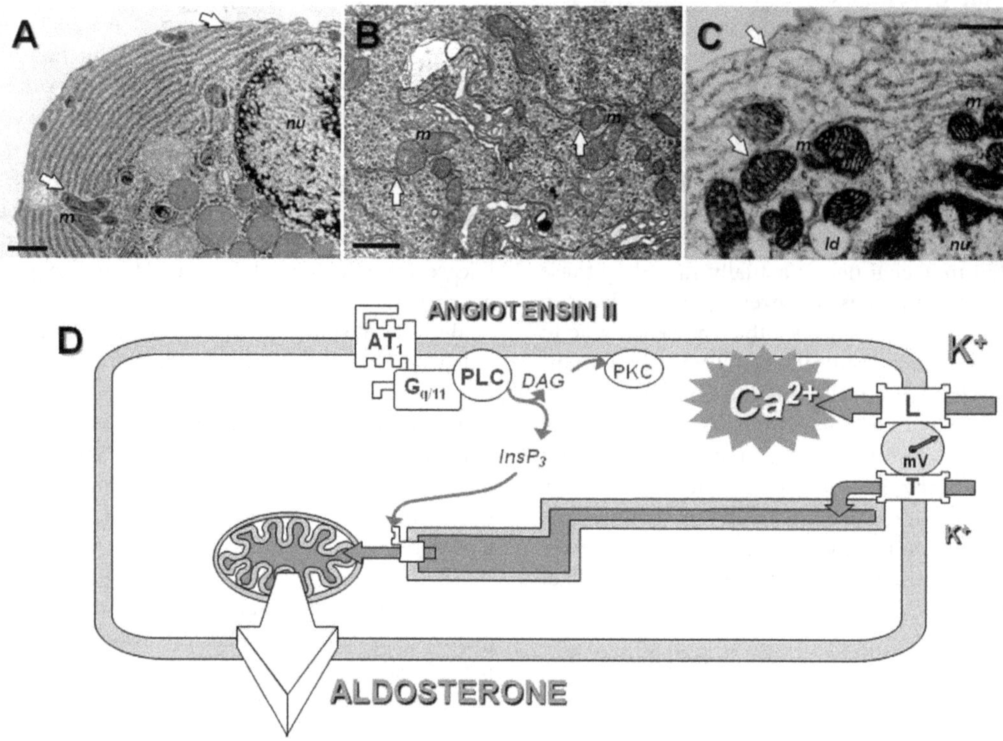

FIGURE 3 | The concept of intracellular calcium pipeline: a model for explaining the selective transport of calcium from the T channels into the mitochondria. Electron microscopy reveals the presence of close apposition in many places of the endoplasmic reticulum (ER) with the plasma membrane or the mitochondria (white arrows), within various cell types, including rat parotid cells **(A)**, rat spinal cord neurons **(B)**, or bovine adrenal glomerulosa cells **(C)**. Scale = 1 μm; *m* indicates mitochondria, *nu* nucleus and *ld* lipid droplets. See Ref. (112) for additional information. **(D)**. A hypothetical model for the cellular transport of calcium into mitochondria. At the pipeline filling site, T-type calcium channels and, to a lesser extent, L-type channels are activated upon cell depolarization by potassium or angiotensin II. Several experimental data suggest that calcium entering the cell through T-type channels could be selectively pumped into the lumen of the ER, while calcium entering through L-type channels would be poured into the cytosol. At the pipeline delivery site, InsP3 receptors are maintained in proximity of the mitochondria within "quasi synaptic" structures. Calcium released upon activation of the InsP3 receptors, due to calcium overloading of the ER and/or to InsP3 production by AT_1 receptor-activated PLC, is rapidly internalized into the very negatively charged matrix, through the mitochondrial inner membrane calcium uniporter. Intramitochondrial calcium elevation then stimulates limiting steps of aldosterone biosynthesis. AT_1, angiotensin II receptor, type 1; $G_{q/11}$, heterotrimeric G protein of the q/11 family; PLC, phospholipase C β; PKC, protein kinase C; $InsP_3$, inositol 1,4,5-trisphosphate.

CONCLUSION

Two properties of T-type calcium channels appear to make them particularly suited for stimulating steroidogenesis: (1) their ability to activate and stay open upon slight depolarization of the cell, and (2) their capacity to convey calcium entering the cell directly to the mitochondria, where regulated steps of steroid biosynthesis occur.

The first property will be particularly favorable in cells displaying a very negative resting potential like glomerulosa cells, because small depolarization induced by physiological concentrations of agonists cannot reach the threshold for activation of L-type channels in these cells. The presence of these channels also renders the cells very sensitive to small changes of the extracellular potassium concentration, which participates, through the modulation of aldosterone secretion, to the maintenance of a normal kalemia. The fact that fasciculata cells have apparently a less negative resting potential probably could explain why steroidogenesis is globally less dependent on T-type channels in these cells and also partly involves L-type channel activity.

Because of calcium toxicity and polyvalence of calcium function, a strong confinement of this cation within the cell is necessary. The functional specificity of some channels is therefore also partly linked to their ability to transport calcium precisely to its site of action. In the case of steroidogenic cells, the mitochondrion is a main target for calcium. Because of the distance between the plasma membrane and these organelles in glomerulosa cells, the availability of intracellular calcium traffic through the lumen of the endoplasmic reticulum presents some advantages. Our working hypothesis is that T-type calcium channels are particularly efficient for stimulating aldosterone biosynthesis in glomerulosa cells because of their ability to load the endoplasmic reticulum with calcium. If the calcium pipeline model is true, one can predict that molecular structures must be maintained at both extremities and that T channels must interact physically with specific proteins. It is therefore conceivable that some mutations of the channel itself (or of the putative protein interacting with the channel) could prevent this interaction and therefore drastically reduce the ability of the channel to modulate steroidogenesis in spite of the fact that its electrophysiological properties are preserved. However, to our knowledge, such a loss of function mutation responsible for a hypoadrenocorticism has not been described.

The gain of function mutations on CACHA1D observed in APA cells could, theoretically, also affect cortisol secretion from fasciculata cells. Indeed, $Ca_V1.3$ channels have been recently shown to be expressed in fasciculata cells and to participate to ACTH- and AngII-stimulated steroidogenic response (75). Similar mutations, shifting the channel permissive window to more negative voltages, would therefore be expected to increase cortisol secretion in an agonist-independent manner. Even if such mutations have not been formally demonstrated, the predicted high sensitivity of these tumors to inhibition by dihydropyridines would be worth of testing. Indeed, an important issue is whether the mutation status may influence the diagnosis, the treatment options, or the therapeutic outcome (32). Moreover, given the ubiquitous role played by calcium in cell biology and the prevalence of the diseases in which a dysfunction of calcium channels has been involved, a detailed understanding of the mechanisms conferring functional specificity to a given class of channels, like T-type channels, provides relevant information for developing strategies in order to get more efficient pharmacological tools in order to treat diseases resulting from calcium deregulation.

AUTHOR CONTRIBUTIONS

MR is responsible for the complete elaboration, writing, and correction of the present manuscript.

ACKNOWLEDGMENTS

This work was supported by a grant from the *Fondation Endocrinologie*.

REFERENCES

1. Tsien RW, Tsien RY. Calcium channels, stores, and oscillations. *Annu Rev Cell Biol* (1990) **6**:715–60. doi:10.1146/annurev.cb.06.110190.003435
2. Trautwein W, Hescheler J. Regulation of cardiac L-type calcium current by phosphorylation and G proteins. *Annu Rev Physiol* (1990) **52**:257–74. doi:10.1146/annurev.ph.52.030190.001353
3. Schulz G, Rosenthal W, Hescheler J, Trautwein W. Role of G proteins in calcium channel modulation. *Annu Rev Physiol* (1990) **52**:275–92. doi:10.1146/annurev.ph.52.030190.001423
4. Rossier MF. Function and differential expression of T-type calcium channels in various pathophysiological states. *Recent Res Dev Biochem* (2003) **4**:13–29.
5. Carbone E, Lux HD. A low voltage-activated, fully inactivating calcium channel in vertebrate sensory neurones. *Nature* (1984) **310**:501–2. doi:10.1038/310501a0
6. Nilius B, Hess P, Lansman JB, Tsien RW. A novel type of cardiac calcium channel in ventricular cells. *Nature* (1985) **316**:443–6. doi:10.1038/316443a0
7. Nowycky MC, Fox AP, Tsien RW. Three types of neuronal calcium channels with different calcium agonist sensitivity. *Nature* (1985) **316**:440–3. doi:10.1038/316440a0
8. Perez-Reyes E, Cribbs LL, Daud A, Lacerda AE, Barclay J, Williamson MP, et al. Molecular characterization of a neuronal low-voltage-activated T-type calcium channel. *Nature* (1998) **391**:896–900. doi:10.1038/36110
9. Perez-Reyes E. Molecular physiology of low-voltage-activated t-type calcium channels. *Physiol Rev* (2003) **83**:117–61. doi:10.1152/physrev.00018.2002
10. Hagiwara N, Irisawa H, Kameyama M. Contribution of two types of calcium currents to the pacemaker potentials of rabbit sino-atrial node cells. *J Physiol* (1988) **395**:233–53. doi:10.1113/jphysiol.1988.sp016916
11. Huguenard JR. Low-threshold calcium currents in central nervous system neurons. *Annu Rev Physiol* (1996) **58**:329–48. doi:10.1146/annurev.ph.58.030196.001553
12. Rossier MF, Burnay MM, Capponi AM. Distinct functions of T- and L-type calcium channels during activation of aldosterone production in adrenal glomerulosa cells. In: Clozel J-P, Nargeot J, Tsien RW, editors. *Low Voltage-Activated T-Type Calcium Channels*. Montpellier: Adis International (1998). p. 176–85.
13. Scholl UI, Goh G, Stolting G, de Oliveira RC, Choi M, Overton JD, et al. Somatic and germline CACNA1D calcium channel mutations in aldosterone-producing adenomas and primary aldosteronism. *Nat Genet* (2013) **45**:1050–4. doi:10.1038/ng.2695
14. Rossier MF, Burnay MM, Vallotton MB, Capponi AM. Distinct functions of T-type and L-type calcium channels during activation of bovine adrenal glomerulosa cells. *Endocrinology* (1996) **137**:4817–26. doi:10.1210/en.137.11.4817
15. Rossier MF, Aptel HBC, Python CP, Burnay MM, Vallotton MB, Capponi AM. Inhibition of low threshold calcium channels by angiotensin II in adrenal glomerulosa cells through activation of protein kinase C. *J Biol Chem* (1995) **270**:15137–42. doi:10.1074/jbc.270.25.15137
16. Quinn SJ, Cornwall MC, Williams GH. Electrical properties of isolated rat adrenal glomerulosa and fasciculata cells. *Endocrinology* (1987) **120**:903–14. doi:10.1210/endo-120-3-903
17. Hu C, Rusin CG, Tan Z, Guagliardo NA, Barrett PQ. Zona glomerulosa cells of the mouse adrenal cortex are intrinsic electrical oscillators. *J Clin Invest* (2012) **122**:2046–53. doi:10.1172/JCI61996
18. Natke E Jr, Kabela E. Electrical response in cat adrenal cortex: possible relation to aldosterone secretion. *Am J Physiol* (1979) **237**:E158–62.
19. Lotshaw DP. Role of membrane depolarization and T-type Ca2+ channels in angiotensin II and K+ stimulated aldosterone secretion. *Mol Cell Endocrinol* (2001) **175**:157–71. doi:10.1016/S0303-7207(01)00384-7
20. Matthews EK, Saffran M. Ionic dependence of adrenal steroidogenesis and ACTH-induced changes in the membrane potential of adrenocortical cells. *J Physiol* (1973) **234**:43–64. doi:10.1113/jphysiol.1973.sp010333
21. Matthews EK. Membrane potential measurement in cells of the adrenal gland. *J Physiol* (1967) **189**:139–48. doi:10.1113/jphysiol.1967.sp008159
22. Quinn SJ, Cornwall MC, Williams GH. Electrophysiological responses to angiotensin II of isolated rat adrenal glomerulosa cells. *Endocrinology* (1987) **120**:1581–9. doi:10.1210/endo-120-3-903
23. Matthews EK, Saffran M. Effect of ACTH on the electrical properties of adrenocortical cells. *Nature* (1968) **219**:1369–70. doi:10.1038/2191369a0
24. Capponi AM, Rossier MF. Regulation of aldosterone secretion. *Curr Opin Endocrinol Diabetes* (1996) **3**:248–57. doi:10.1097/00060793-199606000-00010
25. Capponi AM, Rossier MF. Angiotensin and aldosterone biosynthesis. In: Unger T, Schölkens BA, editors. *Angiotensin*. Berlin: Springer (2004). p. 285–342.
26. Vallotton MB. Primary aldosteronism. Part I diagnosis of primary hyperaldosteronism. *Clin Endocrinol* (1996) **45**:47–52.
27. CONN JW. Primary aldosteronism. *J Lab Clin Med* (1955) **45**:661–4.
28. Rossi GP, Bernini G, Caliumi C, Desideri G, Fabris B, Ferri C, et al. A prospective study of the prevalence of primary aldosteronism in 1,125 hypertensive patients. *J Am Coll Cardiol* (2006) **48**:2293–300. doi:10.1016/j.jacc.2006.07.059
29. Hannemann A, Wallaschofski H. Prevalence of primary aldosteronism in patient's cohorts and in population-based studies – a review of the current literature. *Horm Metab Res* (2012) **44**:157–62. doi:10.1055/s-0031-1295438
30. Fernandes-Rosa FL, Williams TA, Riester A, Steichen O, Beuschlein F, Boulkroun S, et al. Genetic spectrum and clinical correlates of somatic mutations in aldosterone-producing adenoma. *Hypertension* (2014) **64**:354–61. doi:10.1161/HYPERTENSIONAHA.114.03419

31. Choi M, Scholl UI, Yue P, Bjorklund P, Zhao B, Nelson-Williams C, et al. K+ channel mutations in adrenal aldosterone-producing adenomas and hereditary hypertension. *Science* (2011) **331**:768–72. doi:10.1126/science.1198785
32. Zennaro MC, Boulkroun S, Fernandes-Rosa F. An update on novel mechanisms of primary aldosteronism. *J Endocrinol* (2015) **224**:R63–77. doi:10.1530/JOE-14-0597
33. Boulkroun S, Samson-Couterie B, Dzib JF, Lefebvre H, Louiset E, Amar L, et al. Adrenal cortex remodeling and functional zona glomerulosa hyperplasia in primary aldosteronism. *Hypertension* (2010) **56**:885–92. doi:10.1161/HYPERTENSIONAHA.110.158543
34. Fischer E, Beuschlein F. Novel genes in primary aldosteronism. *Curr Opin Endocrinol Diabetes Obes* (2014) **21**:154–8. doi:10.1097/MED.0000000000000060
35. Scholl UI, Stolting G, Nelson-Williams C, Vichot AA, Choi M, Loring E, et al. Recurrent gain of function mutation in calcium channel CACNA1H causes early-onset hypertension with primary aldosteronism. *Elife* (2015) **4**:e06315. doi:10.7554/eLife.06315
36. Matsunaga H, Yamashita N, Maruyama Y, Kojima I, Kurokawa K. Evidence for two distinct voltage-gated calcium channel currents in bovine adrenal glomerulosa cells. *Biochem Biophys Res Commun* (1987) **149**:1049–54. doi:10.1016/0006-291X(87)90514-6
37. Matsunaga H, Maruyama Y, Kojima I, Hoshi T. Transient calcium channel current characterized by a low threshold voltage in zona glomerulosa cells of rat adrenal cortex. *Pflugers Arch* (1987) **408**:351–5. doi:10.1007/BF00581128
38. Cohen CJ, McCarthy RT, Barrett PQ, Rasmussen H. Calcium channels in adrenal glomerulosa cells: potassium and angiotensin II increase T-type calcium current. *Proc Natl Acad Sci USA* (1988) **85**:2412–6. doi:10.1073/pnas.85.7.2412
39. Durroux T, Gallo-Payet N, Payet MD. Three components of the calcium current in cultured glomerulosa cells from rat adrenal gland. *J Physiol* (1988) **404**:713–29. doi:10.1113/jphysiol.1988.sp017315
40. Barrett PQ, Isales CM, Bollag WB, McCarthy RT. Calcium channels and aldosterone secretion: modulation by potassium and atrial natriuretic peptide. *Am J Physiol* (1991) **261**:F706–19.
41. Barrett PQ, Isales CM, Bollag WB, McCarthy RT. Modulation of Ca2+ channels by atrial natriuretic peptide in the bovine adrenal glomerulosa cell. *Can J Physiol Pharmacol* (1991) **69**:1553–60. doi:10.1139/y91-231
42. McCarthy RT, Isales CM, Rasmussen H. T-type calcium channels in adrenal glomerulosa cells: GTP-dependent modulation by angiotensin II. *Proc Nat Acad Sci U S A* (1993) **90**:3260–4. doi:10.1073/pnas.90.8.3260
43. Payet MD, Durroux T, Bilodeau L, Guillon G, Gallo-Payet N. Characterization of potassium and calcium ionic currents in glomerulosa cells from human adrenal glands. *Endocrinology* (1994) **134**:2589–98. doi:10.1210/endo.134.6.7515004
44. Varnai P, Osipenko ON, Vizi ES, Spät A. Activation of calcium current in voltage-clamped rat glomerulosa cells by potassium ions. *J Physiol* (1995) **483**:67–78. doi:10.1113/jphysiol.1995.sp020568
45. Mlinar B, Biagi BA, Enyeart JJ. Voltage-gated transient currents in bovine adrenal fasciculata cells. I. T-type Ca2+ current. *J Gen Physiol* (1993) **102**:217–37.
46. Enyeart JJ, Mlinar B, Enyeart JA. T-type Ca2+ channels are required for adrenocorticotropin-stimulated cortisol production by bovine adrenal zona fasciculata cells. *Mol Endocrinol* (1993) **7**:1031–40. doi:10.1210/me.7.8.1031
47. Barbara JG, Takeda K. Voltage-dependent currents and modulation of calcium channel expression in zona fasciculata cells from rat adrenal gland. *J Physiol* (1995) **488**(Pt 3):609–22. doi:10.1113/jphysiol.1995.sp020994
48. Guyot A, Dupre-Aucouturier S, Ojeda C, Rougier O, Bilbaut A. Two types of pharmacologically distinct Ca(2+) currents with voltage-dependent similarities in zona fasciculata cells isolated from bovine adrenal gland. *J Membr Biol* (2000) **173**:149–63. doi:10.1007/s002320001016
49. Lambert RC, Maulet Y, Mouton J, Beattie R, Volsen S, De Waard M, et al. T-type Ca2+ current properties are not modified by Ca2+ channel beta subunit depletion in nodosus ganglion neurons. *J Neurosci* (1997) **17**:6621–8.
50. Ertel EA, Campbell KP, Harpold MM, Hofmann F, Mori Y, Perez-Reyes E, et al. Nomenclature of voltage-gated calcium channels. *Neuron* (2000) **25**:533–5. doi:10.1016/S0896-6273(00)81057-0
51. Klugbauer N, Marais E, Lacinova L, Hofmann F. A T-type calcium channel from mouse brain. *Pflugers Arch* (1999) **437**:710–5. doi:10.1007/s004240050836
52. Klockner U, Lee JH, Cribbs LL, Daud A, Hescheler J, Pereverzev A, et al. Comparison of the Ca2 + currents induced by expression of three cloned alpha1 subunits, alpha1G, alpha1H and alpha1I, of low-voltage-activated T-type Ca2 + channels. *Eur J Neurosci* (1999) **11**:4171–8. doi:10.1046/j.1460-9568.1999.00849.x
53. Williams ME, Washburn MS, Hans M, Urrutia A, Brust PF, Prodanovich P, et al. Structure and functional characterization of a novel human low-voltage activated calcium channel. *J Neurochem* (1999) **72**:791–9. doi:10.1046/j.1471-4159.1999.0720791.x
54. Lee JH, Daud A, Cribbs LL, Lacerda AE, Pereverzev A, Klockner U, et al. Cloning and expression of a novel member of the low voltage-activated T-type calcium channel family. *J Neurosci* (1999) **19**:1912–21.
55. Lee JH, Gomora JC, Cribbs LL, Perez-Reyes E. Nickel block of three cloned T-type calcium channels: low concentrations selectively block alpha1H. *Biophys J* (1999) **77**:3034–42. doi:10.1016/S0006-3495(99)77134-1
56. Hofmann F, Biel M, Flockerzi V. Molecular basis for calcium channel diversity. *Annu Rev Neurosci* (1994) **17**:399–418. doi:10.1146/annurev.ne.17.030194.002151
57. Catterall WA. Structure and function of voltage-gated ion channels. *Trends Neurosci* (1993) **16**:500–6. doi:10.1016/0166-2236(93)90193-P
58. Cribbs LL, Gomora JC, Daud AN, Lee JH, Perez-Reyes E. Molecular cloning and functional expression of Ca(v)3.1c, a T-type calcium channel from human brain. *FEBS Lett* (2000) **466**:54–8. doi:10.1016/S0014-5793(99)01756-1
59. Tanabe T, Beam KG, Adams BA, Niidome T, Numa S. Regions of the skeletal muscle dihydropyridine receptor critical for excitation-contraction coupling. *Nature* (1990) **346**:567–9. doi:10.1038/346567a0
60. Sheng Z-H, Rettig J, Cook T, Catterall WA. Calcium-dependent interaction of N-type calcium channels with the synaptic core complex. *Nature* (1996) **379**:451–4. doi:10.1038/379451a0
61. Talavera K, Staes M, Janssens A, Klugbauer N, Droogmans G, Hofmann F, et al. Aspartate residues of the Glu-Glu-Asp-Asp (EEDD) pore locus control selectivity and permeation of the T-type Ca(2+) channel alpha(1G). *J Biol Chem* (2001) **276**:45628–35. doi:10.1074/jbc.M103047200
62. Mittman S, Guo J, Agnew WS. Structure and alternative splicing of the gene encoding alpha1G, a human brain T calcium channel alpha1 subunit. *Neurosci Lett* (1999) **274**:143–6. doi:10.1016/S0304-3940(99)00716-8
63. Monteil A, Chemin J, Bourinet E, Mennessier G, Lory P, Nargeot J. Molecular and functional properties of the human alpha(1G) subunit that forms T-type calcium channels. *J Biol Chem* (2000) **275**:6090–100. doi:10.1074/jbc.C000090200
64. Jagannathan S, Punt EL, Gu Y, Arnoult C, Sakkas D, Barratt CLR, et al. Identification and localization of T-type voltage-operated calcium channel subunits in human male germ cells. Expression of multiple isoforms. *J Biol Chem* (2002) **277**:8449–56. doi:10.1074/jbc.M105345200
65. Akaike N, Kanaide H, Kuga T, Nakamura M, Sadoshima J, Tomoike H. Low-voltage-activated calcium current in rat aorta smooth muscle cells in primary culture. *J Physiol* (1989) **416**:141–60. doi:10.1113/jphysiol.1989.sp017754
66. Arnoult C, Cardullo RA, Lemos JR, Florman HM. Activation of mouse sperm T-type Ca2+ channels by adhesion to the egg zona pellucida. *Proc Natl Acad Sci U S A* (1996) **93**:13004–9. doi:10.1073/pnas.93.23.13004
67. Schrier AD, Wang H, Talley EM, Perez-Reyes E, Barrett PQ. The alpha1 H T-type calcium channel is the predominant subtype expressed in bovine and rat zona glomerulosa. *Am J Physiol* (2001) **280**:C265–72.
68. Felizola SJ, Maekawa T, Nakamura Y, Satoh F, Ono Y, Kikuchi K, et al. Voltage-gated calcium channels in the human adrenal and primary aldosteronism. *J Steroid Biochem Mol Biol* (2014) **144**(Pt B):410–6.
69. Lesouhaitier O, Chiappe A, Rossier MF. Aldosterone increases T-type calcium currents in human adrenocarcinoma (H295R) cells by inducing channel expression. *Endocrinology* (2001) **142**:4320–30. doi:10.1210/endo.142.10.8435
70. Rossier MF, Lesouhaitier O, Perrier E, Bockhorn L, Chiappe A, Lalevee N. Aldosterone regulation of T-type calcium channels. *J Steroid Biochem Mol Biol* (2003) **85**:383–8. doi:10.1016/S0960-0760(03)00201-2

71. Liu H, Enyeart JA, Enyeart JJ. ACTH induces Cav3.2 current and mRNA by cAMP-dependent and cAMP-independent mechanisms. *J Biol Chem* (2010) **285**:20040–50. doi:10.1074/jbc.M110.104190
72. Enyeart JJ, Enyeart JA. Ca2+ and K+ channels of normal human adrenal zona fasciculata cells: properties and modulation by ACTH and AngII. *J Gen Physiol* (2013) **142**:137–55. doi:10.1085/jgp.201310964
73. Enyeart JA, Liu H, Enyeart JJ. 8-Phenylthio-adenines stimulate the expression of steroid hydroxylases, $Ca_v3.2$ Ca^{2+} channels, and cortisol synthesis by a cAMP-independent mechanism. *Am J Physiol Endocrinol Metab* (2011) **301**:E941–54. doi:10.1152/ajpendo.00282.2011
74. Quinn SJ, Brauneis U, Tillotson DL, Cornwall MC, Williams GH. Calcium channels and control of cytosolic calcium in rat and bovine zona glomerulosa cells. *Am J Physiol* (1992) **262**:C598–606.
75. Enyeart JJ, Enyeart JA. Adrenal fasciculata cells express T-type and rapidly and slowly activating L-type Ca2+ channels that regulate cortisol secretion. *Am J Physiol Cell Physiol* (2015) **308**:C899–918. doi:10.1152/ajpcell.00002.2015
76. Gomora JC, Xu L, Enyeart JA, Enyeart JJ. Effect of mibefradil on voltage-dependent gating and kinetics of T-type Ca(2+) channels in cortisol-secreting cells. *J Pharmacol Exp Ther* (2000) **292**:96–103.
77. Wolfe JT, Wang H, Perez-Reyes E, Barrett PQ. Stimulation of recombinant Ca(v)3.2, T-type, Ca(2+) channel currents by CaMKIIgamma(C). *J Physiol* (2002) **538**:343–55.
78. Varnai P, Petheo GL, Makara JK, Spat A. Electrophysiological study on the high K+ sensitivity of rat glomerulosa cells. *Pflugers Arch* (1998) **435**:429–31. doi:10.1007/s004240050534
79. Barrett PQ, Ertel EA, Smith MM, Nee JJ, Cohen CJ. Voltage-gated calcium currents have two opposing effects on the secretion of aldosterone. *Am J Physiol* (1995) **268**:C985–92.
80. Chen XL, Bayliss DA, Fern RJ, Barrett PQ. A role for T-type calcium channels in synergistic control of aldosterone production by angiotensin II and potassium. *Am J Physiol* (1999) **276**:F674–83.
81. Spat A, Rohacs T, Horvath A, Szabadkai G, Enyedi P. The role of voltage-dependent calcium channels in angiotensin-stimulated glomerulosa cells. *Endocr Res* (1996) **22**:569–76. doi:10.1080/07435809609043748
82. Spat A, Hunyady L. Control of aldosterone secretion: a model for convergence in cellular signaling pathways. *Physiol Rev* (2004) **84**:489–539. doi:10.1152/physrev.00030.2003
83. Lacinova L, Klugbauer N, Hofmann F. Regulation of the calcium channel alpha(1G) subunit by divalent cations and organic blockers. *Neuropharmacol* (2000) **39**:1254–66. doi:10.1016/S0028-3908(99)00202-6
84. Perchenet L, Benardeau A, Ertel EA. Pharmacological properties of Ca(V)3.2, a low voltage-activated Ca2+ channel cloned from human heart. *Naunyn Schmiedebergs Arch Pharmacol* (2000) **361**:590–9. doi:10.1007/s002100000238
85. Monteil A, Chemin J, Leuranguer V, Altier C, Mennessier G, Bourinet E, et al. Specific properties of T-type calcium channels generated by the human alpha 1I subunit. *J Biol Chem* (2000) **275**:16530–5. doi:10.1074/jbc.C000090200
86. Berthier C, Monteil A, Lory P, Strube C. Alpha(1H) mRNA in single skeletal muscle fibres accounts for T-type calcium current transient expression during fetal development in mice. *J Physiol* (2002) **539**:681–91. doi:10.1113/jphysiol.2001.013246
87. Cribbs LL, Lee JH, Yang J, Satin J, Zhang Y, Daud A, et al. Cloning and characterization of alpha1H from human heart, a member of the T-type calcium channel gene family. *Circ Res* (1998) **83**:103–9. doi:10.1161/01.RES.83.1.103
88. Jimenez C, Bourinet E, Leuranguer V, Richard S, Snutch TP, Nargeot J. Determinants of voltage-dependent inactivation affect Mibefradil block of calcium channels. *Neuropharmacol* (2000) **39**:1–10. doi:10.1016/S0028-3908(99)00153-7
89. Mehrke G, Zong XG, Flockerzi V, Hofmann F. The calcium channel blocker Ro 40-5967 blocks differently T-type and L-type calcium channels. *J Pharmacol Exp Ther* (1994) **271**:1483–8.
90. Martin RL, Lee JH, Cribbs LL, Perez-Reyes E, Hanck DA. Mibefradil block of cloned T-type calcium channels. *J Pharmacol Exp Ther* (2000) **295**:302–8.
91. Todorovic SM, Perez-Reyes E, Lingle CJ. Anticonvulsants but not general anesthetics have differential blocking effects on different T-type current variants. *Mol Pharmacol* (2000) **58**:98–108.
92. Chuang RS, Jaffe H, Cribbs L, Perez-Reyes E, Swartz KJ. Inhibition of T-type voltage-gated calcium channels by a new scorpion toxin. *Nat Neurosci* (1998) **1**:668–74. doi:10.1038/3669
93. Santi CM, Cayabyab FS, Sutton KG, McRory JE, Mezeyova J, Hamming KS, et al. Differential inhibition of T-type calcium channels by neuroleptics. *J Neurosci* (2002) **22**:396–403.
94. Chemin J, Monteil A, Perez-Reyes E, Nargeot J, Lory P. Direct inhibition of T-type calcium channels by the endogenous cannabinoid anandamide. *EMBO J* (2001) **20**:7033–40. doi:10.1093/emboj/20.24.7033
95. Enyeart JA, Liu H, Enyeart JJ. Curcumin inhibits ACTH- and angiotensin II-stimulated cortisol secretion and Cav3.2 current. *J Nat Prod* (2009) **72**:1533–7. doi:10.1021/np900227x
96. Yunker AM. Modulation and pharmacology of low voltage-activated ("T-Type") calcium channels. *J Bioenerg Biomembr* (2003) **35**:577–98. doi:10.1023/B:JOBB.0000008024.77488.48
97. Kaneda M, Akaike N. The low-threshold Ca current in isolated amygdaloid neurons in the rat. *Brain Res* (1989) **497**:187–90. doi:10.1016/0006-8993(89)90987-6
98. Takahashi K, Akaike N. Calcium antagonist effects on low-threshold (T-type) calcium current in rat isolated hippocampal CA1 pyramidal neurons. *J Pharmacol Exp Ther* (1991) **256**:169–75.
99. Ertel SI, Clozel J-P. Mibefradil (Ro 40-5967): the first selective T-type calcium channel blocker. *Exp Opin Investig Drugs* (1997) **6**:569–82. doi:10.1517/13543784.6.5.569
100. Liu JH, Bijlenga P, Occhiodoro T, Fischer-Lougheed J, Bader CR, Bernheim L. Mibefradil (Ro 40-5967) inhibits several Ca2+ and K+ currents in human fusion-competent myoblasts. *Br J Pharmacol* (1999) **126**:245–50. doi:10.1038/sj.bjp.0702321
101. Stengel W, Jainz M, Andreas K. Different potencies of dihydropyridine derivatives in blocking T-type but not L-type Ca2+ channels in neuroblastoma-glioma hybrid cells. *Eur J Pharmacol* (1998) **342**:339–45. doi:10.1016/S0014-2999(97)01495-7
102. Furukawa T, Nukada T, Miura R, Ooga K, Honda M, Watanabe S, et al. Differential blocking action of dihydropyridine Ca2+ antagonists on a T-type Ca2+ channel (alpha1G) expressed in *Xenopus* oocytes. *J Cardiovasc Pharmacol* (2005) **45**:241–6. doi:10.1097/01.fjc.0000154374.88283.15
103. Kau MM, Lo MJ, Tsai SC, Chen JJ, Pu HF, Chien EJ, et al. Effects of prolactin on aldosterone secretion in rat zona glomerulosa cells. *J Cell Biochem* (1999) 72:286–93. doi:10.1002/(SICI)1097-4644(19990201)72:2<286::AID-JCB13>3.0.CO;2-4
104. Rossier MF, Python CP, Capponi AM, Schlegel W, Kwan CY, Vallotton MB. Blocking T-type calcium channels with tetrandrine inhibits steroidogenesis in bovine adrenal glomerulosa cells. *Endocrinology* (1993) **132**:1035–43. doi:10.1210/en.132.3.1035
105. Rossier MF, Ertel EA, Vallotton MB, Capponi AM. Inhibitory action of mibefradil on calcium signaling and aldosterone synthesis in bovine adrenal glomerulosa cells. *J Pharmacol Exp Ther* (1998) **287**:824–31.
106. Python CP, Rossier MF, Vallotton MB, Capponi AM. Peripheral-type benzodiazepines inhibit calcium channels and aldosterone production in adrenal glomerulosa cells. *Endocrinology* (1993) **132**:1489–96. doi:10.1210/endo.132.4.8384990
107. Okayama S, Imagawa K, Naya N, Iwama H, Somekawa S, Kawata H, et al. Blocking T-type Ca2+ channels with efonidipine decreased plasma aldosterone concentration in healthy volunteers. *Hypertens Res* (2006) **29**:493–7. doi:10.1291/hypres.29.493
108. Tanaka T, Tsutamoto T, Sakai H, Fujii M, Yamamoto T, Horie M. Comparison of the effects of efonidipine and amlodipine on aldosterone in patients with hypertension. *Hypertens Res* (2007) **30**:691–7. doi:10.1291/hypres.30.691
109. Burnay MM, Python CP, Vallotton MB, Capponi AM, Rossier MF. Role of the capacitative calcium influx in the activation of steroidogenesis by angiotensin II in adrenal glomerulosa cells. *Endocrinology* (1994) **135**:751–8. doi:10.1210/en.135.2.751
110. Rossier MF, Capponi AM. Antagonistes calciques et inhibition de la sécrétion d'aldostérone. *Métabol Horm Nutr* (2000) **IV**:101–6.

111. Li X, Yang MS. Effects of T-type calcium channel blockers on renal function and aldosterone in patients with hypertension: a systematic review and meta-analysis. *PLoS One* (2014) **9**:e109834. doi:10.1371/journal.pone.0109834
112. Rossier MF. T channels and steroid biosynthesis: in search of a link with mitochondria. *Cell Calcium* (2006) **40**:155–64. doi:10.1016/j.ceca.2006.04.020
113. Hosey MM, Lazdunski M. Calcium channels: molecular pharmacology, structure and regulation. *J Membr Biol* (1988) **104**:81–105. doi:10.1007/BF01870922
114. Hescheler J, Schulz G. G-proteins involved in the calcium channel signalling system. *Curr Opin Neurobiol* (1993) **3**:360–7. doi:10.1016/0959-4388(93)90129-M
115. Lu H-K, Fern RJ, Luthin D, Linden J, Liu L-P, Cohen CJ, et al. Angiotensin II stimulates T-type calcium channel currents *via* activation of a G protein, Gi. *Am J Physiol* (1996) **271**:C1340–9.
116. Lu H-K, Fern RJ, Nee JJ, Barrett PQ. Calcium-dependent activation of T-type calcium channels by calmodulin-dependent protein kinase II. *Am J Physiol* (1994) **267**:F183–9.
117. Fern RJ, Hahm MS, Lu H-K, Liu L-P, Gorelick FS, Barrett PQ. Calcium/calmodulin-dependent protein kinase II activation and regulation of adrenal glomerulosa calcium signaling. *Am J Physiol* (1995) **269**:F751–60.
118. Barrett PQ, Lu HK, Colbran R, Czernik A, Pancrazio JJ. Stimulation of unitary T-type Ca(2+) channel currents by calmodulin-dependent protein kinase II [In Process Citation]. *Am J Physiol Cell Physiol* (2000) **279**:C1694–703.
119. Rossier MF, Burnay MM, Maturana AD, Capponi AM. Duality of the voltage-dependent calcium influx in adrenal glomerulosa cells. *Endocr Res* (1998) **24**:443–7. doi:10.3109/07435809809032631
120. Maturana AD, Burnay MM, Capponi AM, Vallotton MB, Rossier MF. Angiotensin II type 1 receptor activation modulates L- and T-type calcium channel activity through distinct mechanisms in bovine adrenal glomerulosa cells. *J Recept Signal Transduct Res* (1999) **19**:509–20. doi:10.3109/10799899909036668
121. McCarthy RT, Isales CM, Bollag WB, Rasmussen H, Barrett PQ. Atrial natriuretic peptide differentially modulates T- and L-type calcium channels. *Am J Physiol* (1990) **258**:F473–8.
122. Osipenko ON, Varnai P, Mike A, Spät A, Vizi ES. Dopamine blocks T-type calcium channels in cultured rat adrenal glomerulosa cells. *Endocrinology* (1994) **134**:511–4. doi:10.1210/endo.134.1.7903936
123. Drolet P, Bilodeau L, Chorvátová A, Laflamme L, Gallo-Payet N, Payet MD. Inhibition of the T-type calcium current by the dopamine D1 receptor in rat adrenal glomerulosa cells: requirement of the combined action of the G beta gamma protein subunit and cyclic adenosine 3',5'-monophosphate. *Mol Endocrinol* (1997) **11**:503–14. doi:10.1210/me.11.4.503
124. Lenglet S, Louiset E, Delarue C, Vaudry H, Contesse V. Activation of 5-HT(7) receptor in rat glomerulosa cells is associated with an increase in adenylyl cyclase activity and calcium influx through T-type calcium channels. *Endocrinology* (2002) **143**:1748–60. doi:10.1210/endo.143.5.8817
125. Lesouhaitier O, Kodjo MK, Cartier F, Contesse V, Yon L, Delarue C, et al. The effect of the endozepine triakontatetraneuropeptide on corticosteroid secretion by the frog adrenal gland is mediated by activation of adenylyl cyclase and calcium influx through T-type calcium channels. *Endocrinology* (2000) **141**:197–207. doi:10.1210/en.141.1.197
126. Rossier MF, Capponi AM. Angiotensin II and calcium channels. *Vitam Horm* (2001) **60**:229–84. doi:10.1016/S0083-6729(00)60021-3
127. Hunyady L, Rohacs T, Bago A, Deak F, Spät A. Dihydropyridine-sensitive initial component of the angiotensin II-induced calcium response in rat adrenal glomerulosa cells. *Am J Physiol* (1994) **266**:C67–72.
128. Brauneis U, Vassilev PM, Quinn SJ, Williams GH, Tillotson DL. Angiotensin II blocks potassium currents in zona glomerulosa cells from rat, bovine and human adrenals. *Am J Physiol* (1991) **260**:E772–9.
129. Vassilev PM, Kanazirska MV, Quinn SJ, Tillotson DL, Williams GH. Potassium channels in adrenal zona glomerulosa cells: I. *Am J Physiol* (1992) **263**:E752–9.
130. Kanazirska MV, Vassilev PM, Quinn SJ, Tillotson DL, Williams GH. Single potassium channels in adrenal zona glomerulosa cells: II. Inhibition by angiotensin II. *Am J Physiol* (1992) **263**:E760–5.
131. Chorvátová A, Gallo-Payet N, Casanova C, Payet MD. Modulation of membrane potential and ionic currents by the AT1 and AT2 receptors of angiotensin II. *Cell Signal* (1996) **8**:525–32. doi:10.1016/S0898-6568(96)00117-9
132. Lotshaw DP. Characterization of angiotensin II-regulated potassium conductance in rat adrenal glomerulosa cells. *J Membr Biol* (1997) **156**:261–77. doi:10.1007/s002329900206
133. Payet MD, Bilodeau L, Drolet P, Ibarrondo J, Guillon G, Gallo-Payet N. Modulation of a calcium-activated potassium channel by angiotensin II in rat adrenal glomerulosa cells: involvement of a G protein. *Mol Endocrinol* (1995) **9**:935–47. doi:10.1210/me.9.8.935
134. Lobo MV, Marusic ET. Effect of angiotensin II, ATP, and ionophore A23187 on potassium efflux in adrenal glomerulosa cells. *Am J Physiol* (1986) **250**:E125–30.
135. Lobo MV, Marusic ET. Angiotensin II causes a dual effect on potassium permeability in adrenal glomerulosa cells. *Am J Physiol* (1988) **254**:E144–9.
136. Shepherd RM, Fraser R, Nichols DJ, Kenyon CJ. Efflux of potassium ions in angiotensin II-stimulated bovine adrenocortical cells. *J Endocrinol* (1991) **128**:297–304. doi:10.1677/joe.0.1280297
137. Lobo MV, Mendoza RR, Marusic ET. sn-1,2 dioctanoylglycerol mimics the effects of angiotensin II on aldosterone production and potassium permeability in isolated bovine glomerulosa cells. *J Steroid Biochem* (1990) **35**:29–33. doi:10.1016/0022-4731(90)90141-E
138. Shepherd RM, Fraser R, Kenyon CJ. Membrane permeability to potassium and the control of aldosterone synthesis: effects of valinomycin and cromakalim in bovine adrenocortical cells. *J Mol Endocrinol* (1992) **9**:165–73. doi:10.1677/jme.0.0090165
139. Lotshaw DP. Effects of potassium channel blockers on potassium channels, membrane potential, and aldosterone secretion in rat adrenal zona glomerulosa cells. *Endocrinology* (1997) **138**:4167–75. doi:10.1210/en.138.10.4167
140. Hadjokas NE, Goodfriend TL. Inhibition of aldosterone production and angiotensin action by drugs affecting potassium channels. *Pharmacol* (1991) **43**:141–50. doi:10.1159/000138839
141. Chorvátová A, Guyot A, Ojeda C, Rougier O, Bilbaut A. Activation by angiotensin II of calcium-dependent potasium and chloride currents in zona fasciculata cells of bovine adrenal gland. *J Membr Biol* (1998) **162**:39–50. doi:10.1007/s002329900340
142. Mlinar B, Biagi BA, Enyeart JJ. A novel potassium current inhibited by adrenocorticotropic hormone and angiotensin II in adrenal cortical cells. *J Biol Chem* (1993) **268**:8640–4.
143. Wickman K, Clapham DE. Ion channel regulation by G proteins. *Physiol Rev* (1995) **75**:865–79.
144. Aptel HBC, Johnson EIM, Vallotton MB, Rossier MF, Capponi AM. Demonstration of an angiotensin II-induced negative feedback effect on aldosterone synthesis in isolated rat adrenal zona glomerulosa cells. *Mol Cell Endocrinol* (1996) **119**:105–11. doi:10.1016/0303-7207(96)03805-1
145. Louiset E, Contesse V, Groussin L, Cartier D, Duparc C, Barrande G, et al. Expression of serotonin7 receptor and coupling of ectopic receptors to protein kinase A and ionic currents in adrenocorticotropin-independent macronodular adrenal hyperplasia causing Cushing's syndrome. *J Clin Endocrinol Metab* (2006) **91**:4578–86. doi:10.1210/jc.2006-0538
146. Aguilera G, Catt KJ. Dopaminergic modulation of aldosterone secretion in the rat. *Endocrinology* (1984) **114**:176–81. doi:10.1210/endo-114-1-176
147. Rossier MF, Krause K-H, Lew PD, Capponi AM, Vallotton MB. Control of cytosolic free calcium by intracellular organelles in bovine adrenal glomerulosa cells: effects of sodium and inositol 1,4,5-trisphosphate. *J Biol Chem* (1987) **262**:4053–8.
148. Capponi AM, Rossier MF, Davies E, Vallotton MB. Calcium stimulates steroidogenesis in permeabilized bovine adrenal cortical cells. *J Biol Chem* (1988) **263**:16113–7.
149. Rossier MF. Confinement of intracellular calcium signaling in secretory and steroidogenic cells. *Eur J Endocrinol* (1997) **137**:317–25. doi:10.1530/eje.0.1370317
150. Cherradi N, Rossier MF, Vallotton MB, Capponi AM. Calcium stimulates intramitochondrial cholesterol transfer in bovine adrenal glomerulosa cells. *J Biol Chem* (1996) **271**:25971–5. doi:10.1074/jbc.271.42.25971
151. Cherradi N, Rossier MF, Vallotton MB, Timberg R, Friedberg I, Orly J, et al. Submitochondrial distribution of three key steroidogenic proteins (steroidogenic acute regulatory protein, P450 side-chain cleavage and 3β-hydroxysteroid dehydrogenase isomerase enzymes) upon stimulation

by intracellular calcium in adrenal glomerulosa cells. *J Biol Chem* (1997) **272**:7899–907.

152. Brandenburger Y, Kennedy ED, Python CP, Rossier MF, Vallotton MB, Wollheim CB, et al. Possible role for mitochondrial calcium in angiotensin II- and potassium-stimulated steroidogenesis in bovine adrenal glomerulosa cells. *Endocrinology* (1996) **137**:5544–51. doi:10.1210/endo.137.12.8940382
153. Nagai T, Sawano A, Park ES, Miyawaki A. Circularly permuted green fluorescent proteins engineered to sense Ca2+. *Proc Natl Acad Sci U S A* (2001) **98**:3197–202. doi:10.1073/pnas.051636098
154. Lalevee N, Resin V, Arnaudeau S, Demaurex N, Rossier MF. Intracellular transport of calcium from plasma membrane to mitochondria in adrenal H295R cells: implication for steroidogenesis. *Endocrinology* (2003) **144**:4575–85. doi:10.1210/en.2003-0268
155. Putney JW Jr. A model for receptor-regulated calcium entry. *Cell Calcium* (1986) **7**:1–12. doi:10.1016/0143-4160(86)90026-6
156. Putney JW Jr. Capacitative calcium entry revisited. *Cell Calcium* (1990) **11**:611–24. doi:10.1016/0143-4160(90)90016-N
157. Putney JW Jr. "Kissin' cousins": intimate plasma membrane-endoplasmic reticulum interactions underlie capacitative calcium entry. *Cell* (1999) **99**:5–8. doi:10.1016/S0092-8674(00)80056-2
158. Gray LS, Perez-Reyes E, Gomora JC, Haverstick DM, Shattock M, McLatchie L, et al. The role of voltage gated T-type Ca2+ channel isoforms in mediating "capacitative" Ca2+ entry in cancer cells. *Cell Calcium* (2004) **36**:489–97. doi:10.1016/j.ceca.2004.05.001
159. Yanagibashi K, Papadopoulos V, Masaki E, Iwaki T, Kawamura M, Hall PF. Forskolin activates voltage-dependent Ca2+ channels in bovine but not in rat fasciculata cells. *Endocrinology* (1989) **124**:2383–91. doi:10.1210/endo-124-5-2383
160. Yanagibashi K, Kawamura M, Hall PF. Voltage-dependent Ca2+ channels are involved in regulation of steroid synthesis by bovine but not rat fasciculata cells. *Endocrinology* (1990) **127**:311–8. doi:10.1210/endo-127-1-311

17

Adrenocortical Gap Junctions and Their Functions

*Cheryl L. Bell and Sandra A. Murray**

Department of Cell Biology, University of Pittsburgh School of Medicine, Pittsburgh, PA, USA

Correspondence:
Sandra A. Murray
smurray@pitt.edu

Adrenal cortical steroidogenesis and proliferation are thought to be modulated by gap junction-mediated direct cell–cell communication of regulatory molecules between cells. Such communication is regulated by the number of gap junction channels between contacting cells, the rate at which information flows between these channels, and the rate of channel turnover. Knowledge of the factors regulating gap junction-mediated communication and the turnover process are critical to an understanding of adrenal cortical cell functions, including development, hormonal response to adrenocorticotropin, and neoplastic dedifferentiation. Here, we review what is known about gap junctions in the adrenal gland, with particular attention to their role in adrenocortical cell steroidogenesis and proliferation. Information and insight gained from electrophysiological, molecular biological, and imaging (immunocytochemical, freeze fracture, transmission electron microscopic, and live cell) techniques will be provided.

Keywords: ACTH, connexin, gap junction plaques, gap junction vesicles, steroidogenesis

INTRODUCTION

The adrenal is a complex gland that is histologically and functionally two tissues, the cortex and medulla, within a connective tissue capsule (1). Not only the two regions of the adrenal gland are from different embryonic origins but also the cells of the medulla are composed of cells that have a neuroendocrine function, while the cells of the cortex are epithelial cells that function in endocrine metabolism. There is evidence that cells of both the cortex and the medulla are regulated by cell–cell communication of regulatory molecules through membrane channels, called gap junctions (2–8). The efficiency of the adrenal gland, as well as other endocrine glands, to respond to stimulation is thought to depend not only on hormone receptor interaction but also on intercellular communication through gap junctions.

Gap junctions in the adrenal gland, as in other tissues, provide low-resistance pathways for the direct intercellular exchange of small molecules (9, 10). In early years, gap junctions and cell communication were mainly studied with electron microscopic (11–13), electrophysiological (14), and fluorescent dye transfer (15, 16) techniques. More recently, however, the proteins (connexins) composing the gap junction pore have been identified, and the tissue distribution of the different connexin family members has been demonstrated (17–20). Further, the molecular details of the

---

Abbreviations: 18-alpha/beta GA, 18-alpha/beta glycerrhetinic acid; ACTH, adrenocorticotropin hormone; DbcAMP, dibutyryl cyclic adenosine monophosphate; FSH, follicle-stimulating hormone; GFP, green fluorescent protein; LAMP, lysosomal-associated membrane protein; MAPK, mitogen-activated protein kinase; PKA, protein kinase A; PKC, protein kinase C; RNAi, RNA interference; SBAC, bovine adrenal cortical cell line; SW-13, Scott white human adrenal cortical tumor cell line; TEM, transmission electron microscopy; TPA, 12-O-tetradecanoylphorbol-13-acetate; Y-1, mouse adrenal cortical tumor cell line.

assembly of connexins into functional gap junction channels, the involvement of kinases in this assembly, and the architectural arrangement of connexins into functional pore complexes have been described (21, 22).

In this review, we present a historical summary of gap junctions in the adrenal cortex from their discovery with imaging and electrophysiological techniques to current studies of the connexin types, distribution, abundance, and turnover. The role of gap junctions in the adrenal cortical response to adrenocorticotropin (ACTH) will be discussed, and the fundamental concepts and implication of gap junctions in steroidogenesis, proliferation, and cancer will be analyzed. Finally, gap junction-mediated cross talk between the cells of the adrenal cortex and medulla will be discussed, as it relates to adrenocortical function. We will begin with a brief review of gap junctions in the adrenal cortex.

CHARACTERIZATION OF GAP JUNCTIONS IN THE ADRENAL CORTEX

Gap junctions occur between the membranes of two closely opposed cells and are characterized by the pairing of intramembranous connexin complexes across a 2–4 nm gap (**Figures 1** and **2**) (23). The first transmission electron microscopic images of gap junction plaques in the adrenal gland were acquired from fetal rat adrenals in 1970 (24) and more extensively from adult glands of a number of animals in 1972 (11, 25). Gap junctions in the adrenal resembled those of other tissues and were positively identified by the presence of the characteristic pentalaminar membrane and the 2–4 nm gap separating the membrane of two adjacent cells (**Figure 2A**). The area of membrane covered by gap junction plaques (plaque size) and the packing pattern of adrenal cortical cell gap junction channels could be obtained with freeze-fracture electron microscopy (11). With this technique, the adrenal cell membrane bilayer was split in the hydrophobic plane (26), and the typical protoplasmic (P)-fracture face and extracellular (E)-fracture face distribution of membrane particles was used to identify gap junctions (**Figure 2B**). Gap junctions could be distinguished by the observed clustering of 8.5 nm particles on the P-fracture face and pits on the E-fracture face (27, 28) (**Figure 2B**). With freeze-fracture techniques, the size of gap junction plaques was demonstrated in the rat adrenal cortex to be larger and more abundant than those found in most other tissues of the body, especially those plaques in the area of the adrenal cortex near or juxtaposed to the medulla (24). Gap junction plaques have now been described in the adrenal from a vast number of different mammalian species (6, 29–31). An important advantage of freeze-fracture imaging was the capacity to confirm that the adrenal cortical gap junctions were composed of aggregates of intramembranous particles that were paired with one another across the intercellular space. The observation that these paired particles extended across the gap, seen with transmission electron microscopy, provided structural evidence for the existence of channels, which could serve as means for movement of molecules between cells. However, the critical role of gap junctions as channels for communication was established by experiments in which it was demonstrated that hepatocytes and myocardial cells only passed current if gap junctions were observed and if gap junctions were not present, current did not pass between cells (32).

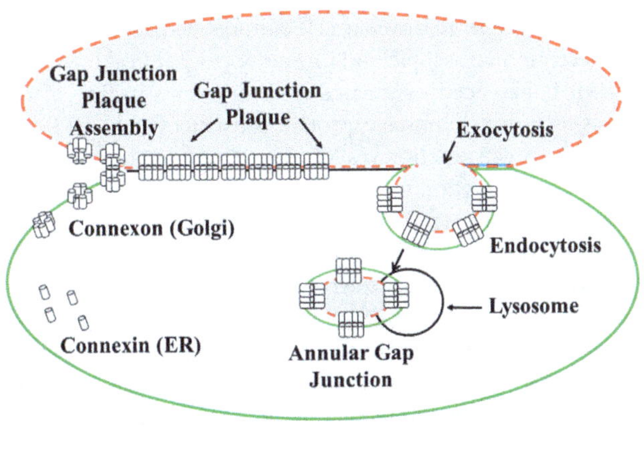

FIGURE 1 | Illustration of the formation and degradation of gap junction plaques and annular gap junctions. Connexin proteins synthesized in the endoplasmic reticulum (ER) oligomerize to form connexon complexes. The connexons are transported to the cell surface and inserted into the plasma membrane where they form hemichannels. These hemichannels can dock with hemichannels of an apposing cell and cluster to form a gap junction plaque, characterized by a 2–4 nm gap between the two cell membranes. Gap junction plaques are removed from the cell surface through endoexocytosis, which results in the formation of an annular gap junction. The annular gap junction is then degraded through lysosomal proteolysis [modified from Ref. (130)].

The movement of current was first demonstrated in the adrenal cortex with electrophysiological techniques in experiments, which used adult and fetal rabbit adrenal gland slices (10). Although such studies confirmed that material was capable of communicating between cells in the adrenal, the function of this movement was not addressed in these early studies. In addition, information on the possible size of molecules that could move between the gap junction channels was provided from dye transfer studies in which molecules smaller than 1,000 Da could communicate between cells while larger molecules were excluded (16, 33, 34). Based mainly on the early electrophysiological and dye transfer studies, as well as transmission electron microscopic and freeze-fracture images, it was hypothesized that gap junctions allowed the passage of molecules between adjacent cells, and thus, modulate adrenal cortical cell population growth and hormonal response (8, 35). However, the molecules composing and regulating the gap junction pore and, more important, the definitive role of gap junction-mediated communication in adrenal cortical function remained to be defined.

Our knowledge concerning the role of gap junctions, in general, was greatly enhanced by the isolation and characterization of the connexin proteins that composed gap junction pores. It has become clear that the particles seen with freeze-fracture electron microscopy are the gap junction channels and that each gap junction channel consists of 12 connexin molecules, 6 from one cell docked to 6 in the adjacent cell. The clustering of these channels forms the gap junction plaque (27, 36).

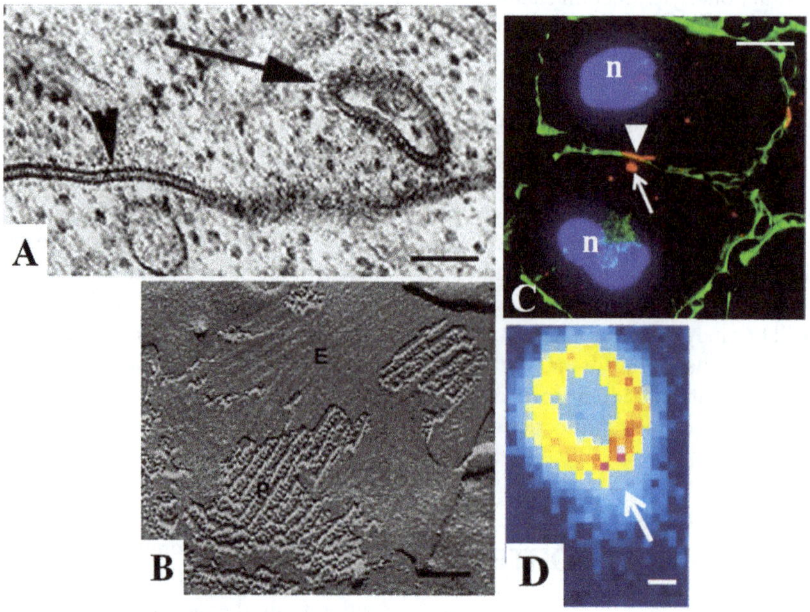

FIGURE 2 | Characterization of gap junctions in SW-13 adrenocortical tumor cells. The size, location, and structure of gap junction plaques (arrowheads) and annular gap junctions (arrows) have been determined with **(A)** transmission electron microscopy, **(B)** freeze-fracture electron microscopy, **(C)** immunofluorescence, and **(D)** confocal microscopy. The protoplasmic (P) and extracellular (E) fracture faces are shown in the freeze-fracture replica of the gap junction plaque in **(B)**. Cell borders are defined by cortical actin (green) in **(C)**. Note the lumen of the annular gap junction revealed with confocal microscopy in **(D)**. n, nucleus. Bars: **(A)** 100 nm, **(B)** 60 nm, **(C)** 10 µm, and **(D)** 0.3 µm. [**(A)** from Ref. (48), **(B)** from Ref. (130), **(C)** from Ref. (131), and **(D)** from Ref. (132)].

The production of antibodies directed at the connexin proteins allowed the detection of gap junction protein types with immunofluorescence and western blot techniques (19, 20, 37). In humans, there are 21 different connexin types that differ by their amino acid sequences and molecular weights (38). Connexin 43 (Cx43) gap junction protein was demonstrated as the major, if not only, connexin gap junction protein type in the adrenal cortex (5, 30, 31, 39, 40). While investigators have also reported Cx26, Cx32, and Cx50 in humans (41), their expression has not been reported in other mammals (3, 6, 7, 42). It should be noted, however, that of the 21 known connexin family members (38), only 6 have been extensively evaluated in the adrenal cortex, and it is possible that others will be detected with further analysis.

With immunofluorescence microscopy, the distribution of Cx43 could be quickly detected and its distribution more reliably compared with adrenal zones than with conventional transmission electron microscopy (5, 30, 40, 43). The Cx43 gap junctions in the adrenal cortex appear as small puncta or longer plaques on the cell surface between contacting cells (**Figures 2C,D**). The cells of the adrenal cortex are polyhedral in shape, and their three-dimensional relationship to one another has been revealed with serial section transmission electron microscopy (44) and scanning electron microscopy of freeze-cracked adrenal glands (45). Based on the three-dimensional imaging provided by these techniques, gap junctions are thought to form at smooth "contact" sites and on facets on microvilli of cells (45). The facets from two cells were observed to be in close apposition, and it is here as well as at the smooth sites on the cell body that the gap junctions most likely are formed (45).

In addition to the typical surface gap junction plaques, cytoplasmic gap junction vesicles have also been reported in the adrenal gland and in adrenal cell cultures with both transmission electron microscopic and immunocytochemical techniques (46–49). It has been confirmed with live cell imaging of cells expressing green fluorescent protein construct (Cx43-GFP) that these annular gap junction vesicles form from a unique process in which the gap junction membrane of one cell is internalized into the cytoplasm of the adjacent cell to form a double-membraned vesicle composed of gap junction protein. This internalization process occurs from the central regions of the gap junction plaques or, in some cases, the entire gap junction plaque membrane is internalized. Once internalized, the annular gap junction vesicle is degraded (50–52), and thus, this is a method for disassembling gap junction plaques and regulating communication. In contrast, gap junction plaque assembly occurs by the addition of new gap junction channels at the gap junction plaque periphery (53). Mechanisms for controlling cell–cell communication are thought to involve both the assembly of gap junction plaques at the cell surface and the disassembly of these plaques by an internalization process that results in annular gap junction vesicle release into the cytoplasm. The capacity to specifically analyze connexin protein distribution within specific compartments is particularly critical for the study of tissues, such as the adrenal, which have cells that express different steroidogenic enzymes and respond differently to stimuli, based on their specific zonal locations.

GAP JUNCTION DISTRIBUTION IN THE ADRENAL CORTEX

In the human, the adrenal cortex can be divided into three morphologically and functionally distinct zones: the outer most zone, zona glomerulosa, and the inner zones, zona fasciculata (ZF) and zona reticularis (ZR). These zones are composed of cells that express different steroidogenic enzymes and thus produce different steroid hormones. Specifically, the ZF produces glucocorticoids, and the ZR produces androgens. Both of these inner zones secrete hormones in response to ACTH. The outer zone, however, produces aldosterone in response to changes in sodium, potassium, and the peptide hormone, angiotensin II.

Just as the three zones of the adrenal have been demonstrated to be morphologically and functionally distinct, the level of expression of gap junction protein in the three zones of the adrenal has been demonstrated to differ using immunocytochemistry (**Figures 3** and **4**). Specifically, a differential distribution of Cx43 has been reported in the adrenal of human (4, 42) as well as a host of other mammals including rat (3, 5), mouse (40, 54), guinea pig (55), rhesus monkey (40), and cow (4, 8). Specifically, little or no Cx43 gap junction protein was detected between adrenal cells in the zona glomerulosa. In contrast, numerous gap junction plaques were evident at areas of cell–cell contact in the inner cortical areas, such as the ZF and ZR (**Figure 3**). The distribution of gap junctions once speculated from transmission electron and freeze-fracture microscopy (29, 55) could be confirmed and, more importantly quantitated, while simultaneously validating which zone was being viewed. With computer-assisted microspectrofluorometric image analysis, it was demonstrated that there were twice as many gap junctions per area between cells in the ZR than between cells in the ZF (6). While the number of gap junctions differed, there were no significant differences in the average size of gap junctions in the rat ZF compared with those in the ZR.

Consistent with the immunocytochemical quantitative analysis, when the expression of Cx43-encoded mRNA was analyzed with Northern Blot techniques in samples prepared from the capsule of the adrenal gland, which contain adherent zona glomerulosa cells, there was little gap junction RNA detected. In contrast, samples prepared from decapsulated glands, which contained mainly the ZF/ZR cells, had an abundance of gap junction RNA. It is thought that the detection of small amounts of Cx43-encoded mRNA in the zona glomerulosa with Northern Blot and almost no Cx43 gap junction proteins detected with immunocytochemical analysis may reflect possible contamination of the zona glomerulosa-enriched samples with cells from the ZF. In addition, some of the mRNA Cx43 detected with Northern Blot in the zona glomerulosa-enriched samples is thought to come from the presence of fibroblastic cells from the connective tissue capsule and trabeculea that project into the substance of the cortex in the sample (**Figure 3D**). In fact, these trabeculea within the substance of the gland were revealed with immunocytochemistry. To increase the accuracy for comparing the distribution of gap junctions with adrenal cortical zones, Oil Red O staining, which detects lipid droplets in the cytoplasm of cells in the ZF and ZR (56), has been used. The Oil Red O stain is much less abundant in zona glomerulosa cells that have few, if any, lipid droplets (56).

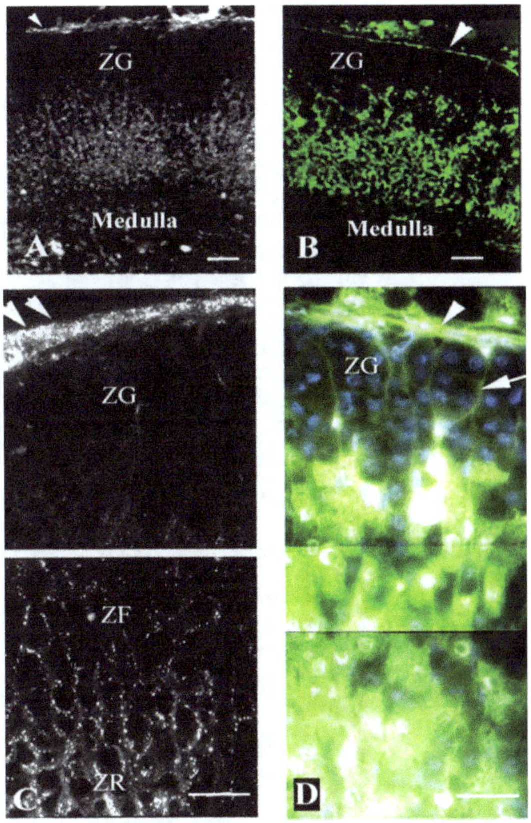

FIGURE 3 | Gap junction (Cx43) localization and dye communication in the intact adrenal gland. Immunohistochemical localization of Cx43 gap junction proteins revealed extensive staining in the zona fasciculata (ZF) and zona reticularis (ZR), while there was limited staining in the zona glomerulosa (ZF) [left panels: **(A,C)**]. Correspondingly, lucifer yellow dye communication between cells was more abundant in the inner zones of the adrenal cortex (ACTH responsive areas) than in the outer zone [right panels: **(B,D)**]. Capsule (arrowheads), connective tissue trabecule (arrow), and Cx43 (white puncta). Bars: **(A,B)** 50 μm and **(C,D)** 30 μm [modified from Ref. (30)].

The pattern of Oil Red O staining distinguished the cells of the zona glomerulosa from cells of ZF and ZR and substantiated that the cells which lack Cx43 gap junction staining are indeed cells of the zona glomerulosa (**Figure 4**) (30).

In parallel to the differential localization of gap junction plaques is the pattern of dye communication in the intact adrenal cortex. Specifically, lucifer yellow dye moved extensively in the inner cortex while dye communication was limited to the capsular projections of connective tissue between the cells of the zona glomerulosa (**Figures 3B,D** and **4B,D**) (5, 30). Dye communication was not observed between cells of the zona glomerulosa. This lack of dye movement would be consistent with the observed absence of Cx43 protein in immunofluorescence studies and would further support the suggestion that other connexin family members do not assemble into functional gap junctions in this zone. In the inner two cortical zones, where gap junctions were plentiful, dye was transferred (30). It should be noted that while Cx43 was found in the inner two zones, it is possible that connexin types, other than Cx43, may be located

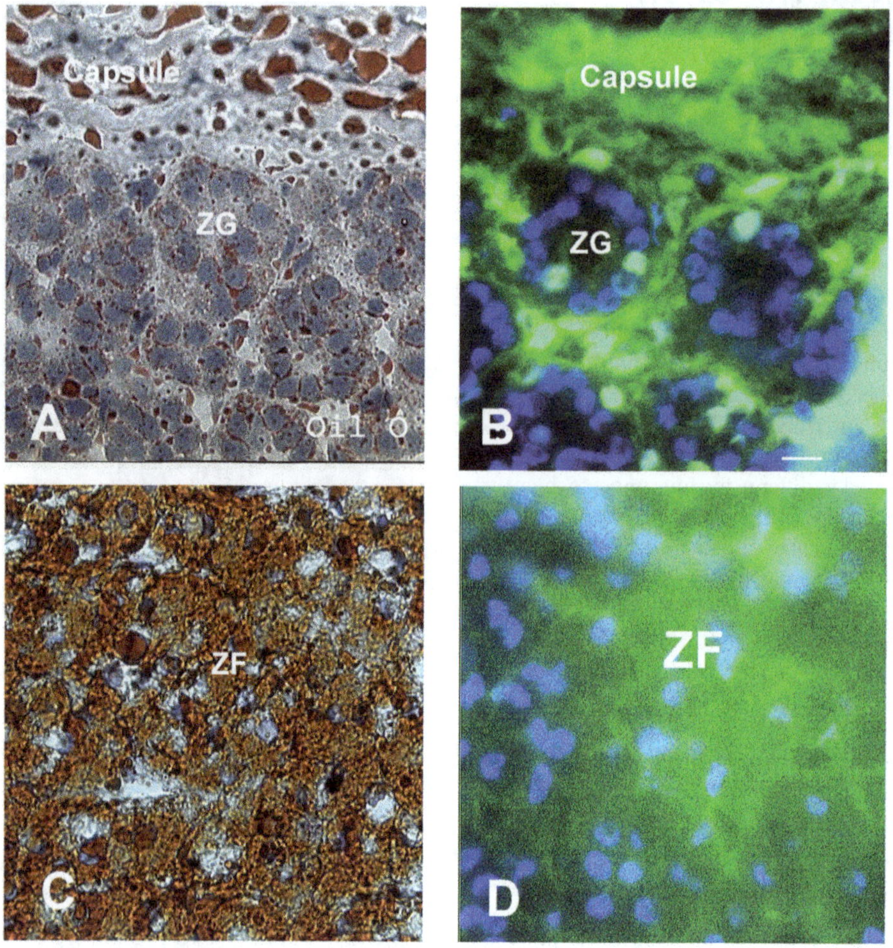

FIGURE 4 | Communication in the intact adrenal cortex. Oil Red O staining was used to distinguish the lipid-rich zona fasciculata and zona reticularis from the zona glomerulosa **(A,C)**. Lucifer yellow dye was transferred between the fibroblasts of the connective tissue capsule and trabeculae; however, communication was absent between cells of the zona glomerulosa **(B)**. The cells of the inner two cortical zones, particularly those in the zona fasciculata, exhibited extensive dye communication **(D)**. Note the Lucifer yellow and Oil Red O staining are diffuse and seen throughout the cytoplasm, which somewhat obscures the cell boundaries and nuclei. Bars: **(A–D)** 30 μm [modified from Ref. (30)].

in these inner two zones since not all of the 21 known connexin family members have been evaluated. In addition, there is a possibility that other, yet to be discovered, connexin type could be detected in the future. It is speculated that while cells of the zona glomerulosa, for reasons yet to be determined, are less dependent on cell–cell communication, the communication of a regulatory molecule between cells of the inner two layers modulates their functions.

ROLE OF GAP JUNCTIONS IN ADRENAL CORTICAL FUNCTION

Steroidogenesis

Gap junctions, for years, have been suggested to play a key role in a number of physiological phenomena (3, 57, 58). However, in early years, this proposed role was solely based on the observations that dye and current could move between cells that had gap junctions and not on experimental evidence that demonstrates actual physiological responses. Adrenal cortical cells were one of the first endocrine cell types in which a direct relationship was established between gap junctions and physiological responses (59). Furthermore, the findings in the adrenal cortex have been used to lend support to the speculations that gap junctions influence physiological events in other cell types (60, 61).

The first set of experiments, which demonstrated functional gap junction-mediated communication, were studies in which adrenal cells were placed into culture with ovarian granulosa cells. It is well documented that cells of the inner adrenal cortical zones possess specific receptors for ACTH and, when bound to its receptor, ACTH elicits a number of responses (62, 63), including an activation of cAMP-dependent protein kinase A (PKA) (59, 64), an increase in steroid synthesis (7, 65, 66), and a decrease in proliferation of cells in culture (2, 8, 67). In the adrenal/granulosa coculture populations, a cytochemical method was used to specifically localize free catalytic subunits (C) of PKA at subcellular, light microscopic levels of resolution

(59, 68). In these studies, heterotypic, adrenal/granulosa, cell pairs were demonstrated to form gap junctions and ACTH treatment activated PKA in the adrenal cell populations (59). Moreover, ACTH stimulation not only, as expected, activated PKA in the adrenal cells but also with time, within the granulosa cells that were in contact with adrenal cells. The ovarian granulosa cells lacked ACTH receptors but had receptors for follicle-stimulating hormone (FSH), which activates PKA (69). Treatment of the coculture cell population with FSH activated PKA in the granulosa cells and in the adrenal cells that formed cell contacts with granulosa cells (**Figure 5**). Importantly, adrenal cell secretion of steroid hormones was increased (59). The finding that hormone treatment stimulated bidirectional exchange of a signal that initiated PKA activation in adrenal/granulosa coculture cell populations provided compelling evidence that the hormone-induced intercellular communication, which activated PKA, could serve a biological role.

In further support of the biological role of gap junctions in adrenal cortical function, inhibition of gap-junctional communication with 18-alpha glycyrrhetinic acid (18-alpha GA) treatment decreased the steroidogenic responsiveness of bovine adrenal cells in culture to ACTH (4). Specifically, it was demonstrated that 18-alpha GA treatment decreased the steroidogenic response to a submaximal dose of ACTH but did not decrease steroidogenesis if cells were treated with saturating doses of ACTH (4). A similar decrease in ACTH-stimulated steroidogenesis was demonstrated in bovine and human cell lines and in rat primary cell populations treated with 18-alpha GA (8). The effects of treatment with this glycyrrhetinic acid derivative were also substantiated in experiments in which Cx43 antisense transfection techniques were used to inhibit gap junction-mediated communication (8). Cell populations expressing Cx43 antisense grew faster, had decreased capacity for cell–cell communication, and had a diminished steroidogenic responsiveness to ACTH treatment compared with null transfected control populations (8). This decrease in ACTH-mediated steroidogenesis following gap junction inhibition by either chemical treatment or Cx43 antisense expression is consistent with the concept that gap junction-mediated communication is a necessary factor in hormonal response. It has been suggested that gap junction communication of cAMP signaling, and subsequent PKA activation in the recipient cell, may increase the efficiency of hormone response by facilitating amplification of ACTH signaling throughout the population. This would be particularly useful at submaximal stimulation doses of the hormone, as suggested by Munari-Silem, when only a small population of the cells may be responding to ACTH (4).

In addition to 18-alpha, 18-beta glycerrhetinic acid (18-beta GA) has also been used in a number of studies to inhibit gap junction communication (70–72). Huang and colleagues found that treatment with 18-beta GA increased the basal levels of steroidogenesis secreted in rat primary adrenal cell cultures (73). These findings are interesting given that the increased steroidogenesis appears to be PKA-independent and would suggest a direct effect of the 18-beta GA on the production of steroidogenic enzymes in addition to their effect on inhibition of gap junction-mediated cell communication. It should be noted that neither cell communication nor the effect of ACTH stimulation was measured in this study. Further investigations are needed to determine if the concentrations of 18-beta GA used in this study eliminated cell–cell communication, and more importantly, if the ACTH-stimulated steroidogenesis at submaximal and saturating treatment doses were altered. It should also be noted that both 18-alpha and 18-beta GA have formulas very similar to that of cortisol and may be mistaken, with some assay methods, for an adrenal steroid (74).

Proliferation

In the intact adrenal gland, it was noted that the cells of the zona glomerulosa, which had few if any gap junctions, divided rapidly. In contrast, cells of the inner zones, where gap junctions were more abundant, proliferated more slowly (6, 40). Based on this inverse relationship between the rate of proliferation in the adrenal zones and the presence of gap junctions, it was suggested that gap junctions play a role in regulating cell proliferation in the adrenal cortex.

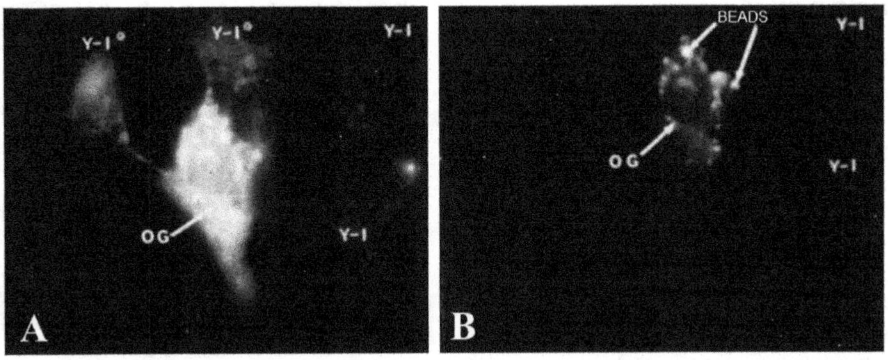

FIGURE 5 | Cocultured adrenal/granulosa cell pairs. Adrenal cell clusters viewed with optics specific for fluorescein isothiocyanate **(A)** or rhodamine isothiocyanate **(B)** were treated with follicle-stimulating hormone (FSH) for 30 min. Abundant protein kinase dissociation was initially observed in granulosa cells (OG) and could be seen, after 5–15 min, in two adrenal cells (Y-1*) that are in contact with the granulosa cell, while two nearby adrenal cells (Y-1) that are not in contact with the granulosa cell failed to dissociate PKA **(A)**. Granulosa cells were identified by pre-labeling them with rhodamine-coated beads **(B)** [modified from Ref. (59)].

In the zona glomerulosa, it has been suggested that the lack of gap junctions and thus capacity for direct communication of growth regulatory molecules would result in more cell proliferation in this zone. Along these same lines of evidence, the slower proliferation rate of cells in the inner zones, where gap junctions are more abundant (5, 40), would be consistent with their greater capacity to communicate growth inhibitory signals. Many factors are known to regulate growth, and gap junction-mediated communication may play a key role by facilitating the movement of these factors between the cells.

In support of the hypothesis that gap junctions contribute to the control of adrenal cell proliferation, possibly by allowing passage of molecules between cells, are the findings that cell proliferation of bovine adrenal cortical cell (SBAC) populations was significantly increased if gap junction protein expression was suppressed by Cx43 gap junction cDNA antisense transfection techniques (8). The average number and size of gap junction plaques decreased while the rate of population growth increased in these studies (8). Conversely, when adrenal cells were treated with ACTH, which increased gap junction protein expression, there was a corresponding decrease in cell population growth (8). Both the ACTH-stimulated increase in gap junction protein expression and decrease in cell population growth were mimicked by treatment with the second messenger, dibutyryl cyclic adenosine monophosphate [DbcAMP (1 mM)]. It is, thus, thought that the ACTH-induced alterations in Cx43 gap junction protein expression and proliferation are modulated by a PKA mechanism. Further, the findings of an inverse relationship between gap junctions and proliferation would suggest that, in the adrenal cortex, along with the multiple mechanisms known to be involved in controlling adrenal gland structure and function, ACTH-stimulated intercellular communication *via* gap junctions may represent an important factor in adrenal gland behavior. However, not only is gap junction-mediated cell communication thought to regulate ACTH-induced changes in steroidogenesis and proliferation but also there is compelling evidence that ACTH serves to regulate gap junction protein expression and stability at the cell surface.

REGULATION OF GAP JUNCTION EXPRESSION

In a number of studies of adrenal cells in culture, ACTH has been demonstrated to increase gap junction protein expression and to increase the size and number of surface gap junction plaques (4, 7, 8). These effects on gap junctions can be mimicked by treatments that increase cAMP levels and activate PKA (59, 64). Specifically, an increase in gap junction plaque size and number at the cell surface as well as the decrease in gap junction plaque disassembly (internalization to form annular gap junctions) was reported following DbcAMP treatment. These results are consistent with the theory that the changes in gap junctions following ACTH treatment were dependent on cAMP and the activation of protein kinase. Conversely, elevation of cAMP and PKA activation has been demonstrated to decrease the number of annular gap junctions in adrenal cortical cells (75). This suggests that PKA activation may decrease gap junction plaque internalization, which would further contribute to the observed increase in gap junction plaques at the cell surface following treatments that elevate cAMP levels in adrenal cell populations.

In addition to the findings made in adrenal cell cultures, the relationship between gap junction protein expression, occurrence, distribution, and ACTH levels in the body have been evaluated in studies in which the tropic state of the adrenal gland was altered by surgical removal of the pituitary (46). The removal of the pituitary, termed hypophysectomy, eliminates the source of ACTH since the pituitary secretes this as well as a variety of other hormones that are either produced by cells of the anterior pituitary (growth hormone, gonadotrophins, prolactin, and thyroid stimulating hormone) or by cells of the hypothalamus and then stored in the pituitary (antidiuretic hormone and oxytocin) (1, 76). The elimination of ACTH by hypophysectomy led to a profound atrophy of the cortex, which was more marked in the inner zones (ZF and ZR) than in the zona glomerulosa (46). While increasing ACTH levels increased gap junctions, eliminating ACTH by perturbing the pituitary–adrenal gland axis by hypophysectomy in mice led to diminished Cx43 gap junction expression mainly in the ZF (**Figure 6**) (31). If these hypophysectomized animals were treated with ACTH, Cx43 gap junction plaque size was increased (46). The increase in gap junction protein expression occurred in the ACTH-dependent zones (ZF and ZR) with no change in the ACTH-independent zone (zona glomerulosa). Thus Cx43 gap junction protein expression can be regulated *in vivo* as well as in adrenal cell populations maintained in culture, in further support that ACTH can modulate gap junctions.

The molecular mechanism for how ACTH may modulate gap junctions has not been demonstrated in the adrenal gland. It is well documented, however, that ACTH treatment results in PKA activation (64); reviewed by Ruggiero and Lalli (77), and in a number of other cell types, activation of PKA has been shown to increase gap junction plaque assembly by facilitating the phosphorylation of gap junction protein (78). Specifically, PKA activation results in the phosphorylation of serines (S364, S365,

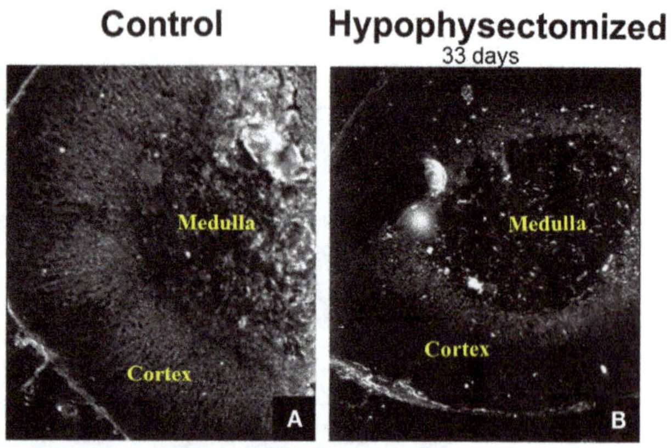

FIGURE 6 | Immunohistochemical demonstration of gap junction (Cx43) distribution in the adrenal gland. Gap junction proteins were abundant in the inner cortex of the mouse adrenal **(A)**. Hypophysectomy led to diminished Cx43 gap junction expression mainly in the zona fasciculata at 33 days post-surgery **(B)** [modified from Ref. (31)].

S369, and S373) on the C-terminal tail of Cx43 (78). Treatment with ACTH, based on this information, would be expected to phosphorylate one or more of these serines. There is a need, however, for increased information on the relationship between ACTH treatment and connexin phosphorylation if we are to fully understand the role of gap junction function in adrenal cell behavior.

To date, the largest increase in information on gap junction regulation and function comes from the knowledge of which Cx43 C-terminal tail amino acids are phosphorylated and dephosphorylated (22, 78–81). Phosphorylation/dephosphorylation events on the C-terminal tail of Cx43 are dependent on activation of PKA, as well as a number of other kinases including protein kinase C (PKC), tyrosine kinase, mitogen-activated protein kinase (MAPK), and casein kinase 1 (22, 82–84). These protein kinases, through triggering the phosphorylation of particular amino acids on the tail of Cx43, regulate gap junctions (assembly into plaques, stability at the cell surface, gap junction plaque disassembly, and cell–cell communication). Specifically, there are at least 11 serine and 2 tyrosine residues on the C-terminal tail of Cx43 (Cx43-C-terminus) that, when phosphorylated, result in either an increase in gap junction function (S325, S328, S330, S364/365, and S373) or the downregulation of gap junction activity (Y247, S255, S262, Y265, S279/282, and S368) (85–87). These observations have been made mainly from studies in clonal lines of murine fibroblasts (L929 cells), fibroblasts derived from Cx43 knockout and wild-type mice, rat liver epithelial cells (T51B), HeLa cells, and rat primary granulosa cells (88). It should be noted that ACTH-mediated activation of either S364, S365, S369, S373, or other possible amino acids of the C-terminal tail of Cx43 has not, to our knowledge, been examined. Furthermore, protein kinase-mediated phosphorylation of the C-terminus of Cx43 has been demonstrated to play a role in gap junction plaque internalization and annular gap junction vesicle formation (89, 90). Specifically, MAPK, casein kinase 1, and PKC activation increases the number of annular gap junction vesicles while decreasing gap junctions on the cell surface (69, 80, 89–92). In the case of PKC-mediated hyperphosphorylation of Cx43, it is thought that phosphorylation makes this connexin more vulnerable to proteolytic degradation, thus decreasing gap junction-mediated communication. The interplay between the various kinase pathways in Cx43 phosphorylation and cell–cell communication have not been elucidated in the adrenal cortex. Such studies, however, are needed if we are to fully understand the role of ACTH in regulating those endocrine cell responses that are dependent on the communication of molecules between cells. Certainly, in the adrenal gland, there is a need for cells to cooperate and get information from one another. Gap junctions provide this function, and when gap junctions are lost from a population, pathological conditions, including cancers, are thought to develop (42, 93, 94).

LOSS OF GAP JUNCTIONS AND ADRENAL CORTEX CANCER

The loss of gap junction function has been implicated in tumor development (93–99). Most tumors associated with the adrenal cortex develop in the ZF (100) where, under normal conditions, gap junctions tend to be large and abundant (6, 40, 42). The most common types of adrenal gland tumors are adrenal adenomas, which are non-cancerous tumors of the cortex (101, 102). Adrenocortical carcinoma, cancer of the adrenal cortex, is rarely observed; however, patients with certain inherited genetic disorders are at a higher risk of developing this cancer (102).

In the adrenal cortex, a decrease in gap junction expression has been correlated with the stage of tumor differentiation/progression (42). Specifically, in studies to characterize gap junctions during tumorigenesis, the number of gap junctions observed per cell was quantitated and compared in normal human cells of the adrenal gland ZF, as well as cells from adenoma and carcinoma adrenal gland tissues. Cells from the ZF of normal adrenal glands displayed a much higher number of gap junctions per cell (13.78 ± 1.93 SEM) than when compared with benign adrenocortical adenomas (4.6 ± 1.17 SEM; $p \leq 0.05$). The number of gap junctions demonstrated between cells of malignant adrenocortical tumors (1.42 ± 0.58 SEM; $p \leq 0.05$) were significantly lower than both the normal and benign cells (42). These observations are consistent with the hypothesis that a capacity for increase in proliferation coupled with the loss of terminal differentiation as the tumor progresses from non-malignant to malignant reflects the loss of gap junction-mediated communication of growth regulatory molecules between cells. Further, it has been suggested that the increased capacity for tumor metastasis may result from the loss of the cell–cell adhesion that is provided not only by adhesion junctions but also by gap junctions (103–105). Interestingly, exogenous Cx43 can decrease cell proliferation and contribute to reversion of the transformed phenotype (106, 107). Both observations are suggestive of a relationship between gap junctions, differentiation, and proliferation. There is a hope that the induction of gap junctions in malignant cells will provide a novel therapeutic strategy for treating adrenal cancer and, in addition, pharmacological methods and manipulations designed to increase gap junctions may someday serve as a therapeutic method.

While some investigators have suggested the loss of gap junctions in adrenal tumor cell populations, others have demonstrated that metastatic tumors are correlated with an increase in the expression of connexins dependent on the tissue type (108–111). In few cases, tumor cells are capable of communication with other tumor cells through gap junctions; however, they do not communicate with normal cells (112). The difference in the detection of changes in some studies compared with others may reflect the complex nature of cancers in addition to the adrenal zones of origin of the various tumors. Further investigations of the relationship between gap junction expression and tumor progression are needed. This is specifically true when studying the adrenal gland, given the number of adrenal incidentalomas that are commonly detected and the need to differentiate benign from malignant detections. The reported lack of gap junctions in the carcinoma cell population, if found to be widespread in different tumor populations, could be used as an additional method of determining the capacity for metastasis and as an indicator of the rate at which the tumor may proliferate. Furthermore, if cancer cells of the adrenal are capable of communicating with one another but not with normal cells as suggested by Yamasaki in other tissues (112), it would be possible to design protocols that use gap junction-mediated communication to selectively kill the cancer cells while leaving the normal healthy cells intact, the bystander effect (113–115).

CROSS TALK BETWEEN CELLS OF THE CORTEX AND MEDULLA

It is becoming clear that the cells of the medulla and the cortical cells are physically interwoven with one another (116) and, thus, the possibility of gap junction-mediated communication between chromaffin cells and adrenocortical cells may exist. In humans, as well as other mammals, for example cortical cells can be found within the medulla in contact with chromaffin cells (116–118). Furthermore, inner cortical cells of the ZR are in direct contact with the chromaffin cells of the medulla (1), and gap junctions between these cells could possibly provide a mechanism for direct communication of information. Certainly, there is a functional relationship between the cortical and medullary cells, since the adrenal androgens, particularly dehydroepiandrosterone (DHEA), which is produced in ZR following ACTH stimulation, can inhibit chromaffin cell proliferation and differentiation (119, 120). In addition, cells of the cortex may influence catecholamine release from chromaffin cells while the chromaffin cells may regulate adrenal cortical steroid hormone production (10, 116, 121). Gap junctions may provide a mechanism for some of the functional interdependency, especially, among those cells at the medullary–cortical interface area and among islands of cortical cells located within the medulla.

In the medulla, several different connexin types (Cx29, Cx36, Cx43, and Cx50) have been reported to be expressed, depending on the species (41, 122). While some investigators have not reported gap junction plaques in the medulla, others have demonstrated clusters of medullary cells that express Cx43 antigens (5). It is thought that gap junctions in the medulla play a role in the catecholamine (epinephrine and norepinephrine) secretory process and, thus, helps in mediating the body's response to stress (54, 123–125). In addition, stress causes a well-orchestrated, cascade of events that result in the release of a number of other hormones, including glucocorticoids from the adrenal cortex (126). Gap-junctional coupling may complement electrical coupling to enhance communication of signals needed for synchronized cellular hormone release in response to ACTH or low synaptic activity during stress (125).

SUMMARY

Gap junctions are thought to be important in regulating cell population growth, cell morphology, differentiation, cell migration, wound healing, and cell function (2, 93, 108). By analyzing the frequency, distribution, and function of these junctions within intact adrenal glands as well as in adrenal cells in culture following ACTH stimulation, the role of connexins in these processes may be clarified. The specific spatial abundance of gap junction proteins in the adrenal cortical zones is intriguing with regard to its functional implications. It can be suggested that cells of the zona glomerulosa, which express fewer gap junctions than the two other cortical zones, may be less dependent on cell–cell communication for normal function than the cells of the ZF or ZR. Further, a relationship between proliferation rates, steroidogenesis, and gap junction presence or absence in the gland has been suggested (**Figure 7**). Studies to demonstrate the effects of gap junction overexpression and inhibition in the adrenal glands are needed, if we are to resolve some of the questions of how gap junctions function as adrenal cells undergo the morphological and proliferative changes associated with the establishment and maintenance of cortical zonation and hormone-mediated steroidogenesis.

Intact adrenal glands and adrenal cell cultures provide us with a valuable paradigm for studying gap junctions and the cellular mechanisms involved in hormone responses. Indeed, study of adrenocortical cells *in vivo* and *in vitro* is important not only for an understanding of adrenal gland function *per se* but also for providing insight into the foundation of cell communication and biological response in other tissues. But, beyond cell communication, it is becoming apparent that gap junctions play a role in providing adhesive forces needed to hold cells together (103–105).

In addition to gap junction-mediated communication and adhesion, the gap junction internalization process that results in increased annular gap junction vesicles within the cytoplasm and fewer surface gap junction plaques could be important to events in the adrenal gland. Annular gap junctions were reported in the adrenal gland as early as 1988 with transmission electron microscopy (49). It has been demonstrated that annular gap junctions undergo degradation (13, 51, 52). Relatively large numbers of annular gap junctions occur in the adrenal gland, and it could be postulated that gap junction turnover is high in this tissue. Rapid turnover could be needed for migration of the cells to maintain the cortical zones during cytogenesis, for example. Such suggestions are not without precedent. In the ovary, for example, gap junctions are thought to allow the movement of molecules to the egg from the follicular granulosa cells (60, 61). In the case of the ovary, phosphorylation of the C-terminal tail of connexin has been demonstrated to be regulated by the peptide hormone, luteinizing hormone (127). Large numbers of annular gap junctions are reported during ovulation, and it is thought that if gap junctions are not internalized from the surface of the granulosa cells that the egg will remain "trapped" within follicle and ovulation will not occur (128). Gap junctions in a similar way could potentially retard the migration of cells from one area to another (centripetal migration) by tethering the cells to one another. Inhibiting cell migration through the granulosa cell layer of the follicle, in the case of the ovary, or as cells migrate in the adrenal gland could keep cells connected to one another if gap junctions fail to internalize. Such possibilities, however, are yet to be demonstrated.

REMAINING QUESTIONS

It is clear from early studies that there is a relationship between gap junctions and ACTH-mediated responses in the adrenal cortex. There are, however, very few recent articles available

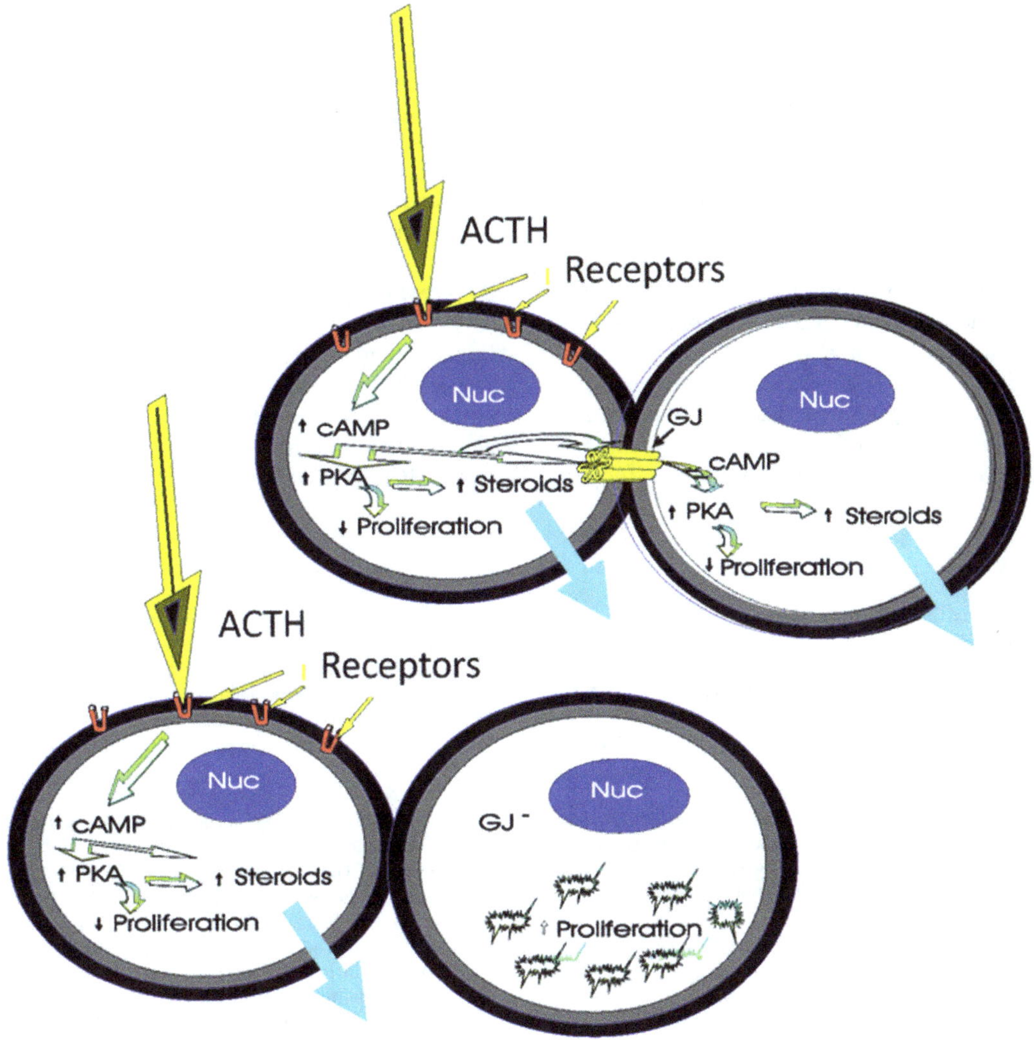

FIGURE 7 | Schematic of the role of gap junctions in steroidogenesis and cell proliferation. The binding of ACTH to its receptors on coupled cortical cells stimulates cyclic adenosine monophosphate (cAMP) to activate protein kinase A (PKA), thereby increasing steroidogenesis and decreasing proliferation. Gap junction-mediated movement of cAMP between cells in the population would amplify hormonal responses in contacting cells, thus increasing ACTH-mediated steroidogenesis. An increase in the number of gap junctions, increases ACTH-mediated steroidogenesis while decreasing proliferation. However, if gap junctions are decreased as a result of molecular manipulations or chemical treatments, for example, ACTH stimulation in one cell does not affect steroidogenesis in the second cell, and there would be a loss in coordinated cell function between cells [modified from Ref. (130)].

on gap junctions in the adrenal cortex. Yet, there are important questions that remain to be answered. For example, in human conditions with diminished circulating ACTH levels, are there changes in the expression or distribution of adrenal cortical gap junctions, as seen following hypophysectomy in rodents (30)? There is dramatic remodeling and relocation of gap junction plaques in the diabetic heart (129). Would the remodeling of gap junctions in the adrenal occur in this and in other endocrine related diseases? Adrenal cortical steroidogenesis is influenced mainly by the activation of PKA (59, 64). In tissues, other than the adrenal, PKA has been shown to phosphorylate the C-terminal tail of Cx43 gap junction proteins (22, 78–81). Such PKA-mediated connexin phosphorylations have been demonstrated to be critical in regulating gap junction assembly and stability (22, 78–81). In the adrenal cortex following ACTH treatment, it is presumed that gap junction protein phosphorylation occurs. However, which Cx43 C-terminal tail amino acids are phosphorylated is unknown. Further, the interplay between PKA and the other protein kinases (PKC, tyrosine kinase, MAPK, and casein kinase 1) in the regulation of gap junctions and adrenal cortical functions needs to be investigated. It has become clear that connexins can have multiple regulatory functions, which depend upon their phosphorylated state (22, 82, 84). Unfortunately, the role of protein kinase-mediated connexin phosphorylation in the adrenal cortex, although described in other tissues, has not been investigated, to our knowledge, in the adrenal cortex. However, one would predict that as cells alter their function that the need for gap junction-mediated cell communication, and thus gap junction expression and phosphorylation, may also change. Moreover, the molecules moving between cells may change. One molecule that has been demonstrated to transfer between gap junctions of adrenal cells to regulate steroidogenesis is cAMP (59, 68). But surely, more than this, one molecule is moving between the cells of the adrenal. The abundance of gap junctions in the inner cortex would suggest a high demand for communication of molecules in these zones. The following question has yet to be answered: how movement of molecules between cells serves to regulate the cascade of events involved in proliferation but more importantly in differentiation of the cells such that transcription factors needed for the production of cortisol in one zone of the adrenal but for androgens in another zone.

The study of adrenocortical cells *in vivo* and *in vitro* is important not only for an understanding of adrenal gland function *per se* but also for providing insight into the foundation of cell communication and biological response in other tissues. Further study will elucidate how gap junctions and cell–cell communication as well as gap junction-mediated adhesion is related to adrenal gland development cell differentiation and steroidogenic function.

AUTHOR CONTRIBUTIONS

CB wrote sections of the manuscript, prepared figures, and edited the manuscript. SM wrote sections of the manuscript, prepared figures, and edited the manuscript.

ACKNOWLEDGMENTS

This review provides only a sampling of the literature that is available on this topic, and we apologize to authors whose original works have not been cited. Work in the authors' laboratory is supported by funds from the National Science Foundation (NSF, grant# MCB-0444398) to SM.

REFERENCES

1. James VHT. *The Adrenal Gland Comprehensive Endocrinology*. New York, NY: Raven Press, Ltd (1992).
2. Decker RS, Donta ST, Larsen WJ, Murray SA. Gap junctions and ACTH sensitivity in Y-1 adrenal tumor cells. *J Supramol Struct* (1978) 9:497–507. doi:10.1002/jss.400090405
3. Meda P, Pepper MS, Traub O, Willecke K, Gros D, Beyer E, et al. Differential expression of gap junction connexins in endocrine and exocrine glands. *Endocrinology* (1993) 133:2371–8. doi:10.1210/en.133.5.2371
4. Munari-Silem Y, Lebrethon MC, Morand I, Rousset B, Saez JM. Gap junction-mediated cell-to-cell communication in bovine and human adrenal cells. A process whereby cells increase their responsiveness to physiological corticotropin concentrations. *J Clin Invest* (1995) 95:1429–39. doi:10.1172/JCI117813
5. Murray SA, Kumar NM, Gilula NB. Gap junction expression in rat adrenal gland. Intercellular communication through gap junctions. *Prog Cell Res* (1995) 4:293–6. doi:10.1016/B978-0-444-81929-1.50059-9
6. Murray SA, Pharrams S. Comparison of gap junction expression in the adrenal gland. *Microsc Res Tech* (1997) 36:510–9. doi:10.1002/(SICI)1097-0029(19970315)36:6<510::AID-JEMT8>3.3.CO;2-S
7. Oyoyo UA, Shah US, Murray SA. The role of alpha1 (connexin-43) gap junction expression in adrenal cortical cell function. *Endocrinology* (1997) 138:5385–97. doi:10.1210/en.138.12.5385
8. Shah US, Murray SA. Bimodal inhibition of connexin 43 gap junctions decreases ACTH-induced steroidogenesis and increases bovine adrenal cell population growth. *J Endocrinol* (2001) 171:199–208. doi:10.1677/joe.0.1710199
9. De Mello WC. The role of cAMP and calcium on the modulation of junctional conductance: an integrated hypothesis. *Cell Biol Int Rep* (1983) 7:1033–40. doi:10.1016/0309-1651(83)90008-5
10. Joseph T, Slack C, Gould RP. Gap junctions and electrotonic coupling in foetal rabbit adrenal cortical cells. *J Embryol Exp Morphol* (1973) 29:681–96.
11. Friend DS, Gilula NB. Variations in tight and gap junctions in mammalian tissues. *J Cell Biol* (1972) 53:758–76. doi:10.1083/jcb.53.3.758
12. Goodenough DA. The structure of cell membranes involved in intercellular communication. *Am J Clin Pathol* (1975) 63:636–45. doi:10.1093/ajcp/63.5.636
13. Murray SA, Larsen WJ, Trout J, Donta ST. Gap junction assembly and endocytosis correlated with patterns of growth in a cultured adrenocortical tumor cell (SW-13). *Cancer Res* (1981) 41:4063–74.
14. Loewenstein WR. Junctional intercellular communication. The cell-to-cell membrane channel. *Physiol Rev* (1981) 61(4):829–913.
15. Meda P, Michaels RL, Halban PA, Orci L, Sheridan JD. In vivo modulation of gap junctions and dye coupling between B-cells of the intact pancreatic islet. *Diabetes* (1983) 32:858–68. doi:10.2337/diabetes.32.9.858
16. Wade MH, Trosko JE, Schindler M. A fluorescence photobleaching assay of gap junction-mediated communication between human cells. *Science* (1986) 232:525–8. doi:10.1126/science.3961495
17. Fried K, Mitsiadis TA, Guerrier A, Haegerstrand A, Meister B. Combinatorial expression patterns of the connexins 26, 32, and 43 during development, homeostasis, and regeneration of rat teeth. *Int J Dev Biol* (1996) 40:985–95.
18. Gimlich RL, Kumar NM, Gilula NB. Sequence and developmental expression of mRNA coding for a gap junction protein in *Xenopus*. *J Cell Biol* (1988) 107:1065–73. doi:10.1083/jcb.107.3.1065
19. Kumar NM, Gilula NB. Cloning and characterization of human and rat liver cDNAs coding for a gap junction protein. *J Cell Biol* (1986) 103:767–76. doi:10.1083/jcb.103.3.767
20. Kumar NM, Gilula NB. Molecular biology and genetics of gap junction channels. *Semin Cell Biol* (1992) 3:3–16. doi:10.1016/S1043-4682(10)80003-0
21. Johnson KE, Mitra S, Katoch P, Kelsey LS, Johnson KR, Mehta PP. Phosphorylation on Ser-279 and Ser-282 of connexin43 regulates endocytosis and gap junction assembly in pancreatic cancer cells. *Mol Biol Cell* (2013) 24:715–33. doi:10.1091/mbc.E12-07-0537
22. Solan JL, Lampe PD. Connexin43 phosphorylation: structural changes and biological effects. *Biochem J* (2009) 419:261–72. doi:10.1042/BJ20082319
23. Yeager M, Nicholson BJ. Structure of gap junction intercellular channels. *Curr Opin Struct Biol* (1996) 6:183–92. doi:10.1016/S0959-440X(96)80073-X
24. McNutt NS, Jones AL. Observations on the ultrastructure of cytodifferentiation in the human fetal adrenal cortex. *Lab Invest* (1970) 22:513–27.
25. Friend DS, Gilula NB. A distinctive cell contact in the rat adrenal cortex. *J Cell Biol* (1972) 53:148–63. doi:10.1083/jcb.53.1.148
26. Branton D, Bullivant S, Gilula NB, Karnovsky MJ, Moor H, Muhlethaler K, et al. Freeze-etching nomenclature. *Science* (1975) 190:54–6. doi:10.1126/science.1166299
27. Amsterdam A, Josephs R, Lieberman ME, Lindner HR. Organization of intramembrane particles in freeze-cleaved gap junctions of rat graafian follicles: optical-diffraction analysis. *J Cell Sci* (1976) 21:93–105.
28. Shivers RR, McVicar LK. Gap junctions revealed by freeze-fracture electron microscopy. *Microsc Res Tech* (1995) 31:437–45. doi:10.1002/jemt.1070310512
29. Decker RS. Gap junctions and steroidogenesis in the fetal mammalian adrenal cortex. *Dev Biol* (1981) 82:20–31. doi:10.1016/0012-1606(81)90425-5
30. Davis K, Prentice N, Gay VL, Murray SA. Gap junction proteins and cell-cell communication in the three functional zones of the adrenal gland. *J Endocrinol* (2002) 173:13–21. doi:10.1677/joe.0.1730013
31. Davis KT, McDuffie I, Mawhinney LA, Murray SA. Hypophysectomy results in a loss of connexin gap junction protein from the adrenal cortex. *Endocr Res* (2000) 26:561–70. doi:10.3109/07435800009048571
32. Hertzberg EL, Spray DC, Bennett MV. Reduction of gap junctional conductance by microinjection of antibodies against the 27-kDa liver gap junction polypeptide. *Proc Natl Acad Sci U S A* (1985) 82:2412–6. doi:10.1073/pnas.82.8.2412

33. el-Fouly MH, Trosko JE, Chang CC. Scrape-loading and dye transfer. A rapid and simple technique to study gap junctional intercellular communication. *Exp Cell Res* (1987) 168:422–30. doi:10.1016/0014-4827(87)90014-0
34. Revel JP, Yancey SB, Meyer DJ, Nicholson B. Cell junctions and intercellular communication. *In Vitro* (1980) 16:1010–7. doi:10.1007/BF02619251
35. Murray SA, Polizotto S. Characterization of the morphological growth, and steroidogenic effect of TPA on mouse Y-1 adrenal cortical tumor cells in culture. *Am J Anat* (1988) 183:166–77. doi:10.1002/aja.1001830207
36. Raviola E, Goodenough DA, Raviola G. Structure of rapidly frozen gap junctions. *J Cell Biol* (1980) 87:273–9. doi:10.1083/jcb.87.1.273
37. Hsieh CL, Kumar NM, Gilula NB, Francke U. Distribution of genes for gap junction membrane channel proteins on human and mouse chromosomes. *Somat Cell Mol Genet* (1991) 17:191–200. doi:10.1007/BF01232976
38. Gilula NB. Topology of gap junction protein and channel function. *Ciba Found Symp* (1987) 125:128–39.
39. Murray SA, Oyoyo UA, Pharrams SY, Kumar NM, Gilula NB. Modulation of gap junction expression in rat and human adrenal cortical cells in culture. *Anat Rec* (1993) 1:86.
40. Murray SA, Oyoyo UA, Pharrams SY, Kumar NM, Gilula NB. Characterization of gap junction expression in the adrenal gland. *Endocr Res* (1995) 21:221–9. doi:10.3109/07435809509030438
41. Willenberg HS, Schott M, Saeger W, Tries A, Scherbaum WA, Bornstein SR. Expression of connexins in chromaffin cells of normal human adrenals and in benign and malignant pheochromocytomas. *Ann N Y Acad Sci* (2006) 1073:578–83. doi:10.1196/annals.1353.060
42. Murray SA, Davis K, Fishman LM, Bornstein SR. Alpha1 Connexin 43 gap junctions are decreased in human adrenocortical tumors. *J Clin Endocrinol Metab* (2000) 85:890–5. doi:10.1210/jc.85.2.890
43. Murray SA, Shakespeare TI. *Immunofluorescence: Applications for Analysis of Connexin Distribution and Trafficking. Gap Junction Channels and Hemichannels.* Boca Raton, FL: CRC Press. Taylor & Francis Group (2016). p. 1–19.
44. Idelman S. Ultrastructure of the mammalian adrenal cortex. *Int Rev Cytol* (1970) 27:181–281. doi:10.1016/S0074-7696(08)61248-6
45. Motta P, Muto M, Fujita T. Three dimensional organization of mammalian adrenal cortex. A scanning electron microscopic study. *Cell Tissue Res* (1979) 196:23–38. doi:10.1007/BF00236346
46. Murray SA, Nickel BM, Gay VL. Endocytosis of connexin protein in adrenal cells. *Endocr Res* (2004) 30:647–54. doi:10.1081/ERC-200043942
47. Nickel B, Boller M, Schneider K, Shakespeare T, Gay V, Murray SA. Visualizing the effect of dynamin inhibition on annular gap vesicle formation and fission. *J Cell Sci* (2013) 126(Pt 12):2607–16. doi:10.1242/jcs.116269
48. Nickel BM, DeFranco BH, Gay VL, Murray SA. Clathrin and Cx43 gap junction plaque endoexocytosis. *Biochem Biophys Res Commun* (2008) 374:679–82. doi:10.1016/j.bbrc.2008.07.108
49. Watanabe H, Washioka H, Tonosaki A. Gap junction and its cytoskeletal undercoats as involved in invagination-endocytosis. *Tohoku J Exp Med* (1988) 156:175–90. doi:10.1620/tjem.156.175
50. Berthoud VM, Tadros PN, Beyer EC. Connexin and gap junction degradation. *Methods* (2000) 20:180–7. doi:10.1006/meth.1999.0935
51. Falk MM, Fong JT, Kells RM, O'Laughlin MC, Kowal TJ, Thevenin AF. Degradation of endocytosed gap junctions by autophagosomal and endo-/lysosomal pathways: a perspective. *J Membr Biol* (2012) 245:465–76. doi:10.1007/s00232-012-9464-0
52. Guan X, Ruch RJ. Gap junction endocytosis and lysosomal degradation of connexin43-P2 in WB-F344 rat liver epithelial cells treated with DDT and lindane. *Carcinogenesis* (1996) 17:1791–8. doi:10.1093/carcin/17.9.1791
53. Lauf U, Giepmans BN, Lopez P, Braconnot S, Chen SC, Falk MM. Dynamic trafficking and delivery of connexons to the plasma membrane and accretion to gap junctions in living cells. *Proc Natl Acad Sci U S A* (2002) 99:10446–51. doi:10.1073/pnas.162055899
54. Desarmenien MG, Jourdan C, Toutain B, Vessieres E, Hormuzdi SG, Guerineau NC. Gap junction signalling is a stress-regulated component of adrenal neuroendocrine stimulus-secretion coupling in vivo. *Nat Commun* (2013) 4:2938. doi:10.1038/ncomms3938
55. Black VH, Robbins D, McNamara N, Huima T. A correlated thin-section and freeze-fracture analysis of guinea pig adrenocortical cells. *Am J Anat* (1979) 156:453–503. doi:10.1002/aja.1001560404
56. Plump AS, Erickson SK, Weng W, Partin JS, Breslow JL, Williams DL. Apolipoprotein A-I is required for cholesteryl ester accumulation in steroidogenic cells and for normal adrenal steroid production. *J Clin Invest* (1996) 97:2660–71. doi:10.1172/JCI118716
57. Larsen WJ, Azarnia R, Loewenstein WR. Intercellular communication and tissue growth: IX. Junctional membrane structure of hybrids between communication-competent and communication-incompetent cells. *J Membr Biol* (1977) 34:39–54. doi:10.1007/BF01870292
58. Loewenstein WR, Rose B. The cell-cell channel in the control of growth. *Semin Cell Biol* (1992) 3:59–79. doi:10.1016/S1043-4682(10)80008-X
59. Murray SA, Fletcher WH. Hormone induced intercellular signal transfer dissociates cyclic AMP-dependent protein kinase. *J Cell Biol* (1984) 98:1710–20. doi:10.1083/jcb.98.5.1710
60. Norris RP, Ratzan WJ, Freudzon M, Mehlmann LM, Krall J, Movsesian MA, et al. Cyclic GMP from the surrounding somatic cells regulates cyclic AMP and meiosis in the mouse oocyte. *Development* (2009) 136:1869–78. doi:10.1242/dev.035238
61. Shuhaibar LC, Egbert JR, Norris RP, Lampe PD, Nikolaev VO, Thunemann M, et al. Intercellular signaling *via* cyclic GMP diffusion through gap junctions restarts meiosis in mouse ovarian follicles. *Proc Natl Acad Sci U S A* (2015) 112:5527–32. doi:10.1073/pnas.1423598112
62. Armato U, Nussdorfer GG, Neri G, Draghi E, Andreis PG, Mazzocchi G, et al. Effects of ACTH and 3', 5'-cyclic purine nucleotides on the morphology and metabolism of normal adult human adrenocortical cells in primary tissue culture. *Cell Tissue Res* (1978) 190:187–205. doi:10.1007/BF00218169
63. Gill GN. Mechanism of ACTH action. *Metabolism* (1972) 21:571–88. doi:10.1016/0026-0495(72)90101-1
64. Murray SA, Byus CV, Fletcher WH. Intracellular kinetics of free catalytic units dissociated from adenosine 3', 5'-monophosphate-dependent protein kinase in adrenocortical tumor cells. *Endocrinology* (1985) 116:364–74. doi:10.1210/endo-116-1-364
65. Ramirez LC, Millot C, Maume BF. Effect of ACTH on endogenous steroid biosynthesis in long-term primary cultures from newborn rat adrenal cells. *Acta Endocrinol (Copenh)* (1984) 107:401–12.
66. Simmonds PJ, Phillips ID, Poore KR, Coghill ID, Young IR, Canny BJ. The role of the pituitary gland and ACTH in the regulation of mRNAs encoding proteins essential for adrenal steroidogenesis in the late-gestation ovine fetus. *J Endocrinol* (2001) 168:475–85. doi:10.1677/joe.0.1680475
67. Murray SA, Nickel BM, Gay VL. Gap junctions as modulators of adrenal cortical cell proliferation and steroidogenesis. *Mol Cell Endocrinol* (2008) 300:51–6. doi:10.1016/j.mce.2008.09.027
68. Murray SA, Fletcher WH. Multiparameter morphology as a means of specifically identifying hormone stimulated adrenal cortical tumor cells (Y-1) and granulosa cells in coculture. *Scan Electron Microsc* (1984) 1:401–7.
69. Yogo K, Ogawa T, Akiyama M, Ishida-Kitagawa N, Sasada H, Sato E, et al. PKA implicated in the phosphorylation of Cx43 induced by stimulation with FSH in rat granulosa cells. *J Reprod Dev* (2006) 52:321–8. doi:10.1262/jrd.17107
70. Michon L, Nlend Nlend R, Bavamian S, Bischoff L, Boucard N, Caille D, et al. Involvement of gap junctional communication in secretion. *Biochim Biophys Acta* (2005) 1719:82–101. doi:10.1016/j.bbamem.2005.11.003
71. Pan F, Mills SL, Massey SC. Screening of gap junction antagonists on dye coupling in the rabbit retina. *Vis Neurosci* (2007) 24:609–18. doi:10.1017/S0952523807070472
72. Xia Y, Nawy S. The gap junction blockers carbenoxolone and 18beta-glycyrrhetinic acid antagonize cone-driven light responses in the mouse retina. *Vis Neurosci* (2003) 20:429–35. doi:10.1017/S0952523803204089
73. Huang SH, Wu JC, Hwang RD, Yeo HL, Wang SM. Effects of 18beta-glycyrrhetinic acid on the junctional complex and steroidogenesis in rat adrenocortical cells. *J Cell Biochem* (2003) 90:33–41. doi:10.1002/jcb.10610
74. Kang L, Li S, Chen C, Wand F. Research progress on structure modification and biological activity of 18 beta-glycyrrhetinic acid. *Curr Opin Complement Alterna Med* (2013) 1:34–44. doi:10.7178/cocam.1
75. Wynn J, Shah U, Murray SA. Redistribution of connexin 43 by cAMP: a mechanism for growth control in adrenal cells. *Endocr Res* (2002) 28:663–8. doi:10.1081/ERC-120016983
76. Melmed S, Polonsky KS, Larsen PR, Kronenberg HM. *Williams Textbook of Endocrinology*. Philadelphia: Elsevier (2016).

77. Ruggiero C, Lalli E. Impact of ACTH signaling on transcriptional regulation of steroidogenic genes. *Front Endocrinol* (2016) 7:24. doi:10.3389/fendo.2016.00024
78. Lampe PD, Lau AF. Regulation of gap junctions by phosphorylation of connexins. *Arch Biochem Biophys* (2000) 384:205–15. doi:10.1006/abbi.2000.2131
79. Cooper CD, Solan JL, Dolejsi MK, Lampe PD. Analysis of connexin phosphorylation sites. *Methods* (2000) 20:196–204. doi:10.1006/meth.1999.0937
80. Lin R, Martyn KD, Guyette CV, Lau AF, Warn-Cramer BJ. v-Src tyrosine phosphorylation of connexin43: regulation of gap junction communication and effects on cell transformation. *Cell Commun Adhes* (2006) 13:199–216. doi:10.1080/15419060600848516
81. TenBroek EM, Lampe PD, Solan JL, Reynhout JK, Johnson RG. Ser364 of connexin43 and the upregulation of gap junction assembly by cAMP. *J Cell Biol* (2001) 155:1307–18. doi:10.1083/jcb.200102017
82. Sirnes S, Kjenseth A, Leithe E, Rivedal E. Interplay between PKC and the MAP kinase pathway in Connexin43 phosphorylation and inhibition of gap junction intercellular communication. *Biochem Biophys Res Commun* (2009) 382:41–5. doi:10.1016/j.bbrc.2009.02.141
83. Thomas MA, Zosso N, Scerri I, Demaurex N, Chanson M, Staub O. A tyrosine-based sorting signal is involved in connexin43 stability and gap junction turnover. *J Cell Sci* (2003) 116:2213–22. doi:10.1242/jcs.00440
84. Wayakanon P, Bhattacharjee R, Nakahama K, Morita I. The role of the Cx43 C-terminus in GJ plaque formation and internalization. *Biochem Biophys Res Commun* (2012) 42:456–61. doi:10.1016/j.bbrc.2012.03.018
85. Nimlamool W, Andrews RM, Falk MM. Connexin43 phosphorylation by PKC and MAPK signals VEGF-mediated gap junction internalization. *Mol Biol Cell* (2015) 26:2755–68. doi:10.1091/mbc.E14-06-1105
86. Pahujaa M, Anikin M, Goldberg GS. Phosphorylation of connexin43 induced by Src: regulation of gap junctional communication between transformed cells. *Exp Cell Res* (2007) 313:4083–90. doi:10.1016/j.yexcr.2007.09.010
87. Solan JL, Lampe PD. Connexin 43 in LA-25 cells with active v-src is phosphorylated on Y247, Y265, S262, S279/282, and S368 *via* multiple signaling pathways. *Cell Commun Adhes* (2008) 15:75–84. doi:10.1080/15419060802014016
88. Lampe PD, Lau AF. The effects of connexin phosphorylation on gap junctional communication. *Int J Biochem Cell Biol* (2004) 36:1171–86. doi:10.1016/S1357-2725(03)00264-4
89. Rivedal E, Leithe E. Connexin43 synthesis, phosphorylation, and degradation in regulation of transient inhibition of gap junction intercellular communication by the phorbol ester TPA in rat liver epithelial cells. *Exp Cell Res* (2005) 302:143–52. doi:10.1016/j.yexcr.2004.09.004
90. Ruch RJ, Trosko JE, Madhukar BV. Inhibition of connexin43 gap junctional intercellular communication by TPA requires ERK activation. *J Cell Biochem* (2001) 83:163–9. doi:10.1002/jcb.1227
91. Ek-Vitorin JF, King TJ, Heyman NS, Lampe PD, Burt JM. Selectivity of connexin 43 channels is regulated through protein kinase C-dependent phosphorylation. *Circ Res* (2006) 98:1498–505. doi:10.1161/01.RES.0000227572.45891.2c
92. Lampe PD, Cooper CD, King TJ, Burt JM. Analysis of Connexin43 phosphorylated at S325, S328 and S330 in normoxic and ischemic heart. *J Cell Sci* (2006) 119:3435–42. doi:10.1242/jcs.03089
93. Azarnia R, Loewenstein WR. Intercellular communication and the control of growth: XII. Alteration of junctional permeability by simian virus 40. Roles of the large and small T antigens. *J Membr Biol* (1984) 82:213–20.
94. Fitzgerald DJ, Yamasaki H. Tumor promotion: models and assay systems. *Teratog Carcinog Mutagen* (1990) 10:89–102. doi:10.1002/tcm.1770100205
95. Eghbali B, Kessler JA, Reid LM, Roy C, Spray DC. Involvement of gap junctions in tumorigenesis: transfection of tumor cells with connexin 32 cDNA retards growth in vivo. *Proc Nat Acad Sci U S A* (1991) 88(23):10701–5. doi:10.1073/pnas.88.23.10701
96. Holder JW, Elmore E, Barrett JC. Gap junction function and cancer. *Cancer Res* (1993) 53:3475–85.
97. Hotz-Wagenblatt A, Shalloway A. Gap junctional communication and neoplastic transformation. *Crit Rev Oncog* (1993) 4:541–58.
98. King TJ, Lampe PD. Mice deficient for the gap junction protein Connexin32 exhibit increased radiation-induced tumorigenesis associated with elevated mitogen-activated protein kinase (p44/Erk1, p42/Erk2) activation. *Carcinogenesis* (2004) 25:669–80. doi:10.1093/carcin/bgh071
99. Tsuchiya T. A useful marker for evaluating tissue-engineered products: gap-junctional communication for assessment of the tumor-promoting action and disruption of cell differentiation in tissue-engineered products. *J Biomater Sci Polym Ed* (2000) 11:947–59. doi:10.1163/156856200744129
100. Macfarlane DA. Cancer of the adrenal cortex; the natural history, prognosis and treatment in a study of fifty-five cases. *Ann R Coll Surg Engl* (1958) 23:155–86.
101. Abecassis M, McLoughlin MJ, Langer JE, Kudlow JE. Serendipitous adrenal masses: prevalence, significance, and management. *Am J Surg* (1985) 149:783–8. doi:10.1016/S0002-9610(85)80186-0
102. Cardoso CC, Bornstein SR, Hornsby PJ. New methods for investigating experimental human adrenal tumorigenesis. *Mol Cell Endocrinol* (2009) 300:175–9. doi:10.1016/j.mce.2008.10.046
103. Saunders MM, Seraj MJ, Li Z, Zhou Z, Winter CR, Welch DR, et al. Breast cancer metastatic potential correlates with a breakdown in homospecific and heterospecific gap junctional intercellular communication. *Cancer Res* (2001) 61:1765–7.
104. Stein LS, Stein DW, Echols J, Burghardt RC. Concomitant alterations of desmosomes, adhesiveness, and diffusion through gap junction channels in a rat ovarian transformation model system. *Exp Cell Res* (1993) 207:19–32. doi:10.1006/excr.1993.1158
105. Tate A, Lung T, Radhakrishnan A, Lim SD, Lin X, Edlund M. Changes in gap junctional connexin isoforms during prostate cancer progression. *Prostate* (2006) 66:19–31. doi:10.1002/pros.20317
106. Naus CC, Bani-Yaghoub M, Rushlow W, Bechberger JF. Consequences of impaired gap junctional communication in glial cells. *Adv Exp Med Biol* (1999) 468:373–81. doi:10.1007/978-1-4615-4685-6_29
107. Naus CC, Bechberger JF, Zhang, Venance L, Yamasaki H, Juneja SC, et al. Altered gap junctional communication, intercellular signaling, and growth in cultured astrocytes deficient in connexin43. *J Neurosci Res* (1997) 49:528–40. doi:10.1002/(SICI)1097-4547(19970901)49:5<528::AID-JNR3>3.0.CO;2-D
108. Kamibayashi Y, Oyamada Y, Mori M, Oyamada M. Aberrant expression of gap junction proteins (connexins) is associated with tumor progression during multistage mouse skin carcinogenesis in vivo. *Carcinogenesis* (1995) 16:1287–97. doi:10.1093/carcin/16.6.1287
109. Koo BK, An JH, Jeon KH, Choi SH, Cho YM, Jang HC, et al. Two cases of ectopic adrenocorticotropic hormone syndrome with olfactory neuroblastoma and literature review. *Endocr J* (2008) 55:469–75. doi:10.1507/endocrj.K07E-005
110. Miekus K, Czernik M, Sroka J, Czyz J, Madeja Z. Contact stimulation of prostate cancer cell migration: the role of gap junctional coupling and migration stimulated by heterotypic cell-to-cell contacts in determination of the metastatic phenotype of Dunning rat prostate cancer cells. *Biol Cell* (2005) 97:893–903. doi:10.1042/BC20040129
111. Zhang W, Nwagwu C, Le DM, Yong VW, Song H, Couldwell WT. Increased invasive capacity of connexin43-overexpressing malignant glioma cells. *J Neurosurg* (2003) 99:1039–46. doi:10.3171/jns.2003.99.6.1039
112. Yamasaki H. Role of cell-cell communication in tumor suppression. *Immunol Ser* (1990) 51:245–66.
113. Cottin S, Ghani K, Caruso M. Bystander effect in glioblastoma cells with a predominant cytoplasmic localization of connexin43. *Cancer Gene Ther* (2008) 15:823–31. doi:10.1038/cgt.2008.49
114. Carystinos GD, Katabi MM, Laird DW, Galipeau J, Chan H, Alaoui-Jamali MA, et al. Cyclic-AMP induction of gap junctional intercellular communication increases bystander effect in suicide gene therapy. *Clin Cancer Res* (1999) 5:61–8.
115. Thuringer D, Jego G, Berthenek K, Hammann A, Solary E, Garrido C. Gap junction-mediated transfer of miR-145-5p from microvascular endothelial cells to colon cancer cells inhibits angiogenesis. *Oncotarget* (2016) 7: 281260–8. doi:10.18632/oncotarget.8583
116. Ehrhart-Bornstein M, Bornstein SR. Cross-talk between adrenal medulla and adrenal cortex in stress. *Ann N Y Acad Sci* (2008) 1148:112–7. doi:10.1196/annals.1410.053
117. Bornstein SR, González-Hernández JA, Ehrhart-Bornstein M, Adler G, Scherbaum WA. Intimate contact of chromaffin and cortical cells within the human adrenal gland forms the cellular basis for important intraadrenal

interactions. *J Clin Endocrinol Metab* (1994) 78:225–32. doi:10.1210/jcem.78.1.7507122

118. Ehrhart-Bornstein M, Hinson JP, Bornstein SR, Scherbaum WA, Vinson GP. Intraadrenal interactions in the regulation of adrenocortical steroidogenesis. *Endocr Rev* (1998) 19:101–43. doi:10.1210/edrv.19.2.0326
119. Sicard F, Ehrhart-Bornstein M, Corbeil D, Sperber S, Krug AW, Ziegler CG, et al. Age-dependent regulation of chromaffin cell proliferation by growth factors, dehydroepiandrosterone (DHEA), and DHEA sulfate. *Proc Natl Acad Sci U S A* (2007) 104:2007–12. doi:10.1073/pnas.0610898104
120. Ziegler CG, Sicard F, Lattke P, Bornstein SR, Ehrhart-Bornstein M, Krug AW. Dehydroepiandrosterone (DHEA) induces a neuroendocrine phenotype in nerve growth factor (NGF)-stimulated chromaffin pheochromocytoma PC12 cells. *Endocrinology* (2008) 149:320–8. doi:10.1210/en.2007-0645
121. Schinner S, Bornstein SR. Cortical-chromaffin cell interactions in the adrenal gland. *Endocr Pathol* (2005) 16:91–8. doi:10.1385/EP:16:2:091
122. Hodson DJ, Legros C, Desarmenien MG, Guerineau NC. Roles of connexins and pannexins in (neuro) endocrine physiology. *Cell Mol Life Sci* (2015) 72:2911–28. doi:10.1007/s00018-015-1967-2
123. Colomer C, Lafont C, Guerineau NC. Stress-induced intercellular communication remodeling in the rat adrenal medulla. *Ann N Y Acad Sci* (2008) 1148:106–11. doi:10.1196/annals.1410.040
124. Colomer C, Olivos Ore LA, Coutry N, Mathieu MN, Arthaud S, Fontanaud P, et al. Functional remodeling of gap junction-mediated electrical communication between adrenal chromaffin cells in stressed rats. *J Neurosci* (2008) 28:6616–26. doi:10.1523/JNEUROSCI.5597-07.2008
125. Martin AO, Mathieu MN, Chevillard C, Guerineau NC. Gap junctions mediate electrical signaling and ensuing cytosolic Ca2+ increases between chromaffin cells in adrenal slices: a role in catecholamine release. *J Neurosci* (2001) 21:5397–405. doi:10.1038/ncomms3938
126. Ranabir S, Reetu K. Stress and hormones. *Indian J Endocrinol Metab* (2011) 15:18–22. doi:10.4103/2230-8210.77573
127. Granot I, Dekel N. Phosphorylation and expression of connexin-43 ovarian gap junction protein are regulated by luteinizing hormone. *J Biol Chem* (1994) 269:30502–9.
128. Simon AM, Goodenough DA, Li E, Paul DL. Female infertility in mice lacking connexin 37. *Nature* (1997) 385:525–9. doi:10.1038/385525a0
129. Lin H, Ogawa K, Imanaga I, Tribulova N. Remodeling of connexin 43 in the diabetic rat heart. *Mol Cell Biochem* (2006) 290:69–78. doi:10.1007/s11010-006-9166-y
130. Murray S, Davis K, Gay V. ACTH and adrenocortical gap junctions. *Microsc Res Tech* (2003) 61:240–6. doi:10.1002/jemt.10332
131. Falk MM, Bell CL, Kells Andrews RM, Murray SA. Molecular mechanisms regulating the formation, trafficking and processing of annular gap junctions. *BMC Cell Biol* (2016) 17(Suppl 1):22. doi:10.1186/s12860-016-0087-7
132. Murray SA, Williams SY, Dillard CY, Narayanan SK, McCauley J. Relationship of cytoskeletal filaments to annular gap junction expression in human adrenal cortical tumor cells in culture. *Exp Cell Res* (1997) 234:398–404. doi:10.1006/excr.1997.3628

18

ACTH Action on StAR Biology

Barbara J. Clark*****

Department of Biochemistry and Molecular Genetics, University of Louisville, Louisville, KY, USA

***Correspondence:**
Barbara J. Clark
bjclark@louisville.edu

Adrenocorticotropin hormone (ACTH) produced by the anterior pituitary stimulates glucocorticoid synthesis by the adrenal cortex. The first step in glucocorticoid synthesis is the delivery of cholesterol to the mitochondrial matrix where the first enzymatic reaction in the steroid hormone biosynthetic pathway occurs. A key response of adrenal cells to ACTH is activation of the cAMP-protein kinase A (PKA) signaling pathway. PKA activation results in an acute increase in expression and function of the Steroidogenic Acute Regulatory protein (StAR). StAR plays an essential role in steroidogenesis- it controls the hormone-dependent movement of cholesterol across the mitochondrial membranes. Currently StAR's mechanism of action remains a major unanswered question in the field. However, some insight may be gained from understanding the mechanism(s) controlling the PKA-dependent phosphorylation of StAR at S194/195 (mouse/human StAR), a modification that is required for function. This mini-review provides a background on StAR's biology with a focus on StAR phosphorylation. The model for StAR translation and phosphorylation at the outer mitochondrial membrane, the location for StAR function, is presented to highlight a unifying theme emerging from diverse studies.

Keywords: StAR, adrenal, ACTH, translation, phosphorylation

STAR (STARD1) DISCOVERY AND FUNCTION

The study of steroid hormone production has origins in work on adrenocorticotropin hormone (ACTH)-stimulated adrenal steroid synthesis (Macchi and Hechter, 1954a,b,c; Stone and Hechter, 1954). ACTH binds to its cognate 7-transmembrane G-protein coupled receptor, the melanocortin 2 receptor (encoded by the MC2R gene) that is located at the plasma membrane of adrenal fasciculata cells. ACTH binding to MC2R results in activation of multiple signal transduction pathways with the cAMP-dependent protein kinase A (cAMP-PKA) pathway being central to hormone-dependent activation of adrenal glucocorticoid and androgen synthesis (reviewed in Gallo-Payet and Payet, 2003; Spat et al., 2016). All steroid hormones are produced from cholesterol and the steroidogenic enzymes in cortisol synthesis, the major adrenal steroid produced in response to ACTH, have been reviewed in detail (Miller and Auchus, 2011). This mini-review focuses on the rapid or acute response to tropic hormonal stimulation- the movement of cholesterol into mitochondria. The first enzymatic reaction is the conversion of cholesterol to pregnenolone by the cytochrome P450 side chain cleavage enzyme (P450scc). P450scc is located in the mitochondrial matrix and work from the 1950s–1970s laid a solid foundation that cholesterol transport into mitochondria for access to P450scc was a key control point in steroidogenesis (Ferguson, 1962, 1963). The prevailing model at that time was that *de novo* synthesis of a protein factor upon hormonal stimulation was necessary for the cholesterol transfer. Furthermore, this factor needed to fulfill the following criteria: be newly synthesized upon hormonal stimulation in a time- and dose-dependent manner, be localized at the mitochondria, and have a short-half (reviewed in

Clark and Stocco, 2014; Stocco et al., 2016). Here, I will highlight the studies which demonstrated that the Steroidogenic Acute Regulatory protein (StAR) fulfills the criteria for the acute regulator of steroidogenesis.

The first characterization of StAR was as phosphoproteins (pp with MW in kDa) pp37, pp32, and pp30 that appeared in rat adrenal after ACTH stimulation (Krueger and Orme-Johnson, 1983; Pon and Orme-Johnson, 1986; Pon et al., 1986; Alberta et al., 1989; Epstein and Orme-Johnson, 1991). Both *in vivo* and cell culture approaches provided strong correlative data that ACTH-cAMP-PKA induction of these proteins coincided with steroid production. In addition, the proteins were shown to be associated with mitochondria, and the pp32 and pp30 forms were processed forms of pp37 (Alberta et al., 1989; Epstein and Orme-Johnson, 1991; Krueger and Orme-Johnson, 1983; Pon and Orme-Johnson, 1986; Pon et al., 1986). Similar hormonal responsive protein(s) were characterized in the MA-10 mouse Leydig tumor cells, and ultimately the StAR protein was purified and cDNA cloned from this cell line (Clark et al., 1994). The deduced amino acid sequence encodes a protein with estimated molecular weight of 31.6 kDa with the amino-terminal region containing a classical mitochondrial targeting sequence (Clark et al., 1994). Expression of the cDNA in steroidogenic cells or *in vitro* in the presence of isolated mitochondria followed by Western blot analysis confirmed the cDNA encoded the pp37 protein previously characterized (Clark et al., 1994; King et al., 1995; Lin et al., 1995). The cDNA encoded a functional protein based on assays that measured increased steroid production in COS-1 cells or steroidogenic cells after transient expression of the cDNA. As anticipated, the 37 kDa StAR protein was imported and processed by mitochondria to generate the 30 kDa StAR protein (King et al., 1995). However, steroidogenesis ceases with removal of tropic hormone stimuli yet the 30 kDa form of StAR localized in the mitochondrial matrix is present with an estimated half-life of 4–5 h (Stocco and Sodeman, 1991; Granot et al., 2003). Thus, the requirement for a labile, short half-life criteria for the acute regulator of steroidogenesis required subsequent structure-function studies. Database searches using the cDNA and protein sequences revealed that StAR represented a novel protein (Clark et al., 1994). Shortly after the initial reports on StAR appeared, a conserved protein domain named the START domain (for steroidogenic acute regulatory protein (StAR)-related lipid-transfer domain), was identified using Web-based resources for predicting putative functional domains based on primary sequence data (Ponting and Aravind, 1999). Members of the START domain protein superfamily share a 210 amino acid region that folds into an α/β helix-grip fold structure containing a long hydrophobic cleft for lipid binding (reviewed in Stocco, 2001; Clark, 2012). The START domain within the StAR protein spans amino acids 65–285, which encodes the processed 30 kDa form, and binds cholesterol. Key studies showed that only the START domain is required for StAR's function: (1) addition of the 30 kDa StAR protein to isolated mitochondria promotes cholesterol transfer and pregnenolone production; and (2) expression of a cDNA encoding only the START domain, e.g., lacking the N-terminal mitochondrial targeting sequence (N62StAR), is capable of stimulating steroid production in steroidogenic cells or heterologous COS-1 cells (Arakane et al., 1996; Wang et al., 1998). Furthermore, mutations in the human *STAR* gene (*STARD1*) were identified in patients with congenital lipoid adrenal hyperplasia (lipoid CAH), a disorder marked by a lack of adrenal and gonadal steroidogenesis due to the inability to move cholesterol into the mitochondria [(Lin et al., 1995; Bose et al., 2000); reviewed in (Miller, 2014)]. The finding that *STAR* mutations are the genetic basis for lipoid CAH was key to establishing the essential role for StAR in ACTH-stimulated steroidogenesis as well as gonadotropin-stimulated steroidogenesis (Lin et al., 1995; Caron et al., 1997). A common mutation found in the *STAR* gene is a nonsense mutation, Q258X, which results in truncation of the last 28 amino acids (Nakae et al., 1997; Kim et al., 2011). Expression of C-terminal truncated forms of StAR in COS-1 cells confirmed that the loss of C-terminal helix, within the START domain, results in an inactive protein (Arakane et al., 1996; Wang et al., 1998).

The finding that N-terminal truncated StAR (N62StAR) was functional in cell-based assays, indicated that mitochondrial import was not required for function. However, the targeting of StAR to mitochondria may be important for efficient cholesterol transfer and steroid production *in vivo*. A mouse model of lipoid CAH was generated by "knocking out" StAR expression and, as anticipated, the animals lacked steroid production and significant amounts of cholesterol accumulated in the adrenals and gonads (Caron et al., 1997). Expression of a full-length *STAR* transgene in the StAR knockout mice restored adrenal and gonadal steroidogenesis while expression of the N62*STAR* transgene only partially restored steroidogenesis in a tissue- and gender-specific manner (Sasaki et al., 2008). The mice with the N62StAR transgene retained modest lipid accumulation in the adrenal and gonads. These data support that StAR is capable of functioning without the N-terminal mitochondrial targeting sequence, but highlight the importance of correct and efficient subcellular localization of the protein for full function *in vivo*. In the absence of mitochondrial import, N62StAR still associates with mitochondria outer membrane (Arakane et al., 1996; Wang et al., 1998).

STAR PHOSPHORYLATION AND FUNCTION

Early studies proposed an association between StAR phosphorylation and function (Pon et al., 1986; Chaudhary and Stocco, 1991; Clark et al., 1995; Hartigan et al., 1995). A PKA-dependent phosphorylation at S194 (mouse) or S195 (human) was validated as an important post-translational modification required for StAR's function in cell-based and *in vitro* assays (Arakane et al., 1996; Jo et al., 2005; Baker et al., 2007). StAR-S194/195 nomenclature reflects the deletion of 3 nucleotides in exon 2 that eliminates a residue which lies within the cleavable mitochondrial signal sequence in mouse StAR. A key study confirmed the relevance for StAR-S194 phosphorylation *in vivo*; StAR knock-out mice were used to demonstrate that re-expression of wild-type StAR but not StAR-S194A restored steroidogenesis in the adrenal and testis

(Sasaki et al., 2014). The newborn StAR-S194A transgenic male mice had lipid accumulation in the adrenal and testis, and circulating hormone levels (high ACTH and low corticosterone and testosterone) similar to StAR knock-out mice. Thus, StAR phosphorylation at S194/195 is critical for function *in vivo*.

The molecular mechanism of action for StAR-mediated cholesterol transport across the mitochondrial membranes is not fully defined, therefore it remains a challenge to define the role of S194/195 phosphorylation in StAR's function. The current model for StAR-mediated cholesterol transport asserts that protein-protein interactions between StAR and OMM protein(s) triggers cholesterol transfer (Bose et al., 1999; Mathieu et al., 2002; Baker et al., 2007; Roostaee et al., 2008; Rajapaksha et al., 2013). Structural changes in the START domain induced by cholesterol binding and by interaction with the OMM as well as the kinetics of cholesterol transfer across the mitochondrial membranes have been reviewed elsewhere (Miller, 2007). Precursor StAR processing to the mitochondrial 30 kDa form is reported to be very efficient, stoichiometric, and dependent upon cholesterol-induced structural changes (Artemenko et al., 2001; Rajapaksha et al., 2013). Import of StAR is proposed to be the "off switch" for cholesterol transfer due to loss of StAR interaction with an OMM protein complex (Bose et al., 1999; Miller, 2007). However, the transit time at the OMM contributes to StAR function with slower mitochondrial import associated with greater activity (Bose et al., 2002). Does StAR phosphorylation affect cholesterol binding or mitochondrial import? Purified hStAR START domain containing the S195A mutation was shown to have the same cholesterol binding kinetics as wild-type StAR START domain, indicating that phosphorylation is not required for cholesterol binding (Baker et al., 2007). StAR-S194A/S195A or non-phosphorylated forms of wild-type StAR are efficiently processed to the 30 kDa mitochondrial matrix form both in cell culture and *in vivo* studies, thus phosphorylation doesn't appear necessary for StAR import (Arakane et al., 1997; Jo et al., 2005; Sasaki et al., 2014; Clark and Hudson, 2015). The region that slows StAR import is a protease-resistant domain that spans amino acids 63–188 (Bose et al., 1999, 2002), therefore, it is unlikely that S194/195 phosphorylation alters StAR import rates, although this has not been directly tested.

While StAR phosphorylation doesn't appear to be required for mitochondrial import, understanding the import mechanism may provide insight into StAR-OMM interactions that are required for function. TOM20 and TOM22 are the receptor components of the Translocase of the outer membrane (TOM) complex that function with the pore-forming TOM40 complex to control protein import into mitochondria (Becker et al., 2012; Harbauer Angelika et al., 2014). Classically, post-translational protein import via a TOM20/22-TOM40 pathway is associated with proteins that are synthesized in the cytoplasm with a cleavable amino-terminal amphipathic helix that serves as a mitochondrial matrix targeting sequence, such as StAR (reviewed in Harbauer Angelika et al., 2014, **Figure 1**). The proteins are in complex with chaperones to maintain an unfolded state for import while the amino terminal sequence binds TOM20/22 receptors (Harbauer Angelika et al., 2014). However, a co-translational mechanism for import of matrix-localized proteins with amino-terminal cleavable signal sequences was proposed over 40 years ago (Kellems et al., 1974) and recent data in yeast support this model. mRNAs co-purify with isolated mitochondria in wild-type yeast strains but not TOM20 deficient strains following cycloheximide (CHX) treatment (Eliyahu et al., 2010). These data indicate that blocking translation and stabilizing polysomes by CHX enhances ribosome-mRNA interactions with mitochondria in a TOM20-dependent manner. StAR has been shown to co-purify with TOM22 and siRNA knock-down of TOM22 in MA-10 cells results in diminished cholesterol metabolism by isolated mitochondria (Prasad et al., 2015, 2016). Since the StAR import mechanism is incompletely described, I use TOM20/22 to reflect both receptors work together for preprotein import in the classical mitochondrial import model. However, it may be that TOM20 and TOM22 can serve redundant functions for StAR import while TOM22 is required for StAR function (Rajapaksha et al., 2013, 2016).

Localized translation and post-translational modification of StAR at the mitochondria is an attractive model for the acute control of steroidogenesis (Dyson et al., 2008; Eliyahu et al., 2010; Lesnik et al., 2015). This model is supported by data that show StAR mRNA was associated with mitochondrial A-kinase anchoring protein 121 (AKAP121) and type II PKA in MA-10 mouse Leydig cells (Dyson et al., 2008, 2009). Independent studies have also demonstrated a PKA-dependent co-localization of AKAP121, acyl-CoA, and upstream ERK1/2 kinases with StAR at the mitochondria (reviewed in Poderoso et al., 2009; Paz et al., 2016). Thus, the co-localization of PKA and AKAP proteins at the mitochondria is emerging as a consistent theme. siRNA-mediated silencing of AKAP121 in MA-10 Leydig cells resulted in loss of PKA (PKAR2) association with mitochondria, independent of Bt_2cAMP treatment, indicating that an AKAP121-PKAR2 complex is constitutively poised at the OMM (Dyson et al., 2008). Immunofluorescence-based detection of AKAP1 in H295R human adrenocortical cell line showed co-localization with TOM20, indicating localization with mitochondria in an adrenal cell line (Grozdanov and Stocco, 2012). Furthermore, a portion of StAR 3′UTR mRNA was shown to directly bind to AKAP1 and in H295R cells and StAR mRNA was recovered following AKAP1 immunoprecipitation (Grozdanov and Stocco, 2012). The StAR mRNA-AKAP1 interaction was detected only after Bt_2cAMP treatment of H295R cells suggesting that newly transcribed StAR mRNA associates with AKAP1. Our earlier work demonstrated that StAR mRNA levels and endogenous protein levels are greatly diminished in the PKA deficient mouse Kin-8 adrenocortical cells following Bt_2cAMP treatment compared to the PKA responsive Y1 adrenocortical cells (Clark et al., 1997; Clark and Hudson, 2015). Yet despite the lower StAR mRNA levels, the mRNA was associated with actively transcribing ribosomes and StAR protein synthesis rates were the same in both cell lines, indicating translation is intact in the absence of PKA signaling (Clark and Hudson, 2015; Clark et al., 1997). Conversely, in MA-10 cells that lack AKAP1 via siRNA-mediated silencing, Bt_2cAMP treatment increased StAR steady-state mRNA levels but StAR protein levels were diminished. Together the data support that newly transcribed StAR mRNA associates with AKAP1 in adrenocortical cells (Kin8

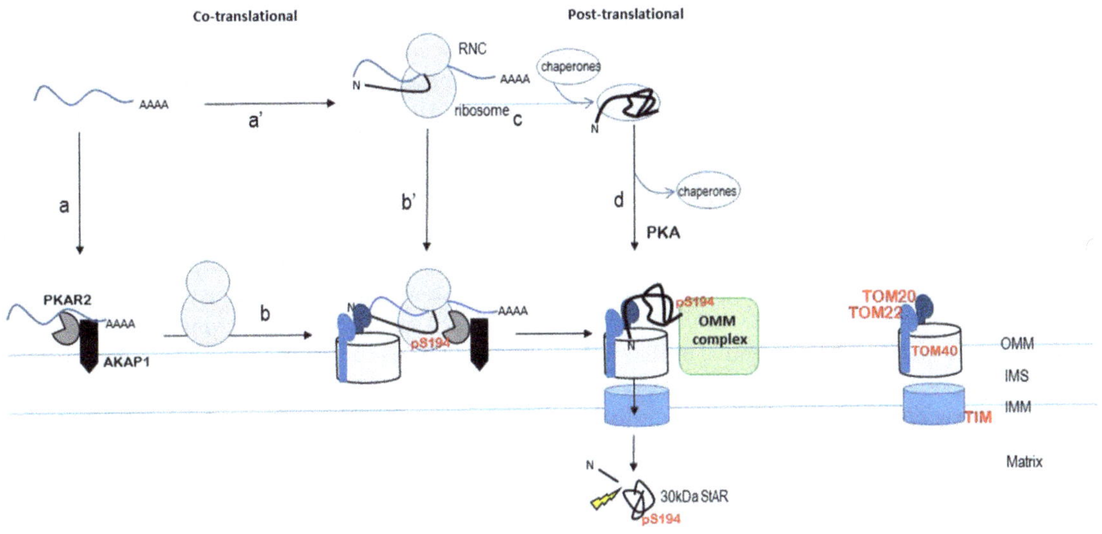

FIGURE 1 | Model for localized StAR translation and phosphorylation at mitochondria. The TOM20/22-40 complex is an established pathway for import of matrix-localized proteins that contain an N-terminal cleavable signal peptide. StAR is modeled within this import pathway, although the import pathway for StAR remains to be determined. The ribosome nascent chain complex (RNC) is shown as StAR mRNA bound by the ribosome and protein depicted as black line with the N-terminus denoted (N). The START domain is depicted by the "folded" black line. StAR translation is modeled on both free ribosomes (steps c and d) and mitochondria-associated ribosomes (steps a to b or a' to b') as described in the text. Cleavage of the N-terminal signal sequence by matrix metalloproteases (indicated by the thunderbolt) produces the 30 kDa STAR protein (START domain) in the matrix. The import of StAR is the "off switch" for cholesterol transfer due to loss of interaction with an OMM protein complex. The OMM protein complex (indicated here as a green rectangle) that facilitates the StAR-dependent cholesterol transfer from the OMM to the matrix remains to be determined. Proposed OMM components of this complex include StAR, AKAP, PKA, VDAC1/2, TOM22, PCP, TSPO, and ACBD3. The OMM protein that interacts specifically with phosphoStAR to trigger complex formation for cholesterol transfer across the mitochondrial membranes remains to be identified. TIM (Translocase of the inner membrane) complex; IMS, intermembrane space; OMM, outer mitochondrial membrane; IMM, inner mitochondrial membrane. Concepts of this model have been presented by others in Dyson et al. (2008), Poderoso et al. (2009), Grozdanov and Stocco (2012), Aghazadeh et al. (2015), Prasad et al. (2015), Lee et al. (2016b), Midzak and Papadopoulos (2016), and Paz et al. (2016).

and H295R cells) and that the AKAP1-StAR mRNA association contributes to translation efficiency. The model that AKAP1 localizes PKAR2 at the OMM provides a platform for localized phosphorylation of StAR (Grozdanov and Stocco, 2012; Merrill and Strack, 2014, **Figure 1**). Recently StAR mRNA association with mitochondria in MA-10 cells was demonstrated using high resolution fluorescence *in situ* hybridization (Lee et al., 2016a). Key findings from this work indicate that StAR mRNA-mitochondrial interactions are dynamic, and suggest that when StAR transcription is maximally activated, newly transcribed and processed StAR mRNA is delivered to the cytoplasm and mitochondria for efficient translation.

The prevailing concept is that StAR phosphorylation influences key interactions with OMM proteins that promote cholesterol transfer. The challenge is that several StAR-interacting complexes at the OMM have been proposed yet the identity of the functional StAR cholesterol transfer complex remains to be validated (Bose et al., 2008; Rone et al., 2012; Issop et al., 2015). Early work characterized a OMM protein complex that included 18 kDa translocator protein (TSPO) and voltage-dependent anion channels 1 (VDAC1) (Liu et al., 2006). The working model was that upon hormonal stimulation StAR is expressed and associates with acyl-coenzyme A binding domain containing 3 protein (ACBD3), previously referred to as TSPO-associated protein (PAP7), leading to a StAR-PKA-ACBD3-TSPO-VDAC1 complex at the OMM (reviewed in Papadopoulos et al., 2015; Midzak and Papadopoulos, 2016). *In vitro* studies using mitochondria isolated from sheep adrenal incubated with radiolabeled, *in vitro* synthesized StAR protein identified VDAC1 and phosphate carrier protein (PCP, SLC25A3) as components of a StAR-containing complex (Bose et al., 2008). VDAC1, VDAC2, TOM22, and StAR have been shown to be part of large multiprotein complexes purified from mitochondria or mitochondria-associated endoplasmic reticulum (ER) membrane (MAM) regions isolated from rat testes and MA-10 mouse Leydig tumor cells (Prasad et al., 2015). The functional significance for these proposed complexes is based on data that demonstrated siRNA-mediated silencing and/or pharmacological inhibition of TSPO, VDAC1, VDAC2, or ACBD3 decreased or blocked cAMP-PKA-mediated steroid production in steroidogenic cells or StAR-mediated steroid production in COS-1 cells. However, mouse models lacking either TSPO or VDAC1 expression are viable and fertile (Weeber et al., 2002; Sileikyte et al., 2014; Tu et al., 2014), although VDAC1$^{-/-}$ mice present with mitochondrial alterations in a strain-dependent manner. Loss of VDAC2 results in embryonic lethality (Anflous et al., 2001; Craigen and Graham, 2008). These studies indicate that TSPO and VDAC1 are not obligatory for steroidogenesis, and suggest a redundancy of function for cholesterol transfer may occur in the absence of these factors. The question is whether StAR phosphorylation drives interaction with any of these OMM proteins. siRNA-mediated silencing of VDAC1 or PCP protein expression in COS-1 cells resulted in decreased vector-driven StAR protein levels with a corresponding decrease in phosphoStAR levels and steroidogenic response (Bose et al., 2008). The 30 kDa StAR was detected by Western blot analysis indicating that mitochondrial import of StAR was intact in VDAC1 null cells. However, 30 kDa phosphoStAR was greatly diminished indicating that in the absence of VDAC1, import of phosphorylated StAR into mitochondria was blocked. Addition of cysteine protease inhibitors to the VDAC1 deficient cells restored StAR phosphorylation and phosphoStAR mitochondrial import and steroid production to levels observed in control cells (Bose et al., 2008). One interpretation of these data is that VDAC1 may help stabilize precursor StAR allowing for StAR phosphorylation and enhanced cholesterol transport function. In a separate study, COS-1 cells with siRNA-mediated loss of VDAC2 expression retained vector-driven StAR synthesis and phosphorylation but there was no steroidogenic response (Prasad et al., 2015). In the absence of VDAC2, as with VDAC1, no mitochondrial import of phosphoStAR was detected (unphosphorylated StAR was not measured) (Prasad et al., 2015). Furthermore, a StAR-VDAC2 complex was immunoprecipitated from COS-1 cells overexpressing VDAC2 and N62StAR, providing the first evidence for a possible direct interaction between StAR and an OMM protein (Prasad et al., 2015). These data suggest that synthesis of phosphorylated precursor StAR is not sufficient for function, and support a role for specific phosphoStAR-OMM interactions mediating cholesterol transfer. The authors propose that StAR is synthesized at MAM regions and interacts with VDAC2 for subsequent mitochondrial import and StAR processing (Prasad et al., 2015). Perhaps the loss of phosphoStAR import in the absence of either VDAC1 or VDAC2 reflects a loss of StAR's N-terminal interaction with the TOM20/22-TOM40 complex, leading to loss of StAR structure which is necessary for cholesterol transfer function of StAR (Rajapaksha et al., 2013; Prasad et al., 2015, **Figure 1**).

In summary, ACTH action on StAR biology requires an immediate response to hormone stimulation, which is seen in a rapid increase in StAR transcription. StAR translation, phosphorylation, and mitochondrial import are likely coordinated processes, but the mechanisms regulating these steps are lacking. Nevertheless, the work over the past decade supports a model for localized translation at the mitochondria. One proposed scenario is the newly transcribed StAR mRNA binds AKAP1 through 3′UTR-driven interactions localizing the mRNA to the mitochondria where it is bound by ribosomes and translated (**Figure 1**, step a and b). Alternatively, cytoplasmic StAR mRNA is bound by ribosomes and the ribosome-nascent-chain is directed to mitochondria where the interaction is stabilized by 3′UTR mRNA-AKAP1 interaction, similar to co-translational models described for yeast (**Figure 1**, step a' and b'). StAR mRNA 3′UTR driving mitochondrial location and localized translation could explain the amino-terminal truncated form of StAR (N62StAR), which lacks the signal sequence, being localized to the OMM and functional. Translation of the amino-terminal mitochondrial signal sequence, on the other hand, could lead to recognition by the TOM20/22-TOM40 complex, thereby tethering StAR to the TOM complex. StAR translation continues and phosphorylation of S194/195 of the START domain occurs in a co-translational process by the mitochondrial localized PKA. Post-translational mitochondrial targeting of StAR would follow the classical pathway; StAR is synthesized on cytoplasmic polysomes, bound by chaperones, and targeted to TOM20/22 by the N-terminal signal sequence (**Figure 1**, steps c and d). StAR phosphorylation could occur at any step in this classical pathway. In both the co- and post-translational models, there must be a mechanism allowing for folding of the START domain and phosphorylation of S194/195 that are necessary for interactions at the OMM that promote cholesterol transfer. StAR import is slowed by a pause domain (Bose et al., 1999, 2002), and this could permit time necessary to generate phosphoStAR by mitochondrial localized PKA. The retention of phosphoStAR's START domain at the OMM signals for cholesterol transfer. Thus, studies directed at testing StARS194/195-OMM protein interactions may help uncover the ACTH-dependent phosphoStAR-OMM protein interaction specific for cholesterol transfer.

AUTHOR CONTRIBUTIONS

BC reviewed the literature, generated the figure, and wrote the mini-review.

REFERENCES

1. Aghazadeh, Y., Zirkin, B. R., and Papadopoulos, V. (2015). Pharmacological regulation of the cholesterol transport machinery in steroidogenic cells of the testis. *Vitam. Horm.* 98, 189–227. doi: 10.1016/bs.vh.2014.12.006
2. Alberta, J. A., Epstein, L. F., Pon, L. A., and Orme-Johnson, N. R. (1989). Mitochondrial localization of a phosphoprotein that rapidly accumulates in adrenal cortex cells exposed to adrenocorticotropic hormone or to cAMP. *J. Biol. Chem.* 264, 2368–2372.
3. Anflous, K., Armstrong, D. D., and Craigen, W. J. (2001). Altered mitochondrial sensitivity for ADP and maintenance of creatine-stimulated respiration in oxidative striated muscles from VDAC1-deficient mice. *J. Biol. Chem.* 276, 1954–1960. doi: 10.1074/jbc.M006587200
4. Arakane, F., King, S. R., Du, Y., Kallen, C. B., Walsh, L. P., Watari, H., et al. (1997). Phosphorylation of steroidogenic acute regulatory protein (StAR) modulates its steroidogenic activity. *J. Biol. Chem.* 272, 32656–32662. doi: 10.1074/jbc.272.51. 32656
5. Arakane, F., Sugawara, T., Nishino, H., Liu, Z., Holt, J. A., Pain, D., et al. (1996). Steroidogenic acute regulatory protein (StAR) retains activity in the absence of its mitochondrial import sequence: implications for the mechanism of StAR action. *Proc. Natl. Acad. Sci. U.S.A.* 93, 13731–13736. doi: 10.1073/pnas.93.24. 13731
6. Artemenko, I. P., Zhao, D., Hales, D. B., Hales, K. H., and Jefcoate, C. R. (2001). Mitochondrial processing of newly synthesized steroidogenic acute regulatory protein (StAR), but not total StAR, mediates cholesterol transfer to cytochrome P450 side chain cleavage enzyme in adrenal cells. *J. Biol. Chem.* 276, 46583–46596. doi: 10.1074/jbc.M107815200

7. Baker, B. Y., Epand, R. F., Epand, R. M., and Miller, W. L. (2007). Cholesterol binding does not predict activity of the steroidogenic acute regulatory protein, StAR. *J. Biol. Chem.* 282, 10223–10232. doi: 10.1074/jbc.M611221200
8. Becker, T., Böttinger, L., and Pfanner, N. (2012). Mitochondrial protein import: from transport pathways to an integrated network. *Trends Biochem. Sci.* 37, 85–91. doi: 10.1016/j.tibs.2011.11.004
9. Bose, H. S., Lingappa, V. R., and Miller, W. L. (2002). Rapid regulation of steroidogenesis by mitochondrial protein import. *Nature* 417, 87–91. doi: 10. 1038/417087a
10. Bose, H. S., Sato, S., Aisenberg, J., Shalev, S. A., Matsuo, N., and Miller, W. L. (2000). Mutations in the steroidogenic acute regulatory protein (StAR) in six patients with congenital lipoid adrenal hyperplasia. *J. Clin. Endocrinol. Metab.* 85, 3636–3639. doi: 10.1210/jc.85.10.3636
11. Bose, H. S., Whittal, R. M., Baldwin, M. A., and Miller, W. L. (1999). The active form of the steroidogenic acute regulatory protein, StAR, appears to be a molten globule. *Proc. Natl. Acad. Sci. U.S.A.* 96, 7250–7255. doi: 10.1073/pnas.96. 13.7250
12. Bose, M., Whittal, R. M., Miller, W. L., and Bose, H. S. (2008). Steroidogenic activity of StAR requires contact with mitochondrial VDAC1 and phosphate carrier protein. *J. Biol. Chem.* 283, 8837–8845. doi: 10.1074/jbc. M709221200
13. Caron, K. M., Soo, S. C., Wetsel, W. C., Stocco, D. M., Clark, B. J., and Parker, K. L. (1997). Targeted disruption of the mouse gene encoding steroidogenic acute regulatory protein provides insights into congenital lipoid adrenal hyperplasia. *Proc. Natl. Acad. Sci. U.S.A.* 94, 11540–11545. doi: 10.1073/pnas.94.21.11540
14. Chaudhary, L. R., and Stocco, D. M. (1991). Effect of different steroidogenic stimuli on protein phosphorylation and steroidogenesis in MA-10 mouse Leydig tumor cells. *Biochim. Biophys. Acta* 1094, 175–184. doi: 10.1016/0167-4889(91) 90006-J
15. Clark, B. J., and Hudson, E. A. (2015). StAR protein stability in Y1 and Kin-8 mouse adrenocortical cells. *Biology (Basel)* 4:200. doi: 10.3390/biology4010200
16. Clark, B. J. (2012). The mammalian START domain protein family in lipid transport in health and disease. *J. Endocrinol.* 212, 257–275. doi: 10.1530/JOE- 11-0313
17. Clark, B. J., Combs, R., Hales, K. H., Hales, D. B., and Stocco, D. M. (1997). Inhibition of transcription affects synthesis of steroidogenic acute regulatory protein and steroidogenesis in MA-10 mouse Leydig tumor cells. *Endocrinology* 138, 4893–4901. doi: 10.1210/en.138.11.4893
18. Clark, B. J., Pezzi, V., Stocco, D. M., and Rainey, W. E. (1995). The steroidogenic acute regulatory protein is induced by angiotensin II and K+ in H295R adrenocortical cells. *Mol. Cell. Endocrinol.* 115, 215–219. doi: 10.1016/0303- 7207(95)03683-0
19. Clark, B. J., Wells, J., King, S. R., and Stocco, D. M. (1994). The purification, cloning, and expression of a novel luteinizing hormone-induced mitochondrial protein in MA-10 mouse Leydig tumor cells. Characterization of the steroidogenic acute regulatory protein (StAR). *J. Biol. Chem.* 269, 28314–28322.
20. Clark, J. B., and Stocco, M. D. (2014). "The Steroidogenic Acute Regulatory Protein (StAR)," in Cholesterol Transporters of the START Domain Protein Family in Health and Disease: START Proteins - Structure and Function, eds J. B. *Clark and M. D. Stocco (New York, NY: Springer New York)*, 15–47.
21. Craigen, W. J., and Graham, B. H. (2008). Genetic strategies for dissecting mammalian and Drosophila voltage-dependent anion channel functions. *J. Bioenerg. Biomembr.* 40, 207–212. doi: 10.1007/s10863-008-9146-x
22. Dyson, M. T., Jones, J. K., Kowalewski, M. P., Manna, P. R., Alonso, M., Gottesman,
A. A. E., et al. (2008). Mitochondrial A-kinase anchoring protein 121 binds type II protein kinase A and enhances steroidogenic acute regulatory protein-mediated steroidogenesis in MA-10 mouse leydig tumor cells. *Biol. Reprod.* 78, 267–277. doi: 10.1095/biolreprod.107.064238
23. Dyson, M. T., Kowalewski, M. P., Manna, P. R., and Stocco, D. M. (2009). The differential regulation of steroidogenic acute regulatory protein-mediated steroidogenesis by type I and type II PKA in MA-10 cells. *Mol. Cell. Endocrinol.* 300, 94–103. doi: 10.1016/j.mce.2008.11.029
24. Eliyahu, E., Pnueli, L., Melamed, D., Scherrer, T., Gerber, A. P., Pines, O., et al. (2010). Tom20 mediates localization of mRNAs to mitochondria in a translation-dependent manner. *Mol. Cell. Biol.* 30, 284–294. doi: 10.1128/MCB. 00651-09
25. Epstein, L. F., and Orme-Johnson, N. R. (1991). Regulation of steroid hormone biosynthesis. Identification of precursors of a phosphoprotein targeted to the mitochondrion in stimulated rat adrenal cortex cells. *J. Biol. Chem.* 266, 19739–19745.
26. Ferguson, J. J., Jr. (1962). Puromycin and adrenal responsiveness to adrenocorticotropic hormone. *Biochim. Biophys. Acta* 57, 616–617. doi: 10. 1016/0006-3002(62)91176-9
27. Ferguson, J. J. Jr. (1963). Protein synthesis and adrenocorticotropin responsiveness. *J. Biol. Chem.* 238, 2754–2759.
28. Gallo-Payet, N., and Payet, M. D. (2003). Mechanism of action of ACTH: beyond cAMP. *Microsc. Res. Tech.* 61, 275–287. doi: 10.1002/jemt.10337
29. Granot, Z., Geiss-Friedlander, R., Melamed-Book, N., Eimerl, S., Timberg, R., Weiss, A. M., et al. (2003). Proteolysis of normal and mutated steroidogenic acute regulatory proteins in the mitochondria: the fate of unwanted proteins. *Mol. Endocrinol.* 17, 2461–2476. doi: 10.1210/me.2003-0074
30. Grozdanov, P. N., and Stocco, D. M. (2012). Short RNA molecules with high binding affinity to the KH motif of A-kinase anchoring protein 1 (AKAP1): implications for the regulation of steroidogenesis. *Mol. Endocrinol.* 26, 2104–2117. doi: 10.1210/me.2012-1123
31. Harbauer Angelika, B., Zahedi René P., Sickmann, A., Pfanner, N., and Meisinger, (2014). The protein import machinery of mitochondria—a regulatory hub in metabolism, stress, and disease. *Cell Metab.* 19, 357–372. doi: 10.1016/j.cmet. 2014.01.010
32. Hartigan, J. A., Green, E. G., Mortensen, R. M., Menachery, A., Williams, G. H., and Orme-Johnson, N. R. (1995). Comparison of protein phosphorylation patterns produced in adrenal cells by activation of cAMP-dependent protein kinase and Ca-dependent protein kinase. *J. Steroid Biochem. Mol. Biol.* 53, 95–101. doi: 10. 1016/0960-0760(95)00026-V
33. Issop, L., Fan, J., Lee, S., Rone, M. B., Basu, K., Mui, J., et al. (2015). Mitochondria-associated membrane formation in hormone-stimulated Leydig cell steroidogenesis: role of ATAD3. *Endocrinology* 156, 334–345. doi: 10.1210/ en.2014-1503
34. Jo, Y., King, S. R., Khan, S. A., and Stocco, D. M. (2005). Involvement of protein kinase C and cyclic adenosine 3',5'-monophosphate-dependent kinase in steroidogenic acute regulatory protein expression and steroid biosynthesis in Leydig cells. *Biol. Reprod.* 73, 244–255. doi: 10.1095/biolreprod.104. 037721
35. Kellems, R. E., Allison, V. F., and Butow, R. A. (1974). Cytoplasmic type 80 S ribosomes associated with yeast mitochondria. II. Evidence for the association of cytoplasmic ribosomes with the outer mitochondrial membrane *in situ*. *J. Biol. Chem.* 249, 3297–3303.
36. Kim, J. M., Choi, J. H., Lee, J. H., Kim, G. H., Lee, B. H., Kim, H. S., et al. (2011).
37. High allele frequency of the p.Q258X mutation and identification of a novel mis-splicing mutation in the STAR gene in Korean patients with congenital lipoid adrenal hyperplasia. *Eur. J. Endocrinol.* 165, 771–778. doi: 10.1530/EJE- 11-0597
38. King, S. R., Ronen-Fuhrmann, T., Timberg, R., Clark, B. J., Orly, J., and Stocco,
A. A. M. (1995). Steroid production after *in vitro* transcription, translation, and mitochondrial processing of protein products of complementary deoxyribonucleic acid for steroidogenic acute regulatory protein. *Endocrinology* 136, 5165–5176. doi: 10.1210/endo.136.11.7588255
39. Krueger, R. J., and Orme-Johnson, N. R. (1983). Acute adrenocorticotropic hormone stimulation of adrenal corticosteroidogenesis. Discovery of a rapidly induced protein. *J. Biol. Chem.* 258, 10159–10167.
40. Lee, J., Foong, Y. H., Musaitif, I., Tong, T., and Jefcoate, C. (2016a). Analysis of specific RNA in cultured cells through quantitative integration of q-PCR and N-SIM single cell FISH images: application to hormonal stimulation of StAR transcription. *Mol. Cell. Endocrinol.* 429, 93–105. doi: 10.1016/j. mce.2016. 04.001
41. Lee, J., Tong, T., Duan, H., Foong, Y. H., Musaitif, I., Yamazaki, T., et al. (2016b). Regulation of StAR by the N-terminal domain and coinduction of SIK1 and TIS11b/Znf36l1 in single cells. *Front. Endocrinol. (Lausanne)* 7:107. doi: 10. 3389/fendo.2016.00107
42. Lesnik, C., Golani-Armon, A., and Arava, Y. (2015). Localized translation near the mitochondrial outer membrane: an update. *RNA Biol.* 12, 801–809. doi: 10. 1080/15476286.2015.1058686
43. Lin, D., Sugawara, T., Strauss, J. F. III., Clark, B. J., Stocco, D. M., Saenger, P., et al. (1995). Role of steroidogenic acute regulatory protein in adrenal

and gonadal steroidogenesis. *Science* 267, 1828–1831. doi: 10.1126/science.7892608

44. Liu, J., Rone, M. B., and Papadopoulos, V. (2006). Protein-protein interactions mediate mitochondrial cholesterol transport and steroid biosynthesis. *J. Biol. Chem.* 281, 38879–38893. doi: 10.1074/jbc.M608820200
45. Macchi, I. A., and Hechter, O. (1954a). Studies of ACTH action upon perfused bovine adrenals; duration of ACTH action. *Endocrinology* 55, 434–438. doi: 10. 1210/endo-55-4-434
46. Macchi, I. A., and Hechter, O. (1954b). Studies of ACTH action upon perfused bovine adrenals; minimal ACTH concentration requisite for maximal glandular response. *Endocrinology* 55, 426–433. doi: 10.1210/endo-55-4-426
47. Macchi, I. A., and Hechter, O. (1954c). Studies of ACTH action upon perfused bovine adrenals; corticosteroid biosynthesis in isolated glands maximally stimulated with ACTH. *Endocrinology* 55, 387–402. doi: 10.1210/endo- 55-4-387
48. Mathieu, A. P., Fleury, A., Ducharme, L., Lavigne, P., and LeHoux, J. G. (2002). Insights into steroidogenic acute regulatory protein (StAR)-dependent cholesterol transfer in mitochondria: evidence from molecular modeling and structure-based thermodynamics supporting the existence of partially unfolded states of StAR. *J. Mol. Endocrinol.* 29, 327–345. doi: 10.1677/jme.0. 0290327
49. Merrill, R. A., and Strack, S. (2014). Mitochondria: a kinase anchoring protein 1, a signaling platform for mitochondrial form and function. *Int. J. Biochem. Cell Biol.* 48, 92–96. doi: 10.1016/j.biocel.2013.12.012
50. Midzak, A., and Papadopoulos, V. (2016). Adrenal mitochondria and steroidogenesis: from individual proteins to functional protein assemblies. *Front. Endocrinol. (Lausanne).* 7:106.doi: 10.3389/fendo.2016.00106
51. Miller, L. W. (2014). "Congenital lipoid adrenal hyperplasia," in Cholesterol Transporters of the START Domain Protein Family in Health and Disease: START Proteins - Structure and Function, eds J. B. *Clark and M. D. Stocco (New York, NY: Springer New York),* 73–97.
52. Miller, W. L. (2007). Steroidogenic acute regulatory protein (StAR), a novel mitochondrial cholesterol transporter. *Biochim. Biophys. Acta* 1771, 663–676. doi: 10.1016/j.bbalip.2007.02.012
53. Miller, W. L., and Auchus, R. J. (2011). The molecular biology, biochemistry, and physiology of human steroidogenesis and its disorders. *Endocr. Rev.* 32, 81–151. doi: 10.1210/er.2010-0013
54. Nakae, J., Tajima, T., Sugawara, T., Arakane, F., Hanaki, K., Hotsubo, T., et al. (1997). Analysis of the steroidogenic acute regulatory protein (StAR) gene in Japanese patients with congenital lipoid adrenal hyperplasia. *Hum. Mol. Genet.* 6, 571–576. doi: 10.1093/hmg/6.4.571
55. Papadopoulos, V., Aghazadeh, Y., Fan, J., Campioli, E., Zirkin, B., and Midzak, A. (2015). Translocator protein-mediated pharmacology of cholesterol transport and steroidogenesis. *Mol. Cell. Endocrinol.* 408, 90–98. doi: 10.1016/j.mce.2015. 03.014
56. Paz, C., Cornejo Maciel, F., Gorostizaga, A., Castillo, A. F., Mori Sequeiros Garcia, M. M., Maloberti, P. M., et al. (2016). Role of protein phosphorylation and tyrosine phosphatases in the adrenal regulation of steroid synthesis and mitochondrial function. *Front. Endocrinol.* 7:60. doi: 10.3389/fendo.2016. 00060
57. Poderoso, C., Maloberti, P., Duarte, A., Neuman, I., Paz, C., Maciel, F. C., et al. (2009). Hormonal activation of a kinase cascade localized at the mitochondria is required for StAR protein activity. *Mol. Cell. Endocrinol.* 300, 37–42. doi: 10. 1016/j.mce.2008.10.009
58. Pon, L. A., Hartigan, J. A., and Orme-Johnson, N. R. (1986). Acute ACTH regulation of adrenal corticosteroid biosynthesis. Rapid accumulation of a phosphoprotein. *J. Biol. Chem.* 261, 13309–13316.
59. Pon, L. A., and Orme-Johnson, N. R. (1986). Acute stimulation of steroidogenesis in corpus luteum and adrenal cortex by peptide hormones. Rapid induction of a similar protein in both tissues. *J. Biol. Chem.* 261, 6594–6599.
60. Ponting, C. P., and Aravind, L. (1999). START: a lipid-binding domain in StAR, HD-ZIP and signalling proteins. *Trends Biochem. Sci.* 24, 130–132. doi: 10. 1016/S0968-0004(99)01362-6
61. Prasad, M., Kaur, J., Pawlak, K. J., Bose, M., Whittal, R. M., and Bose, H. S. (2015). Mitochondria-associated endoplasmic reticulum membrane (MAM) regulates steroidogenic activity via steroidogenic acute regulatory protein (StAR)-voltage-dependent anion channel 2 (VDAC2) interaction. *J. Biol. Chem.* 290, 2604–2616. doi: 10.1074/jbc.M114.605808
62. Prasad, M., Walker, A. N., Kaur, J., Thomas, J. L., Powell, S. A., Pandey, A. V., et al. (2016). Endoplasmic reticulum stress enhances mitochondrial metabolic activity in mammalian adrenals and gonads. *Mol. Cell. Biol.* 36, 3058–3074. doi: 10.1128/MCB.00411-16
63. Rajapaksha, M., Kaur, J., Bose, M., Whittal, R. M., and Bose, H. S. (2013). Cholesterol-mediated conformational changes in the steroidogenic acute regulatory protein are essential for steroidogenesis. *Biochemistry* 52, 7242–7253. doi: 10.1021/bi401125v
64. Rajapaksha, M., Kaur, J., Prasad, M., Pawlak, K. J., Marshall, B., Perry, E. W., et al. (2016). An outer mitochondrial translocase, Tom22, is crucial for inner mitochondrial steroidogenic regulation in adrenal and gonadal tissues. *Mol. Cell. Biol.* 36, 1032–1047. doi: 10.1128/MCB.01107-15
65. Rone, M. B., Midzak, A. S., Issop, L., Rammouz, G., Jagannathan, S., Fan, J., et al. (2012). Identification of a dynamic mitochondrial protein complex driving cholesterol import, trafficking, and metabolism to steroid hormones. *Mol. Endocrinol.* 26, 1868–1882. doi: 10.1210/me.2012-1159
66. Roostaee, A., Barbar, E., Lehoux, J. G., and Lavigne, P. (2008). Cholesterol binding is a prerequisite for the activity of the steroidogenic acute regulatory protein (StAR). *Biochem. J.* 412, 553–562. doi: 10.1042/BJ20071264
67. Sasaki, G., Ishii, T., Jeyasuria, P., Jo, Y., Bahat, A., Orly, J., et al. (2008). Complex role of the mitochondrial targeting signal in the function of steroidogenic acute regulatory protein revealed by bacterial artificial chromosome transgenesis *in vivo*. *Mol. Endocrinol.* 22, 951–964. doi: 10.1210/me.2007-0493
68. Sasaki, G., Zubair, M., Ishii, T., Mitsui, T., Hasegawa, T., and Auchus, R. J. (2014). The contribution of serine 194 phosphorylation to steroidogenic acute regulatory protein function. *Mol. Endocrinol.* 28, 1088–1096. doi: 10.1210/me. 2014-1028
69. Sileikyte, J., Blachly-Dyson, E., Sewell, R., Carpi, A., Menabo, R., Di Lisa, F., et al. (2014). Regulation of the mitochondrial permeability transition pore by the outer membrane does not involve the peripheral benzodiazepine receptor (Translocator Protein of 18 kDa (TSPO)). *J. Biol. Chem.* 289, 13769–13781. doi: 10.1074/jbc.M114.549634
70. Spät, A., Hunyady, L., and Szanda, G. (2016). Signaling Interactions in the adrenal cortex. *Front. Endocrinol. (Lausanne)* 7:17. doi: 10.3389/fendo.2016.00017 Stocco, D. M. (2001). StAR protein and the regulation of steroid hormone biosynthesis. *Annu. Rev. Physiol.* 63, 193–213. doi: 10.1146/annurev.physiol.63. 1.193
71. Stocco, D. M., and Sodeman, T. C. (1991). The 30-kDa mitochondrial proteins induced by hormone stimulation in MA-10 mouse Leydig tumor cells are processed from larger precursors. *J. Biol. Chem.* 266, 19731–19738.
72. Stocco, D. M., Zhao, A. H., Tu, L. N., Morohaku, K., and Selvaraj, V. (2016). A brief history of the search for the protein(s) involved in the acute regulation of steroidogenesis. *Mol. Cell. Endocrinol.* doi: 10.1016/j.mce.2016.07.036. [Epub ahead of print].
73. Stone, D., and Hechter, O. (1954). Studies on ACTH action in perfused bovine adrenals: the site of action of ACTH in corticosteroidogenesis. *Arch. Biochem. Biophys.* 51, 457–469. doi: 10.1016/0003-9861(54)90501-9
74. Tu, L. N., Morohaku, K., Manna, P. R., Pelton, S. H., Butler, W. R., Stocco, D. M., et al. (2014). Peripheral benzodiazepine receptor/translocator protein global knock-out mice are viable with no effects on steroid hormone biosynthesis. *J. Biol. Chem.* 289, 27444–27454. doi: 10.1074/jbc.M114.578286
75. Wang, X., Liu, Z., Eimerl, S., Timberg, R., Weiss, A. M., Orly, J., et al. (1998). Effect of truncated forms of the steroidogenic acute regulatory protein on intramitochondrial cholesterol transfer. *Endocrinology* 139, 3903–3912. doi: 10. 1210/en.139.9.3903
76. Weeber, E. J., Levy, M., Sampson, M. J., Anflous, K., Armstrong, D. L., Brown, S. E., et al. (2002). The role of mitochondrial porins and the permeability transition pore in learning and synaptic plasticity. *J. Biol. Chem.* 277, 18891–18897. doi: 10.1074/jbc.M201649200

19

Molecular Mechanisms of Stem/Progenitor Cell Maintenance in the Adrenal Cortex

*Antonio Marcondes Lerario[1], Isabella Finco[1], Christopher LaPensee[1] and Gary Douglas Hammer[1,2,3]**

[1] *Department of Internal Medicine, Division of Metabolism, Endocrinology, and Diabetes, University of Michigan, Ann Arbor, MI, USA,* [2] *Endocrine Oncology Program, Comprehensive Cancer Center, University of Michigan, Ann Arbor, MI, USA,* [3] *Center for Organogenesis, University of Michigan, Ann Arbor, MI, USA*

Correspondence:
Gary Douglas Hammer
ghammer@med.umich.edu

The adrenal cortex is characterized by three histologically and functionally distinct zones: the outermost zona glomerulosa (zG), the intermediate zona fasciculata, and the innermost zona reticularis. Important aspects of the physiology and maintenance of the adrenocortical stem/progenitor cells have emerged in the last few years. Studies have shown that the adrenocortical cells descend from a pool of progenitors that are localized in the subcapsular region of the zG. These cells continually undergo a process of centripetal displacement and differentiation, which is orchestrated by several paracrine and endocrine cues, including the pituitary-derived adrenocorticotrophic hormone, and angiotensin II. However, while several roles of the endocrine axes on adrenocortical function are well established, the mechanisms coordinating the maintenance of an undifferentiated progenitor cell pool with self-renewal capacity are poorly understood. Local factors, such as the composition of the extracellular matrix (ECM) with embedded signaling molecules, and the activity of major paracrine effectors, including ligands of the sonic hedgehog and Wnt signaling pathways, are thought to play a major role. Particularly, the composition of the ECM, which exhibits substantial differences within each of the three histologically distinct concentric zones, has been shown to influence the differentiation status of adrenocortical cells. New data from other organ systems and different experimental paradigms strongly support the conclusion that the interactions of ECM components with cell-surface receptors and secreted factors are key determinants of cell fate. In this review, we summarize established and emerging data on the paracrine and autocrine regulatory loops that regulate the biology of the progenitor cell niche and propose a role for bioengineered ECM models in further elucidating this biology in the adrenal.

Keywords: adrenal cortex, paracrine signaling, stem cells, organogenesis, extracellular matrix, tissue homeostasis

INTRODUCTION

In vertebrates, adrenal steroid hormones are effectors of different adaptive responses to oscillations in the organism's internal and external environment, broadly referred as *stress*. Adrenal steroid hormones serve to modulate a wide range of processes that are central to physiologic response to stress, including energy metabolism, immune response, electrolyte homeostasis, and fluid balance. The three main classes of adrenal steroid hormones, mineralocorticoids, glucocorticoids, and androgens, are produced by the adrenal cortex under the tight regulation of distinct and independent endocrine regulatory loops: the renin–angiotensin–aldosterone system (RAAS) and the hypothalamus–pituitary–adrenal (HPA) axis. The ability of the adrenal gland to respond independently to these endocrine signals is dependent upon subpopulations of steroidogenic cells with distinct morphological and functional characteristics that are localized in specific concentric compartments (zones) of the cortex. In humans, three histologically distinct zones are evident: the outermost *zona glomerulosa* (zG), the intermediate *zona fasciculata* (zF), and the innermost *zona reticularis* (zR), which are responsible for the production of mineralocorticoids, glucocorticoids, and androgens, respectively (1). Although the morphological and physiological aspects of the adrenal cortex have been relatively well characterized, the regulatory mechanisms responsible for the establishment and maintenance of the three zones are not fully understood.

In the last few years, sophisticated molecular techniques, such as lineage tracing, and genetically modified animals have significantly contributed to our understanding of the embryonic development and homeostasis of the adrenal cortex, illuminating key molecules and signaling pathways that are implicated in these processes (discussed below in Sections "Progenitor Populations in the Adrenal Gland" and "Signaling Pathways and Adrenal Progenitors"). Accordingly, the Wnt and the hedgehog pathways have emerged as major paracrine factors that regulate both organogenesis and homeostasis of the gland. Both are essential for the establishment and maintenance of an undifferentiated population of steroidogenic precursor cells in the periphery of the organ that continuously replenish the cortical cells of the three zones throughout life (discussed below in Sections "Progenitor Populations in the Adrenal Gland" and "Signaling Pathways and Adrenal Progenitors"). While the effectors of the RAAS and the HPA axis [angiotensin 2 and adrenocorticotrophic hormone (ACTH), respectively] are considered primary endocrine mediators that promote activity of adrenocortical steroidogenic cells (2–4), recent data support that the *microenvironment*, comprised of the extracellular matrix (ECM), its associated proteins, and several paracrine and autocrine factors, are also major determinants of cell behavior and fate (discussed below in Sections "Signaling Pathways and Adrenal Progenitors" and "The Adrenocortical Progenitor Niche"). Emerging data support an important role for non-steroidogenic/mesenchymal-like cells that lie in the adrenal capsule in the maintenance of the adrenocortical progenitor pool (5–8). This review focuses on the role of microenvironmental factors and signaling pathways that contribute to the maintenance of the adrenal cortex. We will discuss emerging data on the role of specific paracrine and autocrine loops between capsular/stromal cells and cortical cells in establishing a specialized microenvironment that supports and maintains the adrenal progenitors throughout the life—the *niche*—and how this signaling contributes to the anatomical and functional zonation of the adrenal cortex.

DEVELOPMENTAL ORIGINS OF THE ADRENAL CORTEX

The adrenal cortex originates from cells of the celomic epithelium, which in the mammalian embryo is composed of a single squamous cell layer that covers the external surface of the viscera and the inner surface of the body wall. Around embryonic day 9.5 (E9.5) in mice, and during the fourth to sixth weeks of human gestation, a thickening of the celomic epithelium between the urogenital ridge and the dorsal mesentery forms the adrenogonadal *primordium* (AGP). At the eighth week of human gestation (E10.5 in mice), the AGP divides into dorsomedial and ventrolateral portions, giving rise to the adrenal and gonadal *primordia*, respectively (1, 9–11).

Between the weeks 8 and 9 of human gestation (E13 in mice), the *adrenal primordium* is invaded by cells of the neural crest that coalesce centrally to form the adrenal medulla (12). Subsequently, the *adrenal primordium* is surrounded by mesenchymal cells, which will ultimately form the adrenal capsule (13). At this point, compartmentalization of the adrenal cortex into two structurally distinct areas is evident: a central area, comprised of large polyhedric eosinophilic cells referred as the "fetal zone," and a peripheral zone adjacent to the newly formed capsule comprised of small and basophilic cells, referred to as "the definitive zone." While in mice this compartmentalization is subtle, in humans, the fetal zone predominates over the definitive zone, constituting up to 80% of the adrenal mass by the end of the gestation (9, 14). In addition, ultrastructural studies in humans have demonstrated the presence of a third zone, referred as the "transitional" or "intermediate zone," which has intermediate morphologic characteristics between the fetal and the definitive zones (9). It has been suggested that after mid-gestation the transitional zone has the capacity to synthesize cortisol (9, 15). By the week 30 of human gestation, the definitive and the transitional zones have morphological features that resemble the adult zG and zF, respectively (16). In humans, the fetal cortex starts to regress by apoptosis soon after birth, completely disappearing after a few weeks (9). In mice, definitive evidence about the presence of a transient fetal zone was provided by the identification of the fetal adrenal-specific enhancer (FAdE), which is only active during early fetal development (see below). The differentiation process of the human adrenal cortex continues until the onset of puberty, when the definitive cortex completes its organization into the three distinct histologic zones that characterize the adult cortex of human and higher primates (14). While the zG and the zF are evident at birth, the androgen-producing zR only starts to form a few years later, marking the onset of the adrenarche, which is the earliest stage of sexual maturation and a precursor of puberty (17).

A transcription factor critical for adrenocortical development and homeostasis is steroidogenic factor 1 (SF1, also known as adrenal four-binding protein or nuclear hormone receptor Ad4BP, encoded by the gene *NR5A1*). All cells that belong to steroidogenic lineages of the adrenal and gonads express SF1, including subpopulations of long-term retained progenitor cells in each organ (8, 18). Therefore, SF1 expression defines the identity of these cells and commitment to steroidogenic differentiation (14, 19, 20). The expression of SF1 is detectable early in fetal life, between the AGP formation and the ultimate establishment of the adrenal *primordium* (14, 18). Genetic loss of *Nr5a1* or its upstream transcriptional regulators *Pbx1*, *Wt1*, and *Cited2*, interferes with AGP formation leading to various degrees of adrenal hypoplasia in mice (12, 14, 21–23). While *Nr5a1* is continuously expressed from the time of *adrenal primordium* formation throughout the adult life, during embryonic stages and early fetal life in mice, the *Nr5a1* expression is driven by the fetal adrenal-specific enhancer (FAdE), which becomes inactive when the definitive cortex forms, suggesting that distinct mechanisms sustain *Nr5a1* expression in the fetal and in the definitive cortex (14).

While the enhancer that is responsible for initiation and maintenance of *Nr5a1* expression in the definitive zone is currently not known, lineage-tracing experiments performed by Zubair et al. have shown that *FAdE*-driven-*Ad4bp*-expressing cells are indeed precursors of most, if not all, Sf1-expressing cells of the definitive cortex (14). It has since been demonstrated that after extinguishing FAdE-dependent SF1 expression, some cells become embedded within the coalescing capsule and later reemerge as FAdE-independent SF1-expressing cells during the formation of the definitive cortex (24).

Steroidogenic factor 1 not only defines the identity/specification of the cells of the definitive cortex but also serves as a key regulator of hormone-dependent steroidogenesis, the hallmark of a differentiated adrenocortical cell. In this regard, the effects of ACTH on differentiation and steroidogenesis are partially mediated by an SF1-induced transcription of steroidogenic enzymes that defines a cortisol-producing cell (25). It remains unclear, however, how a subpopulation of SF1-expressing cells are spared from the pro-differentiation effects of ACTH, preserving their undifferentiated state. One clue to such regulation comes from studies of DAX1, an atypical nuclear receptor that is encoded by the gene *NR0B1* and expressed preferentially in the peripheral/subcapsular cortex. DAX1 functions as a repressor of SF1-mediated transcription and has been shown to have an important role in the maintenance of the undifferentiated state (lack of steroidogenesis) of the adrenocortical progenitor population (26). Studies examining the consequences of genetic loss of DAX1 in the adrenal revealed an unexpectedly hyper-functional zF in younger mice, characterized by an increase in cell proliferation and steroid production. Surprisingly, as the animals aged, they developed adrenal hypofunction consistent with an abnormal premature differentiation of the progenitor cell pool that ultimately resulted in its exhaustion (27, 28). In the next section, we will briefly summarize studies that have begun to explore the molecular and cellular processes that underlie the homeostasis of the progenitor cell population.

PROGENITOR POPULATIONS IN THE ADRENAL GLAND

One of the first reports regarding adrenal regeneration in rats describes the restoration of the adrenal cortex 6 weeks after unilateral adrenal enucleation, a process that involves the removal of the inner content of the adrenal gland (including the medulla), while leaving the capsule and underlying subcapsular cells intact. This observation suggested the presence of an adrenocortical stem and/or progenitor cell population located in the periphery of the adrenal gland (29). The notion of a renewing progenitor population in the adrenal cortex was corroborated by the observation that transplants of bovine adrenocortical cells underneath the kidney capsules of adrenalectomized immunocompromised mice can give rise to adrenocortical tissue with steroidogenic properties (30, 31).

The presence of a progenitor cell population in the periphery in the adrenal gland that gives rise to all the differentiated cell types within the different cortical zones is consistent with a homeostatic model of centripetal migration and differentiation. This idea was first hypothesized in the 19th century, based on histological observations of gradual changes in morphology observed in cells between the capsule and the medulla (32, 33) [reviewed in Ref (34)]. Over the years, different studies have shown that, under physiological conditions, proliferating cells are located preferentially in the outermost layers of the cortex, in the subcapsular region (35, 36). Also, it has been demonstrated that peripheral cortical cells are centripetally displaced until they reach the cortical–medullary boundary and become apoptotic (35, 37). Moreover, studies performed in chimeric and transgenic mosaic rats and mice have shown a radial variegated pattern of the reporters extending from the outer cortex to the cortico-medullary boundary. This observation is consistent with a peripheral clonal origin (38–40). Definitive genetic evidence for a centripetal conversion of adrenocortical cells between concentric zones was finally provided by cell-lineage tracing (8, 41). In one of these studies, transgenic mice were created with a Cre recombinase gene inserted at the *Cyp11b2* locus, in which *Cre* was expressed only in terminally differentiated zG cells (41). When these mice were crossed with mice expressing the *R26R*$^{mT/mG}$ reporter, GFP-positive cells that occupied the zG upon *Cyp11b2-Cre* expression, eventually populated the entire cortex. Over time, an increasing number of centripetally located *Cyp11b1*-expressing cells were found to express GFP, indicating that peripheral zG cells underwent lineage conversion to more centripetal zF cells. In 12-week old mice, nearly the entire cortex was comprised of GFP-positive cells. Although these existing data strongly support the existence of a progenitor population localized in the periphery of the gland that gives rise to all the steroidogenic cells types of the cortex through a process of centripetal displacement/migration and differentiation, the molecular mechanisms that govern this process are not completely understood.

Further studies have provided clues on the molecular fingerprint of the progenitor cell populations and the signaling pathways that regulate their renewal and differentiation. Specific paracrine/autocrine signaling pathways are activated in zonally restricted patterns that reflect the different cell subpopulations that are hypothesized to play an active role in organ homeostasis. The most important and well characterized are the Wnt and the hedgehog pathways. Additionally, a cross-talk between cortical cells and capsular stromal cells regulates the activity of these pathways. Below, we briefly summarize these findings.

SIGNALING PATHWAYS AND ADRENAL PROGENITORS

Wnt Signaling Pathway

The mammalian wingless-type MMTV integration site (Wnt) signaling pathway is one of the most studied pathways in developmental biology, playing important roles in organogenesis, homeostasis, and stem cell biology (42). Wnt ligands represent a large family of highly conserved morphogens that are characterized by repetitive cysteine residues. Secreted Wnt ligands bind to receptors of the Frizzled and lipoprotein receptor-related protein families on the cell surface. Through several cytoplasmic components, the signal is either transduced through β-catenin, which enters the cell nucleus and complexes with T-cell factor/lymphocyte enhancer factor (TCF/LEF) family of transcription factors to activate transcription of Wnt target genes (canonical pathway), and/or activates the non-canonical Wnt pathway to regulate planar cell polarity and calcium signaling (42). In the mouse adrenal gland, β-catenin expression is first observed at E12.5 in Sf1+ cells of the definitive cortex in a scattered fashion beneath the newly formed capsule (43). After E18.5 and throughout life, β-catenin protein expression becomes more enriched in cells of the zG, which have also been demonstrated to bear active canonical Wnt signaling (43, 44).

Canonical Wnt signaling plays several roles in the adrenal cortex. Recent evidence demonstrates that the population of Wnt-responsive cells is heterogeneous and contains small clusters of Shh-producing cells (considered to be adrenal progenitors, as it will be discussed later) and separate differentiated Cyp11b2-expressing cell clusters (44). Interestingly, despite the well-known role of Wnt signaling pathway in promoting cell proliferation in a variety of organ systems, the Wnt-responsive cells do not appear to be heavily proliferating, implying that any role of Wnt signaling in adrenal homeostatic growth might involve a potential cell non-autonomous mechanism (44).

The Wnt pathway is essential for the establishment and maintenance of the subcapsular progenitor cell population. However, it does not appear to play a role in the early formation of the AGP since expression of Ctnnb1 is first detectable in mesothelial cells overlying the indifferent gonad at around E11.5 and in the adrenal primordium at around E12.5, following their separation from the AGP (43, 45). Studies performed in a *Nr5a1/Cre*-mediated *Ctnnb1* conditional knockout mouse model (*Ctnnb1tm2kem* mice crossed into *Sf1/Cre-high* mice), in which canonical Wnt signaling to adrenal primordium SF1-expressing cells from around E12.5 is reduced or absent reveal a marked decrease in cortical cell proliferation which ultimately results in the complete regression of the adrenal gland by E18.5, despite normal formation of the adrenal primordium at earlier time points (43, 46). Loss of β-catenin in approximately 50% of Sf1-expressing cells and hence a resultant ~50% decrease in β-catenin-mediated Wnt signaling (induced by a low efficiency Sf1/Cre-low driver that allows for a subset of cells to escape recombination) results in a histologically normal adrenal through 15 weeks of age, after which the adrenal cortex undergoes progressive thinning over time and ultimate adrenal failure (43, 46). Consistent with a primordial role of the Wnt signaling in maintaining the progenitor cell population, it has been demonstrated that *Nr0b1 (Dax1)* is a transcriptional target of β-catenin, suggesting that both proteins synergistically act to maintain the undifferentiated state that characterizes the progenitor cell population (28). Together, these evidences suggest that canonical Wnt signaling has a role in establishing and maintaining a pool of adrenocortical progenitors throughout life.

Hedgehog Signaling Pathway

The hedgehog signaling pathway (Hh) is a conserved evolutionary pathway that is essential for embryonic development and adult tissue maintenance, renewal, and regeneration. Three secreted hedgehog proteins have been described: sonic hedgehog (SHH), desert hedgehog, and Indian hedgehog. These proteins function in a concentration- and time-dependent fashion, controlling several processes ranging from survival and proliferation to cell fate specification and differentiation (47).

Shh is the only Hh family member that is present in the murine adrenal gland, being detected as early as E12.5 and later expressed in a restricted manner in a subpopulation of cells in the outer zG (8). These cells are Sf1-positive and do not express Cyp11b2 or Cyp11b1, the enzymes necessary for terminal reactions that lead to aldosterone and corticosterone production, respectively. While in the mouse adrenal the Shh+ cells are localized in clusters under the capsule, in the rat these cells form a continuous layer localized between the zG and the zF, known as the *undifferentiated zone* (zU) (48).

Lineage-tracing studies that mark all Shh-expressing cells and their descendants reveal that, by postnatal day 12 (P12), virtually all cells of the cortex are derived from *Shh*-expressing cells, consistent with a role for Shh in the peripheral stem/progenitor cells (8). Studies utilizing an inducible *Shh*-Cre recombinase have demonstrated that shortly after recombination in adult mice, Shh-expressing cells, and their immediate descendants are restricted to the periphery of the cortex. Over time, these cells and their descendants form centripetally expanding radial stripes, supporting the hypothesis that the Shh-expressing cells are a progenitor population that gives rise to all other cortical cell populations (8). BrdU-labeling experiments carried out on rat adrenals identified two sites of proliferation in the outer zF and inner zU and between the zG and zU, suggesting that cell proliferation at the periphery of the zU provides cells to both zG and zF (36). However, the proliferative capacity of these cells is more consistent with their identification as progenitors rather than as stem cells as suggested by the authors. Another study on mouse adrenocortical cell proliferation used BrdU pulse-chase labeling to identify a small population of quiescent non-steroidogenic cells located in the outer cortex that may represent a quiescent progenitor population, which is prompted to divide following ACTH stimulation (35). Additionally, this study suggested that two distinct subpopulations of rapidly cycling cells emerged from the progenitor population—the first constituted by cells that proliferate in response to ACTH and migrate inwards and the second constituted by cells that migrate outwards and are less responsive to ACTH. The authors have suggested that these distinct subgroups of cells are committed transient-amplifying cells that are responsible for the maintenance of the zF and zG, respectively (35). Interestingly, another study has shown that Cyp11b2-expressing cells in the zG derived from the Shh-expressing cells undergo lineage interconversion, differentiating into Cyp11b1-expresing cells in the zF as they migrate inwards, suggesting that cells from both zones are in fact derived from the same lineage (41).

In addition to serving as a progenitor cell population in the cortex, Shh-positive cells presumably signal to Gli1-expressing cells that lie within the capsule (48, 49). Interestingly, the capsular Gli1-expressing cells are a mesenchymal-like population that do not express Sf1 (Gli1+/Sf1−) but descends from the fetal FAdE-utilizing Sf1+ cells of the adrenal *primordium* (24). The fate of the descendants of these *Gli1*-expressing cells has been investigated in a transgenic mouse model with an inducible *Gli1-CreERT2* allele. It has been demonstrated that during adrenal development, *Gli1+* capsular cells behave as stem or precursor cells since they give rise to Sf1+ cells of the early definitive cortex that later become the Sf1+/Shh+ progenitor cell pool (8).

Other Signaling Pathways

In addition to the Gli+/Sf1− cell population, other mesenchymal-like cell lineages have also been identified in the capsule and the stroma. These cells may also have important roles in the adrenal gland maintenance. Bandiera and colleagues observed a long-retained pool of cells expressing the Wilms tumor protein homolog (WT1) in the adrenal capsule that originates from capsular mesenchymal cells and is characterized by AGP features (50). WT1 is a transcriptional regulator that has important roles in organogenesis of different organs, including the adrenals and gonads. Using a Wt1-Cre recombinase line crossed with a reporter line, Bandiera et al. demonstrated that WT1-expressing cells could give rise to steroidogenic cortical cells in the adult adrenal and the Gli1+ population as well, lending support for a role for WT1 in the activation of *Gli1* transcription.

Wood et al. identified a population of cells in the mouse adrenal that starts to express the transcription factor 21 (*Tcf21,* also known as *Pod1*/capsuling/epicardin) at E9.5 onward. After E14.5, Tcf21 expression becomes predominately restricted to the capsule and further diminishes over time, leaving only a small population of capsular Tcf21+ cells through adulthood. Lineage-tracing experiments revealed that before adrenal encapsulation, *Tcf21*-expressing cells and/or their descendants give rise to both non-steroidogenic capsular cells and steroidogenic cortical cells. On the other hand, the population of Tcf21-expressing capsular cells only gives rise to a population of Sf1− stromal cells that express collagen, desmin, and Pdgfrα and persist throughout adult life within the cortex (24).

Taken together, these studies provide evidence that the capsule is a complex niche comprised of multiple long-term retained cell lineages. The roles of each of these populations in the adult adrenal remain unknown, but recent evidence suggests that signaling coming from the capsule is required for the long-term maintenance of the adrenocortical progenitor cells.

THE ADRENOCORTICAL PROGENITOR NICHE

The proper balance of progenitor proliferation and differentiation is crucial, as dysregulation of the mechanisms that regulate the differentiation, proliferation, and self-maintenance of progenitor cells throughout life can result in organ failure. Stem and progenitor cells from different organs and tissues are embedded within a specialized microenvironment, termed the *niche.* Niches are protective locations that support stem cell residence and maintenance. Several components of the niche have been identified, including bioactive compounds, such as Wnt ligands, growth factors [e.g., fibroblast growth factors (FGFs) and epidermal growth factor], chemokines, and a distinct ECM composition that sequesters growth factor signaling and spatially restricts cell movement for appropriate cell–cell interactions. While well-defined niches characterized in different organs vary in size and complexity, most are maintained by a small set of fundamental regulatory signaling loops (51). Although several studies have revealed the importance of these signaling pathways in the adrenal biology as coordinators of stem/progenitor cell specification and differentiation, the formal structural and molecular definition of an adrenocortical progenitor niche remains elusive (52). ECM components are predicted to provide additional structural context to zone-specific signaling pathways discussed in the previous section. Below, we discuss these regulatory mechanisms in further details.

Components of the Adrenocortical Niche

Soluble Factors

Wnt Ligands

As previously discussed, the canonical Wnt/β catenin signaling pathway is considered to be a crucial pathway for the maintenance of the subcapsular stem/progenitor pool (44, 46, 53). While the source and the contribution of different Wnt ligands to Wnt signaling are not currently known, previous observations based on adrenal tumors expression profiles, human clinical syndromes, and mouse models suggest that WNT4 is an important Wnt regulatory paracrine factor in the adrenal cortex. In humans, *WNT4* mutations underlie the defects in Serkal syndrome, an autosomal recessive disorder characterized by multiple malformations including adrenal hypoplasia and male-to-female sexual reversion (54). In mice, while Wnt4 expression is observed in the developing adrenal glands as early as E11.5, by E14.5 it is restricted to the outer cortex (46, 55). Additionally, a mouse model of Wnt4 inactivation suggests that this ligand is required for proper zG differentiation and aldosterone production. In these mice, genetic loss of *Wnt4* decreases *Cyp11b2* expression, leading to a diminished production of aldosterone (55). Interestingly, the anterior tips of the developing gonads of these mice exhibit a steroidogenic enzyme expression pattern similar to adrenocortical cells, suggesting an abnormal differentiation process or a defect in adrenal cell specification during the separation of the AGP (55, 56).

WNT4 is a known transcriptional target of Wnt/β catenin signaling (55). In the adrenal cortex, WNT4 expression is restricted to the zG, precisely where canonical Wnt pathway is known to be active. Additionally, according to our own analysis on a recently published molecular profiling study on adrenocortical carcinomas (57), samples with activating exon 3 *CTNNB1* mutations exhibit increased expression of *WNT4* in comparison to samples without somatic alterations in components of the Wnt pathway (fold change = 17.5, FDR-adjusted p-value <0.001). More recently, it has been demonstrated that the expression levels of canonical Wnt target genes are significantly reduced in the adrenals of a mouse model of *Sf1-Cre* mediated *Wnt4* knockout (*Sf1:Cre;Wnt4Fl/Fl*) (58). Interestingly, it has also been shown that the activation of the protein kinase A pathway enables a zG-to-zF lineage conversion by antagonizing canonical Wnt signaling, which is partially mediated by repression of *Wnt4* expression (58). Together, these data support a model whereby WNT4 serves as an autocrine activator of Wnt signaling, amplifying canonical (β catenin-dependent) Wnt activation within the zG, which is essential for proper zonation. However, whether WNT4 downstream signaling also induces a non-canonical (β catenin-independent) effect is currently not known. In other systems, WNT4 is described preferentially as a non-canonical ligand (59, 60). Last, the roles and the sources of other Wnt ligands that are expressed in the adrenal are yet to be determined.

Other Wnt Pathway-Related Soluble Factors

Bone Morphogenetic Protein-4 (BMP4) is a ligand of the TGF-β superfamily that plays essential roles in embryonic development, stem cell biology, and tissue regeneration (61). Recently, Rege et al. have demonstrated that this protein, its receptors, and downstream molecules are expressed and have functional roles in the human adrenal cortex and in the H295R adrenocortical carcinoma cell line. Interestingly, mRNA expression of *BMP4* follows a zonal distribution gradient, with the highest levels in the zG, suggesting that *BMP4* is a Wnt target gene. *In vitro*, BMP4 actively inhibits the expression of 17,20-lyase and DHEA secretion, possibly serving to prevent a zR fate (62). Consistent with the observed zonal distribution in the adrenal cortex, *BMP4* has been reported as a Wnt target gene in a colorectal cancer cell line (63). Moreover, according to our own analysis on two independent datasets (57, 64), *BMP4* mRNA is upregulated in ACC samples with nuclear immunostaining for β-catenin or with an activating mutation of *CTNNB1* in comparison to those with membranous immunostaining or wild-type for *CTNNB1* somatic mutations (fold change >3.21–6.76, FDR-adjusted *p*-value <0.001). These observations suggest that *BMP4* is a paracrine factor regulated by the Wnt pathway that may have a role in functional zonation by inhibiting a zR fate.

Coiled-coil domain containing 80 (*CCDC80*) has recently been described as a novel Wnt target gene in the adrenal cortex. *In situ* hybridization has shown that it is expressed in cells within the zG. Functional studies have shown that CCDC80 decreases steroidogenesis *in vitro*, suggesting, as for BMP4, a role in cell differentiation or fate. The molecular pathway by which CCDC80 regulates steroidogenesis is yet to be determined in the adrenal gland (44). In the chick embryo, the *CCDC80* homolog equarin regulates FGF signaling by increasing its local availability and by facilitating the interactions of FGF ligands with FGF receptors and proteoglycans (65). Further studies in *CCDC80* null mice aiming to characterize the overall mechanism of action of *CCDC80* in the adrenal gland are ongoing.

Sonic Hedgehog

Sonic hedgehog-expressing cells serve as a *bona fide* progenitor population that contributes to the adrenal cortex homeostasis in adult life, as previously described. Mice with global genetic deletion of *Shh* exhibit severe adrenal hypoplasia during embryonic development due to a reduction in both cortical and capsular cell proliferation (8, 66, 67). However, these animals also have severe malformations in other organs, including pituitary defects that impair ACTH production, making the adrenal phenotype difficult to interpret. Moreover, targeted deletion of *Shh* in Sf1-expressing cells in mice also causes adrenal abnormalities, indicating that Shh is indeed essential for intrinsic (ACTH-independent) adrenal development. While AGP separation, neural crest migration, and encapsulation occur normally, these animals have a hypoplastic adrenal cortex and diminished mitotic activity by E13.5. As age increases, progressive cortical thinning with an apparent defect in steroidogenesis is observed as reflected by a compensatory increase in ACTH levels. Also, an overall thinner capsule is also seen (66). The mechanisms by which Shh deficiency causes this capsular phenotype are not known, but is predicted to result from a defective cortical Shh signaling to the capsular Gli1-expressing cells.

Shh is a secreted ligand that binds to the cell-surface receptor patched homolog 1 (Ptch1). Shh binding relieves Ptch1-mediated inhibition of Smoothened homolog (Smo). Smo stimulates intracellular downstream Shh signaling that, when activated, inhibits the otherwise proteolytic degradation of Gli transcription factors, resulting in Gli-mediated transcriptional activation of Hh target genes (8, 47, 66, 67). Whether a secreted factor produced by Shh-responsive Gli+ capsular cells is required for maintaining the subcapsular progenitor population is currently unknown. Together, these observations indicate that the Shh-expressing subcapsular progenitor cells and the capsular Gli-expressing cells are integral components of the adrenocortical progenitor cell niche.

Fibroblast Growth Factors

The FGFs are a family of secreted signaling proteins that bind to a subclass of membrane-bound tyrosine kinase-coupled receptors (FGFRs 1–4) and intracellular non-signaling proteins (iFGFs) that work as cofactors for other membrane-associated proteins. With few exceptions, FGFs are ubiquitous paracrine/autocrine factors with essential roles in embryogenesis, organogenesis, and tissue homeostasis. FGFs regulate fundamental cellular processes, including proliferation (both promoting and inhibiting), survival, differentiation, migration, and metabolism. FGFs routinely bind to heparin sulfate proteoglycans, which limit their diffusion through the ECM and serve as cofactors that regulate FGF specificity and affinity to different types of FGFRs (68, 69).

Early studies have demonstrated that FGFs exhibit a potent mitogenic effect both in the murine-derived Y1 adrenocortical cell line and primary cultures of bovine and human adrenocortical cells. Interestingly, this effect can be antagonized by ACTH, which promotes cell differentiation by inducing cell cycle arrest and steroidogenesis *in vitro* (70–74). *In vivo*, different combinations of FGF ligands and receptors are expressed in the adrenal capsule and cortex, consistent with a proposed role in homeostasis. RT-PCR analysis from laser capture microdissected adrenals from E15.5 mouse embryos have shown that *Fgf1*, *Fgf2*, and *Fgf9* are the only FGF ligands that are expressed in the embryonic adrenal gland. While *Fgf1* is expressed in the cortex, *Fgf2* and *Fgf9* are expressed preferentially in the capsule. Additionally,

Fgfr1-IIIc, *Fgfr2*-IIIb, and *Fgfr2*-IIIc are expressed in cells of both the capsule and the cortex. Interestingly, the cortical cells that express *Fgfr2* are the also Shh-positive (48, 75, 76).

The importance of FGF signaling in adrenal maintenance has been revealed through several *in vivo* studies. FGF2 encapsulated in poly-lactic-co-glycolic acid enhances the growth of adrenocortical cells implanted under the kidney capsule of mice by fivefold to eightfold (74). Additionally, engineered deletion of the FGF ligand, FGF2 or the FGF receptor *Fgfr2*, results in various degrees of adrenal hypoplasia after birth. The global *Fgfr2*-IIIb knockout results in embryonic lethality due to severe malformations, including adrenal hypoplasia (7). The same adrenal phenotype was recapitulated by a *Sf1*-driven specific knockout of both *Fgfr2*-IIIb and *Fgfr2*-IIIc (77). Evaluation of the embryonic adrenal gland of *Fgfr2*-IIIb global knockout mice at E15.5 revealed a marked capsular defect, characterized by thickening and disorganization of the mesenchymal capsule, with increased mitotic activity and increased number of Gli1-positive cells. Meanwhile, the underlying cortex was hypoplastic with a decrease in both steroidogenic differentiation and mitotic activity. An unexpected, decrease in capsular delta-like protein 1 (Dlk1) suggests that, together with Shh and FGFs, Dlk1 is a mediator of the proposed homeostatic cross-talk between cortical and capsular cells (75).

Delta-Like Protein 1 (DLK1)

Delta-like protein 1 (also known as preadipocyte factor 1—*Pref1*) is a paternally expressed imprinted gene that encodes an epidermal growth factor repeat-containing transmembrane protein. Dlk1 is cleaved by the TNF-alpha-converting enzyme (TACE or ADAM17) to generate a soluble, secreted, and biologically active protein (78, 79). In adipose tissue, DLK1 negatively regulates proliferation and terminal differentiation of adipocyte progenitors (80–83). Mechanistically, DLK1 interacts with fibronectin and facilitates downstream integrin signaling, which includes MEK/ERK activation (80). While the human adrenal cortex expresses high levels of the *DLK1* transcript (the highest levels among all human tissues according to the GTEx portal database), little is known about its downstream signaling and overall function in adrenocortical cells (84). However, *in vivo* studies in rat reveal that *Dlk1* expression is markedly decreased in the regeneration process following enucleation, suggesting a role in adrenal remodeling and zonation. The Dlk1 expression is restricted to a subcapsular population in the rat zU (6, 85, 86). Indeed, the Dlk1+ cells do not express Cyp11b1 and are rarely positive for Cyp11b2. They do, however, express Shh, indicating that they are indeed the progenitor population (48, 87). A low-sodium diet induces a marked downregulation of both Dlk1 and Shh, with a proportional increase in the expression of Cyp11b2. Blocking the RAAS with captopril induces the opposite effect—expansion of Dlk1 and Shh-expressing cells. Additionally, a population of capsular cells responds directly to Dlk1 signaling by increasing the levels of both p-ERK and Gli1, consistent with a role in regulating hedgehog signaling (6). These results predict that in the rat adrenal, Dlk1 is expressed by the cortical progenitor cell population and acts in concert with Shh to activate capsular Gli1, modulating differentiation, remodeling, and zonation (6). However, it should be noted that these conclusions are based on studies in rat, which express Dlk1 in the subcapsular cells whereas, in mice, Dlk1/Pref1 is expressed in the capsule (6, 75).

R-Spondin Family Member 3 (RSPO3)

R-spondins are secreted proteins that have been recently described as important positive regulators of the canonical Wnt pathway (88). R-Spondins are paracrine factors that exhibit a very low diffusion gradient since these proteins firmly binds to certain ECM components such as syndecan-4, remaining close to its secretory source (89). In organs, such as the liver and the gastrointestinal tract, RSPO3 gradients are a critical determinant of regions of active canonical Wnt signaling, being a crucial regulator of the stem/progenitor cell compartment, cell differentiation, and functional compartmentalization (90). R-Spondins interact with members of the leucine-rich-repeat-containing G-protein-coupled receptor (Lgr), which have recently been described as surface stem cell markers (91). Clinical evidence suggests an important role of R-Spondins in stem cell biology and morphogenesis since inactivating mutations in R-Spondin genes are associated with syndromes characterized by stem cell failure and developmental abnormalities (89). The interaction of R-Spondins with the Lgr receptors results in the inactivation of the U3-ubiquitin ligases RNF43 and ZNRF3, which are negative regulators of Wnt signaling by promoting internalization of the *Frizzled* receptors. Consequently, in the presence of R-Spondins, the *Frizzled* receptor will remain on the membrane allowing for Wnt signaling activation (91, 92). A recent paper explores the roles of R-Spondins in the regulation of the canonical Wnt signaling, functional zonation, and progenitor cell activity in the adrenal cortex (5). By using *in situ* hybridization, the authors demonstrated the expression of *Rspo1* and *Rspo3* in the adrenal capsule of the mouse from E12.5 onward. While *Rspo1* co-localized with the *Wt1* mesodermal-like expressing cells, *Rspo3* was preferentially co-expressed with *Nr2f2* and *Gli1*-expressing cells. Additionally, the mRNA abundance of *Rspo3* was significantly higher than *Rspo1*. Interestingly, while the genetic loss of *Rspo1* had no observable effects on the adrenals, loss of *Rspo3* was associated with remarkable phenotypes. By using different crosses of a *Rspo3^{flox}* allele and several CreERT drivers, the authors demonstrated that (a) loss of *Rspo3* results in cortical atrophy both during development and postnatally; (b) these changes are accompanied by a dramatic decrease in canonical Wnt signaling, which results in loss of the expression of canonical Wnt target genes such as *Axin2* and *Wnt4*; (c) loss of a functional zG, characterized by profound morphological changes and loss of expression of zG markers (while retaining zF differentiation); (d) loss of cortical Shh-expressing cells and capsular Gli1-expressing cells; and (e) a significant decrease in the mitotic activity of the cortex. The authors concluded that capsular-derived Rspo3 is a key regulator of both Wnt and Hedgehog signaling in the adrenal cortex, having determinant roles in the establishment and the maintenance of the stem/progenitor cell populations, and in functional zonation (5).

These above findings support a general model whereby several autocrine/paracrine mediators from different sources play regulatory roles in the major signaling pathways that control the progenitor cell compartment and fate determination in the adrenal cortex (**Figure 1**). Some are known to interact with ECM components, indicating that the ECM composition may play a role in these regulatory loops. However, several gaps in the knowledge about the role of the adrenal ECM in paracrine/autocrine signaling and cell fate determination remain. In the following sections, we summarize the main findings that support a regulatory role for the adrenal ECM.

The ECM and Associated Proteins

The ECM is a three-dimensional meshwork of extracellular proteins and polysaccharides that supports cells in each tissue (93). Among its components are included fibrous proteins such as collagens, laminin, fibronectin, and several types of bioactive compounds, such as latent growth factors, enzymes, chemoattractants, and morphogens (94). Therefore, in addition to its role in providing the physical scaffold that shapes the different tissues in an organism, the ECM is a reservoir of several biologically active compounds of different sources that are delivered to the cells in a spatially controlled manner (93, 94). Cells attach to the ECM through a special type of membrane-bound adhesion molecule known as integrins, which are comprised of two interacting subunits. The vertebrate integrin family contains 18 α and 8 β subunits that can assemble into 24 different receptor complexes, each with unique binding properties for different ECM components (93). In the context of the stem cell niche of a variety of organ systems, the interactions between ECM proteins and integrins are fundamental for establishing a balance between self-renewal and differentiation. By forming complexes with different membrane receptors and ECM components, integrins facilitate a strict compartmentalization of cellular responses to different factors on a cell-by-cell basis. Such highly precise control is fundamental to the process of asymmetric division, a fundamental characteristic of self-renewing cells. The complexes that contain integrins, ECM components, and other receptors induce the establishment of cell polarity, restricting fate-determinant molecules to one pole and directing the plane of cell cleavage in such a way that signaling molecules will be asymmetrically distributed between the daughter cells (95). In fact, certain types of integrins have been recognized as crucial for stem cell maintenance in different tissues (96). Supporting this observation, genetic ablation of β1 integrin favors a symmetric pattern of cell division in the mammary stem cell niche, leading to exhaustion of the stem cell compartment (97). Finally, biophysical and biochemical properties of the substrate, such as shape, stiffness, and protein composition, can trigger different transcriptional programs that support either stem cell maintenance or differentiation (98, 99).

Despite the emerging importance of ECM in tissue homeostasis and stem cell biology, few studies have addressed its roles in the adrenal. Early studies in different species have shown that several ECM components and integrins follow a zonal distribution in the adrenal cortex (100, 101). Furthermore, *in vitro* studies on primary adrenal cultures grown on different substrates suggest that different ECM components affect cellular responses to ACTH. For instance, it has been demonstrated in primary cultures from human fetal adrenals that laminin exerts an inhibitory effect on basal and ACTH-induced steroidogenesis, and a positive effect on cell proliferation (102). On the other hand, collagen IV and fibronectin increased cortisol and DHEAS production, respectively (102). While collagen IV is expressed throughout the human fetal adrenal gland, laminin and fibronectin follow a

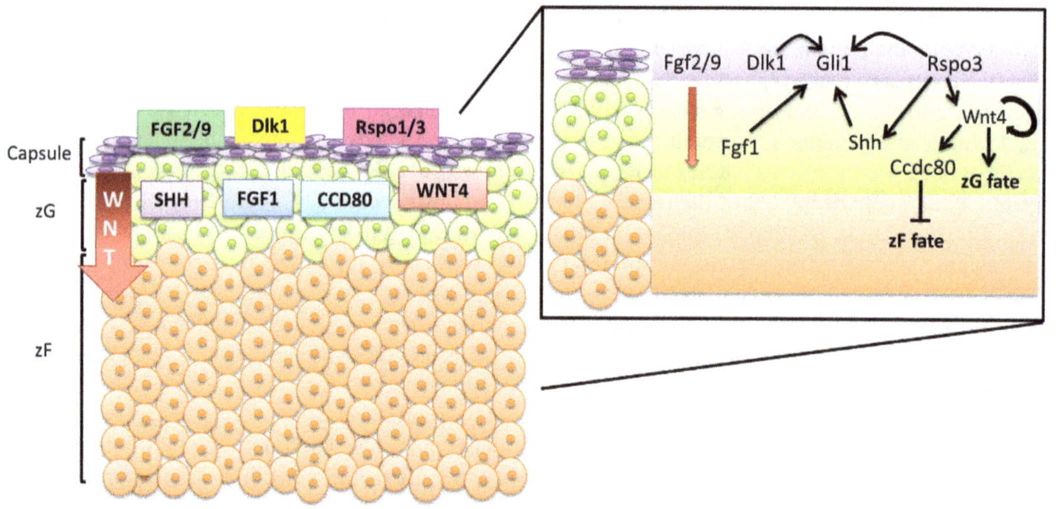

FIGURE 1 | Schematic figure representing paracrine signaling in the adrenal cortex. Adrenal zonation is established and maintained by a compartmentalized secretion of paracrine factors. The zG is characterized by activation of canonical Wnt signaling, which is dependent on the presence of RSPO3 secreted by Gli1-expressing capsular cells. Wnt-expressing cells secrete other paracrine factors that regulate the differentiation of cortical cells. Wnt4 amplifies the activation of canonical Wnt signaling within the zG, helping in maintaining the zonation. Ccdc80 and is a canonical Wnt target gene that prevents zF differentiation. By unknown mechanisms, a small proportion of Wnt-active zG cells, which is a long-living progenitor cell population, secretes Shh, which activates Gli1-dependent signaling on the capsular cells. Other paracrine factors, such as Dlk1 and fibroblast growth factors, also have regulatory roles in the maintenance of the cortical progenitor cells, presumably by regulating Gli1 expression in the capsule.

zonal distribution, being preferentially expressed in cells of the definitive and the fetal zones, respectively (101). Therefore, the differences in cellular responses *in vitro* induced by these different ECM components parallel the functional zonation observed in the fetal gland: laminin suppresses differentiation and promotes proliferation (consistent with the cellular phenotype of the newly forming definitive zone), collagen IV promotes *HSD3B2* expression and cortisol production (resembling the fetal adrenal transitional zone), and fibronectin supports *CYP17A1* expression and DHEAS production. Indeed, primary cultures from zG and zF cells from the adult rat adrenal grown on laminin-coated plates exhibited increased proliferation and reduced basal and ACTH-stimulated aldosterone and cortisol production, respectively (103). Taken together, these results support the hypothesis that the ECM composition modulates cellular responses to hormone and growth factor stimulation, providing an additional mechanism by which the niche itself regulates the balance between self-renewal and differentiation.

CONCLUDING REMARKS AND FUTURE PERSPECTIVES

In the last decade, several important aspects of the physiology of the adrenal cortex have been characterized, including the developmental origins of the different progenitor populations and the molecular pathways that are essential for self-renewal, organ remodeling, and differentiation. Additionally, several paracrine/autocrine bioactive compounds that initiate and maintain these signaling pathways have been identified. However, while the progenitor niche populations of other tissues, such as the skin and the gastrointestinal tract, are clearly defined, the progenitor niche of the adrenal cortex is just beginning to be characterized. Many features of the molecular mechanisms that govern the fate of the adrenocortical progenitor cells are still unknown. As discussed in the previous sections, several studies involving transgenic animal models have illuminated important observations and concepts central to the field. However, these studies are complex and time-consuming. Furthermore, studying such a small yet complex organ like the adrenal gland imposes additional challenges. In the near future, innovative techniques that allow investigators to engage in more complex *in vitro* studies have the potential to move the field forward greatly. Among these, organoid culture and engineered ECM are promising approaches.

Organoid culture has emerged in recent years as a valuable tool to study several aspects of stem cell biology, tissue morphogenesis, and lineage specification (104, 105). Organoids are self-organizing three-dimensional structures that are derived from stem cells and exhibit organotypic anatomic and functional features, including spatially restricted lineage commitment (106, 107). Organoids can be grown *in vitro* from pluripotent stem cells (embryonic stem cells and induced pluripotent stem cells) or organ-specific stem cells (105). Organoid cultures have been established for different mouse and human tissues, including intestines, stomach, lungs, mammary gland, and prostate (108–114). A crucial requirement for establishing an organoid culture is the supplementation of organ-specific and well-defined stem cell niche factors in the culture medium. For example, to culture intestinal organoids, culture medium is supplemented with Wnt3a, EGF, Noggin, and R-spondin 1 (108). Organoids have been proven to be valuable models for studying different aspects developmental biology and stem cell research such as tissue morphogenesis, organogenesis, differentiation, heterotypic interactions between different cell types, and the effects of the ECM on cell differentiation and behavior. However, a current limitation of organoid cultures is the organoid dependence on a suitable three-dimensional matrix. Among the most commonly used scaffolds are collagen and Matrigel. These substrates, however, feature variable compositions and physical properties, which limits studies aiming to characterize the influence of the microenvironment on the organoid properties (105). Furthermore, these substrates pose risks of immunologic reactions and pathogen transfer and are, therefore, unsuitable for clinical applications. Engineered synthetic ECM has emerged as an attractive approach to circumvent these limitations (115).

Engineered ECM, constructed as an artificial substrate, acts to mimic the original three-dimensional microenvironment of a given organ or tissue. Increasingly, sophisticated scaffolds comprised of materials, such as synthetic hydrogels and nanofibers, are frequently employed as artificial ECM substitutes. In addition to biochemical interactions in cell–cell and cell–ECM signaling, mechanical stimuli such as substrate stiffness, and tension forces can also be modeled in engineered ECM (115). In a recent publication Gjorevski et al. studied the effects of stiffness on the dynamics of single cell-derived intestinal organoid formation (116). While intermediate to high stiffness and the presence of fibronectin sustained the expansion of intestinal LGR5-positive stem cells, differentiation and organoid formation required softer matrices and the presence of laminin.

We believe that, in the near future, organoid culture and tissue engineering techniques will increase our power to understand the molecular interactions that regulate the adrenal cortex stem cell niche. Protocols to establish normal adrenocortical and cancer organoid cultures in bioengineered matrices are currently under development in our laboratory.

AUTHOR CONTRIBUTIONS

All authors equally contributed to this manuscript.

FUNDING

AL is supported by CAPES, grant number BEX 8726/13-2.

REFERENCES

1. Yates R, Katugampola H, Cavlan D, Cogger K, Meimaridou E, Hughes C, et al. Adrenocortical development, maintenance, and disease. *Curr Top Dev Biol* (2013) 106:239–312. doi:10.1016/B978-0-12-416021-7.00007-9
2. Chan LF, Metherell LA, Clark AJ. Effects of melanocortins on adrenal gland physiology. *Eur J Pharmacol* (2011) 660(1):171–80. doi:10.1016/j.ejphar.2010.11.041
3. Kramer RE, Gallant S, Brownie AC. Actions of angiotensin II on aldosterone biosynthesis in the rat adrenal cortex. Effects on cytochrome

P-450 enzymes of the early and late pathway. *J Biol Chem* (1980) 255(8): 3442–7.
4. Fujita K, Aguilera G, Catt KJ. The role of cyclic AMP in aldosterone production by isolated zona glomerulosa cells. *J Biol Chem* (1979) 254(17):8567–74.
5. Vidal V, Sacco S, Rocha AS, da Silva F, Panzolini C, Dumontet T, et al. The adrenal capsule is a signaling center controlling cell renewal and zonation through Rspo3. *Genes Dev* (2016) 30(12):1389–94. doi:10.1101/gad.277756.116
6. Guasti L, Cavlan D, Cogger K, Banu Z, Shakur A, Latif S, et al. Dlk1 up-regulates Gli1 expression in male rat adrenal capsule cells through the activation of beta1 integrin and ERK1/2. *Endocrinology* (2013) 154(12):4675–84. doi:10.1210/en.2013-1211
7. Revest JM, Spencer-Dene B, Kerr K, De Moerlooze L, Rosewell I, Dickson C, et al. Fibroblast growth factor receptor 2-IIIb acts upstream of Shh and Fgf4 and is required for limb bud maintenance but not for the induction of Fgf8, Fgf10, Msx1, or Bmp4. *Dev Biol* (2001) 231(1):47–62. doi:10.1006/dbio.2000.0144
8. King P, Paul A, Laufer E. Shh signaling regulates adrenocortical development and identifies progenitors of steroidogenic lineages. *Proc Natl Acad Sci U S A* (2009) 106(50):21185–90. doi:10.1073/pnas.0909471106
9. Mesiano S, Jaffe RB. Developmental and functional biology of the primate fetal adrenal cortex. *Endocr Rev* (1997) 18(3):378–403. doi:10.1210/edrv.18.3.0304
10. Morohashi K. The ontogenesis of the steroidogenic tissues. *Genes Cells* (1997) 2(2):95–106. doi:10.1046/j.1365-2443.1997.1060304.x
11. Ikeda Y, Shen WH, Ingraham HA, Parker KL. Developmental expression of mouse steroidogenic factor-1, an essential regulator of the steroid hydroxylases. *Mol Endocrinol* (1994) 8(5):654–62. doi:10.1210/mend.8.5.8058073
12. Val P, Martinez-Barbera JP, Swain A. Adrenal development is initiated by Cited2 and Wt1 through modulation of Sf-1 dosage. *Development* (2007) 134(12):2349–58. doi:10.1242/dev.004390
13. Keegan CE, Hammer GD. Recent insights into organogenesis of the adrenal cortex. *Trends Endocrinol Metab* (2002) 13(5):200–8. doi:10.1016/S1043-2760(02)00602-1
14. Zubair M, Parker KL, Morohashi K. Developmental links between the fetal and adult zones of the adrenal cortex revealed by lineage tracing. *Mol Cell Biol* (2008) 28(23):7030–40. doi:10.1128/MCB.00900-08
15. Narasaka T, Suzuki T, Moriya T, Sasano H. Temporal and spatial distribution of corticosteroidogenic enzymes immunoreactivity in developing human adrenal. *Mol Cell Endocrinol* (2001) 174(1–2):111–20. doi:10.1016/S0303-7207(00)00445-7
16. Sucheston ME, Cannon MS. Development of zonular patterns in the human adrenal gland. *J Morphol* (1968) 126(4):477–91. doi:10.1002/jmor.1051260408
17. Conley AJ, Bernstein RM, Nguyen AD. Adrenarche in nonhuman primates: the evidence for it and the need to redefine it. *J Endocrinol* (2012) 214(2):121–31. doi:10.1530/JOE-11-0467
18. Luo X, Ikeda Y, Parker KL. A cell-specific nuclear receptor is essential for adrenal and gonadal development and sexual differentiation. *Cell* (1994) 77(4):481–90. doi:10.1016/0092-8674(94)90211-9
19. Lala DS, Rice DA, Parker KL. Steroidogenic factor I, a key regulator of steroidogenic enzyme expression, is the mouse homolog of fushi tarazu-factor I. *Mol Endocrinol* (1992) 6(8):1249–58. doi:10.1210/mend.6.8.1406703
20. Honda S, Morohashi K, Nomura M, Takeya H, Kitajima M, Omura T. Ad4BP regulating steroidogenic P-450 gene is a member of steroid hormone receptor superfamily. *J Biol Chem* (1993) 268(10):7494–502.
21. Bamforth SD, Bragança J, Eloranta JJ, Murdoch JN, Marques FI, Kranc KR, et al. Cardiac malformations, adrenal agenesis, neural crest defects and exencephaly in mice lacking Cited2, a new Tfap2 co-activator. *Nat Genet* (2001) 29(4):469–74. doi:10.1038/ng768
22. Moore AW, McInnes L, Kreidberg J, Hastie ND, Schedl A. YAC complementation shows a requirement for Wt1 in the development of epicardium, adrenal gland and throughout nephrogenesis. *Development* (1999) 126(9):1845–57.
23. Schnabel CA, Selleri L, Cleary ML. Pbx1 is essential for adrenal development and urogenital differentiation. *Genesis* (2003) 37(3):123–30. doi:10.1002/gene.10235
24. Wood MA, Acharya A, Finco I, Swonger JM, Elston MJ, Tallquist MD, et al. Fetal adrenal capsular cells serve as progenitor cells for steroidogenic and stromal adrenocortical cell lineages in *M. musculus*. *Development* (2013) 140(22):4522–32. doi:10.1242/dev.092775
25. Sewer MB, Nguyen VQ, Huang CJ, Tucker PW, Kagawa N, Waterman MR. Transcriptional activation of human CYP17 in H295R adrenocortical cells depends on complex formation among p54(nrb)/NonO, protein-associated splicing factor, and SF-1, a complex that also participates in repression of transcription. *Endocrinology* (2002) 143(4):1280–90. doi:10.1210/endo.143.4.8748
26. Ito M, Yu R, Jameson JL. DAX-1 inhibits SF-1-mediated transactivation via a carboxy-terminal domain that is deleted in adrenal hypoplasia congenita. *Mol Cell Biol* (1997) 17(3):1476–83. doi:10.1128/MCB.17.3.1476
27. Babu PS, Bavers DL, Beuschlein F, Shah S, Jeffs B, Jameson JL, et al. Interaction between Dax-1 and steroidogenic factor-1 in vivo: increased adrenal responsiveness to ACTH in the absence of Dax-1. *Endocrinology* (2002) 143(2):665–73. doi:10.1210/endo.143.2.8658
28. Scheys JO, Heaton JH, Hammer GD. Evidence of adrenal failure in aging Dax1-deficient mice. *Endocrinology* (2011) 152(9):3430–9. doi:10.1210/en.2010-0986
29. Ingle D, Higgins G. Autotransplantation and regeneration of the adrenal gland. *Endocrinology* (1938) 22:458–64. doi:10.1210/endo-22-4-458
30. Thomas M, Hornsby PJ. Transplantation of primary bovine adrenocortical cells into scid mice. *Mol Cell Endocrinol* (1999) 153(1–2):125–36. doi:10.1016/S0303-7207(99)00070-2
31. Thomas M, Northrup SR, Hornsby PJ. Adrenocortical tissue formed by transplantation of normal clones of bovine adrenocortical cells in scid mice replaces the essential functions of the animals' adrenal glands. *Nat Med* (1997) 3(9):978–83. doi:10.1038/nm0997-978
32. Gottschau M. Struktur und embryonale Entwicklung der Nebennieren bei Säugetieren. *Archiv Anatomie Physiologie* (1883) 412–458:412–58.
33. Arnold J. Ein beitrag zu der feineren structur und demchemismus der nenemmieren. *Virchows Arch* (1866) 39:64–117. doi:10.1007/BF01979887
34. Vinson GP. Functional zonation of the adult mammalian adrenal cortex. *Front Neurosci* (2016) 10:238. doi:10.3389/fnins.2016.00238
35. Chang SP, Morrison HD, Nilsson F, Kenyon CJ, West JD, Morley SD. Cell proliferation, movement and differentiation during maintenance of the adult mouse adrenal cortex. *PLoS One* (2013) 8(12):e81865. doi:10.1371/journal.pone.0081865
36. Miyamoto H, Mitani F, Mukai K, Suematsu M, Ishimura Y. Studies on cytogenesis in adult rat adrenal cortex: circadian and zonal variations and their modulation by adrenocorticotropic hormone. *J Biochem* (1999) 126(6):1175–83. doi:10.1093/oxfordjournals.jbchem.a022564
37. Bertholet JY. Proliferative activity and cell migration in the adrenal cortex of fetal and neonatal rats: an autoradiographic study. *J Endocrinol* (1980) 87(1):1–9. doi:10.1677/joe.0.0870001
38. Iannaccone PM, Weinberg WC. The histogenesis of the rat adrenal cortex: a study based on histologic analysis of mosaic pattern in chimeras. *J Exp Zool* (1987) 243(2):217–23. doi:10.1002/jez.1402430207
39. Hu MC, Chou SJ, Huang YY, Hsu NC, Li H, Chung BC. Tissue-specific, hormonal, and developmental regulation of SCC-LacZ expression in transgenic mice leads to adrenocortical zone characterization. *Endocrinology* (1999) 140(12):5609–18. doi:10.1210/endo.140.12.7177
40. Morley SD, Viard I, Chung BC, Ikeda Y, Parker KL, Mullins JJ. Variegated expression of a mouse steroid 21-hydroxylase/beta-galactosidase transgene suggests centripetal migration of adrenocortical cells. *Mol Endocrinol* (1996) 10(5):585–98. doi:10.1210/mend.10.5.8732689
41. Freedman BD, Kempna PB, Carlone DL, Shah MS, Guagliardo NA, Barrett PQ, et al. Adrenocortical zonation results from lineage conversion of differentiated zona glomerulosa cells. *Dev Cell* (2013) 26(6):666–73. doi:10.1016/j.devcel.2013.07.016
42. Nusse R. Wnt signaling. *Cold Spring Harb Perspect Biol* (2012) 4(5):a011163. doi:10.1101/cshperspect.a011163
43. Kim AC, Reuter AL, Zubair M, Else T, Serecky K, Bingham NC, et al. Targeted disruption of beta-catenin in Sf1-expressing cells impairs development and maintenance of the adrenal cortex. *Development* (2008) 135(15):2593–602. doi:10.1242/dev.021493
44. Walczak EM, Kuick R, Finco I, Bohin N, Hrycaj SM, Wellik DM, et al. Wnt signaling inhibits adrenal steroidogenesis by cell-autonomous and

non-cell-autonomous mechanisms. *Mol Endocrinol* (2014) 28(9):1471–86. doi:10.1210/me.2014-1060
45. Usongo M, Farookhi R. beta-catenin/Tcf-signaling appears to establish the murine ovarian surface epithelium (OSE) and remains active in selected post-natal OSE cells. *BMC Dev Biol* (2012) 12:17. doi:10.1186/1471-213X-12-17
46. Walczak EM, Hammer GD. Regulation of the adrenocortical stem cell niche: implications for disease. *Nat Rev Endocrinol* (2015) 11(1):14–28. doi:10.1038/nrendo.2014.166
47. Finco I, LaPensee CR, Krill KT, Hammer GD. Hedgehog signaling and steroidogenesis. *Annu Rev Physiol* (2015) 77:105–29. doi:10.1146/annurev-physiol-061214-111754
48. Guasti L, Paul A, Laufer E, King P. Localization of Sonic hedgehog secreting and receiving cells in the developing and adult rat adrenal cortex. *Mol Cell Endocrinol* (2011) 336(1–2):117–22. doi:10.1016/j.mce.2010.11.010
49. Laufer E, Kesper D, Vortkamp A, King P. Sonic hedgehog signaling during adrenal development. *Mol Cell Endocrinol* (2012) 351(1):19–27. doi:10.1016/j.mce.2011.10.002
50. Bandiera R, Vidal VP, Motamedi FJ, Clarkson M, Sahut-Barnola I, von Gise A, et al. WT1 maintains adrenal-gonadal primordium identity and marks a population of AGP-like progenitors within the adrenal gland. *Dev Cell* (2013) 27(1):5–18. doi:10.1016/j.devcel.2013.09.003
51. Morrison SJ, Spradling AC. Stem cells and niches: mechanisms that promote stem cell maintenance throughout life. *Cell* (2008) 132(4):598–611. doi:10.1016/j.cell.2008.01.038
52. Simon DP, Hammer GD. Adrenocortical stem and progenitor cells: implications for adrenocortical carcinoma. *Mol Cell Endocrinol* (2012) 351(1):2–11. doi:10.1016/j.mce.2011.12.006
53. Kim A, Giordano TJ, Kuick R, Serecky K, Hammer GD. Wnt/betacatenin signaling in adrenocortical stem/progenitor cells: implications for adrenocortical carcinoma. *Ann Endocrinol (Paris)* (2009) 70(3):156. doi:10.1016/j.ando.2009.02.006
54. Mandel H, Shemer R, Borochowitz ZU, Okopnik M, Knopf C, Indelman M, et al. SERKAL syndrome: an autosomal-recessive disorder caused by a loss-of-function mutation in WNT4. *Am J Hum Genet* (2008) 82(1):39–47. doi:10.1016/j.ajhg.2007.08.005
55. Heikkilä M, Peltoketo H, Leppäluoto J, Ilves M, Vuolteenaho O, Vainio S. Wnt-4 deficiency alters mouse adrenal cortex function, reducing aldosterone production. *Endocrinology* (2002) 143(11):4358–65. doi:10.1210/en.2002-220275
56. Jeays-Ward K, Hoyle C, Brennan J, Dandonneau M, Alldus G, Capel B, et al. Endothelial and steroidogenic cell migration are regulated by WNT4 in the developing mammalian gonad. *Development* (2003) 130(16):3663–70. doi:10.1242/dev.00591
57. Zheng S, Cherniack AD, Dewal N, Moffitt RA, Danilova L, Murray BA, et al. Comprehensive pan-genomic characterization of adrenocortical carcinoma. *Cancer Cell* (2016) 29(5):723–36. doi:10.1016/j.ccell.2016.04.002
58. Drelon C, Berthon A, Sahut-Barnola I, Mathieu M, Dumontet T, Rodriguez S, et al. PKA inhibits WNT signalling in adrenal cortex zonation and prevents malignant tumour development. *Nat Commun* (2016) 7:12751. doi:10.1038/ncomms12751
59. Tanigawa S, Wang H, Yang Y, Sharma N, Tarasova N, Ajima R, et al. Wnt4 induces nephronic tubules in metanephric mesenchyme by a non-canonical mechanism. *Dev Biol* (2011) 352(1):58–69. doi:10.1016/j.ydbio.2011.01.012
60. Heinonen KM, Vanegas JR, Lew D, Krosl J, Perreault C. Wnt4 enhances murine hematopoietic progenitor cell expansion through a planar cell polarity-like pathway. *PLoS One* (2011) 6(4):e19279. doi:10.1371/journal.pone.0019279
61. Bakrania P, Efthymiou M, Klein JC, Salt A, Bunyan DJ, Wyatt A, et al. Mutations in BMP4 cause eye, brain, and digit developmental anomalies: overlap between the BMP4 and hedgehog signaling pathways. *Am J Hum Genet* (2008) 82(2):304–19. doi:10.1016/j.ajhg.2007.09.023
62. Rege J, Nishimoto HK, Nishimoto K, Rodgers RJ, Auchus RJ, Rainey WE. Bone morphogenetic protein-4 (BMP4): a paracrine regulator of human adrenal C19 steroid synthesis. *Endocrinology* (2015) 156(7):2530–40. doi:10.1210/en.2014-1942
63. Kim JS, Crooks H, Dracheva T, Nishanian TG, Singh B, Jen J, et al. Oncogenic beta-catenin is required for bone morphogenetic protein 4 expression in human cancer cells. *Cancer Res* (2002) 62(10):2744–8.
64. Heaton JH, Wood MA, Kim AC, Lima LO, Barlaskar FM, Almeida MQ, et al. Progression to adrenocortical tumorigenesis in mice and humans through insulin-like growth factor 2 and beta-catenin. *Am J Pathol* (2012) 181(3):1017–33. doi:10.1016/j.ajpath.2012.05.026
65. Song X, Sato Y, Felemban A, Ito A, Hossain M, Ochiai H, et al. Equarin is involved as an FGF signaling modulator in chick lens differentiation. *Dev Biol* (2012) 368(1):109–17. doi:10.1016/j.ydbio.2012.05.029
66. Huang CC, Miyagawa S, Matsumaru D, Parker KL, Yao HH. Progenitor cell expansion and organ size of mouse adrenal is regulated by sonic hedgehog. *Endocrinology* (2010) 151(3):1119–28. doi:10.1210/en.2009-0814
67. Ching S, Vilain E. Targeted disruption of Sonic Hedgehog in the mouse adrenal leads to adrenocortical hypoplasia. *Genesis* (2009) 47(9):628–37. doi:10.1002/dvg.20532
68. Ornitz DM, Itoh N. The fibroblast growth factor signaling pathway. *Wiley Interdiscip Rev Dev Biol* (2015) 4(3):215–66. doi:10.1002/wdev.176
69. Rodems TS, Iida M, Brand TM, Pearson HE, Orbuch RA, Flanigan BG, et al. Adaptive responses to antibody based therapy. *Semin Cell Dev Biol* (2016) 50:153–63. doi:10.1016/j.semcdb.2016.01.001
70. Gospodarowicz D, Handley HH. Stimulation of division of Y1 adrenal cells by a growth factor isolated from bovine pituitary glands. *Endocrinology* (1975) 97(1):102–7. doi:10.1210/endo-97-1-102
71. Gospodarowicz D, Ill CR, Hornsby PJ, Gill GN. Control of bovine adrenal cortical cell proliferation by fibroblast growth factor. Lack of effect of epidermal growth factor. *Endocrinology* (1977) 100(4):1080–9. doi:10.1210/endo-100-4-1080
72. Crickard K, Ill CR, Jaffe RB. Control of proliferation of human fetal adrenal cells in vitro. *J Clin Endocrinol Metab* (1981) 53(4):790–6. doi:10.1210/jcem-53-4-790
73. Lepique AP, Moraes MS, Rocha KM, Eichler CB, Hajj GN, Schwindt TT, et al. c-Myc protein is stabilized by fibroblast growth factor 2 and destabilized by ACTH to control cell cycle in mouse Y1 adrenocortical cells. *J Mol Endocrinol* (2004) 33(3):623–38. doi:10.1677/jme.1.01485
74. Chu Y, Ho WJ, Dunn JC. Basic fibroblast growth factor delivery enhances adrenal cortical cellular regeneration. *Tissue Eng Part A* (2009) 15(8):2093–101. doi:10.1089/ten.tea.2008.0305
75. Guasti L, Candy Sze WC, McKay T, Grose R, King PJ. FGF signalling through Fgfr2 isoform IIIb regulates adrenal cortex development. *Mol Cell Endocrinol* (2013) 371(1–2):182–8. doi:10.1016/j.mce.2013.01.014
76. Ornitz DM, Xu J, Colvin JS, McEwen DG, MacArthur CA, Coulier F, et al. Receptor specificity of the fibroblast growth factor family. *J Biol Chem* (1996) 271(25):15292–7. doi:10.1074/jbc.271.25.15292
77. Kim Y, Bingham N, Sekido R, Parker KL, Lovell-Badge R, Capel B. Fibroblast growth factor receptor 2 regulates proliferation and Sertoli differentiation during male sex determination. *Proc Natl Acad Sci U S A* (2007) 104(42):16558–63. doi:10.1073/pnas.0702581104
78. Smas CM, Sul HS. Pref-1, a protein containing EGF-like repeats, inhibits adipocyte differentiation. *Cell* (1993) 73(4):725–34. doi:10.1016/0092-8674(93)90252-L
79. Laborda J, Sausville EA, Hoffman T, Notario V. dlk, a putative mammalian homeotic gene differentially expressed in small cell lung carcinoma and neuroendocrine tumor cell line. *J Biol Chem* (1993) 268(6):3817–20.
80. Wang Y, Hudak C, Sul HS. Role of preadipocyte factor 1 in adipocyte differentiation. *Clin Lipidol* (2010) 5(1):109–15. doi:10.2217/clp.09.80
81. Wang Y, Sul HS. Pref-1 regulates mesenchymal cell commitment and differentiation through Sox9. *Cell Metab* (2009) 9(3):287–302. doi:10.1016/j.cmet.2009.01.013
82. Floridon C, Jensen CH, Thorsen P, Nielsen O, Sunde L, Westergaard JG, et al. Does fetal antigen 1 (FA1) identify cells with regenerative, endocrine and neuroendocrine potentials? A study of FA1 in embryonic, fetal, and placental tissue and in maternal circulation. *Differentiation* (2000) 66(1):49–59. doi:10.1046/j.1432-0436.2000.066001049.x
83. Mortensen SB, Jensen CH, Schneider M, Thomassen M, Kruse TA, Laborda J, et al. Membrane-tethered delta-like 1 homolog (DLK1) restricts adipose tissue size by inhibiting preadipocyte proliferation. *Diabetes* (2012) 61(11):2814–22. doi:10.2337/db12-0176
84. Carithers LJ, Ardlie K, Barcus M, Branton PA, Britton A, Buia SA, et al. A novel approach to high-quality postmortem tissue procurement: the GTEx project. *Biopreserv Biobank* (2015) 13(5):311–9. doi:10.1089/bio.2015.0032

85. Halder SK, Takemori H, Hatano O, Nonaka Y, Wada A, Okamoto M. Cloning of a membrane-spanning protein with epidermal growth factor-like repeat motifs from adrenal glomerulosa cells. *Endocrinology* (1998) 139(7):3316–28. doi:10.1210/endo.139.7.6081
86. Okamoto M, Takemori H, Halder SK, Nonaka Y, Hatano O. Implication of ZOG protein (zona glomerulosa-specific protein) in zone development of the adrenal cortex. *Endocr Res* (1998) 24(3–4):515–20. doi:10.3109/07435809809032640
87. Mitani F, Mukai K, Miyamoto H, Suematsu M, Ishimura Y. The undifferentiated cell zone is a stem cell zone in adult rat adrenal cortex. *Biochim Biophys Acta* (2003) 1619(3):317–24. doi:10.1016/S0304-4165(02)00490-7
88. Kim KA, Zhao J, Andarmani S, Kakitani M, Oshima T, Binnerts ME, et al. R-Spondin proteins: a novel link to beta-catenin activation. *Cell Cycle* (2006) 5(1):23–6. doi:10.4161/cc.5.1.2305
89. de Lau WB, Snel B, Clevers HC. The R-spondin protein family. *Genome Biol* (2012) 13(3):242. doi:10.1186/gb-2012-13-3-242
90. Rocha AS, Vidal V, Mertz M, Kendall TJ, Charlet A, Okamoto H, et al. The angiocrine factor rspondin3 is a key determinant of liver zonation. *Cell Rep* (2015) 13(9):1757–64. doi:10.1016/j.celrep.2015.10.049
91. Barker N, Tan S, Clevers H. Lgr proteins in epithelial stem cell biology. *Development* (2013) 140(12):2484–94. doi:10.1242/dev.083113
92. Hao HX, Xie Y, Zhang Y, Charlat O, Oster E, Avello M, et al. ZNRF3 promotes Wnt receptor turnover in an R-spondin-sensitive manner. *Nature* (2012) 485(7397):195–200. doi:10.1038/nature11019
93. Hynes RO, Naba A. Overview of the matrisome – an inventory of extracellular matrix constituents and functions. *Cold Spring Harb Perspect Biol* (2012) 4(1):a004903. doi:10.1101/cshperspect.a004903
94. Hynes RO. The extracellular matrix: not just pretty fibrils. *Science* (2009) 326(5957):1216–9. doi:10.1126/science.1176009
95. Brizzi MF, Tarone G, Defilippi P. Extracellular matrix, integrins, and growth factors as tailors of the stem cell niche. *Curr Opin Cell Biol* (2012) 24(5):645–51. doi:10.1016/j.ceb.2012.07.001
96. Ellis SJ, Tanentzapf G. Integrin-mediated adhesion and stem-cell-niche interactions. *Cell Tissue Res* (2010) 339(1):121–30. doi:10.1007/s00441-009-0828-4
97. Taddei I, Deugnier MA, Faraldo MM, Petit V, Bouvard D, Medina D, et al. Beta1 integrin deletion from the basal compartment of the mammary epithelium affects stem cells. *Nat Cell Biol* (2008) 10(6):716–22. doi:10.1038/ncb1734
98. Qiu Y, Bayomy AF, Gomez MV, Bauer M, Du P, Yang Y, et al. A role for matrix stiffness in the regulation of cardiac side population cell function. *Am J Physiol Heart Circ Physiol* (2015) 308(9):H990–7. doi:10.1152/ajpheart.00935.2014
99. Ahmed M, Ffrench-Constant C. Extracellular matrix regulation of stem cell behavior. *Curr Stem Cell Rep* (2016) 2:197–206. doi:10.1007/s40778-016-0056-2
100. Campbell S, Otis M, Côté M, Gallo-Payet N, Payet MD. Connection between integrins and cell activation in rat adrenal glomerulosa cells: a role for Arg-Gly-Asp peptide in the activation of the p42/p44(mapk) pathway and intracellular calcium. *Endocrinology* (2003) 144(4):1486–95. doi:10.1210/en.2002-220903
101. Chamoux E, Bolduc L, Lehoux JG, Gallo-Payet N. Identification of extracellular matrix components and their integrin receptors in the human fetal adrenal gland. *J Clin Endocrinol Metab* (2001) 86(5):2090–8. doi:10.1210/jcem.86.5.7462
102. Chamoux E, Narcy A, Lehoux JG, Gallo-Payet N. Fibronectin, laminin, and collagen IV interact with ACTH and angiotensin II to dictate specific cell behavior and secretion in human fetal adrenal cells in culture. *Endocr Res* (2002) 28(4):637–40. doi:10.1081/ERC-120016978
103. Otis M, Campbell S, Payet MD, Gallo-Payet N. Expression of extracellular matrix proteins and integrins in rat adrenal gland: importance for ACTH-associated functions. *J Endocrinol* (2007) 193(3):331–47. doi:10.1677/JOE-07-0055
104. Shamir ER, Ewald AJ. Three-dimensional organotypic culture: experimental models of mammalian biology and disease. *Nat Rev Mol Cell Biol* (2014) 15(10):647–64. doi:10.1038/nrm3873
105. Kretzschmar K, Clevers H. Organoids: modeling development and the stem cell niche in a dish. *Dev Cell* (2016) 38(6):590–600. doi:10.1016/j.devcel.2016.08.014
106. Eiraku M, Sasai Y. Self-formation of layered neural structures in three-dimensional culture of ES cells. *Curr Opin Neurobiol* (2012) 22(5):768–77. doi:10.1016/j.conb.2012.02.005
107. Lancaster MA, Knoblich JA. Organogenesis in a dish: modeling development and disease using organoid technologies. *Science* (2014) 345(6194):1247125. doi:10.1126/science.1247125
108. Sato T, Vries RG, Snippert HJ, van de Wetering M, Barker N, Stange DE, et al. Single Lgr5 stem cells build crypt-villus structures in vitro without a mesenchymal niche. *Nature* (2009) 459(7244):262–5. doi:10.1038/nature07935
109. Sato T, Stange DE, Ferrante M, Vries RG, Van Es JH, Van den Brink S, et al. Long-term expansion of epithelial organoids from human colon, adenoma, adenocarcinoma, and Barrett's epithelium. *Gastroenterology* (2011) 141(5):1762–72. doi:10.1053/j.gastro.2011.07.050
110. Karthaus WR, Iaquinta PJ, Drost J, Gracanin A, van Boxtel R, Wongvipat J, et al. Identification of multipotent luminal progenitor cells in human prostate organoid cultures. *Cell* (2014) 159(1):163–75. doi:10.1016/j.cell.2014.08.017
111. Linnemann JR, Miura H, Meixner LK, Irmler M, Kloos UJ, Hirschi B, et al. Quantification of regenerative potential in primary human mammary epithelial cells. *Development* (2015) 142(18):3239–51. doi:10.1242/dev.123554
112. Barker N, Huch M, Kujala P, van de Wetering M, Snippert HJ, van Es JH, et al. Lgr5(+ve) stem cells drive self-renewal in the stomach and build long-lived gastric units in vitro. *Cell Stem Cell* (2010) 6(1):25–36. doi:10.1016/j.stem.2009.11.013
113. Bartfeld S, Bayram T, van de Wetering M, Huch M, Begthel H, Kujala P, et al. In vitro expansion of human gastric epithelial stem cells and their responses to bacterial infection. *Gastroenterology* (2015) 148(1):126–136e6. doi:10.1053/j.gastro.2014.09.042
114. Desai TJ, Brownfield DG, Krasnow MA. Alveolar progenitor and stem cells in lung development, renewal and cancer. *Nature* (2014) 507(7491):190–4. doi:10.1038/nature12930
115. Magin CM, Alge DL, Anseth KS. Bio-inspired 3D microenvironments: a new dimension in tissue engineering. *Biomed Mater* (2016) 11(2):022001. doi:10.1088/1748-6041/11/2/022001
116. Gjorevski N, Sachs N, Manfrin A, Giger S, Bragina ME, Ordóñez-Morán P, et al. Designer matrices for intestinal stem cell and organoid culture. *Nature* (2016) 539(7630):560–4. doi:10.1038/nature20168

20

Adrenal Gland Microenvironment and its Involvement in the Regulation of Stress-Induced Hormone Secretion during Sepsis

Waldemar Kanczkowski[1], Mariko Sue[1] and Stefan R. Bornstein[1,2]*

[1] *Department of Internal Medicine III, Technische Universität Dresden, Dresden, Germany,* [2] *Department of Endocrinology and Diabetes, King's College London, London, UK*

Correspondence:
Waldemar Kanczkowski
waldemar.kanczkowski@uniklinikum-dresden.de

Survival of all living organisms depends on maintenance of a steady state of homeostasis, which process relies on its ability to react and adapt to various physical and emotional threats. The defense against stress is executed by the hypothalamic–pituitary–adrenal axis and the sympathetic–adrenal medullary system. Adrenal gland is a major effector organ of stress system. During stress, adrenal gland rapidly responds with increased secretion of glucocorticoids (GCs) and catecholamines into circulation, which hormones, in turn, affect metabolism, to provide acutely energy, vasculature to increase blood pressure, and the immune system to prevent it from extensive activation. Sepsis resulting from microbial infections is a sustained and extreme example of stress situation. In many critical ill patients, levels of both corticotropin-releasing hormone and adrenocorticotropin, the two major regulators of adrenal hormone production, are suppressed. Levels of GCs, however, remain normal or are elevated in these patients, suggesting a shift from central to local intra-adrenal regulation of adrenal stress response. Among many mechanisms potentially involved in this process, reduced GC metabolism and activation of intra-adrenal cellular systems composed of adrenocortical and adrenomedullary cells, endothelial cells, and resident and recruited immune cells play a key role. Hence, dysregulated function of any of these cells and cellular compartments can ultimately affect adrenal stress response. The purpose of this mini review is to highlight recent insights into our understanding of the adrenal gland microenvironment and its role in coordination of stress-induced hormone secretion.

Keywords: stress system, hypothalamic–pituitary–adrenal axis, immune–adrenal crosstalk, ACTH, glucocorticoids

INTRODUCTION

In order to survive all, living organisms must maintain a steady state of homeostasis. This unique capacity to react and adapt to various physical and emotional threats in higher vertebrates is mediated by a coordinated action of the nervous, endocrine, and immune systems, known as stress system (1). Activation of the stress system, which is composed of the hypothalamic–pituitary–adrenal (HPA) axis and the sympathetic–adrenal medullary system, leads to increased synthesis and release of glucocorticoids (GCs) and catecholamines (CAs) from the adrenal cortex and medulla, respectively (2–4). The main function of these hormones is maintenance and restoration of basal and stress-related body homeostasis. This protective action of adrenal hormones is mostly accomplished by their metabolic, cardioprotective, and anti-inflammatory actions. In particular, both GCs and CAs are known to acutely enhance plasma glucose levels and promote an increased cardiac output and high blood pressure, while protecting against excessive inflammation (5–8).

Secretion of adrenal hormones during stress-free conditions is regulated centrally and is characterized by ultradian rhythms (9). An early morning release of adrenocorticotropic hormone (ACTH) into circulation is enhanced by increased concentrations of corticotropin-releasing hormone (CRH) and arginine vasopressin (AVP) in the hypophyseal portal system of anterior pituitary (10, 11). Consequently, elevated plasma levels of ACTH stimulate adrenocortical cells to produce and release GC hormones. In turn, as a part of negative feedback, GCs act directly on the pituitary gland to reduce ACTH secretion and on hypothalamic neurons to reduce CRH release (11, 12). Systemic rise in CA levels is in turn initiated by activation of the sympathetic nervous system and splenic nerves innervating the adrenal medulla (13, 14).

One of the extreme examples of sustained and severe physical stress is sepsis syndrome. It is characterized by abnormal host response to infection, resulting in systemic inflammation that frequently culminates in a life-threatening dysfunction of multiple organs (15, 16). Severe sepsis remains the leading cause of mortality worldwide, and its incidence is increasing (17, 18). An intact function of the stress system, and in particular the activation of GC and CA production, is critical to survive this adverse condition (19, 20). During sepsis, this homeostatic function of the stress system is frequently impaired with mechanisms remaining largely unknown (21, 22). Consequently, many critically ill patients demonstrate suppressed ACTH and CRH levels while having normal or elevated cortisol levels (22). Hence, a key involvement of pituitary-independent factors was proposed (2). Among these, reduced GC metabolism and activation of local adrenal microenvironment seem to play crucial role (23, 24) (**Figure 1**).

As regulation of the stress system and importance of impaired metabolism of GCs during sepsis were recently presented and discussed in many review articles (25–27), the main purpose of this mini review is to highlight recent insights into our understanding of the role local adrenal gland microenvironment in the regulation of stress-induced hormone secretion during sepsis.

ADRENAL GLAND MICROENVIRONMENT

Within adrenal gland, two embryonically different tissues coexist: mesodermally derived, steroid-producing cortex and ectodermally derived, CA-producing medulla. Within these two environmental niches, interplay between various cells takes place including adrenocortical and chromaffin cells, neuronal cells, immune cells, endothelial cells, and glia cells (28). The adrenal gland is a source of many bioactive substances including steroid hormones, CAs, cytokines, neurotransmitters, and neuropeptides (**Table 1**). These substances are known to interact with various cell types within adrenal gland itself, thereby influencing its function during stress conditions and disease (24, 28).

Adrenal Cortex and Medulla Interactions during Sepsis

Ample evidence exists suggesting a bidirectional interaction between adrenal cortex and the medulla (28). Despite a classical view on the adrenal gland anatomy, demonstrating a clear separation of the cortex and medulla, it has been well documented that these two endocrine tissues are morphologically intermingled (29, 30). This close localization, in turn, enables direct cell–cell and paracrine interactions between adrenocortical and chromaffin cells involving their secretory products.

Consequently, the adrenal cortex-derived GCs were found to enhance synthesis of CAs both *in vitro* (31) and *in vivo* (32–34). GCs were found to execute these effects by upregulating expression of phenylethanolamine *N*-methyltransferase (PNMT), which gene encodes for an enzyme that catalyzes the synthesis of epinephrine from norepinephrine. Furthermore, studies using various knockout mice, which were deficient in steroidogenic factor-1, glucocorticoid receptor, or corticotropin-releasing hormone type 1 receptor, clearly demonstrated that lack of one of the these key steroidogenic regulators impair PNMT gene expression and thus basal and stress-induced epinephrine production (35–38). Similarly, an intact function of adrenal medulla is important to maintain adrenocortical function. It has been shown that coculture of bovine adrenocortical cells with chromaffin cells enhanced a basal GC secretion by 10-fold (39). Furthermore, CAs were found to enhance production of various steroids including cortisol, aldosterone, and androstenedione, through mechanism involving upregulation of steroidogenic acute regulatory protein (28, 40, 41).

During sepsis, an enhanced production of epinephrine and norepinephrine (42–44) and increased secretory capacity of adrenal chromaffin cells were reported (45). Unlike expression of tyrosine hydroxylase, which enzyme is involved in first step of CA biosynthesis, upregulation of PNMT gene expression in adrenal medulla was found to be regulated independently of splanchnic nerve stimulation (28). Instead, an extremely high concentration of GCs was reported to be involved in regulation of PNMT expression during sepsis (46). Consequently, stress-induced expression of PNMT is strongly attenuated in CRH-deficient mice (47).

In addition, adrenal chromaffin cells release many active neuropeptides and transmitters, including neuropeptide Y (NPY), vasoactive intestinal peptide (VIP), or substance P, with known stimulatory action on GCs production (48, 49). For example, VIP, which levels increase during experimental endotoxemia in adrenal medulla, was found to stimulate DHEA, testosterone, androstenedione, cortisol, and aldosterone secretion in adrenocortical cells (48–52). Among other mediators found in adrenal medulla, which may influence GC production during sepsis, are angiotensin, AVP, CRH, ACTH, and apelin (53–55). Although direct stimulatory effects of angiotensin 2, CRH, and ACTH on adrenal hormone production are well described, the degree to which each of these peptides contributes to hormone production during sepsis conditions has not been fully elucidated yet (2, 56). Another interesting peptide found recently to be expressed in the adrenal medulla is apelin. Apelin is a neurohormone, which acts through its receptor APJ expressed in various organs including

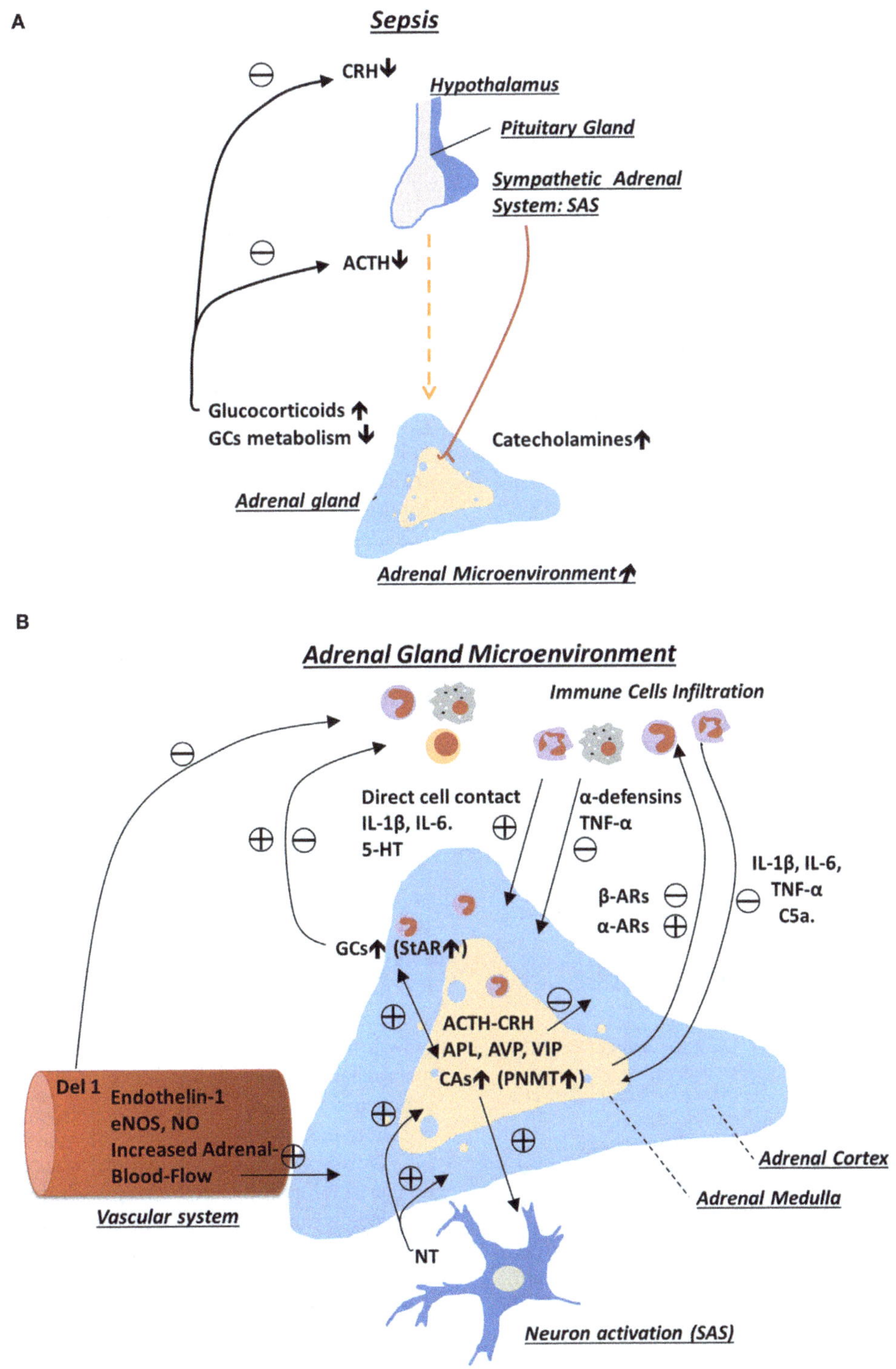

FIGURE 1 | Schematic representation of regulatory mechanisms involved in adrenal gland stress response during sepsis. (A) Sepsis activates the hypothalamic–pituitary–adrenal axis and sympathetic–adrenal medullary system, which in turn enhances production of glucocorticoids (GCs) and catecholamines from the adrenal gland. During chronic phase of sepsis, production of corticotropin-releasing hormone and adrenocorticotropic hormone (ACTH) is inhibited as a result of increased negative feedback from the elevated levels of GCs. High level of adrenal GCs in plasma is sustained due to stimulatory effects provided by intra-adrenal microenvironment and reduced GCs metabolism. **(B)** In the adrenal gland, many cell types including resident and infiltrating immune cells, sympathetic neurons, endothelial cells, and adrenal chromaffin and adrenocortical cells interact with each other. This interaction occurs through a direct cell–cell contact and in a paracrine way, which ultimately leads to sustained production of adrenal hormones. Among many mediators produced in adrenal gland, which are reported to modulate adrenal hormone production, are adrenocortical steroids, catecholemines, and various cytokines such as interleukin (IL)-1β, IL-6, tumor necrosis factor-α, serotonin (5-HT), neurotransmitters, and neurohormones (e.g., APL, ACTH, and vasoactive intestinal peptide).

TABLE 1 | Intra-adrenal interaction involved in a regulation of adrenal stress response.

Cell interactions	Mediators	Action
Immune–adrenal crosstalk (macrophages, neutrophils, mast cells, lymphocytes)	Glucocorticoids (GCs)	Stimulatory effects on naïve and inhibitory actions on activated immune cells
	Cytokines	Stimulatory [interleukin (IL)-1β, IL6] or inhibitory action [tumor necrosis factor (TNF)-α] on adrenal steroidogenesis
	Catecholamine (CA)	Anti-inflammatory effects through activation of β-adrenergic receptors (ARs) (increase IL-10, decrease TNF-α in macrophage, and decrease NO and ROS in neutrophils) Pro-inflammatory effects through activation of α-ARs
	Direct contact	Stimulatory effects on adrenal DHEA synthesis
	α-Defensins	Inhibitory effects on steroidogenesis through decreased sensitivity of adrenal cells to adrenocorticotropic hormone (ACTH)
	Neutrophil extracellular traps	Destruction of adrenal cells and promotion of hemorrhages
Adrenocortical–adrenomedullary interactions (adrenocortical cells and chromaffin cells)	GCs	Stimulatory action on CA synthesis (through PNMT upregulation)
	CAs	Stimulatory action on adrenal steroidogenesis
	Neurotransmitters (NT) (substance P, vasoactive intestinal peptide, neuropeptide Y, etc.)	Stimulatory and inhibitory action on adrenal steroidogenesis
	Local corticotropin-releasing hormone–ACTH system	Stimulatory action on adrenal steroidogenesis
	Apelinergic system	Stimulatory action on adrenal steroidogenesis
Vasculature (endothelial cells)	Endothelin-1	Direct stimulatory effect on GC production
	eNOS and NO	Possible stimulatory effect on steroidogenesis
	Developmental endothelial locus 1	Regulation of immune cells recruitment into adrenal gland
	Adrenal blood flow	Stimulatory effect on steroidogenesis
Innervation (sympathetic neurons)	NT (acetylcholine)	Increased steroidogenesis *via* enhanced sensitivity of adrenal cells to ACTH Increased production and secretion of CAs

hypothalamic neurons, anterior pituitary, and adrenal gland. It was recently found to modulate neuroendocrine response to stress through stimulation of secretion of both ACTH and corticosterone directly and *via* AVP- and CRH-dependent pathways (54, 55, 57).

Recently, a population of nestin-positive glia-like multipotent stem cells was identified in adrenal medulla of nestin-GFP transgenic mice (58). Interestingly, when subjected to chronic stress, this population was able to give rise to new chromaffin cells, suggesting a direct involvement of these cells in the adrenal stress adaptation (58–60). It is therefore very interesting to investigate the fate of this cells and their potential interaction with adrenocortical cells during sepsis conditions.

In summary, an intact function of both adrenal cortex and adrenal medulla is of pivotal importance in the regulation of adrenal stress response. Consequently, any disorders or medications that can attenuate adrenal cortex function will also ultimately affect CAs production by chromaffin cells and *vice versa* potentially impacting the outcome of many stress-related disorders (19).

Immune–Adrenal Crosstalk

In the last 40 years, it has become evident that immune and endocrine systems interact with each other at the level of adrenal gland and that this interaction is crucially involved in the regulation of adrenal gland function during normal and stress conditions (61). This immune–endocrine crosstalk is mostly executed by bidirectional action of paracrine factors, such as steroid hormones, CAs, and various vasoactive or proteolytic enzymes, as well as by direct cell–cell contacts and activation of toll-like receptors (TLRs) (28, 62).

Immune–Adrenal Interaction at the Level of Adrenal Cortex

During non-stress conditions, many immune cells can be found in the innermost zone of adrenal cortex known as *zona reticularis*; these are particularly tissue macrophages (63), dendritic cells (64), mast cells (65), and lymphocytes (66). However, some of them, especially macrophages and mast cells, were also reported in other parts of the adrenal gland including subcapsular region and in the adrenal medulla (64). In non-stress conditions, adrenal-resident immune cells play important homeostatic functions by sensing pathogens, removing apoptotic cells, and promoting tissue remodeling through, e.g., secretion of growth factors (24, 67). Recently, a new population of adrenal macrophages was identified based on the high expression of a complement receptor immunoglobulin, CRIg, which molecule is known to mediate phagocytosis of pathogens and apoptotic cells (68). During systemic inflammation induced either by LPS injection or CLP, highly dynamic changes within adrenal immune cell populations can be observed. For instance, it has been shown that already within first 3 h after administration of LPS or induction of peritonitis in rodents, a rapid infiltration of neutrophils takes place, while the number of local dendritic cells and macrophages declines (69–71).

Using electron microscopy, close cell–cell localization between local immune cells and surrounding adrenocortical, chromaffin, or endothelial cells was demonstrated (64, 66). This in turn enables various bidirectional and direct interactions between each cell type. For example, a functional crosstalk between adrenocortical cells, expressing major histocompatibility complex class II molecules (MHC/HLA), and leukocytes was described. Indeed, a co-incubation of T cells with primary cultures of human adrenocortical cells promoted adrenal androgen and cortisol secretion (66). Besides direct interaction, various immune cells were found to regulate adrenal hormone production in a paracrine way through secretion of cytokines, such as interleukins (IL) 1 and 6 (72), and pro-opiomelanocortin (POMC)-derived peptides, e.g., ACTH and biogenic amines (28, 73).

The ample experimental evidence exists demonstrating that cytokines are critically involved in ACTH-independent activation of GC production during sepsis (72). For example, injection of IL-1β enhanced GC production in hypophysectomized rats (74). Furthermore, an impaired synthesis of GCs after LPS injection was observed in mice receiving sera against tumor necrosis factor (TNF)-α and IL-6 and, to a lesser extent, IL-1β- or in IL-6-deficient mice (75, 76). However, it has been demonstrated that cytokine levels found normally in plasma are far too low to induce hormone production from adrenocortical cells. Therefore, the main source of cytokines must come from the adrenal gland itself (28). Sustained production of cytokines in highly anti-inflammatory environment of the adrenal gland during systemic inflammation was found to be enabled by increased expression of migration inhibitory factor (77). During sepsis, various cell types present within adrenal gland microenvironment may be a potential source of pro-inflammatory cytokines. For example, adrenocortical cells were found to express several TLRs and secrete several cytokines in response to bacterial ligands (78, 79). However, in a recent study, inactivation of myeloid but not adrenocortical TLR signaling resulted in significant reduction of intra-adrenal cytokine levels and activation of the HPA axis after LPS administration (80). The latter observation suggests that immune cells are the key sources of cytokines in the adrenal gland during sepsis. Due to high expression of both cytokine and GC receptors in adrenocortical and immune cells, respectively, cytokines and adrenal hormones are known to regulate production in each other. For example, IL-1β or IL-6 was found to increase adrenal hormone production, whereas TNF stimulation demonstrated rather opposite effect (81–83). In turn, adrenal steroid hormones are known to influence immune cells function. In particular, it has been demonstrated that in naïve immune cells, GCs can activate several inflammatory-related genes, e.g., TLRs, yet in cells treated with LPS, they inhibit inflammation (6). In a recent study, a chronic exposure to GCs was found to cause a shift in the innate–adaptive balance of the immune response, particularly, influencing the chemokine–chemokine receptor networks (84). Besides cytokines, other biologically active substances, such as serotonin (5-HT) or histamine, which are stored by mast cells show stimulatory effects on adrenal steroidogenesis (85, 86).

During prolonged sepsis, the immune–adrenal interaction may also result in the suppression of adrenal hormone production. Despite their important role in host defenses against bacterial infections limiting bacterial spread in circulation (87), a prolonged exposure of adrenal cells to neutrophil-derived antimicrobial agents, such as ROS and proteolytic enzymes secreted during formation of neutrophil extracellular traps, results in tissue damage (88). In addition, neutrophils were found to secrete corticostatins, e.g., α-defensins, which substances are known to interfere with ACTH-mediated increase in adrenocortical hormone production (89). In a recent study using developmental endothelial locus 1 (Del-1)-deficient mice (90), an association between higher amount of infiltrating neutrophils and impaired adrenal corticosterone production after systemic LPS administration was found (91).

Immune–Adrenal Interaction at the Level of Adrenal Medulla

Activation of the sympathetic nerve system during sepsis results in enhanced production and secretion of CAs from the adrenal chromaffin cells (44) through a mechanism involving an increased release of Ca^{2+} from endothelial reticulum (45). An early increase in endogenous CA level plays an important protective role as its absence due to either pharmacological or surgical intervention resulted in induction of hypotension and increased mortality of rats during experimental endotoxemia (20, 43). One of the mechanisms involved in the protective role of CAs, besides well-known vasopressor function, is the anti-inflammatory action on various immune cells. The immunomodulatory effects of CAs are mediated *via* their direct interactions with β-adrenergic receptors (ARs) expressed by a variety of immune cells. In particular, it has been shown that CAs promote IL-10 secretion while decreasing production of pro-inflammatory TNF cytokine in LPS-treated macrophages (92). Furthermore, incubation of neutrophils with CAs decreased NO production and ROS generation (93). However, these immune-suppressive effects of CAs should be carefully interpreted as they may correspond predominantly to the leukocyte populations or be restricted to β-AR activation. In fact, recently both epinephrine and norepinephrine were shown to increase IL-6 production in endothelial cell line: HMEC-1 and in human skin microvascular endothelial cells (94). It has been also found that activation of α-ARs in macrophages by CA may potentiate inflammation by increasing TNF-α production (95). Recently, phagocytes were shown to be able not only to secrete CAs in response to LPS stimulation but also to possess all major CA-generating and -degrading enzymes required for their production and inactivation (96). This discovery adds additional complexity to already complex immune–chromaffin cell interaction. During sepsis, the adrenal medulla shows high degree of immune infiltration (69). This suggests that overactivation of immune cells could potentially impair production and secretion of adrenomedullary hormones or induce structural damage. Indeed, during experimental sepsis induced by CLP, systemic inflammation resulted in a strong apoptosis in the adrenal chromaffin cells, which process required activation of receptors for complement C5a (97). The latter observation suggests that during progression of sepsis, an increased activation of immune system promoting apoptosis of chromaffin cells may impact stress-induced CA production.

Adrenal Vasculature

Vascular system plays a key role in the proper functioning of many vital organs during sepsis. Besides enabling the secretion of steroid hormones and CAs into circulation, adrenal vasculature was found to control leukocyte infiltration through expression of adhesion molecules and Del-1 protein (91).

Adrenal cortex is characterized by high density of endothelial cells that stay in close vicinity with steroid-producing cells. Consequently, both adrenal hormones and endothelial cell-derived products were shown to influence function of adrenal vasculature and steroid-producing cells, respectively. For example, human adrenocortical cells increase production of aldosterone and cortisol once incubated with endothelial cell-conditioned media. Although the exact composition of the latter media was not determined, this stimulatory effect was found to require cAMP, but not PKA, pathway (98). Endothelial cells are known to produce several factors that, e.g., nitric oxide (NO) or endothelin-1, could potentially influence adrenal hormone production. In particular, in rat and human adrenocortical cells, it has been found that endothelin-1 can directly promote GC synthesis and potentiate angiotensin II and ACTH-induced aldosterone production (99). Besides endothelin-1, nitric oxide (NO) was found to exert stimulatory effect on adrenal steroidogenesis by mediating the acute response to ACTH (28). In fact, blocking of NO production either by using NO synthase inhibitor or NO scavengers resulted in decreased ACTH-mediated corticosterone release (100). However, in other studies using perfused adrenal glands administration of L-arginine, the substrate for nitric oxide synthesis did not change corticosterone response to ACTH, suggesting an indirect modulatory action of NO (101).

During sepsis, in many critically ill patients, an increased size of adrenal gland resulting from the hypervascularization and increased blood flow and adrenal hyperplasia were found to positively correlate with survival rate (102). Although an intact activity of splanchnic nerve is crucial in regulation of adrenal blood flow, other factors such as VIP, NPY, or neurotensin were found also to be involved (103, 104). Furthermore, a positive correlation between an increased blood flow and enhanced adrenal steroidogenesis was demonstrated (105). Indeed, an enhanced adrenal blood flow was found to participate in angiotensin II- and ACTH-induced aldosterone and cortisol production. This stimulatory action on adrenal vascular response to angiotensin II and ACTH was found to be mediated by vasoactive substances released from granules of mast cells (106). However, more recently, additional involvement of the cytochrome 450 in controlling the adrenal blood flow after AII and ACTH was demonstrated in rats (24, 107).

SUMMARY

Sepsis and septic shock strongly impacts body homeostasis, which if not sufficiently counteracted by activated stress system results in increased mortality of critically ill patients (56, 108, 109). During chronic phase of sepsis, elevated adrenal hormone secretion was reported to be mediated by pituitary-independent mechanisms including activation of intra-adrenal microenvironment (22, 23). An increasing amount of experimental studies support the key involvement of several cell types and cellular systems present within adrenal gland microenvironment in the sustained production of adrenal hormones during sepsis. Consequently, any impairment in function of these systems can ultimately affect adrenal stress response (2, 24).

AUTHOR CONTRIBUTIONS

WK, MS, and SB have all made substantial, direct, and intellectual contribution to the work and approved it for publication.

FUNDING

This work was supported by grants of the Deutsche Forschungs Gemeinschaft (DFG) to WK (KA 3013/2-2) and SB (BO 1141/11-2).

REFERENCES

1. Nicolaides NC, Kyratzi E, Lamprokostopoulou A, Chrousos GP, Charmandari E. Stress, the stress system and the role of glucocorticoids. *Neuroimmunomodulation* (2015) 22:6–19. doi:10.1159/000362736
2. Bornstein SR, Chrousos GP. Clinical review 104: adrenocorticotropin (ACTH)- and non-ACTH-mediated regulation of the adrenal cortex: neural and immune inputs. *J Clin Endocrinol Metab* (1999) 84:1729–36. doi:10.1210/jcem.84.5.5631
3. Chrousos GP. The hypothalamic-pituitary-adrenal axis and immune-mediated inflammation. *N Engl J Med* (1995) 332:1351–62. doi:10.1056/NEJM199505183322008
4. Chrousos GP. Stress and disorders of the stress system. *Nat Rev Endocrinol* (2009) 5:374–81. doi:10.1038/nrendo.2009.106
5. Bornstein SR, Briegel J. A new role for glucocorticoids in septic shock: balancing the immune response. *Am J Respir Crit Care Med* (2003) 167:485–6. doi:10.1164/rccm.2211010
6. Galon J, Franchimont D, Hiroi N, Frey G, Boettner A, Ehrhart-Bornstein M, et al. Gene profiling reveals unknown enhancing and suppressive actions of glucocorticoids on immune cells. *FASEB J* (2002) 16:61–71. doi:10.1096/fj.01-0245com
7. Ensinger H, Geisser W, Brinkmann A, Wachter U, Vogt J, Radermacher P, et al. Metabolic effects of norepinephrine and dobutamine in healthy volunteers. *Shock* (2002) 18:495–500. doi:10.1097/00024382-200212000-00002
8. Trager K, Radermacher P. Catecholamines in the treatment of septic shock: effects beyond perfusion. *Crit Care Resusc* (2003) 5:270–6.
9. Spiga F, Walker JJ, Terry JR, Lightman SL. HPA axis-rhythms. *Compr Physiol* (2014) 4:1273–98. doi:10.1002/cphy.c140003
10. Gillies GE, Linton EA, Lowry PJ. Corticotropin releasing activity of the new CRF is potentiated several times by vasopressin. *Nature* (1982) 299:355–7. doi:10.1038/299355a0
11. Hinz B, Hirschelmann R. Rapid non-genomic feedback effects of glucocorticoids on CRF-induced ACTH secretion in rats. *Pharm Res* (2000) 17:1273–7. doi:10.1023/A:1026499604848
12. Evans AN, Liu Y, Macgregor R, Huang V, Aguilera G. Regulation of hypothalamic corticotropin-releasing hormone transcription by elevated glucocorticoids. *Mol Endocrinol* (2013) 27:1796–807. doi:10.1210/me.2013-1095
13. Winkler H, Apps DK, Fischer-Colbrie R. The molecular function of adrenal chromaffin granules: established facts and unresolved topics. *Neuroscience* (1986) 18:261–90. doi:10.1016/0306-4522(86)90154-5
14. Elenkov IJ, Wilder RL, Chrousos GP, Vizi ES. The sympathetic nerve – an integrative interface between two supersystems: the brain and the immune system. *Pharmacol Rev* (2000) 52:595–638.
15. Shankar-Hari M, Phillips GS, Levy ML, Seymour CW, Liu VX, Deutschman CS, et al. Developing a new definition and assessing new clinical criteria for septic shock: for the Third International Consensus Definitions for Sepsis and Septic Shock (Sepsis-3). *JAMA* (2016) 315:775–87. doi:10.1001/jama.2016.0289
16. Singer M, Deutschman CS, Seymour CW, Shankar-Hari M, Annane D, Bauer M, et al. The Third International Consensus Definitions for Sepsis and Septic Shock (Sepsis-3). *JAMA* (2016) 315:801–10. doi:10.1001/jama.2016.0287
17. Gaieski DF, Edwards JM, Kallan MJ, Carr BG. Benchmarking the incidence and mortality of severe sepsis in the United States. *Crit Care Med* (2013) 41:1167–74. doi:10.1097/CCM.0b013e31827c09f8
18. Mayr FB, Yende S, Angus DC. Epidemiology of severe sepsis. *Virulence* (2014) 5:4–11. doi:10.4161/viru.27372

19. Chan CM, Mitchell AL, Shorr AF. Etomidate is associated with mortality and adrenal insufficiency in sepsis: a meta-analysis. *Crit Care Med* (2012) 40:2945–53. doi:10.1097/CCM.0b013e31825fec26

20. McKechnie K, Dean HG, Furman BL, Parratt JR. Plasma catecholamines during endotoxin infusion in conscious unrestrained rats: effects of adrenal demedullation and/or guanethidine treatment. *Circ Shock* (1985) 17:85–94.

21. Annane D, Maxime V, Ibrahim F, Alvarez JC, Abe E, Boudou P. Diagnosis of adrenal insufficiency in severe sepsis and septic shock. *Am J Respir Crit Care Med* (2006) 174:1319–26. doi:10.1164/rccm.200509-1369OC

22. Bornstein SR, Engeland WC, Ehrhart-Bornstein M, Herman JP. Dissociation of ACTH and glucocorticoids. *Trends Endocrinol Metab* (2008) 19:175–80. doi:10.1016/j.tem.2008.01.009

23. Boonen E, Bornstein SR, Van den Berghe G. New insights into the controversy of adrenal function during critical illness. *Lancet Diabetes Endocrinol* (2015) 3:805–15. doi:10.1016/S2213-8587(15)00224-7

24. Kanczkowski W, Sue M, Zacharowski K, Reincke M, Bornstein SR. The role of adrenal gland microenvironment in the HPA axis function and dysfunction during sepsis. *Mol Cell Endocrinol* (2015) 408:241–8. doi:10.1016/j.mce.2014.12.019

25. Turrin NP, Rivest S. Unraveling the molecular details involved in the intimate link between the immune and neuroendocrine systems. *Exp Biol Med (Maywood)* (2004) 229:996–1006.

26. Bellavance MA, Rivest S. The HPA-immune axis and the immunomodulatory actions of glucocorticoids in the brain. *Front Immunol* (2014) 5:136. doi:10.3389/fimmu.2014.00136

27. Boonen E, Van den Berghe G. Endocrine responses to critical illness: novel insights and therapeutic implications. *J Clin Endocrinol Metab* (2014) 99:1569–82. doi:10.1210/jc.2013-4115

28. Ehrhart-Bornstein M, Hinson JP, Bornstein SR, Scherbaum WA, Vinson GP. Intraadrenal interactions in the regulation of adrenocortical steroidogenesis. *Endocr Rev* (1998) 19:101–43. doi:10.1210/edrv.19.2.0326

29. Bornstein SR, Gonzalez-Hernandez JA, Ehrhart-Bornstein M, Adler G, Scherbaum WA. Intimate contact of chromaffin and cortical cells within the human adrenal gland forms the cellular basis for important intraadrenal interactions. *J Clin Endocrinol Metab* (1994) 78:225–32. doi:10.1210/jcem.78.1.7507122

30. Gallo-Payet N, Pothier P, Isler H. On the presence of chromaffin cells in the adrenal cortex: their possible role in adrenocortical function. *Biochem Cell Biol* (1987) 65:588–92. doi:10.1139/o87-076

31. Wurtman RJ. Stress and the adrenocortical control of epinephrine synthesis. *Metabolism* (2002) 51:11–4. doi:10.1053/meta.2002.33185

32. Wong DL, Bildstein CL, Siddall B, Lesage A, Yoo YS. Neural regulation of phenylethanolamine N-methyltransferase in vivo: transcriptional and translational changes. *Brain Res Mol Brain Res* (1993) 18:107–14. doi:10.1016/0169-328X(93)90178-R

33. Wong DL. Why is the adrenal adrenergic? *Endocr Pathol* (2003) 14:25–36. doi:10.1385/EP:14:1:25

34. Sharara-Chami RI, Joachim M, Pacak K, Majzoub JA. Glucocorticoid treatment – effect on adrenal medullary catecholamine production. *Shock* (2010) 33:213–7. doi:10.1097/SHK.0b013e3181af0633

35. Gut P, Huber K, Lohr J, Bruhl B, Oberle S, Treier M, et al. Lack of an adrenal cortex in Sf1 mutant mice is compatible with the generation and differentiation of chromaffin cells. *Development* (2005) 132:4611–9. doi:10.1242/dev.02052

36. Yoshida-Hiroi M, Bradbury MJ, Eisenhofer G, Hiroi N, Vale WW, Novotny GE, et al. Chromaffin cell function and structure is impaired in corticotropin-releasing hormone receptor type 1-null mice. *Mol Psychiatry* (2002) 7:967–74. doi:10.1038/sj.mp.4001143

37. Finotto S, Krieglstein K, Schober A, Deimling F, Lindner K, Bruhl B, et al. Analysis of mice carrying targeted mutations of the glucocorticoid receptor gene argues against an essential role of glucocorticoid signalling for generating adrenal chromaffin cells. *Development* (1999) 126:2935–44.

38. Jeong KH, Jacobson L, Pacak K, Widmaier EP, Goldstein DS, Majzoub JA. Impaired basal and restraint-induced epinephrine secretion in corticotropin-releasing hormone-deficient mice. *Endocrinology* (2000) 141:1142–50. doi:10.1210/en.141.3.1142

39. Haidan A, Bornstein SR, Glasow A, Uhlmann K, Lubke C, Ehrhart-Bornstein M. Basal steroidogenic activity of adrenocortical cells is increased 10-fold by coculture with chromaffin cells. *Endocrinology* (1998) 139:772–80. doi:10.1210/en.139.2.772

40. Haidan A, Bornstein SR, Liu Z, Walsh LP, Stocco DM, Ehrhart-Bornstein M. Expression of adrenocortical steroidogenic acute regulatory (StAR) protein is influenced by chromaffin cells. *Mol Cell Endocrinol* (2000) 165:25–32. doi:10.1016/S0303-7207(00)00267-7

41. Guse-Behling H, Ehrhart-Bornstein M, Bornstein SR, Waterman MR, Scherbaum WA, Adler G. Regulation of adrenal steroidogenesis by adrenaline: expression of cytochrome P450 genes. *J Endocrinol* (1992) 135:229–37. doi:10.1677/joe.0.1350229

42. Lukewich MK, Rogers RC, Lomax AE. Divergent neuroendocrine responses to localized and systemic inflammation. *Semin Immunol* (2014) 26:402–6. doi:10.1016/j.smim.2014.01.004

43. Jones SB, Kotsonis P, Majewski H. Endotoxin enhances norepinephrine release in the rat by peripheral mechanisms. *Shock* (1994) 2:370–5. doi:10.1097/00024382-199411000-00012

44. Hahn PY, Wang P, Tait SM, Ba ZF, Reich SS, Chaudry IH. Sustained elevation in circulating catecholamine levels during polymicrobial sepsis. *Shock* (1995) 4:269–73. doi:10.1097/00024382-199510000-00007

45. Lukewich MK, Lomax AE. Endotoxemia enhances catecholamine secretion from male mouse adrenal chromaffin cells through an increase in Ca(2+) release from the endoplasmic reticulum. *Endocrinology* (2014) 155:180–92. doi:10.1210/en.2013-1623

46. Wurtman RJ, Axelrod J. Adrenaline synthesis: control by the pituitary gland and adrenal glucocorticoids. *Science* (1965) 150:1464–5. doi:10.1126/science.150.3702.1464

47. Kvetnansky R, Kubovcakova L, Tillinger A, Micutkova L, Krizanova O, Sabban EL. Gene expression of phenylethanolamine N-methyltransferase in corticotropin-releasing hormone knockout mice during stress exposure. *Cell Mol Neurobiol* (2006) 26:735–54. doi:10.1007/s10571-006-9063-7

48. Ehrhart-Bornstein M, Bornstein SR, Scherbaum WA, Pfeiffer EF, Holst JJ. Role of the vasoactive intestinal peptide in a neuroendocrine regulation of the adrenal cortex. *Neuroendocrinology* (1991) 54:623–8. doi:10.1159/000125969

49. Bornstein SR, Haidan A, Ehrhart-Bornstein M. Cellular communication in the neuro-adrenocortical axis: role of vasoactive intestinal polypeptide (VIP). *Endocr Res* (1996) 22:819–29. doi:10.1080/07435809609043781

50. Cobb VJ, Williams BC, Mason JI, Walker SW. Direct stimulation of cortisol secretion from the human NCI H295 adrenocortical cell line by vasoactive intestinal polypeptide. *J Hypertens* (1997) 15:1735–8. doi:10.1097/00004872-199715120-00081

51. Ait-Ali D, Stroth N, Sen JM, Eiden LE. PACAP-cytokine interactions govern adrenal neuropeptide biosynthesis after systemic administration of LPS. *Neuropharmacology* (2010) 58:208–14. doi:10.1016/j.neuropharm.2010.03.009

52. Haase M, Willenberg HS, Bornstein SR. Update on the corticomedullary interaction in the adrenal gland. *Endocr Dev* (2011) 20:28–37. doi:10.1159/000321211

53. Pope GR, Roberts EM, Lolait SJ, O'Carroll AM. Central and peripheral apelin receptor distribution in the mouse: species differences with rat. *Peptides* (2012) 33(1):139–48. doi:10.1016/j.peptides.2011.12.005

54. Reaux-Le GA, Alvear-Perez R, Zizzari P, Epelbaum J, Bluet-Pajot MT, Llorens-Cortes C. Cellular localization of apelin and its receptor in the anterior pituitary: evidence for a direct stimulatory action of apelin on ACTH release. *Am J Physiol Endocrinol Metab* (2007) 292:E7–15. doi:10.1152/ajpendo.00521.2005

55. Gallo-Payet N, Roussy JF, Chagnon F, Roberge C, Lesur O. Hypothalamic-pituitary-adrenal axis and multiple and organ dysfunction syndrome in critical illness: a special focus on arginine-vasopressin and apelin. *J Organ Dysfunct* (2008) 4:216–29. doi:10.1080/17471060802339711

56. Bornstein SR. Predisposing factors for adrenal insufficiency. *N Engl J Med* (2009) 360:2328–39. doi:10.1056/NEJMra0804635

57. Newson MJ, Roberts EM, Pope GR, Lolait SJ, O'Carroll AM. The effects of apelin on hypothalamic-pituitary-adrenal axis neuroendocrine function are mediated through corticotrophin-releasing factor- and vasopressin-dependent mechanisms. *J Endocrinol* (2009) 202:123–9. doi:10.1677/JOE-09-0093

58. Rubin de Celis MF, Bornstein SR, Androutsellis-Theotokis A, Andoniadou CL, Licinio J, Wong ML, et al. The effects of stress on brain and adrenal stem cells. *Mol Psychiatry* (2016) 21:590–3. doi:10.1038/mp.2015.230
59. Steenblock C, Rubin de Celis MF, Androutsellis-Theotokis A, Sue M, Delgadillo Silva LF, Eisenhofer G, et al. Adrenal cortical and chromaffin stem cells: is there a common progeny related to stress adaptation? *Mol Cell Endocrinol* (2016). doi:10.1016/j.mce.2016.09.011
60. Rubin de Celis MF, Garcia-Martin R, Wittig D, Valencia GD, Enikolopov G, Funk RH, et al. Multipotent glia-like stem cells mediate stress adaptation. *Stem Cells* (2015) 33:2037–51. doi:10.1002/stem.2002
61. Besedovsky H, Sorkin E. Network of immune-neuroendocrine interactions. *Clin Exp Immunol* (1977) 27:1–12.
62. Bornstein SR, Ziegler CG, Krug AW, Kanczkowski W, Rettori V, McCann SM, et al. The role of toll-like receptors in the immune-adrenal crosstalk. *Ann N Y Acad Sci* (2006) 1088:307–18. doi:10.1196/annals.1366.027
63. Schober A, Huber K, Fey J, Unsicker K. Distinct populations of macrophages in the adult rat adrenal gland: a subpopulation with neurotrophin-4-like immunoreactivity. *Cell Tissue Res* (1998) 291:365–73. doi:10.1007/s004410051006
64. Gonzalez-Hernandez JA, Bornstein SR, Ehrhart-Bornstein M, Geschwend JE, Adler G, Scherbaum WA. Macrophages within the human adrenal gland. *Cell Tissue Res* (1994) 278:201–5. doi:10.1007/BF00414161
65. Naccache A, Louiset E, Duparc C, Laquerriere A, Patrier S, Renouf S, et al. Temporal and spatial distribution of mast cells and steroidogenic enzymes in the human fetal adrenal. *Mol Cell Endocrinol* (2016) 434:69–80. doi:10.1016/j.mce.2016.06.015
66. Wolkersdorfer GW, Lohmann T, Marx C, Schroder S, Pfeiffer R, Stahl HD, et al. Lymphocytes stimulate dehydroepiandrosterone production through direct cellular contact with adrenal zona reticularis cells: a novel mechanism of immune-endocrine interaction. *J Clin Endocrinol Metab* (1999) 84:4220–7. doi:10.1210/jcem.84.11.6110
67. Bornstein SR, Rutkowski H, Vrezas I. Cytokines and steroidogenesis. *Mol Cell Endocrinol* (2004) 215:135–41. doi:10.1016/j.mce.2003.11.022
68. Helmy KY, Katschke KJ Jr, Gorgani NN, Kljavin NM, Elliott JM, Diehl L, et al. CRIg: a macrophage complement receptor required for phagocytosis of circulating pathogens. *Cell* (2006) 124:915–27. doi:10.1016/j.cell.2005.12.039
69. Jennewein C, Tran N, Kanczkowski W, Heerdegen L, Kantharajah A, Drose S, et al. Mortality of septic mice strongly correlates with adrenal gland inflammation. *Crit Care Med* (2016) 44:e190–9. doi:10.1097/CCM.0000000000001373
70. Kanczkowski W, Chatzigeorgiou A, Samus M, Tran N, Zacharowski K, Chavakis T, et al. Characterization of the LPS-induced inflammation of the adrenal gland in mice. *Mol Cell Endocrinol* (2013) 371:228–35. doi:10.1016/j.mce.2012.12.020
71. Engstrom L, Rosen K, Angel A, Fyrberg A, Mackerlova L, Pieter KJ, et al. Systemic immune challenge activates an intrinsically regulated local inflammatory circuit in the adrenal gland. *Endocrinology* (2008) 149:1436–50. doi:10.1210/en.2007-1456
72. Bethin KE, Vogt SK, Muglia LJ. Interleukin-6 is an essential, corticotropin-releasing hormone-independent stimulator of the adrenal axis during immune system activation. *Proc Natl Acad Sci U S A* (2000) 97:9317–22. doi:10.1073/pnas.97.16.9317
73. Oates EL, Allaway GP, Armstrong GR, Boyajian RA, Kehrl JH, Prabhakar BS. Human lymphocytes produce pro-opiomelanocortin gene-related transcripts. Effects of lymphotropic viruses. *J Biol Chem* (1988) 263:10041–4.
74. Andreis PG, Neri G, Belloni AS, Mazzocchi G, Kasprzak A, Nussdorfer GG. Interleukin-1 beta enhances corticosterone secretion by acting directly on the rat adrenal gland. *Endocrinology* (1991) 129:53–7. doi:10.1210/endo-129-1-53
75. Fattori E, Cappelletti M, Costa P, Sellitto C, Cantoni L, Carelli M, et al. Defective inflammatory response in interleukin 6-deficient mice. *J Exp Med* (1994) 180:1243–50. doi:10.1084/jem.180.4.1243
76. Hadid R, Spinedi E, Chautard T, Giacomini M, Gaillard RC. Role of several mediators of inflammation on the mouse hypothalamo-pituitary-adrenal axis response during acute endotoxemia. *Neuroimmunomodulation* (1999) 6:336–43. doi:10.1159/000026393
77. Bacher M, Meinhardt A, Lan HY, Mu W, Metz CN, Chesney JA, et al. Migration inhibitory factor expression in experimentally induced endotoxemia. *Am J Pathol* (1997) 150:235–46.
78. Gonzalez-Hernandez JA, Ehrhart-Bornstein M, Spath-Schwalbe E, Scherbaum WA, Bornstein SR. Human adrenal cells express tumor necrosis factor-alpha messenger ribonucleic acid: evidence for paracrine control of adrenal function. *J Clin Endocrinol Metab* (1996) 81:807–13. doi:10.1210/jc.81.2.807
79. Kanczkowski W, Zacharowski K, Wirth MP, Ehrhart-Bornstein M, Bornstein SR. Differential expression and action of toll-like receptors in human adrenocortical cells. *Mol Cell Endocrinol* (2009) 300:57–65. doi:10.1016/j.mce.2008.10.028
80. Kanczkowski W, Alexaki VI, Tran N, Grossklaus S, Zacharowski K, Martinez A, et al. Hypothalamo-pituitary and immune-dependent adrenal regulation during systemic inflammation. *Proc Natl Acad Sci U S A* (2013) 110:14801–6. doi:10.1073/pnas.1313945110
81. Path G, Bornstein SR, Spath-Schwalbe E, Scherbaum WA. Direct effects of interleukin-6 on human adrenal cells. *Endocr Res* (1996) 22:867–73. doi:10.1080/07435809609043788
82. Gonzalez-Hernandez JA, Bornstein SR, Ehrhart-Bornstein M, Gschwend JE, Gwosdow A, Jirikowski G, et al. IL-1 is expressed in human adrenal gland in vivo. Possible role in a local immune-adrenal axis. *Clin Exp Immunol* (1995) 99:137–41. doi:10.1111/j.1365-2249.1995.tb03484.x
83. Judd AM, Call GB, Barney M, McIlmoil CJ, Balls AG, Adams A, et al. Possible function of IL-6 and TNF as intraadrenal factors in the regulation of adrenal steroid secretion. *Ann N Y Acad Sci* (2000) 917:628–37. doi:10.1111/j.1749-6632.2000.tb05428.x
84. van de Garde MD, Martinez FO, Melgert BN, Hylkema MN, Jonkers RE, Hamann J. Chronic exposure to glucocorticoids shapes gene expression and modulates innate and adaptive activation pathways in macrophages with distinct changes in leukocyte attraction. *J Immunol* (2014) 192:1196–208. doi:10.4049/jimmunol.1302138
85. Lefebvre H, Contesse V, Delarue C, Feuilloley M, Hery F, Grise P, et al. Serotonin-induced stimulation of cortisol secretion from human adrenocortical tissue is mediated through activation of a serotonin4 receptor subtype. *Neuroscience* (1992) 47:999–1007. doi:10.1016/0306-4522(92)90047-6
86. Lefebvre H, Prevost G, Louiset E. Autocrine/paracrine regulatory mechanisms in adrenocortical neoplasms responsible for primary adrenal hypercorticism. *Eur J Endocrinol* (2013) 169:R115–38. doi:10.1530/EJE-13-0308
87. Clark SR, Ma AC, Tavener SA, McDonald B, Goodarzi Z, Kelly MM, et al. Platelet TLR4 activates neutrophil extracellular traps to ensnare bacteria in septic blood. *Nat Med* (2007) 13:463–9. doi:10.1038/nm1565
88. von Bruhl ML, Stark K, Steinhart A, Chandraratne S, Konrad I, Lorenz M, et al. Monocytes, neutrophils, and platelets cooperate to initiate and propagate venous thrombosis in mice in vivo. *J Exp Med* (2012) 209:819–35. doi:10.1084/jem.20112322
89. Tominaga T, Fukata J, Naito Y, Nakai Y, Funakoshi S, Fujii N, et al. Effects of corticostatin-I on rat adrenal cells in vitro. *J Endocrinol* (1990) 125:287–92. doi:10.1677/joe.0.1250287
90. Choi EY, Chavakis E, Czabanka MA, Langer HF, Fraemohs L, Economopoulou M, et al. Del-1, an endogenous leukocyte-endothelial adhesion inhibitor, limits inflammatory cell recruitment. *Science* (2008) 322:1101–4. doi:10.1126/science.1165218
91. Kanczkowski W, Chatzigeorgiou A, Grossklaus S, Sprott D, Bornstein SR, Chavakis T. Role of the endothelial-derived endogenous anti-inflammatory factor Del-1 in inflammation-mediated adrenal gland dysfunction. *Endocrinology* (2013) 154:1181–9. doi:10.1210/en.2012-1617
92. Spengler RN, Chensue SW, Giacherio DA, Blenk N, Kunkel SL. Endogenous norepinephrine regulates tumor necrosis factor-alpha production from macrophages in vitro. *J Immunol* (1994) 152:3024–31.
93. Barnett CC Jr, Moore EE, Partrick DA, Silliman CC. Beta-adrenergic stimulation down-regulates neutrophil priming for superoxide generation, but not elastase release. *J Surg Res* (1997) 70:166–70. doi:10.1006/jsre.1997.5118
94. Gornikiewicz A, Sautner T, Brostjan C, Schmierer B, Fugger R, Roth E, et al. Catecholamines up-regulate lipopolysaccharide-induced IL-6 production in human microvascular endothelial cells. *FASEB J* (2000) 14:1093–100.
95. Spengler RN, Allen RM, Remick DG, Strieter RM, Kunkel SL. Stimulation of alpha-adrenergic receptor augments the production of macrophage-derived tumor necrosis factor. *J Immunol* (1990) 145:1430–4.

96. Flierl MA, Rittirsch D, Nadeau BA, Chen AJ, Sarma JV, Zetoune FS, et al. Phagocyte-derived catecholamines enhance acute inflammatory injury. *Nature* (2007) 449:721–5. doi:10.1038/nature06185
97. Flierl MA, Rittirsch D, Gao H, Hoesel LM, Nadeau BA, Day DE, et al. Adverse functions of IL-17A in experimental sepsis. *FASEB J* (2008) 22:2198–205. doi:10.1096/fj.07-105221
98. Ansurudeen I, Willenberg HS, Kopprasch S, Krug AW, Ehrhart-Bornstein M, Bornstein SR. Endothelial factors mediate aldosterone release via PKA-independent pathways. *Mol Cell Endocrinol* (2009) 300:66–70. doi:10.1016/j.mce.2008.11.020
99. Hinson JP, Vinson GP, Kapas S, Teja R. The role of endothelin in the control of adrenocortical function: stimulation of endothelin release by ACTH and the effects of endothelin-1 and endothelin-3 on steroidogenesis in rat and human adrenocortical cells. *J Endocrinol* (1991) 128(2):275–80. doi:10.1677/joe.0.1280275
100. Mohn CE, Fernandez-Solari J, De LA, Prestifilippo JP, de la Cal C, Funk R, et al. The rapid release of corticosterone from the adrenal induced by ACTH is mediated by nitric oxide acting by prostaglandin E2. *Proc Natl Acad Sci U S A* (2005) 102:6213–8. doi:10.1073/pnas.0502136102
101. Cameron LA, Hinson JP. The role of nitric oxide derived from L-arginine in the control of steroidogenesis, and perfusion medium flow rate in the isolated perfused rat adrenal gland. *J Endocrinol* (1993) 139:415–23. doi:10.1677/joe.0.1390415
102. Jung B, Nougaret S, Chanques G, Mercier G, Cisse M, Aufort S, et al. The absence of adrenal gland enlargement during septic shock predicts mortality: a computed tomography study of 239 patients. *Anesthesiology* (2011) 115:334–43. doi:10.1097/ALN.0b013e318225cfd7
103. Breslow MJ. Regulation of adrenal medullary and cortical blood flow. *Am J Physiol* (1992) 262:H1317–30.
104. Engeland WC, Gann DS. Splanchnic nerve stimulation modulates steroid secretion in hypophysectomized dogs. *Neuroendocrinology* (1989) 50:124–31. doi:10.1159/000125211
105. Jones CT, Edwards AV, Bloom SR. The effect of changes in adrenal blood flow on adrenal cortical responses to adrenocorticotrophin in conscious calves. *J Physiol* (1990) 429:377–86. doi:10.1113/jphysiol.1990.sp018262
106. Hinson JP, Vinson GP, Pudney J, Whitehouse BJ. Adrenal mast cells modulate vascular and secretory responses in the intact adrenal gland of the rat. *J Endocrinol* (1989) 121:253–60. doi:10.1677/joe.0.1210253
107. Ansurudeen I, Kopf PG, Gauthier KM, Bornstein SR, Cowley AW Jr, Campbell WB. Aldosterone secretagogues increase adrenal blood flow in male rats. *Endocrinology* (2014) 155:127–32. doi:10.1210/en.2013-1532
108. Cohen J, Vincent JL, Adhikari NK, Machado FR, Angus DC, Calandra T, et al. Sepsis: a roadmap for future research. *Lancet Infect Dis* (2015) 15:581–614. doi:10.1016/S1473-3099(15)70112-X
109. Annane D, Bellissant E, Cavaillon JM. Septic shock. *Lancet* (2005) 365:63–78. doi:10.1016/S0140-6736(04)17667-8

21

The Role of *gsp* Mutations on the Development of Adrenocortical Tumors and Adrenal Hyperplasia

Maria Candida Barisson Villares Fragoso*, Ingrid Quevedo Wanichi, Isadora Pontes Cavalcante and Beatriz Marinho de Paula Mariani

Unidade de Suprarrenal, Disciplina de Endocrinologia e Metabologia, Laboratorio de Hormonios e Genetica Molecular LIM/42, Hospital das Clinicas, Faculdade de Medicina da Universidade de Sao Paulo, Sao Paulo, Brazil

***Correspondence:**
Maria Candida Barisson Villares Fragoso
maria.villares@hc.fm.usp.br

Somatic *GNAS* point mutations, commonly known as *gsp* mutations, are involved in the pathogenesis of McCune–Albright syndrome (MAS) and have also been described in autonomous hormone-producing tumors, such as somatotropinoma, corticotrophoma, thyroid cancer, ovarian and testicular Leydig cell tumors, and primary macronodular adrenocortical hyperplasia (PMAH) (1–3). The involvement of *gsp* mutations in adrenal tumors was first described by Lyons et al. Since then, several studies have detected the presence of *gsp* mutations in adrenal tumors, but none of them could explain its presence along or the mechanism that leads to tumor formation and hormone hypersecretion. As a result, the molecular pathogenesis of the majority of sporadic adrenocortical tumors remains unclear (3). PMAH has also been reported with *gsp* somatic mutations in a few cases. Fragoso et al. identified two distinct *gsp* somatic mutations affecting arginine residues on codon 201 of *GNAS* in a few patients with PMAH who lacked any features or manifestations of MAS. Followed by this discovery, other studies have continued looking for *gsp* mutations based on strong prior evidence demonstrating that increased cAMP signaling is sufficient for cell proliferation and cortisol production (2, 4). With consideration for the previously reported findings, we conjecture that although somatic activating mutations in *GNAS* are a rare molecular event, these mutations could probably be sufficient to induce the development of macronodule hyperplasia and variable cortisol secretion. In this manuscript, we revised the presence of *gsp* mutations associated with adrenal cortical tumors and hyperplasia.

Keywords: *gsp*, *GNAS*, adrenal, tumors, hyperplasia, mutations

INTRODUCTION

Heterotrimeric G proteins are the molecular switches that turn on intracellular signaling cascades in response to the activation of G protein-coupled receptors (GPCRs) by extracellular stimuli. Therefore, G proteins play a crucial role in defining the specificity and temporal characteristics of the cellular response. Heterotrimeric G proteins consist of three subunits, α, β, and γ, and their switching function depends on the ability of the G protein α-subunit (Gα) to cycle between an inactive GDP-bound conformation that is primed to interact with an activated receptor and an active GTP-bound conformation that can modulate the activity of downstream effector proteins. The α subunit is a GTPase; therefore, when the receptor stimulates the G protein, this subunit releases GDP and binds GTP. In this activated state, several α subunit types act directly on effector molecules to modulate their activity. Some α subunits show specificity for effectors; for example, αs activates adenylate cyclases, αi inhibits adenylate cyclases, and αq activates phospholipase C isozymes (5) (**Figure 1**).

The gene encoding the alpha subunit of stimulatory G proteins (GNAS, OMIM 139320) is located on chromosome 20q13.32 (6). Activating somatic mutations of stimulatory G protein called *gsp* mutations can result in the loss of intrinsic GTPase activity of the α subunit with subsequent constitutive activation of adenylate cyclase (7, 8).

gsp mutations are involved in the pathogenesis of McCune–Albright syndrome (MAS), which is an endocrine disorder that is classically defined by the clinical triad of bone fibrous dysplasia, *café-au-lait* skin, and peripheral precocious puberty (1).

Patients with MAS present with a postzygotic *gsp* mutation in a mosaic distribution, resulting in varying degrees of tissue involvement that range from a single site to a widespread distribution. However, if these mutations were germline, they would be lethal. To date, this concept is supported by the absence of any cases resulting from vertical transmission and the discordance in disease among monozygotic twins (9). Adrenal hypercortisolism affects a minority of patients with MAS due to adrenal nodular hyperplasia and around 20 cases were described (8).

Naturally occurring mutations in codons 201 and 227, which alter the GTPase activity in the *GNAS* gene, have been described in autonomous hormone-producing tumors. Mutations involving substitution of either cysteine or histidine and, more rarely, serine for arginine at codon 201 or arginine for glutamine at codon 227 were first described in GH-producing pituitary tumors (10).

The *gsp* mutations have also been described in several tumors, such as somatotropinoma, thyroid tumor, ovarian and testicular Leydig cell tumors, and primary macronodular adrenocortical hyperplasia (PMAH), as well as in rare cases of corticotropinoma, cortisol, and aldosterone-secreting adrenocortical adenoma. All cases described were outside of the classical presentation of MAS (1, 2, 4, 7).

cAMP/PKA Signaling in Adrenocortical Cells

The discovery of the role of cAMP (adenosine 3′5′-cyclic monophosphate) as an intracellular mediator introduced the concept of second messengers in signal transduction. cAMP is a nucleotide synthesized within cells using ATP, and it is under the action of a membrane-bound enzyme, adenylate cyclase. cAMP is continuously produced and inactivated by hydrolysis

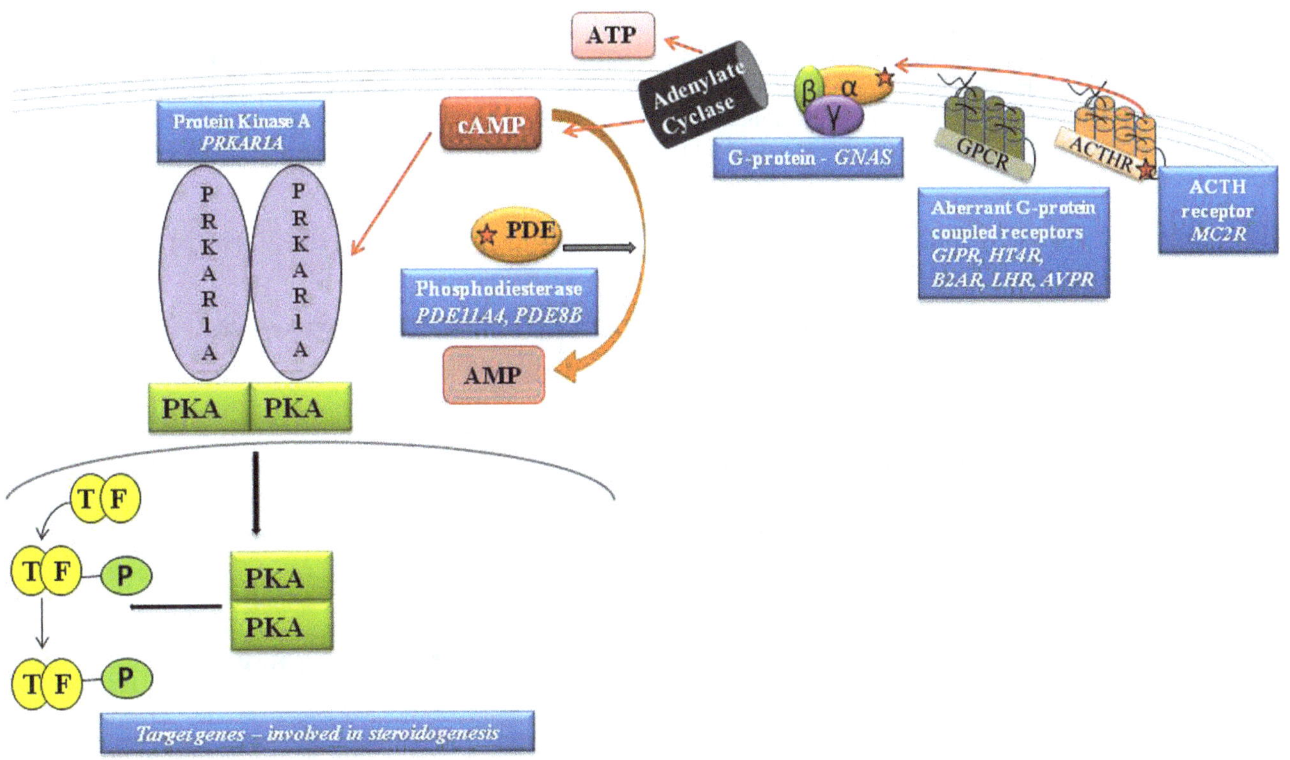

FIGURE 1 | Schematic representation of cAMP pathway. GPCRs cause the activation of G proteins by facilitating the exchange of GTP for GDP on the α subunit. cAMP is degraded to AMP by PDEs. PKA is activated by the rise in cAMP that, by binding both high-affinity cAMP-binding sites of each subunit, leads to the release of active subunits that phosphorylate their substrates, including the nuclear transcription factor, CREB. By inhibiting the intrinsic GTPase activity, *gsp* mutations cause constitutive activation of adenylyl cyclase (AC), leading to increased cAMP; protein kinase A activation. The protein kinase A (PKA) induces phosphorylation of the cAMP-binding protein, CREB, facilitating its traslocation to the nucleus and activation of cAMP-responsive gene transcription. [Adapted from Lacroix et al. (11)].

of 5′-AMP through a family of enzymes known as phosphodiesterase (12–14).

cAMP regulates many aspects of cell function, including enzymes involved in energy metabolism, cell division and differentiation, ion transport, ion channels, and contractile proteins. However, these effects are produced by a common mechanism, the activation of protein kinases by cAMP (**Figure 2**).

Proteins are phosphorylated by various protein kinases. The substrates of protein kinases and phosphatases include enzymes, neurotransmitter receptors, ion channels, and structural proteins, activating or inhibiting through phosphorylation, the target enzymes or ion channels. The increased cAMP production in response to the activation of β-adrenergic receptors affects several enzymes that are involved in glycogen metabolism, adipocytes, and muscle cells. The result consists of a coordinated response in which the energy stored as glycogen and fat becomes available as glucose, acting as a supply for muscle contraction (15).

cAMP, a second messenger, and its effector, protein kinase A (PKA), are key regulators of practically all cellular functions, such as cell growth and cell differentiation, and proliferation, and they mediate the effects of several hormones and neurotransmitters *via* GPCRs. This pathway is one of the major participants in the regulation of growth, proliferation, and hormonal secretion in adrenocortical cells (16, 17).

Once two cAMP molecules bind to each R subunit, the C subunits are released from the holoenzyme and can phosphorylate their targets, which are localized in the cytosol and in the nucleus. In adrenocortical cells, there is stimulation of glucocorticoid synthesis as well as transcriptional induction of steroidogenic enzymes and activation genes that are involved in cell replication (15, 18).

The majority of benign lesions of the adrenal cortex that lead to cortisol overproduction are linked to abnormalities of the cAMP pathway. Genetic defects in the cAMP/PKA that maintain pathway activation have been associated with adrenal disorders as follows:

(1) Ectopic expression of G protein-coupled receptors (19, 20).
(2) Somatic activating mutations in the gene coding for the $G\alpha_s$ protein (*GNAS*) (6, 10, 21).
(3) Somatic activating mutations in the corticotropin receptor gene, *MC2R* (22, 23).
(4) Germline and/or somatic inactivating mutations in the gene coding for the RIα subunit of PKA (*PRKAR1A*) (13, 14, 18).
(5) Inactivating germline mutations in the genes coding two phosphodiesterases (PDE8 and PDE11A) (24, 25).
(6) Activating germline mutations in the gene coding for the Cα subunit of PKA (*PRKACA*) (26).
(7) Somatic mutations in PRKACA, which encodes the catalytic subunit of cyclic AMP-dependent protein kinase (27).
(8) Germline and somatic inactivating mutations of ARMC5 (28, 29).

Nevertheless, because these molecular events are not able to explain all cases of adrenocortical disorders, part of the molecular pathogenesis of the tumors causing Cushing's syndrome remains a challenge to scientific researchers.

gsp Mutations in Adrenal Cortical Tumors

Somatic mutations of genes encoding components of the cAMP/PKA pathway (*GNAS*, *PRKAR1A*, *PDE8B*) and β-catenin (*CTNNB1*) have been reported in a small subset of adrenocortical tumors that produce cortisol (27, 30).

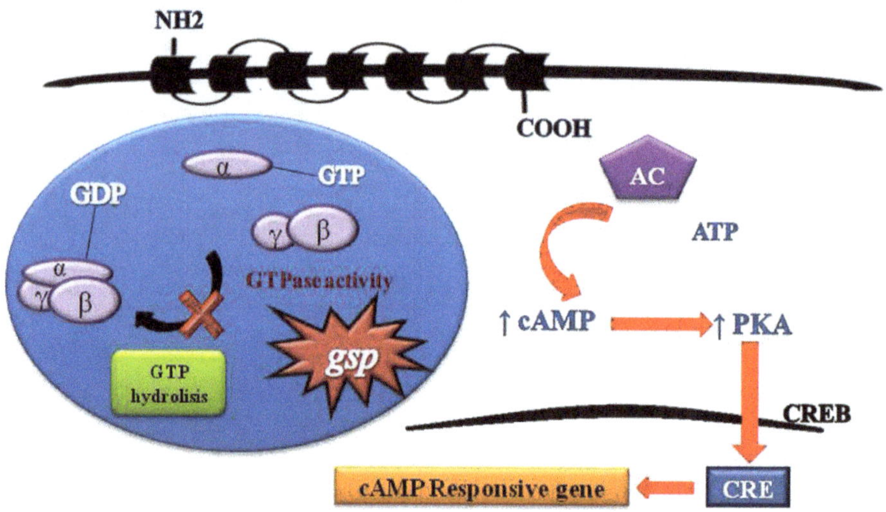

FIGURE 2 | Schematic representation of G protein activation and signaling. Heterotrimeric G proteins are composed of three distinct subunits alpha, beta, and gamma. Activity G protein depends on the alpha subunit. The alpha subunit contains high-affinity binding sites for guanine nucleotides (GDP) and has intrinsic GTPase activity. The GDP-bound form binds tightly to beta and gamma units in its inactive state. The GTP-bound form dissociates from beta and gamma units and serves as a regulator of effectors proteins. The receptor molecules cause the activation of G proteins by facilitating the exchange of GTP for GDP on the alpha subunit. The duration of subunit separation is timed by the rate of alpha subunit-mediated hydrolysis of GTP. The *gsp* mutations Arg201Cys and Gln227Arg at exons 8 and 9, respectively, of GNAS causing a constitutive signal of cAMP pathway.

The first report of the involvement of *gsp* mutations in adrenal tumors was by Lyons et al. In this study, the group tested the gene that encodes the alpha chain of Gi2, and the authors detected mutations that replaced arginine-179 with either cysteine or histidine in 3 of 11 tumors of the adrenal cortex and 3 of 10 endocrine tumors of the ovary (31).

Yoshimoto et al. systemically screened Gs alpha mutations in 197 human endocrine tumors. They included pituitary, thyroid, parathyroid, endocrine pancreas, and (cortex and medulla) adrenal tumors. They identified a unique, 29-year-old female patient with primary aldosteronism associated with a somatic *gsp* mutation in an aldosterone-producing adrenocortical adenoma. The authors commented that when the renin–aldosterone system is suppressed, aldosterone-producing adrenal adenomas become more sensitive to corticotropin stimulation. In this way, corticotropin is transmitted *via* Gs alpha-mediated cyclic AMP production. The study hypothesized that the *gsp* mutations may constitutively stimulate aldosterone synthesis in the glomerulosa zone, transmitting a constitutive signal *via* Gs-mediated cyclic AMP production, which would play an important role in the tumorigenesis of the aldosterone-secreting adenoma (3).

In 2000, Bugalho et al. described the presence of a mutation at codon 201 (CGT to TGT) in a patient with Cushing's syndrome due to a functioning adrenal adenoma (32). In 2004, Dall'Asta et al. also identified *gsp* mutations in one patient with ACTH-independent Cushing's syndrome. The presence of the *gsp* mutation seemed to alter the cortisol responses to agents *via* Gs protein-coupled receptors, whereas these responses are absent in other cases of adenoma-producing Cushing's syndrome without *gsp* mutations (33).

Moreover, Libé and Bertherat investigated the presence of genetic alterations on a series of 10 ACTH-independent Cushing's syndrome cases due to adrenocortical cortisol-secreting adenomas. The *gsp* mutation was identified in only one case, demonstrating that this abnormality is a rare cause of adrenocortical tumors. These findings suggest that different mechanisms are probably involved in adrenal tumorigenesis in primarily benign disorders (34).

A study conducted by Almeida et al. using the whole-genome expression profile (WGEP) of *PRKAR1A* and *GNAS*-mutant analysis revealed that not all cAMP activation is the same. Adrenal lesions harboring *PRKAR1A* or *GNAS* mutations share downstream activation of specific oncogenic signals (such as MAPK and cell cycle genes), but they differ substantially in their effects on others. These results support the hypothesis that several pathways can activate cAMP (13).

In 2013, Sidhu et al. described, for the first time, the presence of the p.R201C, a *GNAS* activating mutation in a malignant pediatric adrenocortical tumor. The malignant features described were as follows: areas of necrosis, microcytic degeneration, and both venous and capsular microinvasion. The tumor tissue also presented with abnormal allele-specific hypomethylation of the *KCNQ1OT1* gene involved in Beckwith–Wiedemann syndrome. Somatic mutations in these genes may constitutively activate the cAMP-protein kinase cascade, leading to cellular proliferation, which may then result in genomic instability and epigenetic alterations that give rise to ACTs and malignancy. This study suggested, for the first time, that activation of the cAMP-PKA cascade alone may not be sufficient to cause malignant transformation in the adrenal cortex without resulting in secondary events (35).

Recently, somatic mutations of *PRKACA* (encoding the catalytic subunit of PKA) have been identified in more than one-third of the patients with Cushing's syndrome from sporadic adrenocortical adenomas; however, the molecular pathogenesis of the majority of sporadic adrenocortical tumors remains unclear (18, 27, 36).

In summary, apart from the known somatic mutations described in the literature, no other recurrent mutation by itself can explain the mechanism of tumor formation and hormone hypersecretion.

gsp Mutations in Primary Macronodular Adrenal Hyperplasia

Over the last two decades, different studies have supported that multiple molecular mechanisms may be involved in the pathogenesis of PMAH (7, 12–14, 37). Several pathways were studied and analyzed for gene alterations, suggesting that there may be a heterogeneous group of diseases with a common presentation, ranging from subclinical hypercortisolism to overt Cushing's syndrome.

Bilateral adrenal hyperplasia may be part of MAS that is associated with hypercortisolism, especially in young children during the first years of age. The adrenal nodules of these patients carried the *gsp* mutation and adrenal cortical cells increased the levels of cAMP (6, 8).

In 2003, Fragoso et al. identified two distinct *gsp* somatic mutations affecting arginine residues in codon 201 of *GNAS* in a few patients with PMAH without any features or manifestations of MAS (2).

Subsequently, Hsiao et al. also reported the presence of *gsp* somatic mutation in one additional patient with PMAH (4). On the other hand, an additional study failed to observe *gsp* mutations in PMAH (37). Technical variations in the methodologies employed for the investigation of *gsp* mutations could explain the discrepancy in these published findings.

Almeida et al. described the analyzed the WGEP of primary pigmented nodular adrenocortical disease (PPNAD) patients associated with gsp mutations. The data indicated that cAMP activation in adrenal lesions harboring *gsp* mutations share the downstream activation of some oncogenic signals but differ significantly in their effects on others (13).

Considering the great variation of MAS, these cases might characterize late *gsp* somatic mutations considering that similar mutations have been described outside the context of MAS (e.g., acromegaly, thyroid cancer, and ovarian–testicular neoplasms) (7).

Based on strong previous evidence implying that increased cAMP signaling is sufficient for cell proliferation and cortisol production, we posit that although these somatic activating mutations in *GNAS* are a rare molecular event, they are probably sufficient to induce the development of macronodule hyperplasia and variable cortisol secretion (12, 38, 39).

Primary macronodular adrenocortical hyperplasia is a heterogeneous disorder that could be associated with genetic defects in both germline and somatic levels. The presence of somatic *gsp* mutations was detected in rare cases with PMAH without MAS features. The role of *gsp* mutations in the development of this adrenal disorder remains partially unclear (2).

Recent studies have now indicated that PMAH is more frequently genetically determined than previously believed (28, 29). Germline mutations of *ARMC5* in ~50% of patients with apparently sporadic PMAH, and also in a large family with genetically transmitted PMAH. The *ARMC5* has no apparent link to the cAMP pathway, but its inactivation decreases the expression of both MC2R and various steroidogenic enzymes (19).

Activation of Cyclic AMP Signaling in Lesions of the Adrenal Cortex due to Somatic GNAS Mutations

Aberrations in cAMP/PKA signaling are essential to the pathogenesis of benign cortisol-producing lesions of the adrenal cortex (40).

An important study by Almeida and coauthors analyzed the WGEP of adrenal lesions harboring somatic *GNAS* mutations in the normal adrenal pool and tissue with somatic *PRKAR1A* genes. They included three microdissected samples from adrenal lesions that were all caused by the same somatic *GNAS* mutation (p.R201H) as follows: a cortisol-producing adenoma from patients with PMAH and Cushing's syndrome and hyperplasia from patients with MAS and Cushing's syndrome. The results of this study showed that the MAPK and p53 signaling pathways were highly overexpressed in all lesions compared with normal tissues. *GNAS*-mutant tissues were significantly enriched for extracellular matrix receptor interaction and focal adhesion pathways compared with *PRKAR1A* mutants. In addition, *NFKB*, *NFKBIA*, and *TNFRSF1A* were overexpressed in *GNAS*-mutant adrenal tissue (13).

NFKB is a transcription activator nuclear factor kappa light-chain enhancer of activated B cells, a complex protein that controls DNA transcription, cytokine production, and cell survival. The nuclear factor kappa–beta controls the expression of various genes that are involved in cancer-related processes, including immune and inflammatory responses; cell adhesion, proliferation, differentiation, and apoptosis; and angiogenesis (13).

TNFRSF1A is a tumor necrosis factor receptor member of the superfamily 1A and the protein encoded by this gene is a member of the TNF-receptor superfamily. This protein is one of the major receptors for tumor necrosis factor-alpha. This receptor can activate NF-kappa–beta and mediate apoptosis, and it functions as a regulator of inflammation (13).

The study of adrenal lesions harboring *PRKAR1A* or *GNAS* mutations, conducted by Almeida et al. suggested that cAMP signaling inhibitors could be used as molecularly designed therapies for subclinical CS in the context of bilateral adrenal hyperplasia (13).

Despite the importance of the cAMP pathway, these molecular events are a rare cause of adrenocortical tumors and adrenal hyperplasia, showing that several other genes should be involved in the cAMP pathway as long as other genes are involved in adrenal tumorigenesis and hyperplastic development.

NEW INSIGHTS

This review aimed to provide a summary of the main studies on the role of cAMP and *gsp* mutations on the development of adrenocortical tumors and adrenal hyperplasia. Throughout this review, we showed that *gsp* mutations are a rare cause of adrenal disorders and involvement of *gsp* mutations in increasing the cAMP levels is not always detected.

The molecular pathogenesis of cortisol-producing adrenal adenomas and adrenal hyperplasia is not well understood.

Somatic mutations in the gene encoding beta-catenin (*CTNNB1*) have primarily been found in non-secreting adrenocortical adenomas, and there is some evidence that increased endocrine activity may be linked to aberrant cAMP signaling.

Tumor suppressor genes point mutations (such as *CTNNB1*) and alterations in the cortisol producing (*ARMC5* and *PKC* mutations) could lead to alterations in cAMP pathway.

Mutations in the genes *PDE11A*, *PDE8B*, and *PRKAR1A* have also been identified in patients with adrenal disorders related to cortisol production (14).

Nevertheless, lesions of the adrenal gland that are associated with adrenal Cushing syndrome, independent of their *GNAS*, *PRKAR1A*, *PDE11A*, and *PDE8B* mutations, have functional abnormalities in cAMP signaling. It is hypothesized that epigenetic events or additional genetic defects of the regulatory molecules in this pathway exist and have yet to be identified (41).

CONCLUSION

The genetic analyses of the molecular pathogenesis of sporadic cortisol-secreting adrenocortical adenomas confirm the key role of the cAMP/PKA-signaling pathway in stimulating both the function and proliferation of adrenocortical cells. They provide insights into the development of adrenal hormonal autonomy and may provide the basis for novel advances in the diagnosis and therapy of adrenal Cushing's syndrome.

In conclusion, this review demonstrates that not all increased cAMP/PKA signaling has the same effect on adrenocortical tumor formation. The role of non-PKA-dependent functions of cAMP in the adrenal cortex has not been adequately investigated.

Based on strong previous evidence implying that increased cAMP signaling is sufficient for cell proliferation and cortisol production (38), we surmise that although really rare, these *gsp* mutations are probably sufficient for macronodule formation and the hypercortisolism status.

AUTHOR CONTRIBUTIONS

MCBVF, IQW, IPC, BMPM: All authors contributed equally for the article.

REFERENCES

1. Dumitrescu CE, Collins MT. McCune-Albright syndrome. *Orphanet J Rare Dis* (2008) 3:12. doi:10.1186/1750-1172-3-12
2. Fragoso MC, Domenice S, Latronico AC, Martin RM, Pereira MA, Zerbini MC, et al. Cushing's syndrome secondary to adrenocorticotropin-independent macronodular adrenocortical hyperplasia due to activating mutations of GNAS1 gene. *J Clin Endocrinol Metab* (2003) 88(5):2147–51. doi:10.1210/jc.2002-021362
3. Yoshimoto K, Iwahana H, Fukuda A, Sano T, Itakura M. Rare mutations of the Gs alpha subunit gene in human endocrine tumors. Mutation detection by polymerase chain reaction-primer-introduced restriction analysis. *Cancer* (1993) 72(4):1386–93. doi:10.1002/1097-0142(19930815)72:4<1386::AID-CNCR2820720439>3.0.CO;2-J
4. Hsiao HP, Kirschner LS, Bourdeau I, Keil MF, Boikos SA, Verma S, et al. Clinical and genetic heterogeneity, overlap with other tumor syndromes, and atypical glucocorticoid hormone secretion in adrenocorticotropin-independent macronodular adrenal hyperplasia compared with other adrenocortical tumors. *J Clin Endocrinol Metab* (2009) 94(8):2930–7. doi:10.1210/jc.2009-0516
5. Hamm HE. The many faces of G protein signaling. *J Biol Chem* (1998) 273(2):669–72. doi:10.1074/jbc.273.2.669
6. Weinstein LS, Liu J, Sakamoto A, Xie T, Chen M. Minireview: GNAS: normal and abnormal functions. *Endocrinology* (2004) 145(12):5459–64. doi:10.1210/en.2004-0865
7. Antonini SR, Fragoso MC, Lacroix A. [Clinical and molecular aspects of the ACTH-independent bilateral macronodular adrenal hyperplasia]. *Arq Bras Endocrinol Metabol* (2004) 48(5):620–36. doi:10.1590/S0004-27302004000500006
8. Brown RJ, Kelly MH, Collins MT. Cushing syndrome in the McCune-Albright syndrome. *J Clin Endocrinol Metab* (2010) 95(4):1508–15. doi:10.1210/jc.2009-2321
9. Happle R. The McCune-Albright syndrome: a lethal gene surviving by mosaicism. *Clin Genet* (1986) 29(4):321–4. doi:10.1111/j.1399-0004.1986.tb01261.x
10. Landis CA, Masters SB, Spada A, Pace AM, Bourne HR, Vallar L. GTPase inhibiting mutations activate the alpha chain of Gs and stimulate adenylyl cyclase in human pituitary tumours. *Nature* (1989) 340(6236):692–6. doi:10.1038/340692a0
11. Lacroix A, Bourdeau I, Lampron A, Mazzuco TL, Tremblay J, Hamet P. Aberrant G-protein coupled receptor expression in relation to adrenocortical overfunction. *Clin Endocrinol* (2010) 73(1):1–15. doi:10.1111/j.1365-2265.2009.03689.x
12. de Joussineau C, Sahut-Barnola I, Levy I, Saloustros E, Val P, Stratakis CA, et al. The cAMP pathway and the control of adrenocortical development and growth. *Mol Cell Endocrinol* (2012) 351(1):28–36. doi:10.1016/j.mce.2011.10.006
13. Almeida MQ, Azevedo MF, Xekouki P, Bimpaki EI, Horvath A, Collins MT, et al. Activation of cyclic AMP signaling leads to different pathway alterations in lesions of the adrenal cortex caused by germline PRKAR1A defects versus those due to somatic GNAS mutations. *J Clin Endocrinol Metab* (2012) 97(4):E687–93. doi:10.1210/jc.2011-3000
14. Bimpaki EI, Nesterova M, Stratakis CA. Abnormalities of cAMP signaling are present in adrenocortical lesions associated with ACTH-independent Cushing syndrome despite the absence of mutations in known genes. *Eur J Endocrinol* (2009) 161(1):153–61. doi:10.1530/EJE-09-0027
15. Almeida MQ, Stratakis CA. How does cAMP/protein kinase A signaling lead to tumors in the adrenal cortex and other tissues? *Mol Cell Endocrinol* (2011) 336(1–2):162–8. doi:10.1016/j.mce.2010.11.018
16. Bertherat J, Groussin L, Sandrini F, Matyakhina L, Bei T, Stergiopoulos S, et al. Molecular and functional analysis of PRKAR1A and its locus (17q22-24) in sporadic adrenocortical tumors: 17q losses, somatic mutations, and protein kinase A expression and activity. *Cancer Res* (2003) 63(17):5308–19.
17. Lefebvre H, Duparc C, Prévost G, Bertherat J, Louiset E. Cell-to-cell communication in bilateral macronodular adrenal hyperplasia causing hypercortisolism. *Front Endocrinol* (2015) 6:34. doi:10.3389/fendo.2015.00034
18. Bourdeau I, Matyakhina L, Stergiopoulos SG, Sandrini F, Boikos S, Stratakis CA. 17q22-24 chromosomal losses and alterations of protein kinase a subunit expression and activity in adrenocorticotropin-independent macronodular adrenal hyperplasia. *J Clin Endocrinol Metab* (2006) 91(9):3626–32. doi:10.1210/jc.2005-2608
19. Assie G, Louiset E, Sturm N, René-Corail F, Groussin L, Bertherat J, et al. Systematic analysis of G protein-coupled receptor gene expression in adrenocorticotropin-independent macronodular adrenocortical hyperplasia identifies novel targets for pharmacological control of adrenal Cushing's syndrome. *J Clin Endocrinol Metab* (2010) 95(10):E253–62. doi:10.1210/jc.2009-2281
20. Lacroix A, Tremblay J, Rousseau G, Bouvier M, Hamet P. Propranolol therapy for ectopic beta-adrenergic receptors in adrenal Cushing's syndrome. *N Engl J Med* (1997) 337(20):1429–34. doi:10.1056/NEJM199711133372004
21. Levine MA, Jap TS, Mauseth RS, Downs RW, Spiegel AM. Activity of the stimulatory guanine nucleotide-binding protein is reduced in erythrocytes from patients with pseudohypoparathyroidism and pseudopseudohypoparathyroidism: biochemical, endocrine, and genetic analysis of Albright's hereditary osteodystrophy in six kindreds. *J Clin Endocrinol Metab* (1986) 62(3):497–502.
22. Almeida MQ, Kaupert LC, Brito LP, Lerario AM, Mariani BM, Ribeiro M, et al. Increased expression of ACTH (MC2R) and androgen (AR) receptors in giant bilateral myelolipomas from patients with congenital adrenal hyperplasia. *BMC Endocr Disord* (2014) 14:42. doi:10.1186/1472-6823-14-42
23. Swords FM, Noon LA, King PJ, Clark AJ. Constitutive activation of the human ACTH receptor resulting from a synergistic interaction between two naturally occurring missense mutations in the MC2R gene. *Mol Cell Endocrinol* (2004) 213(2):149–54. doi:10.1016/j.mce.2003.10.052
24. Horvath A, Boikos S, Giatzakis C, Robinson-White A, Groussin L, Griffin KJ, et al. A genome-wide scan identifies mutations in the gene encoding phosphodiesterase 11A4 (PDE11A) in individuals with adrenocortical hyperplasia. *Nat Genet* (2006) 38(7):794–800. doi:10.1038/ng1809
25. Horvath A, Mericq V, Stratakis CA. Mutation in PDE8B, a cyclic AMP-specific phosphodiesterase in adrenal hyperplasia. *N Engl J Med* (2008) 358(7):750–2. doi:10.1056/NEJMc0706182
26. Calebiro D, Hannawacker A, Lyga S, Bathon K, Zabel U, Ronchi C, et al. PKA catalytic subunit mutations in adrenocortical Cushing's adenoma impair association with the regulatory subunit. *Nat Commun* (2014) 5:5680. doi:10.1038/ncomms6680
27. Beuschlein F, Fassnacht M, Assié G, Calebiro D, Stratakis CA, Osswald A, et al. Constitutive activation of PKA catalytic subunit in adrenal Cushing's syndrome. *N Engl J Med* (2014) 370(11):1019–28. doi:10.1056/NEJMoa1310359
28. Assié G, Libé R, Espiard S, Rizk-Rabin M, Guimier A, Luscap W, et al. ARMC5 mutations in macronodular adrenal hyperplasia with Cushing's syndrome. *N Engl J Med* (2013) 369(22):2105–14. doi:10.1056/NEJMoa1304603
29. Alencar GA, Lerario AM, Nishi MY, Mariani BM, Almeida MQ, Tremblay J, et al. ARMC5 mutations are a frequent cause of primary macronodular adrenal Hyperplasia. *J Clin Endocrinol Metab* (2014) 99(8):E1501–9. doi:10.1210/jc.2013-4237
30. Durand J, Lampron A, Mazzuco TL, Chapman A, Bourdeau I. Characterization of differential gene expression in adrenocortical tumors harboring beta-catenin (CTNNB1) mutations. *J Clin Endocrinol Metab* (2011) 96(7):E1206–11. doi:10.1210/jc.2010-2143
31. Lyons J, Landis CA, Harsh G, Vallar L, Grünewald K, Feichtinger H, et al. Two G protein oncogenes in human endocrine tumors. *Science* (1990) 249(4969):655–9. doi:10.1126/science.2116665
32. Bugalho MJ, Li X, Rao CV, Soares J, Sobrinho LG. Presence of a Gs alpha mutation in an adrenal tumor expressing LH/hCG receptors and clinically associated with Cushing's syndrome. *Gynecol Endocrinol* (2000) 14(1):50–4. doi:10.3109/09513590009167660
33. Dall'Asta C, Ballarè E, Mantovani G, Ambrosi B, Spada A, Barbetta L, et al. Assessing the presence of abnormal regulation of cortisol secretion by membrane hormone receptors: in vivo and in vitro studies in patients with functioning and non-functioning adrenal adenoma. *Horm Metab Res* (2004) 36(8):578–83. doi:10.1055/s-2004-825797
34. Libé R, Bertherat J. Molecular genetics of adrenocortical tumours, from familial to sporadic diseases. *Eur J Endocrinol* (2005) 153(4):477–87. doi:10.1530/eje.1.02004
35. Sidhu A, Debelenko L, Misra VK. Infantile adrenocortical tumor with an activating GNAS1 mutation. *J Clin Endocrinol Metab* (2013) 98(1):E115–8. doi:10.1210/jc.2012-2933

36. Libé R, Mantovani G, Bondioni S, Lania AG, Pedroni C, Beck-Peccoz P, et al. Mutational analysis of PRKAR1A and Gs(alpha) in sporadic adrenocortical tumors. *Exp Clin Endocrinol Diabetes* (2005) 113(5):248–51. doi:10.1055/s-2005-837651
37. Christopoulos S, Bourdeau I, Lacroix A. Clinical and subclinical ACTH-independent macronodular adrenal hyperplasia and aberrant hormone receptors. *Horm Res* (2005) 64(3):119–31. doi:10.1159/000088818
38. Lania AG, Mantovani G, Spada A. Mechanisms of disease: mutations of G proteins and G-protein-coupled receptors in endocrine diseases. *Nat Clin Pract Endocrinol Metab* (2006) 2(12):681–93. doi:10.1038/ncpendmet0324
39. Meoli E, Bossis I, Cazabat L, Mavrakis M, Horvath A, Stergiopoulos S, et al. Protein kinase A effects of an expressed PRKAR1A mutation associated with aggressive tumors. *Cancer Res* (2008) 68(9):3133–41. doi:10.1158/0008-5472.CAN-08-0064
40. Boston BA, Mandel S, LaFranchi S, Bliziotes M. Activating mutation in the stimulatory guanine nucleotide-binding protein in an infant with Cushing's syndrome and nodular adrenal hyperplasia. *J Clin Endocrinol Metab* (1994) 79(3):890–3. doi:10.1210/jcem.79.3.8077378
41. Fragoso MC, Alencar GA, Lerario AM, Bourdeau I, Almeida MQ, Mendonca BB, et al. Genetics of primary macronodular adrenal hyperplasia. *J Endocrinol* (2015) 224(1):R31–43. doi:10.1530/JOE-14-0568

22

New Directions for the Treatment of Adrenal Insufficiency

Gerard Ruiz-Babot, Irene Hadjidemetriou, Peter James King and Leonardo Guasti *

Centre for Endocrinology, William Harvey Research Institute, Barts and the London School of Medicine and Dentistry, Queen Mary University of London, London, UK

***Correspondence:**
*Leonardo Guasti, Centre for Endocrinology, William Harvey Research Institute, Barts and the London School of Medicine and Dentistry, Queen Mary University of London, Charterhouse Square, London EC1M 6BQ, UK
l.guasti@qmul.ac.uk*

Adrenal disease, whether primary, caused by defects in the hypothalamic–pituitary–adrenal (HPA) axis, or secondary, caused by defects outside the HPA axis, usually results in adrenal insufficiency, which requires lifelong daily replacement of corticosteroids. However, this kind of therapy is far from ideal as physiological demand for steroids varies considerably throughout the day and increases during periods of stress. The development of alternative curative strategies is therefore needed. In this review, we describe the latest technologies aimed at either isolating or generating *de novo* cells that could be used for novel, regenerative medicine application in the adrenocortical field.

Keywords: regeneration, adrenal cortex, stem cells, transplantation, encapsulation, steroidogenesis, zonation, SF1

The adrenal cortex is the primary site of steroid synthesis, producing glucocorticoids under the control of the hypothalamic–pituitary–adrenal (HPA) axis and mineralocorticoids under the control of the renin–angiotensin system. Glucocorticoids affect carbohydrate metabolism and mediate the mammalian stress response, while mineralocorticoids control blood volume and salt homeostasis. For this reason, the adrenal cortex is essential for life.

The adrenal cortex originates in a group of mesoderm-derived cells lying between the urogenital ridge and the dorsal aorta, forming the precursors of the adrenal glands and the gonads, the adrenogonadal primordium (AGP) (1). At around embryonic day (e)9.0 in the mouse, these cells begin to express the transcription factor steroidogenic factor 1 (SF1), which is essential for both adrenal and gonadal development (2). SF1 not only binds to response elements in the promoter regions of steroidogenic genes to positively regulate their transcription but can also be considered a true effector of cell fate as it starts a genetic program driving embryonic mesenchymal cells toward a steroidogenic phenotype/lineage (3, 4); its absolute requirement for steroidogenesis has been recently demonstrated *in vivo* (5). Other than SF1, at least four additional transcription factors have been shown to be key determinants of adrenal cortex development: Wilms tumor 1 (WT1), a zinc finger protein, and CBP/p300-interacting transactivator 2 (CITED2), which are both expressed at early stages in the urogenital ridge and synergistically promote adrenal development through induction of SF1 transcription (6, 7); pre-B-cell leukemia transcription factor 1 (PBX1), a homeodomain protein, which has been proposed to facilitate the access of important developmental factors (such as SF1) to chromatin to induce differentiation (8, 9); dosage-sensitive sex reversal, adrenal hypoplasia critical region, on chromosome X, gene 1 (DAX1) (10), whose mutations are associated with a variety of developmentally relevant conditions in the adrenal and gonads (11), such as adrenal hypoplasia congenita. Moreover, multiple pathways have been implicated in the fine-tuned regulation of adrenal cortex development and function [reviewed in Ref. (12–15)]. The contribution of each of these signaling pathways has been studied by employing either *in vitro* systems or animal models, such as genetic lineage tracing (16, 17). Not surprisingly, the alteration of some of these pathways, such as the WNT pathway, results in adrenal cancer [reviewed in Ref. (18)].

The adult gland is divided into at least three distinct zones arranged concentrically around the medulla; the zona glomerulosa (ZG, which synthesizes mineralocorticoids), which lies just underneath the capsule, the zona fasciculata (ZF, which synthesizes glucocorticoids), and then the zona reticularis (which synthesizes adrenal androgens in humans and primates). Zonation occurs around birth [for review, see Ref. (12)].

Primary adrenal insufficiency is due to a number of adrenal disorders, and management of these patients can be challenging (19). Current treatments entail lifelong replacement with exogenous steroids. None suitably mimic the diurnal pattern of cortisol noted in healthy individuals, and objective variables to measure quality of replacement are lacking. Fine-tuning of replacement leaves only a narrow margin for improvement. Under-replacement can result in severe impairment of well-being and incipient crisis. Conversely, chronic over-replacement can lead to substantial morbidity including obesity, osteoporosis, and impaired glucose tolerance. Furthermore, despite attention to detail with regards to replacement regimens, overall standardized mortality ratio for patients with adrenal failure is ~2.1.

Transplantation of Adrenal Glands and Cells

Adrenal autotransplantation in humans is poorly characterized. A few surgeons tested the potential benefits of adrenal autotransplantation in patients with Cushing's disease since the early 1960s. At that time, replacement therapy with synthetic steroids was becoming the gold standard for patients with Cushing's disease but they hypothesized that autotransplantation would be an effective alternative to lifelong therapy (20–26). Adrenals were mainly transplanted in the thigh, because it is an easily accessible site should the transplant become not viable and need removal. The degree of autotransplant survival was, however, questionable, at least in those cases where follow-up is available (27). More recently, a successful mother-to-daughter allograft has been reported in a pediatric patient who developed adrenal insufficiency following fulminant meningococcemia (28). Allotransplantations of whole adrenal–kidney or adrenal–kidney–pancreas have also been described in clinical reports (29, 30); however, these multiple organ transplants are only feasible and/or recommended when the recipients have severe co-morbidities.

The refinement of allotransplantation and xenotransplantation has been the focus of more recent research, where a variety of animal models have been employed. Hornsby and colleagues performed initial work, demonstrating that transplantation of human adrenocortical cells into adrenalectomized severe combined immunodeficiency (scid) mice could be an effective technique for the treatment of adrenal insufficiency (31). They also developed a model, in which they showed that co-transplantation in a polycarbonate cylinder of clonal or primary bovine adrenocortical cells with 3T3 fibroblasts into scid mice could rescue them from developing adrenal insufficiency (32, 33). 3T3 cells were either treated with mitomycin C or lethally irradiated (to prevent proliferation upon implantation) and were overexpressing FGF1 (to aid vascularization).

Through their work, they also showed that transplanted adrenocortical cells (of either human or bovine origin) could survive and form a functional, vascularized tissue that was able to replace the host animal's organ. The newly formed tissue was able to produce and secrete the necessary amounts of cortisol, albeit aldosterone was only produced by primary bovine adrenocortical cells, but not from clonal cells (32). One possible reason for this might be that bovine adrenocortical cells preparations, albeit derived from the ZF, could contain some ZG cells or that some ZF cells could transdifferentiate to a ZG phenotype. It was later shown, however, that ZF cells are incapable of giving rise to ZG cells (34). In the same study, Teebken and Scheumann showed that transplanting ZG cells can give rise to both ZG and ZF, thus making ZG cells more suitable for transplantation (34). This is presumable because the harvest of ZG cells might result in the inclusion of progenitor cells with bi-potency, given their location in the subcapsular region close to fully mature ZG cells in mouse (16, 35) and rat (36, 37). More recently, using mouse cell fate mapping and gene-deletion tools, Freedman and colleagues demonstrated that ZF cells indeed derive from fully differentiated ZG cells through lineage conversion (38). Similar results were observed during adrenal autotransplantation in the spleen of adrenalectomized rats (39).

Furthermore, genetic modifications such as immortalization of bovine primary adrenocortical cultures with telomerase reverse transcriptase (hTERT) have been shown to be very effective in xenotransplantation procedures. This technique aids the expansion of adrenocortical cells *in vitro* leading to improved efficacy (40, 41). Although hTERT is known to be a key-tumorigenic factor, when expressed on its own it did not alter the properties of the donor's adrenocortical cell (42).

Possible Platforms for Cell Transplantation

Other groups looked into harnessing the properties of the adrenal cortex extracellular matrix (ECM). It is well established that the ECM plays a significant role in organ growth and development, as well as function, by providing structural support and by regulating cell signaling and cell-to-cell interactions (43). The ECM of the adrenal cortex is quite complex, mainly composed of collagen IV, fibronectin, and laminin and it was postulated that different ECM components might affect the biological activity of cortical cells (44). In fact, primary cultures of human fetal adrenal cells seeded on collagen IV or laminin were found to be more proliferative, as opposed to fibronectin, which enhanced cell apoptosis. In addition, collagen increased cell sensitivity to ACTH, whereas fibronectin and laminin had the opposite effect (45).

Further work to assess the function of implanted cells seeded on a collagen matrix, using a mouse model with adrenal insufficiency, determined that treatment involving staged bilateral adrenalectomy of the animals and implantation of collagen sponges each time was the most beneficial. This protocol lead to a 100% survival rate (up from 42% in mice with only one implant and 0% in animal receiving the graft without cells) and reversal of adrenal insufficiency, supported by restoration of corticosterone levels and the expression of adrenal markers by the transplanted cells (46).

Some researchers focused on the use of the native organ's own decellularized ECM to act as a scaffold in transplantation procedures to regenerate various organs, including the heart, liver, and lungs (47). *In vitro* studies, using porcine decellularized adrenal ECM as a scaffold for human fetal adrenal cells, resulted in successful cell attachment and a good cell function, the latter assessed by cell proliferation and cortisol secretion (48). Therefore, decellularized adrenal ECM could represent an improved scaffold for transplanted cells, providing a native three-dimensional structure that would support growth and incorporation of transplanted cells into the native environment to form a fully functional adrenal tissue.

Stem Cells and Reprograming Strategies

An ever-increasing number of translational scientists are striving to take advantage of the remarkable properties of stem cells that are not only offering an unparalleled opportunity to study human biology and disease processes *in vitro* but also to translate basic scientific discoveries to therapeutic applications. The development of cell therapy has, however, been overlooked to date in field of endocrinology, with the exception of the worldwide effort to generate functional pancreatic beta cells to cure type-I diabetes. Indeed, the Californian company Viacyte has been granted FDA approval to launch the first clinical evaluation of a stem-cell-derived islet replacement therapy for the treatment of patients with type-I diabetes in 2015 (http://viacyte.com/clinical/clinical-trials/). Other clinical trials are in the pipeline, a culmination of decades of intense *in vitro* and animal studies carried out by dozens of laboratories (49). Despite the fact that the morbidity of diabetes vs. adrenal insufficiency is clearly not comparable, conceivably the search for alternative treatments for adrenal insufficiency has been neglected, except for a few important discoveries (see below).

Cellular reprograming describes the process where a fully differentiated, specialized cell type is induced to transform into a different cell type that it would not otherwise become under normal physiological conditions. Sir John Gurdon of Britain and Shinya Yamanaka of Japan were awarded the Nobel Prize in 2012 for their groundbreaking discoveries in the field. Gurdon's research showed that it was possible to reverse the specialization of cells. By transferring a nucleus from a frog's intestinal cell into a frog's egg cell that had its nucleus removed, he was able to obtain a tadpole. Building on Gurdon's work, Yamanaka published a paper in 2006 demonstrating that mature murine cells can become immature stem cells (called inducible pluripotent stem cells, IPSCs) by expressing genes encoding four transcription factors (50). IPSCs can then be differentiated to several tissues using specific cocktails of growth factors/cytokines/chemical compounds. Yamanaka's breakthrough opened the door to studying tissue-specific diseases and developing diagnosis and treatments. Reprograming is not only achieved through the generation of IPSCs but also through direct reprograming (also known as lineage conversion). Lineage conversion, which is usually achieved by forced expression of lineage-determining factors, is a recently developed and attractive alternative to obtain cells of a given lineage [reviewed in Ref. (51, 52)]. Lineage conversion into several clinically relevant cell types might also prove to be a safer alternative to IPSCs; in fact, genetic (copy number variation, chromosome duplication) and epigenetic variations, which have been described in IPSCs lines and that have raised a number of questions regarding the functional relevance as well as patient safety in potential translational applications, are uncommon during lineage conversion (51).

In recent years, several studies have shown the possibility of obtaining cells with steroidogenic properties resembling adrenocortical cells from murine and human cell sources (**Table 1**). Pioneering studies in mouse embryonic stem cells (ESCs) showed that the ectopically stable expression of SF1 in the presence of cAMP resulted in a dramatic change of cell morphology and subsequent upregulation of *Cyp11a1* together with an induction of steroidogenesis. However, these cells were incapable of producing different steroid hormones *de novo*, since only progesterone was detected after treatment with 20α-hydroxycholesterol, a freely diffusible form of cholesterol (53).

TABLE 1 | Details of published studies on adrenocortical or adrenogonwadal reprograming.

PMID	Article	Cells	Origin	Methodology
9199334	Crawford PA, et al. *Mol Cell Biol* (1997)	Embryonic stem cells (ESC)	Mouse (RW4 129/SvJ)	Stable transfection of SF1
15569155	Gondo S, et al. *Genes Cells* (2004)	Bone marrow stem cells (BMCs)	Mouse [C57BL/6Tg14 (act-EGFP)osbY01]	Adenovirus SF1
16728492	Yazawa T, et al. *Endocrinology* (2006)	Bone marrow stem cells (BMCs)	Human (hMSChTERT-E6/E7)	Stable transfection of SF1
17975261	Tanaka T, et al. *J Mol Endocrinol* (2007)	Bone marrow stem cells (BMCs)	Human (commercial cell line)	Adenovirus SF1
18566117	Gondo S, et al. *Endocrinology* (2008)	Adipose mesenchymal cells (AMCs)	Mouse (C57BL/6J) (B6)	Adenovirus SF1
19359379	Yazawa T, et al. *Endocrinology* (2009)	Bone marrow stem cells (BMCs)	Human (hMSChTERT-E6/E7)	Retrovirus SF1/LRH-1
20133449	Yazawa T, et al. *Mol Endocrinol* (2010)	Umbilical cord blood (UCB-MSCs)	Human (umbilical cord blood)	Retrovirus SF1
21129436	Yazawa T, et al. *Mol Cell Endocrinol* (2011)	Embryonic stem cells (ESC)	Mouse (EBRTcH3)	Retrovirus (inducible SF1)
21610156	Jadhav U, et al. *Endocrinology* (2011)	Embryonic stem cells (ESC)	Mouse (R1 ES cell line)	Stable transfection of SF1
21764617	Mazilu JK, et al. *Mol Genet Metab* (2011)	Mesoderm-derived cells	Human	Adenoviral SF1/Dax1/Cited2/ Pbx1/WT1
22324479	Wei X, et al. *Cell Prolif* (2012)	Umbilical cord mesenchymal stem cells (UC-MSCs)	Human (umbilical cord)	Adenovirus SF1
22778223	Sonoyama T, et al. *Endocrinology* (2012)	Embryonic Stem cell (ESC) iPS (from fibroblasts)	Human (H9 and KhES1) human (201B7)	Mesoderm diff. and nucleofection SF1

In 2004, Gondo and colleagues described the capacity of long-term cultured mouse bone marrow cells (BMCs) to differentiate into a steroidogenic lineage using adenoviral-mediated SF1 overexpression (54). In this study, the authors were able to detect several steroidogenic enzymes and quantify the levels of all steroid hormones except aldosterone; further study showed that the cells failed to express *Cyp11b2*. Interestingly, reprogramed cells were responsive to ACTH, resulting in enhanced steroidogenic enzyme upregulation and hormone production. Despite the improvement in the steroidogenic profiling compared with the previous study, these cells showed a mixed pattern of adrenal and gonadal phenotypes. Moreover, only supraphysiological concentrations of ACTH were able to significantly induce progesterone and deoxycortisone secretion. It also raises the question of the function of MC2R in BMCs physiology, as the authors found the receptor to be expressed in non-reprogramed cells.

The same group later obtained steroidogenic cells from mouse adipose tissue-derived mesenchymal cells (AMCs), using a similar strategy (55). Remarkably, when the steroidogenic gene expression profile and hormone production of AMCs and BMCs were compared, AMCs showed an enhanced cortisol/testosterone ratio compared with BMCs. This enrichment of the adrenocortical vs. gonadal phenotype was further potentiated by treatment with all-trans retinoic acid (ATRA), suggesting that the tissue/cell source and the culture conditions are essential to determine the resultant phenotype during reprograming.

The first studies describing the generation of steroidogenic cells from human origin were from Miyamoto's research group. In this work, human mesenchymal stem cells (hMSCs) stably expressing SF1 (as well as hTERT, E6, and E7) were able to upregulate steroidogenic enzymes and produce both adrenal and gonadal steroids after treatment with cAMP. Immunohistochemical analysis of rat GFP$^+$ BMCs injected into rat testes showed upregulation of steroidogenic enzymes in the engrafted cells (56). Taken together, these studies demonstrated that MSCs have the ability to differentiate into steroidogenic cells both *in vivo* and *in vitro*.

Since then, several groups have succeeded in differentiating human cells to a steroidogenic phenotype. Tanaka et al. efficiently reprogramed human BMCs upon overexpression of SF1 with adenovirus (57) and more recently this was achieved by retroviral overexpression of LRH-1 [like SF1, a member of the NR5A nuclear receptor family (58)]. However, it is likely that LRH-1 has a more prominent role in gonadal steroidogenesis *in vivo*, since LRH-1 is barely detectable in the adrenal cortex but highly expressed in the gonads, while SF1 is abundantly expressed in both adrenals and gonads (59, 60), and actually at higher levels in cells of the AGP destined to form the adrenal cortex (7).

Human steroidogenic-like cells were also successfully reprogramed from umbilical cord blood mesenchymal stem cells (UCB-MSCs) (61) and umbilical cord Wharton's jelly-derived MSC (UC-MSCs) (62) through retroviral or adenoviral overexpression of SF1. In the latter study, the authors compared UC-MSCs with BM-MSCs and concluded that UCS-MSCs are the better cell sources since, after reprograming, these cells had a higher proliferative potential, expressed higher levels of steroidogenic enzymes, secreted more steroid hormones, and had a significantly higher cell viability.

Recently, several groups have changed their focus onto ESCs, as the first attempts to reprogram these cells were only partially successful (53). Yazawa et al. reported that to efficiently reprogram mouse ESCs (mESCs) to a steroidogenic phenotype, an initial differentiation to a mesenchymal lineage is needed (63). Once differentiation was achieved (using pulse exposures to ATRA and plating cells into collagen IV-coated dishes), cells became steroidogenic upon overexpression of SF1, resulting in an upregulation of steroidogenic enzymes as well as steroid hormone production. Interestingly, the gene expression profile of these cells was similar to that of the zona fasciculata. Alternatively, Jadhav and Jameson provided evidence that steroidogenic cells can be produced from mESCs using different protocols, the most efficient involving the withdrawal of leukemia inhibitory factor from the ESC medium followed by treatment with cAMP. Using this protocol, steroid-producing reprogramed ESCs appear to acquire a gonadal-like cell type lineage (64). Again, these works highlight the importance of the reprograming strategy/protocol to obtain a specific adrenal/gonadal-like cell type.

Sonoyama et al. demonstrated the capacity of human ES cells (hESCs) to become steroidogenic (65). Using a similar approach as previously reported (63, 64), after differentiation of hESCs to a mesodermal lineage (in this case using a GSK3β inhibitor) and upon overexpression of SF1 and cAMP treatment, hESCs showed overexpression of steroidogenic enzymes as well as hormone production. The authors also obtained the first steroidogenic cells reprogramed from an IPSC line (201B7, obtained from human fibroblasts).

Despite none of the strategies described above have been tested in *in vivo* models of adrenal insufficiency (i.e., adrenalectomized animals), they provide strong evidence that cells can be reprogramed to a steroidogenic phenotype through overexpression of SF1 and cAMP treatment. The choice of the most appropriate source of cells as substrates for reprograming is still debated and might differ depending on downstream applications. Differences in species, cell/tissue source, cellular development stage, epigenetic landscape, SF1/transcription factors dosage (66), regulatory feedbacks of activators/repressors, culture conditions, and timings of reprograming might affect the final phenotype of the reprogramed cells. In this regard, one cannot rule out the possibility that in order to generate fully functional adrenocortical cells, other transcriptions factors might be needed. Factors, such as Dax1, Pbx1, Cited2, WT1, or WNT4, known to be associated with adrenal and gonadal development have been used in reprograming strategies with minor effects on steroidogenic outcome (57, 58, 67). However, given the importance of dosage and regulatory feedback between these key transcription factors, reprograming strategies using a combination of them at specific dosages might be indispensible to obtain cells with a steroidogenic pattern resembling the one found *in vivo*.

There are still several hurdles to overcome to efficiently reprogram human cells to be used for personalized cell-based therapies in patients with adrenal insufficiency in clinics: (1) the conditions to obtain cells with restricted adrenocortical-specific gene expression and hormone production are far from optimized (see above). (2) In most of the protocols, upon overexpression of SF1, cells terminally differentiate with a consequent growth arrest. This makes it difficult to prepare the large amount of cells needed for cell therapy. The use of inducible vectors should allow the expression of SF1 (and/or other factors) at a desired culture time-point when there are enough cells for clinical purposes. (3) The methodologies used until now are all based on the overexpression of SF1 exogenously, either episomally or virally. Optimization of the culture conditions in a gene delivery-free model of reprograming might help to avoid the

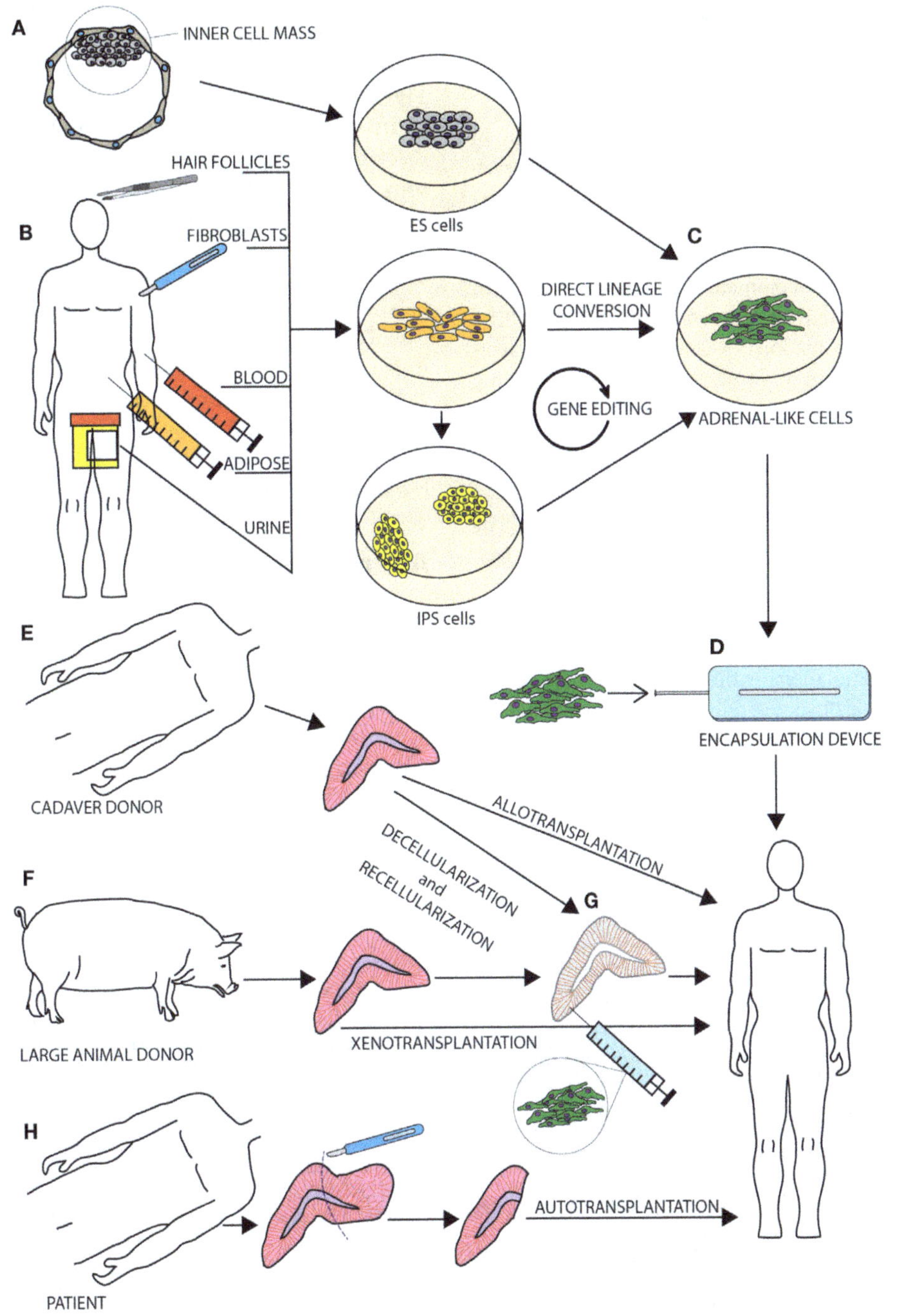

FIGURE 1 | This figure outlines novel and tested strategies for the treatment of adrenal insufficiency. Human embryonic stem (ES) cells **(A)** as well as somatic cells (such as fibroblasts, hair follicle dermal papillae, adipose tissue-derived stem cells, and urine-derived stem cells) established from human donors **(B)** can be cultured *in vitro* and induced to acquire an adrenocortical phenotype **(C)** through specific differentiation protocols. A gene-editing step can be included in case of monogenic disorders. Reprogramed cells that have successfully acquired an adrenocortical phenotype could then be implanted back into a donor, either inside an encapsulation device **(D)** or inside a decellularized adrenal of human or large-animal origin **(G)**. While autotransplantation **(H)** has been trailed in humans in pioneering surgery during the 1960s (see text) and allotransplantation **(E)** has been a poorly tested option, xenotransplantation **(F)** has never been tested in humans.

safety concerns about these cells. The use of excisable vectors together with the new CRISPR-dCasVP64 technology to activate specific transgenes without the use of transcription factors (68) might reduce the safety concerns of this method of obtaining reprogramed steroidogenic cells *in vitro*.

Recent Breakthroughs in Overcoming Rejection and the Treatment of Monogenic Diseases

A major factor limiting the application of stem-cell therapy in patients transplanted with ECs-derived adrenocortical cells or even autologous IPSCs-derived adrenocortical cells (i.e., in those individuals affected by autoimmune Addison's) is the recipient's need to adhere to lifelong immunosuppression. An effort going back a couple of decades in the field of biomaterials is providing us with the technology, which can make an impact in the clinical setting today; in fact, several encapsulation devices (endowed with excellent biocompatibility) have been developed and are undergoing clinical testing in patients with type-I diabetes. Animal studies (49) and published preliminary human studies (69) have demonstrated that the device's semipermeable membranes can tightly immune isolate transplanted cells while allowing diffusion of nutrients, such as glucose. Therefore, encapsulating adrenocortical cells is a strategy that should prevent rejection of the grafted tissue, whichever the source of it.

In recent times, a fast-paced development of gene-editing technologies using different approaches has made it possible to correct known disease-causing mutations without leaving any footprint (70). This technology could be successfully applicable to monogenic conditions causing adrenal insufficiency (such as congenital adrenal hyperplasia or familial glucocorticoid deficiency). For example, cultures of reprogrammable cell sources such as skin fibroblasts or urine-derived cells could be established and the mutated gene reverted to a wild-type status via gene editing; after successful reprograming to an adrenocortical phenotype (via IPSCs generation or via lineage conversion), cells could be reimplanted back into the donor, housed either inside an encapsulation device or a decellularized adrenal gland obtained from cadaver or large animal.

Potential future strategies, as well as pioneering past and present attempts to cure adrenal insufficiency are outlined in **Figure 1**.

In conclusion, while autotransplantation has long been discarded, allotransplantation is currently being considered only in specific clinical settings and xenotransplantation has not reached the bedside, stem-cell biology has granted great promise for tissue engineering and regenerative medicine. Treatments employing stem cells offer the potential to successfully treat patients with new modalities in the future, by essentially regenerating and replacing non-functional tissues or organs. A permanent collaborative and multidisciplinary effort carried out by translational scientists with expertise in stem cells, bioengineering, and material science is undeniably necessary to fully develop alternative treatments for adrenal insufficiency that have true clinical relevance.

Acknowledgments

The following funding bodies supported this work: Biotechnology and Biological Sciences Research Council (BBSRC BB/L00267/1, to LG), Rosetrees Trust (to LG), Barts and The London Charity (417/2235, to LG), EU COFUND (PCOFUND-GA-2013-608765, to LG and GRB). IH is supported by a Medical Research Council (MRC, G0802796) PhD studentship.

References

1. Hatano O, Takakusu A, Nomura M, Morohashi K. Identical origin of adrenal cortex and gonad revealed by expression profiles of Ad4BP/SF-1. *Genes Cells* (1996) **1**(7):663–71. doi:10.1046/j.1365-2443.1996.00254.x
2. Luo X, Ikeda Y, Parker KL. A cell-specific nuclear receptor is essential for adrenal and gonadal development and sexual differentiation. *Cell* (1994) **77**(4):481–90. doi:10.1016/0092-8674(94)90211-9
3. Schimmer BP, White PC. Minireview: steroidogenic factor 1: its roles in differentiation, development, and disease. *Mol Endocrinol* (2010) **24**(7):1322–37. doi:10.1210/me.2009-0519
4. Wong M, Ikeda Y, Luo X, Caron KM, Weber TJ, Swain A, et al. Steroidogenic factor 1 plays multiple roles in endocrine development and function. *Recent Prog Horm Res* (1997) **52**:167–82.
5. Buaas FW, Gardiner JR, Clayton S, Val P, Swain A. In vivo evidence for the crucial role of SF1 in steroid-producing cells of the testis, ovary and adrenal gland. *Development* (2012) **139**(24):4561–70. doi:10.1242/dev.087247
6. Wilhelm D, Englert C. The Wilms tumor suppressor WT1 regulates early gonad development by activation of Sf1. *Genes Dev* (2002) **16**(14):1839–51. doi:10.1101/gad.220102
7. Val P, Martinez-Barbera JP, Swain A. Adrenal development is initiated by Cited2 and Wt1 through modulation of Sf-1 dosage. *Development* (2007) **134**(12):2349–58. doi:10.1242/dev.004390
8. Schnabel CA, Selleri L, Cleary ML. Pbx1 is essential for adrenal development and urogenital differentiation. *Genesis* (2003) **37**(3):123–30. doi:10.1002/gene.10235
9. Berkes CA, Bergstrom DA, Penn BH, Seaver KJ, Knoepfler PS, Tapscott SJ. Pbx marks genes for activation by MyoD indicating a role for a homeodomain protein in establishing myogenic potential. *Mol Cell* (2004) **14**(4):465–77. doi:10.1016/S1097-2765(04)00260-6
10. Clipsham R, McCabe ER. DAX1 and its network partners: exploring complexity in development. *Mol Genet Metab* (2003) **80**(1–2):81–120. doi:10.1016/j.ymgme.2003.08.023
11. El-Khairi R, Martinez-Aguayo A, Ferraz-de-Souza B, Lin L, Achermann JC. Role of DAX-1 (NR0B1) and steroidogenic factor-1 (NR5A1) in human adrenal function. *Endocr Dev* (2011) **20**:38–46. doi:10.1159/000321213
12. Kim AC, Barlaskar FM, Heaton JH, Else T, Kelly VR, Krill KT, et al. In search of adrenocortical stem and progenitor cells. *Endocr Rev* (2009) **30**(3):241–63. doi:10.1210/er.2008-0039
13. Walczak EM, Hammer GD. Regulation of the adrenocortical stem cell niche: implications for disease. *Nat Rev Endocrinol* (2015) **11**(1):14–28. doi:10.1038/nrendo.2014.166
14. Laufer E, Kesper D, Vortkamp A, King P. Sonic hedgehog signaling during adrenal development. *Mol Cell Endocrinol* (2012) **351**(1):19–27. doi:10.1016/j.mce.2011.10.002
15. Gallo-Payet N, Battista MC. Steroidogenesis-adrenal cell signal transduction. *Compr Physiol* (2014) **4**(3):889–964. doi:10.1002/cphy.c130050
16. King P, Paul A, Laufer E. Shh signaling regulates adrenocortical development and identifies progenitors of steroidogenic lineages. *Proc Natl Acad Sci U S A* (2009) **106**(50):21185–90. doi:10.1073/pnas.0909471106
17. Walczak EM, Kuick R, Finco I, Bohin N, Hrycaj SM, Wellik DM, et al. Wnt signaling inhibits adrenal steroidogenesis by cell-autonomous and non-cell-autonomous mechanisms. *Mol Endocrinol* (2014) **28**(9):1471–86. doi:10.1210/me.2014-1060
18. Else T, Kim AC, Sabolch A, Raymond VM, Kandathil A, Caoili EM, et al. Adrenocortical carcinoma. *Endocr Rev* (2014) **35**(2):282–326. doi:10.1210/er.2013-1029

19. Bancos I, Hahner S, Tomlinson J, Arlt W. Diagnosis and management of adrenal insufficiency. *Lancet Diabetes Endocrinol* (2015) **3**(3):216–26. doi:10.1016/S2213-8587(14)70142-1
20. Hardy JD. Surgical management of Cushing's syndrome with emphasis on adrenal autotransplantation. *Ann Surg* (1978) **188**(3):290–307. doi:10.1097/00000658-197809000-00004
21. Hardy JD. Autotransplantation of adrenal remnant to high in Cushing's disease. Preserving residual cortical activity while avoiding laparotomy. *JAMA* (1963) **185**:134–6. doi:10.1001/jama.1963.03060020094036
22. Hardy JD, Langford HG. Adrenal autotransplantation in Cushing's disease. *Ann N Y Acad Sci* (1964) **120**:667–8. doi:10.1111/j.1749-6632.1965.tb30692.x
23. Ibbertson HK, O'Brien KP. Adrenal autografts in treatment of Cushing's disease. *Br Med J* (1962) **2**(5306):703–6. doi:10.1136/bmj.2.5306.703
24. Franksson C, Birke G, Plantin LO. Adrenal autotransplantation in Cushing's syndrome. *Acta Chir Scand* (1959) **117**:409–15.
25. Birke G, Franksson C, Moberger G, Plantin LO. Storage and autotransplantation of human adrenal tissue. *Acta Chir Scand* (1956) **111**(2):113–23.
26. Drucker WD, Localio SA, Becker MH, Bergman B. Autotransplantation of hyperplastic human adrenal tissue. *Arch Intern Med* (1967) **120**(2):185–92. doi:10.1001/archinte.1967.00300020057007
27. Hardy JD, Moore DO, Langford HG. Cushing's disease today. Late follow-up of 17 adrenalectomy patients with emphasis on eight with adrenal autotransplants. *Ann Surg* (1985) **201**(5):595–603. doi:10.1097/00000658-198505000-00008
28. Grodstein E, Hardy MA, Goldstein MJ. A case of human intramuscular adrenal gland transplantation as a cure for chronic adrenal insufficiency. *Am J Transplant* (2010) **10**(2):431–3. doi:10.1111/j.1600-6143.2009.02929.x
29. Vouillarmet J, Buron F, Houzard C, Carlier MC, Chauvet C, Brunet M, et al. The first simultaneous kidney-adrenal gland-pancreas transplantation: outcome at 1 year. *Am J Transplant* (2013) **13**(7):1905–9. doi:10.1111/ajt.12296
30. Dubernard JM, Cloix P, Tajra LC, Alduglihan W, Borson F, Lefrancois N, et al. Simultaneous adrenal gland and kidney allotransplantation after synchronous bilateral renal cell carcinoma: a case report. *Transplant Proc* (1995) **27**(1):1320–1.
31. Thomas M, Northrup SR, Hornsby PJ. Adrenocortical tissue formed by transplantation of normal clones of bovine adrenocortical cells in scid mice replaces the essential functions of the animals' adrenal glands. *Nature* (1997) **3**(9):978–83.
32. Thomas M, Hornsby PJ. Transplantation of primary bovine adrenocortical cells into scid mice. *Mol Cell Endocrinol* (1999) **153**:125–36. doi:10.1016/S0303-7207(99)00070-2
33. Thomas M, Wang X, Hornsby PJ. Human adrenocortical cell xenotransplantation: model of cotransplantation of human adrenocortical cells and 3T3 cells in scid mice to form vascularized tissue and prevent adrenal insufficiency. *Xenotransplantation* (2002) **9**:58–67. doi:10.1046/j.0908-665x.2001.00138.x
34. Teebken OE, Scheumann GFW. Differentiated corticosteroid production and regeneration after selective transplantation of cultured and noncultured adrenocortical cells in the adrenalectomized rat. *Transplantation* (2000) **70**(5):836–43. doi:10.1097/00007890-200009150-00022
35. Huang CC, Miyagawa S, Matsumaru D, Parker KL, Yao HH. Progenitor cell expansion and organ size of mouse adrenal is regulated by sonic hedgehog. *Endocrinology* (2010) **151**(3):1119–28. doi:10.1210/en.2009-0814
36. Guasti L, Paul A, Laufer E, King P. Localization of Sonic hedgehog secreting and receiving cells in the developing and adult rat adrenal cortex. *Mol Cell Endocrinol* (2011) **336**(1–2):117–22. doi:10.1016/j.mce.2010.11.010
37. Guasti L, Candy Sze WC, McKay T, Grose R, King PJ. FGF signalling through Fgfr2 isoform IIIb regulates adrenal cortex development. *Mol Cell Endocrinol* (2013) **371**(1–2):182–8. doi:10.1016/j.mce.2013.01.014
38. Freedman BD, Kempna PB, Carlone DL, Shah MS, Guagliardo NA, Barrett PQ, et al. Adrenocortical zonation results from lineage conversion of differentiated zona glomerulosa cells. *Dev Cell* (2013) **26**(6):666–73. doi:10.1016/j.devcel.2013.07.016
39. Allende G, Chavira R, Quintanar-Stephano A. Biochemical evidence of the functional recovery and regeneration of adrenal autotransplants in the rat spleen. *Endocrine* (2001) **16**(3):173–9. doi:10.1385/ENDO:16:3:173
40. Thomas M, Yang L, Hornsby PJ. Formation of functional tissue from transplanted adrenocortical cells expressing telomerase reverse transcriptase. *Nat Biotechnol* (2000) **18**:39–42. doi:10.1038/71894
41. Huang Q, Chen M, Liang S, Acha V, Liu D, Yuan F, et al. Improving cell therapy – experiments using transplanted telomerase-immortalized cells in immunodeficient mice. *Mech Ageing Dev* (2007) **128**(1):25–30. doi:10.1016/j.mad.2006.11.006
42. Thomas M, Suwa T, Yang L, Zhao L, Hawks CL, Hornsby PJ. Cooperation of hTERT, SV40 T Antigen and oncogenic Ras in tumorigenesis: a cell transplantation model using bovine adrenocortical cells. *Neoplasia* (2002) **4**(6):493–500. doi:10.1038/sj.neo.7900262
43. Badylak SF. The extracellular matrix as a scaffold for tissue reconstruction. *Cell Dev Biol* (2002) **13**:377–83. doi:10.1016/S1084952102000940
44. Chamoux E, Bolduc L, Lehoux JG, Gallo-Payet N. Identification of extracellular matrix components and their integrin receptors in the human fetal adrenal gland. *J Clin Endocrinol Metab* (2001) **86**(5):2090–8. doi:10.1210/jcem.86.5.7462
45. Chamoux E, Narcy A, Lehoux J-G, Gallo-Payet N. Fibronectin, laminin and collagen IV as modulators of cell behaviour during adrenal gland development in the human fetus. *J Clin Endocrinol Metab* (2002) **87**(4):1819–28. doi:10.1210/jcem.87.4.8359
46. Zupekan T, Dunn JCY. Adrenocortical cell transplantation reverses a murine model of adrenal failure. *J Pediatr Surg* (2011) **46**(6):1208–13. doi:10.1016/j.jpedsurg.2011.03.057
47. Faulk DM, Johnson SA, Zhang L, Badylak SF. Role of the extracellular matrix in whole organ engineering. *J Cell Physiol* (2014) **229**(8):984–9. doi:10.1002/jcp.24532
48. Allen RA, Seltz LM, Jiang BSH, Kasick RT, Sellaro TL, Badylak SF, et al. Adrenal extracellular matrix scaffolds support adrenocortical cell proliferation and function in vitro. *Tissue Eng* (2010) **16**(11):3363–74. doi:10.1089/ten.TEA.2010.0005
49. Cogger K, Nostro MC. Recent advances in cell replacement therapies for the treatment of type 1 diabetes. *Endocrinology* (2015) **156**(1):8–15. doi:10.1210/en.2014-1691
50. Takahashi K, Yamanaka S. Induction of pluripotent stem cells from mouse embryonic and adult fibroblast cultures by defined factors. *Cell* (2006) **126**(4):663–76. doi:10.1016/j.cell.2006.07.024
51. Vierbuchen T, Wernig M. Molecular roadblocks for cellular reprogramming. *Mol Cell* (2012) **47**(6):827–38. doi:10.1016/j.molcel.2012.09.008
52. Sancho-Martinez I, Baek SH, Izpisua Belmonte JC. Lineage conversion methodologies meet the reprogramming toolbox. *Nat Cell Biol* (2012) **14**(9):892–9. doi:10.1038/ncb2567
53. Crawford PA, Sadovsky Y, Milbrandt J. Nuclear receptor steroidogenic factor 1 directs embryonic stem cells toward the steroidogenic lineage. *Mol Cell Biol* (1997) **17**(7):3997–4006.
54. Gondo S, Yanase T, Okabe T, Tanaka T, Morinaga H, Nomura M, et al. SF-1/Ad4BP transforms primary long-term cultured bone marrow cells into ACTH-responsive steroidogenic cells. *Genes Cells* (2004) **9**(12):1239–47. doi:10.1111/j.1365-2443.2004.00801.x
55. Gondo S, Okabe T, Tanaka T, Morinaga H, Nomura M, Takayanagi R, et al. Adipose tissue-derived and bone marrow-derived mesenchymal cells develop into different lineage of steroidogenic cells by forced expression of steroidogenic factor 1. *Endocrinology* (2008) **149**(9):4717–25. doi:10.1210/en.2007-1808
56. Yazawa T, Mizutani T, Yamada K, Kawata H, Sekiguchi T, Yoshino M, et al. Differentiation of adult stem cells derived from bone marrow stroma into Leydig or adrenocortical cells. *Endocrinology* (2006) **147**(9):4104–11. doi:10.1210/en.2006-0162
57. Tanaka T, Gondo S, Okabe T, Ohe K, Shirohzu H, Morinaga H, et al. Steroidogenic factor 1/adrenal 4 binding protein transforms human bone marrow mesenchymal cells into steroidogenic cells. *J Mol Endocrinol* (2007) **39**(5):343–50. doi:10.1677/JME-07-0076
58. Yazawa T, Inanoka Y, Mizutani T, Kuribayashi M, Umezawa A, Miyamoto K. Liver receptor homolog-1 regulates the transcription of steroidogenic enzymes and induces the differentiation of mesenchymal stem cells into steroidogenic cells. *Endocrinology* (2009) **150**(8):3885–93. doi:10.1210/en.2008-1310
59. Parker KL, Schimmer BP. Steroidogenic factor 1: a key determinant of endocrine development and function. *Endocr Rev* (1997) **18**(3):361–77. doi:10.1210/edrv.18.3.0301
60. Fayard E, Auwerx J, Schoonjans K. LRH-1: an orphan nuclear receptor involved in development, metabolism and steroidogenesis. *Trends Cell Biol* (2004) **14**(5):250–60. doi:10.1016/j.tcb.2004.03.008
61. Yazawa T, Inaoka Y, Okada R, Mizutani T, Yamazaki Y, Usami Y, et al. PPAR-gamma coactivator-1alpha regulates progesterone production in ovarian granulosa cells with SF-1 and LRH-1. *Mol Endocrinol* (2010) **24**(3):485–96. doi:10.1210/me.2009-0352
62. Wei X, Peng G, Zheng S, Wu X. Differentiation of umbilical cord mesenchymal stem cells into steroidogenic cells in comparison to bone marrow mesenchymal stem cells. *Cell Prolif* (2012) **45**(2):101–10. doi:10.1111/j.1365-2184.2012.00809.x

63. Yazawa T, Kawabe S, Inaoka Y, Okada R, Mizutani T, Imamichi Y, et al. Differentiation of mesenchymal stem cells and embryonic stem cells into steroidogenic cells using steroidogenic factor-1 and liver receptor homolog-1. *Mol Cell Endocrinol* (2011) **336**(1–2):127–32. doi:10.1016/j.mce.2010.11.025
64. Jadhav U, Jameson JL. Steroidogenic factor-1 (SF-1)-driven differentiation of murine embryonic stem (ES) cells into a gonadal lineage. *Endocrinology* (2011) **152**(7):2870–82. doi:10.1210/en.2011-0219
65. Sonoyama T, Sone M, Honda K, Taura D, Kojima K, Inuzuka M, et al. Differentiation of human embryonic stem cells and human induced pluripotent stem cells into steroid-producing cells. *Endocrinology* (2012) **153**(9):4336–45. doi:10.1210/en.2012-1060
66. Val P, Swain A. Gene dosage effects and transcriptional regulation of early mammalian adrenal cortex development. *Mol Cell Endocrinol* (2010) **323**(1):105–14. doi:10.1016/j.mce.2009.12.010
67. Mazilu JK, McCabe ER. Moving toward personalized cell-based interventions for adrenal cortical disorders: part 2 – human diseases and tissue engineering. *Mol Genet Metab* (2011) **104**(1–2):80–8. doi:10.1016/j.ymgme.2011.06.011
68. Kearns NA, Genga RM, Enuameh MS, Garber M, Wolfe SA, Maehr R. Cas9 effector-mediated regulation of transcription and differentiation in human pluripotent stem cells. *Development* (2014) **141**(1):219–23. doi:10.1242/dev.103341
69. Ludwig B, Reichel A, Steffen A, Zimerman B, Schally AV, Block NL, et al. Transplantation of human islets without immunosuppression. *Proc Natl Acad Sci U S A* (2013) **110**(47):19054–8. doi:10.1073/pnas.1317561110
70. Cox DB, Platt RJ, Zhang F. Therapeutic genome editing: prospects and challenges. *Nat Med* (2015) **21**(2):121–31. doi:10.1038/nm.3793

23

The Herbicide Atrazine Potentiates Angiotensin II-Induced Aldosterone Synthesis and Release From Adrenal Cells

*Arthur D. Zimmerman, Laci Mackay, Robert J. Kemppainen, Melaney A. Jones, Casey C. Read, Dean Schwartz and Chad D. Foradori**

Department of Anatomy, Physiology and Pharmacology, College of Veterinary Medicine, Auburn University, Auburn, AL, United States

***Correspondence:**
Chad D. Foradori
foradori@auburn.edu

Atrazine is one of the most commonly used pre-emergence and early post-emergence herbicides in the world. We have shown previously that atrazine does not directly stimulate the pituitary or adrenal to trigger hormone release but acts centrally to activate a stress-like activation of the hypothalamic-pituitary-adrenal axis. In doing so, atrazine treatment has been shown to cause adrenal morphology changes characteristic of repeated stress. In this study, adrenals from atrazine treated and stressed animals were directly compared after 4 days of atrazine treatment or restraint stress. Both atrazine and stressed animals displayed reduced adrenocortical zona glomerulosa thickness and aldosterone synthase (CYP11B2) expression, indicative of repeated adrenal stimulation by adrenocorticotropic hormone. To determine if reduced CYP11B2 expression resulted in attenuated aldosterone synthesis, stressed and atrazine treated animals were challenged with angiotensin II (Ang II). As predicted, stressed animals produced less aldosterone compared to control animals when stimulated. However, atrazine treated animals had higher circulating aldosterone concentrations compared to both stressed and control groups. Ang II-induced aldosterone release was also potentiated in atrazine pretreated human adrenocortical carcinoma cells (H295R). Atrazine pretreated did not alter the expression of the rate limiting steroidogenic StAR protein or angiotensin II receptor 1. Atrazine treated animals also presented with higher basal blood pressure than vehicle treated control animals suggesting sustained elevations in circulating aldosterone levels. Our results demonstrate that treatment with the widely used herbicide, atrazine, directly increases stimulated production of aldosterone in adrenocortical cells independent of expression changes to rate limiting steroidogenic enzymes.

Keywords: atrazine, herbicide, adrenal, aldosterone, angiotensin II, H295R

INTRODUCTION

Atrazine (2-chloro-4-ethylamino-6-isopropylamino-s-triazine) is one of the most commonly used herbicides worldwide (1). Atrazine is used to control annual grasses and broadleaf weeds in agricultural crops such as corn, sugarcane, and sorghum, as well as on urban golf courses with an estimated annual application of 80 million pounds (2). Atrazine's widespread use and relatively long half-life makes it the most commonly detected herbicide in water sources (3, 4). In plants, atrazine inhibits photosynthesis in plants by binding to the D1 protein located in the thylakoid membrane of chloroplasts, thereby blocking electron transport necessary for photosynthesis (5, 6).

In rats, the effects of atrazine exposure on the hypothalamic-pituitary-gonadal (HPG) axis have been well documented. In particular, we have shown that atrazine will inhibit both pulsatile and preovulatory surge release of gonadotropin releasing hormone (GnRH) and the subsequent release of luteinizing hormone (LH) from the pituitary (7–9). The mechanism by which atrazine inhibits GnRH and LH release is not fully understood. It is possible that the inhibitory effects of atrazine and its chlorometabolites on gonadotropins (8–10) is partially due to the interaction between the chlorotriazine and the hypothalamic-pituitary-adrenal (HPA) axis. All evidence suggests, atrazine acts centrally in the brain to induce this response. Central infusion of atrazine or molar equivalent doses of its primary metabolites, results in a rapid rise in stress hormones. Atrazine does not induce adrenocorticotropic hormone (ACTH) release in pituitary cell cultures. Additionally, the blockade of corticotropin-releasing hormone (CRH) receptors inhibits atrazine-induced elevation in corticosterone *in vivo*. This suggests that atrazine does not directly stimulate ACTH release from the pituitary, but requires CRH receptor activation, presumably from hypothalamic derived CRH. Likewise, the concurrent rise in plasma ACTH and corticosterone concentrations after atrazine treatment, and the lack of atrazine-induced corticosterone in animals under dexamethasone suppression or in animals without a pituitary, does not support a direct action of atrazine on adrenal gland steroidogenesis. However, we have termed atrazine's effects on the HPA axis as "stress-like" since, although CRH receptor activation is required for atrazine-induced ACTH release, CRH cells of the hypothalamic paraventricular nucleus fail to display markers of activation after atrazine treatment (cFos and P-CREB) (11). Likewise, animals do not perceive atrazine as a stressor. Animals do not respond to atrazine treatment with hyperthermia or display avoidance behavior common in stressed animals (12).

Through our previous investigation, the zona glomerulosa (zG) of the adrenal cortex was found to be reduced in thickness after 4 days of atrazine treatment (11). As mentioned, atrazine treatment results in elevated concentrations in circulating ACTH similar to those found in restraint stressed animals (11, 13). ACTH treated or restraint stressed rats have similar reductions in zG thickness to atrazine treated animals (14, 15). We hypothesized that the changes in adrenal morphology induced by atrazine treatment would mimic those in restraint stressed animals (14). In addition, we investigated the ability of atrazine or stressed animals to mobilize aldosterone production in response to angiotensin II stimulation and possible effects on blood pressure. We hypothesized that rats exposed to repeated (4 days) atrazine treatment or stress (restraint) would display lower aldosterone plasma concentrations compared to control animals. While our findings do not support this hypothesis, it identified novel and profound effects of exposure to the ubiquitous herbicide, atrazine, on aldosterone synthesis and release both *in vitro* and *in vivo*.

METHODS

Animals

All animal surgeries and experimental protocols were approved by the Animal Care and Use Committee of Auburn University (2015-2729) and were carried out in accordance with National Institutes of Health and Association for Assessment and Accreditation of Laboratory Animal Care guidelines. Young adult female Sprague Dawley rats (age 60 to 90 days) were obtained from Charles River Laboratories (Wilmington, MA). Animals were single- or double-housed and maintained on a 10-hour dark:14-hour light photoperiod (lights on at 0700 hours) with *ad libitum* access to food and water. The number of signal housed animals were distributed equally across treatment groups and the basal stress hormones from these animals were not statically different to pair-housed animals. All treatments were given within 2 hours of lights on. All blood sampling was completed within 5 hours of lights on. After ≥4 days to acclimate to the vivarium, all animals were bilaterally ovariectomized under 4% isoflurane followed by carprofen (Zoetis, Kalamazoo, MI) 2.2 mg/kg subcutaneously every 24 hours for 72 hours. Animals were allowed 7 to 10 days to recover before additional procedures were conducted. Ovarectomized-female rats were used in the current experiments to be consistent with our previous findings of atrazine-induced reduction in zG morphology (11). To reduce nonspecific stress associated with handling and gavage, animals used for all experiments were habituated for 4 to 7 days before treatment was initiated. A total of 135 animals were used in the described experiments.

Test Substances

For animal studies, atrazine (45330; Sigma-Aldrich, Burlington, MA; certified, 98.8% pure) was prepared weekly as a suspension in 1% carboxymethylcellulose (CMC) sodium salt (9004-32-4; Alfa Aesar, Haverhill, MA) and deionized water. Suspensions were stored refrigerated (at 2°C to 8°C) until use. For cell culture studies, atrazine was dissolved in Dimethyl sulfoxide (DMSO; Sigma-Aldrich; 276855) and stored at -20°C until diluted into media. The *in vivo* dose and *in vitro* concentration selections were predicated on previous reports from our laboratories and others that reported repeatable and robust elevations in stress hormones after oral gavage of atrazine. The *in vivo* no effect level for the atrazine-induced activation of the HPA axis is 5 mg/kg in male rats (13), and the lowest observed effect level reported for female rats is 12.5 mg/kg (16). However, to characterize the effects of atrazine on adrenal morphology and activation, doses at the higher end of the known effective range to elicit a rise in stress hormone concentrations were used (11).

Experiment 1: Effects of Atrazine or Restraint Stress Treatment on Adrenal Morphology

Animals were administered atrazine [100 mg/kg of body weight (BW)] in CMC by gavage once daily, CMC alone, or restraint stressed for 30 minutes in Plas-Labs Scientific restraint stress (Lansing, MI; 553-BSRR) for 4 consecutive days. Previous reports involving repeated stress and changes to adrenal morphology used 30 mins or 2 hours of daily restraint stress (14, 15). In the present studies, 30 mins of restraint stress was used because the hormone response (amplitude and duration of ACTH and corticosterone) to 30 mins of restraint is similar to that of atrazine (100mg/kg) treatment (11, 13). Animals were weighed daily. After completion of the last treatment, animals were euthanized by carbon dioxide inhalation, and the right adrenal gland was collected, weighed, and placed in 10% neutral-buffered formalin for immunohistochemical processing. Eight animals were used per treatment group.

Experiment 2: Effects of Atrazine or Restraint Stress on Angiotensin II Induced Aldosterone Release

Animals were administered atrazine (100 mg/kg BW) in CMC by gavage once daily, CMC alone, or restraint stressed for 30 minutes in Plas-Labs Scientific restraint stress (Lansing, MI; 553-BSRR) for 4 consecutive days. On the 4th day, but before the final treatment, animals were injected with dexamethasone (100 μg/kg in safflower oil, subcutaneously; 50-02-2; Sigma-Aldrich, St. Louis, MO). Atrazine and restraint stress have been shown to induce a rise in blood ACTH concentrations. Dexamethasone pretreatment was given on the final day of treatment to suppress ACTH release, to avoid ACTH-induced rise in aldosterone concentrations. 90 mins after dexamethasone, the gavage or restraint stress was administered. 45 minutes post treatment, animals were anesthetized with 4% isoflurane and an intra-atrial cannula was inserted for blood sampling, as described previously (17). Heparin saline (10 U) was injected *via* the jugular catheter. Approximately 60 min after final treatment, a baseline blood sample (50 μL) was taken and placed in heparin- and EDTA-treated tube on ice. Following the baseline sample, animals were treated with angiotensin II (Ang II, 5 μg/kg of BW; 4474-91-3; Alfa Aesar, Ward Hill, MA). From baseline sample (timepoint 0 min), samples were taken every 10 min for 40 min. Samples were spun at 1500 rpm for 15 minutes at 4°C. Plasma was frozen at −20°C until assayed for aldosterone. Seven animals were used per treatment group.

Experiment 3: Effects of Atrazine Treatment Duration on Angiotensin II-Induced Aldosterone Release

Animals were administered atrazine in CMC (100 mg/kg BW), or CMC only for 1, 2, 3, or 4 consecutive days. On the final day of treatment animals were injected with vehicle (safflower oil, subcutaneously) or dexamethasone (100 μg/kg in safflower oil, subcutaneously; 50-02-2; Sigma-Aldrich, St. Louis, MO) and returned to their home cage. After 90 mins, the animals were anesthetized with 4% isoflurane. An intra-atrial cannula was inserted for blood sampling. Heparin saline (10 U) was injected *via* the jugular catheter. Forty-five minutes later a baseline blood sample (50 μL) was removed and placed in heparin- and EDTA-treated tube on ice. Following the baseline sample, animals were treated with angiotensin II (Ang II, 5 μg/kg of BW; 4474-91-3; Alfa Aesar, Ward Hill, MA). From baseline sample (timepoint 0 min), samples were taken every 10 min for 40 min. Samples were spun at 1500 rpm for 15 minutes at 4°C. Plasma was frozen at −20°C until assayed for aldosterone. Eight animals were used per treatment group.

Experiment 4: Effects of Atrazine Treatment on Aldosterone Production in Human Adrenocortical Cells

NCl-H295R (H295R) cells were purchased through American Type Culture collection (ATCC CRL-2128; Manassas, VA). H295R cells were grown at 37°C and 5% CO_2 in DMEM/F12 medium (Gibco Invitrogen, Carlsbad, CA) containing 2.5% FBS (HyClone, South Logan, UT), 2 mM L-glutamine (BioWhittaker Cambrex, East Rutherford, NJ), 1% ABAM (A5955, Sigma-Aldrich) and 1% ITS+ Premix Universal Culture Supplement (354352, Corning, Cleveland, TN). For analysis of response to atrazine and Ang II, cells were sub-cultured onto 12-well dishes at a density of 1.5×10^5 cells/well.

Experiment 4a

One day before the experiment, cells were changed to low-serum experimental medium (1% FBS). After 16 hours, cells were changed to low-serum media containing 0.1, 1.0, or 10 μM of atrazine or the DMSO vehicle (final concentration <0.1%). After 24 hours of pretreatment, cultures were treated with 0.1 nM Ang II in fresh low-serum experimental medium containing the same atrazine or vehicle treatments. Post 24 hours of Ang II treatment, media was collected for aldosterone measurement and cells were collected for protein determination. Three biological replicates across 2-3 passages were used per treatment.

Experiment 4b

One day before the experiment, cells were changed to low-serum experimental medium (1% FBS). After 16 hours, cells were changed to media containing 10 μM of atrazine or the DMSO vehicle (final concentration <0.1%). After 1, 3, 6, 24, or 48 hours, cultures were treated with 0.1 nM Ang II in fresh low-serum experimental medium not containing atrazine. Post 24 hours of Ang II treatment, media was collected for aldosterone measurement and cells were collected for protein determination. Three biological replicates across 2-3 passages replicates were used per treatment.

Experiment 5. Effects of Atrazine Treatment on Blood Pressure

Animals were administered atrazine in CMC (100 mg/kg BW), or CMC only for 4 consecutive days. Animals were weighed daily. On the final day of treatment, rats were maintained under 1.5% isoflurane in 3 liters/min oxygen throughout experiment. Carotid artery was cannulated for arterial pressure measurement, electrocardiographic wires attached to record Lead II ECG and the jugular vein was cannulated for fluid and drug infusion. Angiotensin II was infused at a rate of 0.1 ml/min at doses of 10, 30, 100, 300, 1000 ng/kg/min for 5 min or until arterial pressure stabilized. Phosphate buffered saline was then infused until arterial pressure returned to baseline before next infusion of angiotensin II. At the completion of the experiment, isoflurane was increased to 5% and heart and kidney removed and frozen in liquid nitrogen. Baseline values represent values before angiotensin II infusion. Increases in pressure represent the maximum increase in pressure in response to angiotensin II infusion. Eight animals were used per treatment group.

Experiment 6. Effects of Atrazine Treatment on Select Gene Expression and Blood Electrolyte Levels

Animals were administered atrazine in CMC (100 mg/kg BW), or CMC only for 4 consecutive days. On the final day of treatment, animals were euthanized by cervical dislocation. Within 2 mins, blood samples were collected and analyzed with the iSTAT Portable Clinical Analyzer using the iSTAT CG8+ cartridge (03M86-01, iSTAT, Princeton, NJ). The iSTAT has previously been validated for rodent use (18, 19). Heart, kidney, and left adrenal tissue were collected and kept at -80°C until gene analysis. Five animals were used per treatment group.

Immunohistochemistry

To determine the changes to adrenal morphology after repeated atrazine treatment, right adrenal glands were embedded in paraffin and 6-μm sections were placed on HistoBond slides. Slides were warmed at 55°C for 45 minutes, deparaffinized and rehydrated though xylene and graded ethanol. Sections were then antigen-unmasked by boiling in Tris buffer (10 mM Tris, 1 mM EDTA) at pH 9.0 for 15 minutes. Slides were washed in PBS (pH 7.2) and then placed in blocking solution (1% BSA in PBS) for 20 minutes. Slides were incubated in hybridization chambers overnight in a primary antibody cocktail in blocking solution [1:100 mouse anti–cytochrome P450 aldosterone synthase (Millipore, Billerica, MA; MAB6021; RRID: AB_95224) and 1:500 goat anti–11β-hydroxylase (Santa Cruz Biotechnology, Dallas, TX; sc-47652, RRID: AB_2088384)]. After incubation in primary antibody, slides were washed three times in PBS and then incubated in a fluorescent secondary antibody cocktail for 1 hour [1:250 Alexa Fluor 488 donkey–anti-mouse (Invitrogen; A21202) and 1:250 Alexa Fluor 594 donkey–anti-goat (A11058)]. After incubation in secondary antibody, slides were rinsed in phosphate buffer (pH 7.2) and then coverslipped with hardset mounting media with 4′,6-diamidino-2-phenylindole counterstain (Vector Laboratories, Inc., Burlingame, CA; H-1500). Slides were then imaged at ×20 magnification with a Perkin Elmer Cri-Nuance fluorescent multispectral imaging camera (Model FX; Perkin Elmer, Waltham, MA) in conjunction with a Zeiss Axioskop microscope (Carl Zeiss Microscopy, LLC, Thornwood, NY). With tunable filters matched to the bandwidths of molecular markers, the camera acquired spectral information from each sample, resulting in component images. The various signals from multiple labels in the resulting image were "unmixed" by the software, and a composite image was produced, allowing spectral characterization and quantitation for each of the multi-labeled components in an image while removing any autofluorescence. Immunofluorescent controls included the omission of the primary antibody from the immunostaining protocol and pre-adsorption with the respective antigens for each primary antibody, which completely eliminated staining for the corresponding antigen.

Slides were analyzed in ImageJ Software (National Institutes of Health, Bethesda, MD) to measure the length of each adrenal cortical layer. Layers were measured in microns, with the immunofluorescence and 4′,6-diamidino-2-phenylindole counterstain used to distinguish the morphological differences in each layer (*zona glomerulosa* (zG), *zona fasciculata* (zF), and *zona reticularis* (zR)).

Aldosterone Analysis

Aldosterone was measured using an EIA kit (ENZO® Life Sciences; ADI-900-173). The optical density of each sample was read at 405 nm using the Molecular Devices SpectraMax ID5. The concentration of aldosterone (pg/mL) was determined using the Softmax Pro microplate data software and presented as a ratio of cell protein level.

RNA Extraction

RNA extraction was performed using the Qiagen (Valencia, CA) RNeasy Microarray Tissue kit (73304). Tissue was placed in QIAzol lysis reagent and homogenized for 30-40 seconds. Following homogenization, the homogenate was placed on the bench top at room temperature for 5 minutes to promote dissociation of the nucleoprotein complexes. Chloroform (200 μL) was added, mixed and allowed to sit at room temperature for 3 minutes. Homogenates were then centrifuged at 12,000 x g for 15 minutes at 4°C. The upper aqueous layer was removed and mixed with 600 μL of 70% ethanol. A RNA easy Mini spin column along with DNAse digestion set (Qiagen; 79254) were used for purification. Concentration (ng/μL) and purity (260/280 ratio) were determined using the Thermo Scientific (Pittsburgh, PA) NanoDrop ND-1000 Spectrophotometer. cDNA synthesis was performed using the Bio-Rad iScript cDNA synthesis kit (Hercules, CA; 170-88912).

Real-Time PCR Analysis

PCR analysis was performed for angiotensin II type 1 receptor (AT_1R), 11β- hydroxylase (CYP11B1), aldosterone synthase (CYP11B2), steroidogenic acute regulatory protein (StAR) and glyceraldyhyde 3-phosphate dehydrogenase (GAPDH) was used as the housekeeping gene. The DNA sequence for each gene was obtained from the National Center for Biotechnology Information (NCBI). The primer pair products were validated by gel electrophoresis and DNA sequence analysis to original gene (**Table 1**). PCR was carried out using the Bio-rad iCycler iQ real-time detection system with Bio-Rad iQ SYBR Green Supermix. One cycle was performed at 95°C for 10 minutes to activate polymerase and denature the DNA. Fluorescence data collection was performed for 40 cycles at 95°C for 15 seconds and 40 cycles at 58°C for 1 minute. The fold change of each target mRNA expression relative to GAPDH under experimental and control conditions were calculated based on the threshold cycle

TABLE 1 | Primer squences.

Gene	Forward primer (5'- 3')	Reverse primer (5'- 3')	Amplificate size (bp)	Reference Sequence
GAPDH	GGTGATGCTGGTGCTGAGTA	GGATGCAGGGATGATGTTCT	369	NM_017008.4
CYP11B1	TTACCCAAGAGCTTGACTCGTTGGAC	ACCATCTCGGATATGACACTCCAG	161	XM_039079756.1
CYP11B2	ACGAGGTAGCAAGGGACTTCTTGGA	GCATGGATGAACTTCAGGCTACCA	193	XM_039078395.1
StAR	AAGAAGGAAAGCCAGCAGGAGAATGGA	TGCGGTCCACCAGTTCTTCATAGAGTC	133	NM_031558.3
AT1R	GCTAAGCAGCTCACTCACTAC	AACTCTTGACCTCCCATCTC	363	NM_031009.2

GAPDH, Glyceraldehyde-3-Phosphate Dehydrogenase; CYP11B1, 11-beta hydroxylase; CYP11B2, aldosterone synthase; StAR, Steroidogenic acute regulatory protein; AT1R, Angiotensin II receptor type 1.

(C_T) asr = $2^{-\Delta(\Delta C_T)}$, where $\Delta C_T = C_T(\text{target}) - C_T(\text{GAPDH})$ and $\Delta(\Delta C_T) = \Delta C_T(\text{experimental}) - \Delta C_T(\text{control})$. The amplicons for all primer sets were sequenced and validated.

Protein Extraction and Quantification

Media was removed and saved for aldosterone analysis. Cells were rinsed with PBS and put on ice. While remaining on ice, 50 µL of RIPA buffer with Halt was added to each of the twelve wells and cells were harvested and homogenized while on ice. The protein content of samples was then determined by the Bio-Rad protein assay (Bradford and Lowry) by following the manufacturer recommendation (20).

Statistical Analysis

One-way ANOVA were performed in experiments 1, and 2 for adrenal morphology and peak/AUC aldosterone plasma concentrations. A 2-way ANOVA followed by post-hoc Bonferroni paired-comparisons were performed in experiments 2, 3, 4 and 5 for aldosterone plasma concentrations over timed samples, peak/AUV aldosterone across days of treatment, culture media aldosterone concentrations across atrazine concentrations or duration and angiotensin II treatment, and blood pressure parameters. Cardiac mechanical parameters are presented as either baseline values (values before angiotensin II administration) or as a change from baseline (peak response to an angiotensin II). Multiple t tests were performed on the effect of each angiotensin II dose in vehicle and atrazine treated rats. Statistical analysis for the real-time PCR data was performed using a modification of the ΔCt (21). The level of statistical significance was set at $P \leq 0.05$ for all statistical tests. All values were reported as the mean ± SEM. Prism 8 for Mac was used for all analysis (GraphPad Software, Inc., La Jolla, CA).

RESULTS

Experiment 1: Effects of Atrazine or Restraint Stress Treatment on Adrenal Morphology

Atrazine treatment had no statistically significant effects on adrenal cortical or medulla thickness (**Table 2**; $F_{(2, 21)} = 0.91$, $P = 0.91$; $F_{(2, 21)} = 0.136$, $P = 0.874$, respectively). When adrenal cortical zones were analyzed, the zG was found to be reduced in thickness after 4 days of treatment with 100 mg/kg BW of atrazine or 30 min of restraint stress when compared with vehicle-treated animals (**Table 2**, **Figure 1A**; $F_{(2, 21)} = 20.8$, $P < 0.001$). Atrazine or restraint stress treatments had no effect on the thickness of the zF or zR ($F_{(2, 21)} = 3.09$, $P = 0.066$; $F_{(2, 21)} = 0.85$, $P = 0.44$, respectively). There was no treatment effect on cell density in the zG or zF ($F_{(2, 21)} = 1.37$, $P = 0.277$; $F_{(2, 21)} = 2.09$, $P = 0.149$). Cell density was lower in the zR of atrazine treated animals compared to vehicle treated animals ($F_{(2, 21)} = 9.00$, $P < 0.005$). There were no differences in adrenal weights (% BW) between treatment groups ($F_{(2, 21)} = 0.437$, $P = 0.652$). Along with decreased zG layer thickness (**Figure 1B**), atrazine and stressed animals had less immunoreactivity (**Figure 1C**, $F_{(2, 21)} = 5.10$, $P = 0.016$) and expression (**Figure 1D**, $F_{(2, 21)} = 20.87$, $P < 0.001$) for aldosterone

TABLE 2 | Effects of atrazine or stress treatment on adrenal morphology.

Adrenal Metrics	Vehicle			Atrazine			Stress		
zG Thickness (µm)	111.90	4.60	8	71.74	3.76	8*	77.41	5.73	8*
zF Thickness (µm)	729.01	18.50	8	778.33	27.73	8	819.83	29.92	8
zR Thickness (µm)	477.87	28.51	8	346.74	14.53	8	433.24	28.81	8
Cortical Thickness (µm)	1318.78	49.04	8	1305.81	34.09	8	1330.48	32.75	8
Medulla (µm)	1022.77	67.22	8	1060.67	75.38	8	1013.63	59.80	8
zG Cell Density	40.23	0.99	8	43.77	1.06	8	42.77	1.22	8
zF Cell Density	12.66	0.59	8	11.63	0.40	8	12.93	0.41	8
zR Cell Density	27.27	0.85	8	22.53	0.88	8*	25.17	0.62	8
Adrenal Weight (% BW)	0.0152	0.00091	8	0.0156	0.00097	8	0.0164	0.00089	8

Data presented as the mean ± SEM. Asterisk signifies difference from control group (P < 0.05).

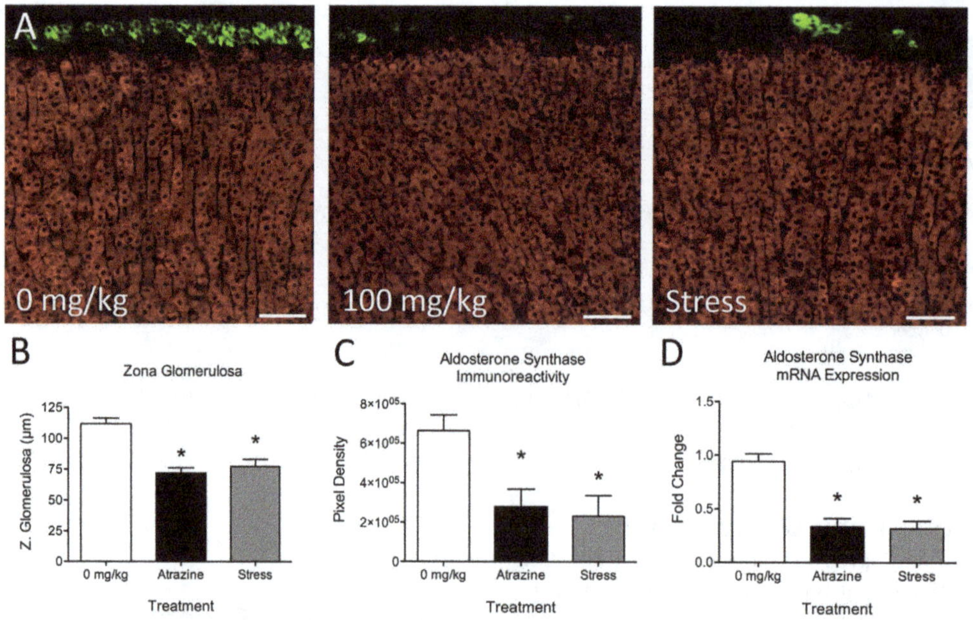

FIGURE 1 | Atrazine treatment and repeated restraint stress reduce zona glomerulosa thickness and aldosterone synthase immunoreactivity and expression. **(A)** Representative images of the adrenal cortex of vehicle, atrazine (100 mg/kg), and restraint stressed animals displaying aldosterone synthase (green) and 11β-Hydroxylase immunofluorescence. **(B–D)** Histograms depicting **(B)** mean zona glomerulosa thickness, mean aldosterone synthase **(C)** immunoreactivity and **(D)** expression in adrenals of vehicle, atrazine (100mg/kg), and restraint stressed animals after 4 days of treatment. Data presented as the mean ± SEM. Asterisks signify difference from vehicle group ($P < 0.05$).

synthase There was no significant effect of treatment on animal body weight (**Supplementary Table 1**, $F_{(2, 84)} = 1.56$, $P = 0.217$).

Experiment 2: Effects of Atrazine or Restraint Stress on Angiotensin II Induced Aldosterone Release

Intravenous infusion of angiotensin II resulted in higher plasma aldosterone levels in all treatment groups (**Figure 2A**, $F_{(1, 38)} = 14.0$, $P = 0.0005$). There was no significant difference in baseline aldosterone levels. At the 10 min timepoint, atrazine treated animals had a higher concentration of aldosterone compared to vehicle and stress treated groups ($F_{(8, 76)} = 3.47$, $P = 0.0019$). Atrazine treated animals displayed a higher peak plasma aldosterone concentration after Ang II treatment compared to vehicle and restraint stressed animals, independent of timepoint of peak aldosterone (**Figure 2B**; $F_{(2, 18)} = 6.8$, $P = 0.0068$). The stressed animals had a delayed time to peak compared to both vehicle and atrazine treated groups (vehicle=12.22 min, atrazine=10.0 min, stressed=21.67; $F_{(2, 18)} = 5.1$, $P = 0.02$). The area under the curve (AUC) levels were significantly different between all groups (**Figure 2C**; $F_{(2, 18)} = 10.5$, $P = 0.0009$). The mean AUC for atrazine treated animals was significantly higher than vehicle animals and stressed animals had significantly lower AUC levels compared to vehicle treated animals. There was no

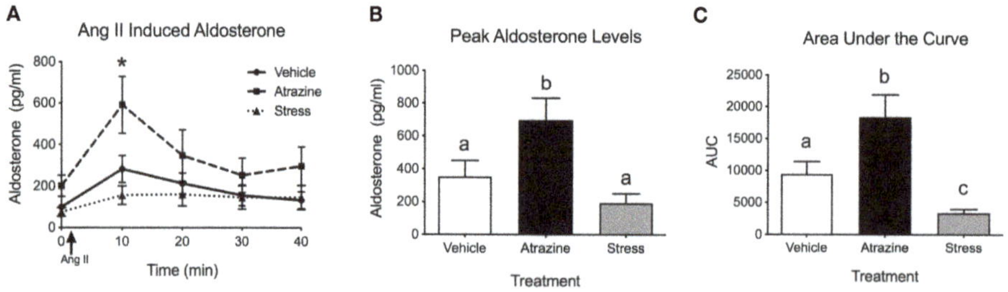

FIGURE 2 | Atrazine treatment increases circulating aldosterone concentrations after angiotensin II (Ang II). **(A)** Line graph depicting aldosterone concentrations before and after infusion of Ang II in vehicle, atrazine (100mg/kg), and restraint stressed animals after 4 days of treatment. Arrow indicates timing of Ang II (5 µg/kg of BW). Histograms depicting **(B)** peak aldosterone concentrations and **(C)** area under the curve levels in vehicle, atrazine (100mg/kg), and restraint stressed animals after 4 days of treatment. Data presented as the mean ± SEM. Asterisk signifies difference from control group ($P < 0.05$). Letters denote significant difference between groups.

significant effect of treatment on animal body weight (**Supplementary Table 1**, $F_{(2, 72)} = 0.88$, $P = 0.42$).

Experiment 3: Effects of Atrazine Treatment Duration on Angiotensin II Induced Aldosterone Release

Only animals treated with atrazine for 4 days demonstrated a significantly increased peak Ang II-induced aldosterone (**Figure 3A**; $F_{(1, 40)} = 4.2$, $P = 0.047$). There were no significant differences in peak plasma aldosterone concentration between animals treated with atrazine or vehicle for 1, 2, or 3 days in their response to Ang II. Animals treated with atrazine for 3 or 4 days displayed significantly larger AUC compared to vehicle treated animals (**Figure 3B**; $F_{(1, 40)} = 6.7$, $P = 0.013$). There was no effect of atrazine treatment on AUC after 1 or 2 days of treatment. There was no significant effect of treatment on animal body weight (**Supplementary Table 1**, $F_{(1, 56)} = 2.68$, $P = 0.11$).

Experiment 4: Effects of Atrazine Treatment on Aldosterone Production in Human Adrenocortical Cells

H295R cells were treated with 0.1, 1.0, or 10 μM atrazine for 24 hours then stimulated with Ang II (0.1 nM). Preliminary work demonstrated that 0.1 nM Ang II treatment of cultured H295R cells failed to elicit a significant increase in aldosterone concentrations in culture media (**Supplementary Figure 1**). This dose was used to investigate possible increased response to Ang II due to atrazine. Cultures pretreated with 1.0 or 10 μM of atrazine and then stimulated with Ang II had significantly elevated aldosterone concentrations compared to cultures pretreated with atrazine alone (**Figure 4A**; $F_{(1, 16)} = 29.7$, $P < 0.0001$). Vehicle or 0.1 μM atrazine treated cultures did not display increased aldosterone concentrations in the media after Ang II treatment. H295R cells were subsequently treated with 10 μM atrazine for 1, 3, 6, 24, or 48 hours then treated with Ang II. Cultures treated for 24 or 48 hours displayed a significant increase in media aldosterone concentration (**Figure 4B**; $F_{(1, 20)} = 29.7$, $P < 0.0001$).

Experiment 5. Effects of Atrazine Treatment on Blood Pressure and Heart Rate

Atrazine treatment increased basal systolic arterial pressure in anesthetized rats but had no effect on diastolic arterial pressure, mean arterial pressure, pulse pressure or heart rate. (**Figure 5A**, $t(8) = 3.1$, $P = 0.015$). Ang II infusion caused a dose dependent increase in arterial pressure but atrazine treated animals displayed lower responses to Ang II infusions compared to vehicle treated control animals (**Figure 5B**, $F_{(1, 37)} = 15.3$, $P = 0.0004$),

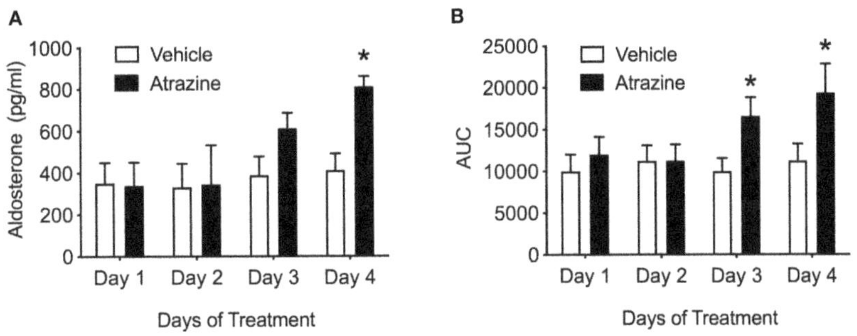

FIGURE 3 | Atrazine treatment increases circulating aldosterone concentrations after angiotensin II over 4 days of treatment. Histograms depicting **(A)** peak aldosterone concentrations and **(B)** area under the curve levels in vehicle (white bars) and atrazine (100mg/kg, black bars) after 1, 2, 3, and 4 days of treatment. Data presented as the mean ± SEM. Asterisk signifies difference from control group ($P < 0.05$).

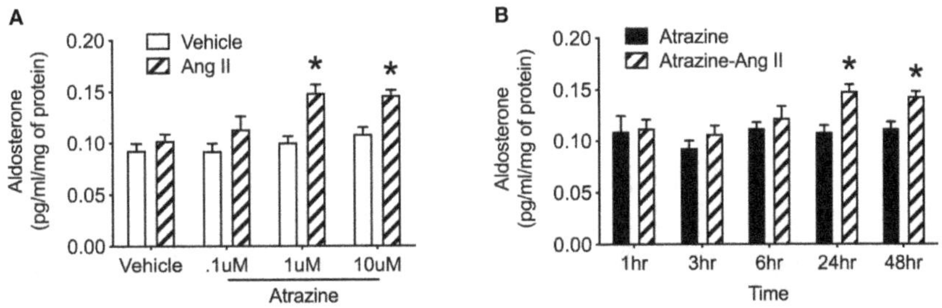

FIGURE 4 | Atrazine increases Ang II-induced aldosterone synthesis in human adrenal cell lines. **(A)** Histogram depicting mean media concentration of aldosterone (pg/ml/mg) in cell cultures treated with atrazine (.1, 1.0, or 10.0 μm) or atrazine plus Ang II (0.1 nM). Atrazine treatment was 24 h in duration. **(B)** Histogram depicting mean media concentration of aldosterone (pg/ml/mg) in media of H295R cell cultures treated with atrazine (1 μm; solid black bars) or atrazine plus Ang II (0.1 nM). Atrazine treatment was 1, 3, 6, 24, or 48 h in duration. Data presented as the mean ± SEM. Asterisk signifies difference from control group ($P < 0.05$).

systolic (**Figure 5C**, $F_{(1, 37)} = 6.03$, $P = 0.019$), and diastolic pressure (**Figure 5D**, $F_{(1, 37)} = 14.4$, $P = 0.0005$). There was no significant effect of treatment on animal body weight (**Supplementary Table 1**, $F_{(1, 32)} = 0.53$, $P = 0.47$).

Experiment 6. Effects of Atrazine Treatment on Select Gene Expression

There was no effect of atrazine treatment on the adrenal expression of CYP11B1, StAR, and AT1R (**Figure 6**, t(8) = 0.32, $P = 0.76$; t(8) = 1.65, $P = 0.138$; t(8) = 0.32, $P = 0.76$; t(8) = 0.2.1, $P = 0.069$). However, aldosterone synthase (CYP11B2) was significantly lower in atrazine treated animals compared to controls (t(8) = 7.43, $P < 0.0001$). In heart and kidney tissues, there was no effect of atrazine treatment on AT1R expression (t(8) = 1.93, $P = 0.088$; t(8) = 1.69, $P = 0.13$, respectively). There was no significant effect of treatment on animal body weight (**Supplementary Table 1**, $F_{(1, 32)} = 0.70$, $P = 0.41$).

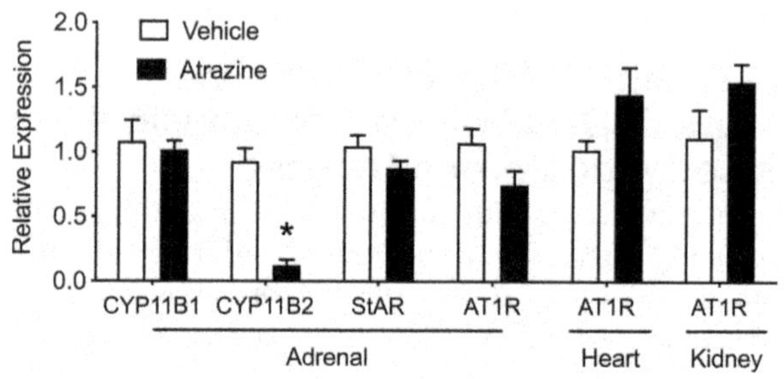

FIGURE 6 | Effects of atrazine treatment on select gene expression of the adrenal, heart and kidney. Histogram depicting the fold change expression of CYP11B1 (11β-Hydroxylase), CYP11B2 (aldosterone synthase), steroidogenic acute regulatory (StAR) protein, angiotensin II receptor type 1 (AT_1R) expression in the adrenal, heart, and kidney of vehicle (clear bar) or atrazine (black bar, 100 mg/kg). Data presented as the mean ± SEM. Asterisk signifies difference from control group ($P < 0.05$).

DISCUSSION

We and others have demonstrated that atrazine acts centrally to induce a "stress-like" response resulting in a rapid rise in ACTH and corticosterone plasma concentrations (11, 13, 16, 22, 23). Prolonged atrazine treatment can lead to altered adrenal and thymus weights (24–26) which are also identified in repeatedly stressed animals with sustained elevated stress hormones (27–30). Specifically, we have demonstrated that repeated atrazine exposure can alter adrenal cortical morphology with a reduction in zG thickness (11). At the time of previous reports, we attributed atrazine-induced adrenal morphology changes to repeated adrenal stimulation *via* ACTH release because the morphology change mimicked those of repeatedly stressed animals and atrazine had no direct, stimulatory effects on the adrenal (11, 14, 31). In the current work, we tested this theory by treating animals with atrazine, vehicle, or restraint stress for 4 days (**Figure 1**, **Table 2**). There was a significant reduction in aldosterone synthase immunoreactivity and expression in both atrazine and stressed groups when compared to control animals.

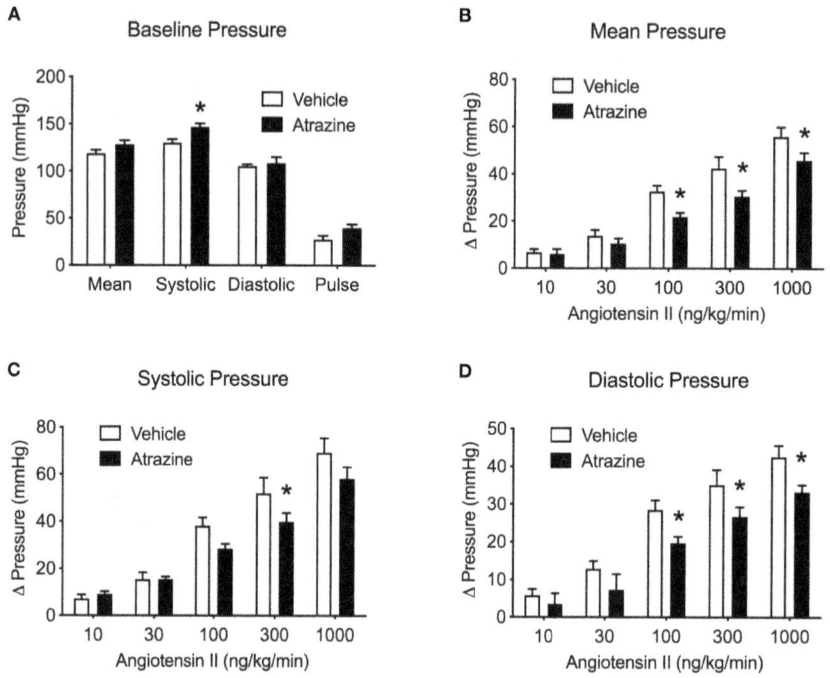

FIGURE 5 | Atrazine treatment alters basal arterial pressure and attenuates pressor effects of Ang II infusion. Histograms depicting the baseline blood pressure **(A)** in vehicle and atrazine (100 mg/kg) treated animals and changes in mean **(B)**, systolic **(C)** and diastolic **(D)** pressures in vehicle or atrazine treated animals during angiotensin infusion (10-1000 ng/kg/min). Data presented as the mean ± SEM. Asterisk signifies difference from control group ($P < 0.05$).

Similarly, there was a significant reduction in the zG thickness in both stressed and atrazine treated groups compared to control animals. Chronically stressed animals present with hyperplasia and hypertrophy in the zF, and reduced cell size in the zona glomerulosa (14). The 4-day treatment duration in the present study did not result in significant zF changes but did reduce zG thickness. The present findings suggest activation of the stress response or ACTH treatment first acts to reduce zG activity then increases zF thickness over a longer time period (32). There was no difference found between stressed and atrazine treated animals except for a reduced cell density in the zF. There was a significant reduction in zona glomerulosa thickness in atrazine and stressed treated animals with no change in other cortical layers or total cortical thickness. The lack of significant change in total cortical thickness is explained by a matter of proportion. The adrenal cortex is approximately 90% zona fasciculata and zona reticularis combined. Therefore, small but significant changes to the zona glomerulosa thickness is insignificant when combined with other cortical zones.

The acute rate-limiting step mediating aldosterone production includes the activation of steroidogenic acute regulatory protein (StAR). StAR regulates the transport of cholesterol from the outer to the inner mitochondrial membrane. The transcriptional and translational regulation of StAR controls the expression level of the 37 kDa StAR protein (33–37). Aldosterone synthase (CYP11B2) present in the zG catalyzes the final steps in the production of aldosterone from cholesterol acetate. This is accomplished in three separate reactions converting 11-deoxycorticosterone to aldosterone *via* intermediates corticosterone and 18-hydroxycorticosterone by aldosterone synthase (38). ACTH in repeatedly stressed animals or cultured zG cells causes regression of the zona glomerulosa and suppression of aldosterone synthase expression (14, 39, 40). Similarly, low-dose infusion of ACTH in human subjects results in an initial increase in plasma aldosterone levels during the first 12–36 h, but a slow decline in these values in subsequent days (41). The mechanism for ACTH-mediated repression of aldosterone production and aldosterone synthase expression remains unknown. One theory postulates that repeated ACTH stimulation induces CYP11B1 and CYP17, the activities of which direct the precursors of the steroidogenic pathway away from the production of aldosterone, and towards that of cortisol or corticosterone (42). CYP11B2 immunoreactivity and expression were significantly lower in atrazine and stressed animals (**Figure 1**).

To determine if the reduction in aldosterone synthase in the zG of stressed and atrazine treated animals would lead to reduced adrenal response to stimulation, animals were restraint stressed or treated with atrazine for 4 days and then challenged with Ang II. As predicted, stressed animals, after Ang II stimulation, had lower AUC aldosterone plasma concentrations when compared to vehicle and atrazine treated groups (**Figure 2**). While this is the first *in vivo* report, attenuated Ang II-induced aldosterone release from adrenal tissue from repeatedly restraint stressed animals has been reported previously (31). In contrast to stressed animals, after Ang II stimulation, atrazine treated animals had higher circulating aldosterone concentrations in both peak levels and AUC when compared to vehicle and stressed animals. This finding led us to reject our original hypothesis, that repeated stress and atrazine treatment would have similar effects on the zG resulting in lowered aldosterone secretion after stimulation.

To better understand the surprising findings of increased aldosterone release in atrazine treated animals, the response to Ang II stimulation was assayed after 1, 2, 3, or 4 days of atrazine treatment. Plasma atrazine concentrations peak 2 hours post gavage in the rat with the majority of atrazine and its metabolites cleared from the animal by 24 hours (43, 44). If atrazine potentiated aldosterone producing cells in a rapid pharmacological manner, aldosterone concentrations would predictably be as high or higher in 1 or 2 day treated groups than animals treated for 4 days because atrazine-induced ACTH would not have driven down aldosterone synthase expression after 1 or 2 exposures. However, there was no difference in aldosterone concentrations between atrazine and vehicle treated groups after 1 or 2 days of treatment (**Figure 3**). After 3 and 4 days of atrazine treatment, the AUC of plasma atrazine concentrations were higher than vehicle treated groups. Peak aldosterone concentrations after Ang II treatment were only significantly above control animals after 4 days of atrazine treatment suggesting the need for multiple exposures and cell physiological changes, most likely, dependent on gene expression changes. While not definitive, our current findings suggest that the increased aldosterone production in atrazine treated animals is not due to a short-term pharmacological action of atrazine but more likely at the level of gene regulation, particularly at the levels of AT1 receptor, StAR or CYP11B2. However, while CYP11B2 was reduced, atrazine treatment had no effect on adrenal AT1 receptor or StAR expression (**Figure 6**).

Aldosterone production is primarily regulated by the renin-angiotensin-aldosterone system which involves multiple organs and organ systems including the kidneys, gastrointestinal tract, and ingestive behavior. To reduce these variables, human adrenocortical carcinoma cells, H295R, were pretreated with atrazine. A dose response experiment identified an Ang II concentration to minimally stimulate aldosterone release in culture. This allowed for the identification of possible atrazine-induced potentiated stimulation (**Supplemental Figure 1**). Adrenal cells pre-treated with 1 or 10 μM of atrazine followed by Ang II stimulation had higher aldosterone concentrations in their media (**Figure 4A**). However, aldosterone concentrations were only elevated in atrazine pre-treated cultures plus Ang II after 24 and 48 hours but not after 1, 3, or 6 hours of atrazine treatment (**Figure 4B**). Similar to *in vivo* findings, atrazine induced-aldosterone potentiation *in vitro* does not occur when extracellular atrazine concentrations are at their highest but after prolonged exposure. This further supports atrazine acting through gene alteration rather than acute pharmacological effects.

Atrazine treated animals presented with significantly higher systolic baseline blood pressure and a significantly reduced response to Ang II in arterial, systolic, and diastolic pressure (**Figure 5**). Atrazine treatment has previously been linked to cardiovascular issues in mice (45) and dogs (46). Treatment with atrazine or its metabolite diaminochlorotriazine (DACT) to male and female beagles results in significant signs of cardiovascular issues including cardiac lesions, cardiac hypertrophy, and atrial fibrillation (46–48). Similarly, male mice treated with atrazine present with cardiac lesions after 21 days of treatment (46).

Although the reported cardiac issues associated with atrazine treatment are vague and not well characterized, prolonged elevated plasma aldosterone concentrations or hyper-aldosteronism resulting in elevated blood pressure can lead to atrial fibrillation, cardiac lesions, and cardiac hypertrophy (49–52).

Atrazine animals had reduced changes in blood pressure in response to Ang II. There was no difference in AT1R expression in heart tissue or kidney tissue (**Figure 6**). The mechanism of reduced response to Ang II stimulated blood pressure in atrazine treated animals is unknown. Perhaps atrazine animals are responding normally to Ang II stimulation but their elevated basal pressure results in a significantly smaller change from basal blood pressure. Atrazine treatment had no effect on blood pH or electrolyte levels suggesting no major alteration of kidney function (**Supplemental Table S2**). However, blood analysis was performed on atrazine and control animals not challenged with Ang II.

While all of our current evidence implicates a direct action of atrazine on aldosterone-producing cells of the adrenal, there are multiple other mediators of the renin-angiotensin-aldosterone system (RAAS) which need to be investigated further such as renin, angiotensin converting enzyme, and endogenous angiotensin concentrations. There may also be an autonomic response to atrazine exposure which could potentiate aldosterone release. The splanchnic innervation of the adrenal acts as an extra-angiotensin mechanism in the control of aldosterone secretion. Splanchnic nerve activation leads to release of catecholamines (epinephrine, norepinephrine, and dopamine). Catecholamines have been shown to directly stimulate aldosterone production (53). Ang II infusion can also potentiate the release of catecholamines from the adrenal medulla during splanchnic nerve stimulation (54). Atrazine could work to potentiate the paracrine stimulatory action of catecholamines on aldosterone release. However, elevated catecholamines are immunosuppressive and our work has demonstrated no immune toxicity in response to similar atrazine treatment (26, 55).

Our original report of atrazine-induced changes in adrenal morphology was performed in ovarectomized females to control for variation in the ovarian cycle and in conjunction to examining atrazine's effects on luteinizing hormone pulsatile and pre-ovulatory surge release. Estrogens elicit direct vasodilatory effects *in vivo*, albeit they may affect blood pressure also through other mechanisms, including inhibition of sympathetic tone (56). In adrenal cells, estradiol, working through ERβ, inhibits CYP11B2 expression (57–59). The use of ovarectomized animals most likely increased the potential synthesis of aldosterone. Preliminary data suggests atrazine potentiation of Ang II-stimulated aldosterone release persists in estradiol treated animals. However, as predicted, treatment with estradiol reduces Ang II-induced aldosterone concentrations equally across treatments (data not shown). It may be more difficult to identify atrazine-induced reduction in zona glomerulosa thickness in intact females. Estrogen reduces zona glomerulosa activity and presumably cell size (60). Males should also be included in future investigations since males present with higher aldosterone levels than females and perhaps are more responsive to endogenous Ang II stimulation (61).

In the current study we have shown that adrenal cells of atrazine treated animals respond to Ang II with increased release of aldosterone compared with stressed or control animals. In addition, atrazine treatment results in enhancement of aldosterone release from cultured human adrenocortical cells. In addition, atrazine treated animals present with higher baseline blood pressure and possessed a lower response to Ang II treatment than vehicle treated control groups. Aldosterone plays a central role in the regulation of systemic arterial pressure through its systemic synthesis *via* the renin-angiotensin aldosterone cascade (62).

Pathological consequences of excess mineralocorticoid activity included high blood pressure and evidence of myocardial necrosis and fibrosis (63, 64). Recent work suggests aldosterone has widespread cardiovascular and metabolic effects, beyond its effects on fluid and electrolyte balance (65). Aldosterone increases superoxide generation (66, 67). This may involve decreases in glucose-6-phosphate dehydrogenase activity and increases in NADPH oxidase. Atrazine treatment has also been linked to increased oxidative stress but the mechanism is not known (21, 68, 69). Atrazine treated animals displayed increased Ang II-induced aldosterone plasma concentrations after 3 and 4 days of treatment but not after 1 or 2 days of atrazine treatment. After 4 days of atrazine treatment, blood pressure was elevated. The required duration of atrazine dosing suggests possible prolonged effects. Roger et al. (2014) reported that rat dams treated with 125 mg/kg of atrazine over gestational days 16 through 20 produced adult offspring with elevated basal blood pressure (70). It is not known how long the atrazine-induced increased aldosterone stimulation will be sustained after treatment termination but the long-term effects on blood pressure after gestational exposure may suggest similar mechanisms at play.

As stated previously, aldosterone synthesis is primarily regulated by the rate limiting enzymatic work of StAR and CYP11B2. While expression of StAR and CYP11B2 levels are correlated with the degree of aldosterone synthesis, there are post-translational modification and phosphorylation events that can mediate their activity. Translational regulation controls the level of expression of the 37 kDa StAR protein, while phosphorylation of StAR is crucial for its activity (33–37). Increased intracellular calcium levels, following Ang II treatment, causes increased StAR activation in the H295R cell line (71–73) as well as primary cultures of bovine adrenocortical cells (74, 75). Atrazine has been shown in multiple cell types to be a specific phosphodiesterase (PDE) inhibitor (76–80). In adrenal cells, inhibition of PDE activity is associated with increased steroidogenesis (81, 82). Some Cushing syndrome cases have been linked to mutations to PDE subtypes (83). Although atrazine treatment does not directly stimulate zG cells, it may inhibit PDE activity and thus allow enhanced stimulation of zG cells in response to Ang II treatment. However, the timing and duration of atrazine treatment (>2 days) required for increased Ang II response does not support a direct pharmacological mechanism on PDE, however, additional work is needed to fully investigate a role for PDE inhibition in atrazine's effects on aldosterone synthesis.

Due to its convenience of use, low cost, weed control efficacy, and relatively long half-life in the environment, atrazine is one of the most commonly identified herbicides in water sources (84, 85). While banned in many countries, atrazine is widely used in the United States and is often found in water sources above the

While banned in many countries, atrazine is widely used in the United States and is often found in water sources above the Environmental Protection Agency's mandated limit (4, 86, 87). Atrazine exposure in humans and animals has been linked to cardiovascular changes with no defined underlining cause (45, 70, 88–91). Future investigations will focus on the long-term effects of atrazine exposure on aldosterone regulation and establishing a No Observed Adverse Effect Level (NOAEL). Indeed, more work is needed to understand the effects of atrazine on aldosterone production and the ramifications of atrazine exposure to the renin-angiotensin-aldosterone system, blood pressure, kidney function, and the possible long-term effects of their disruption.

AUTHOR CONTRIBUTIONS

CF, LM, and AZ contributed to conception and design of the study. DS, CR, RK, and MJ were instrumental in performing experiments. CF and LM performed the statistical analysis. CF and AZ wrote the first draft of the manuscript. All authors contributed to the article and approved the submitted version.

FUNDING

This research was funded by the Animal Health and Disease Research Program, College of Veterinary Medicine, Auburn University.

REFERENCES

1. Benbrook CM. Trends in Glyphosate Herbicide Use in the United States and Globally. *Environ Sci Eur* (2016) 28(1):3. doi: 10.1186/s12302-016-0070-0
2. USGS. *Estimated Annual Agricultural Pesticide Use*. Washington, D.C.: US Geological Survey (2021). Available at: https://water.usgs.gov/nawqa/pnsp/usage/maps/county-level/PreliminaryEstimates/EPest.county.estimates.2013.txt.
3. Comber SDW. Abiotic Persistence of Atrazine and Simazine in Water. *Pesticide Sci* (1999) 55(7):696–702. doi: 10.1002/(SICI)1096-9063(199907)55:7<696::AID-PS11>3.0.CO;2-7
4. EPA. *National Primary Drinking Water Regulations*. Washington, D.C.: Environmental Protection Agency (2021). Available at: https://www.epa.gov/ground-water-and-drinking-water/national-primary-drinking-water-regulations.
5. Tischer W, Strotmann H. Relationship Between Inhibitor Binding by Chloroplasts and Inhibition of Photosynthetic Electron Transport. *Biochim Biophys Acta* (1977) 460(1):113–25. doi: 10.1016/0005-2728(77)90157-8
6. Erickson JM, Pfister K, Rahire M, Togasaki RK, Mets L, Rochaix JD. Molecular and Biophysical Analysis of Herbicide-Resistant Mutants of Chlamydomonas Reinhardtii: Structure-Function Relationship of the Photosystem II D1 Polypeptide. *Plant Cell* (1989) 1(3):361–71. doi: 10.1105/tpc.1.3.361
7. Foradori CD, Hinds LR, Hanneman WH, Handa RJ. Effects of Atrazine and Its Withdrawal on Gonadotropin-Releasing Hormone Neuroendocrine Function in the Adult Female Wistar Rat. *Biol Reprod* (2009) 81(6):1099–105. doi: 10.1095/biolreprod.109.077453
8. Foradori CD, Hinds LR, Hanneman WH, Legare ME, Clay CM, Handa RJ. Atrazine Inhibits Pulsatile Luteinizing Hormone Release Without Altering Pituitary Sensitivity to a Gonadotropin-Releasing Hormone Receptor Agonist in Female Wistar Rats. *Biol Reprod* (2009) 81(1):40–5. doi: 10.1095/biolreprod.108.075713
9. Foradori CD, Zimmerman AD, Hinds LR, Zuloaga KL, Breckenridge CB, Handa RJ. Atrazine Inhibits Pulsatile Gonadotropin-Releasing Hormone (GnRH) Release Without Altering GnRH Messenger RNA or Protein Levels in the Female Rat. *Biol Reprod* (2013) 88(1):9. doi: 10.1095/biolreprod.112.102277
10. Cooper RL, Laws SC, Das PC, Narotsky MG, Goldman JM, Lee Tyrey E, et al. Atrazine and Reproductive Function: Mode and Mechanism of Action Studies. *Birth Defects Res B Dev Reprod Toxicol* (2007) 80(2):98–112. doi: 10.1002/bdrb.20110
11. Foradori CD, Healy JE, Zimmerman AD, Kemppainen RJ, Jones MA, Read CC, et al. Characterization of Activation of the Hypothalamic-Pituitary-Adrenal Axis by the Herbicide Atrazine in the Female Rat. *Endocrinology* (2018) 159(9):3378–88. doi: 10.1210/en.2018-00474
12. Hotchkiss MG, Best DS, Cooper RL, Laws SC. Atrazine Does Not Induce Pica Behavior at Doses That Increase Hypothalamic-Pituitary-Adrenal Axis Activation and Cause Conditioned Taste Avoidance. *Neurotoxicol Teratol* (2012) 34(3):295–302. doi: 10.1016/j.ntt.2012.03.001
13. Laws SC, Hotchkiss M, Ferrell J, Jayaraman S, Mills L, Modic W, et al. Chlorotriazine Herbicides and Metabolites Activate an ACTH-Dependent Release of Corticosterone in Male Wistar Rats. *Toxicol Sci* (2009) 112(1):78–87. doi: 10.1093/toxsci/kfp190
14. Ulrich-Lai YM, Figueiredo HF, Ostrander MM, Choi DC, Engeland WC, Herman JP. Chronic Stress Induces Adrenal Hyperplasia and Hypertrophy in a Subregion-Specific Manner. *Am J Physiol Endocrinol Metab* (2006) 291(5): E965–73. doi: 10.1152/ajpendo.00070.2006
15. Aguilera G, Kiss A, Lu A, Camacho C. Regulation of Adrenal Steroidogenesis During Chronic Stress. *Endocrine Res* (1996) 22(4):433–43. doi: 10.1080/07435809609043729
16. Fraites MJ, Cooper RL, Buckalew A, Jayaraman S, Mills L, Laws SC. Characterization of the Hypothalamic-Pituitary-Adrenal Axis Response to Atrazine and Metabolites in the Female Rat. *Toxicol Sci* (2009) 112(1):88–99. doi: 10.1093/toxsci/kfp194
17. Foradori CD, Hinds LR, Quihuis AM, Lacagnina AF, Breckenridge CB, Handa RJ. The Differential Effect of Atrazine on Luteinizing Hormone Release in Adrenalectomized Adult Female Wistar Rats. *Biol Reprod* (2011) 85(4):684–9. doi: 10.1095/biolreprod.111.092452
18. Tinkey P, Lembo T, Craig S, West C, Van Pelt C. Use of the i-STAT Portable Clinical Analyzer in Mice. *Lab Anim (NY)* (2006) 35(2):45–50. doi: 10.1038/laban0206-45
19. Keiver K, Duggal S, Simpson ME. Ethanol Administration Results in a Prolonged Decrease in Blood Ionized Calcium Levels in the Rat. *Alcohol* (2005) 37(3):173–8. doi: 10.1016/j.alcohol.2005.07.008
20. Bradford MM. A Rapid and Sensitive Method for the Quantitation of Microgram Quantities of Protein Utilizing the Principle of Protein-Dye Binding. *Analytical Biochem* (1976) 72:248–54. doi: 10.1016/0003-2697(76)90527-3
21. Zimmerman AD, Breckenridge CB, Yi KD, Sawhney Coder P, Wanders D, Judd RL, et al. Changes in Hepatic Phase I and Phase II Biotransformation Enzyme Expression and Glutathione Levels Following Atrazine Exposure in Female Rats. *Xenobiotica* (2018) 48(9):867–81. doi: 10.1080/00498254.2017.1374486
22. Tinfo NS, Hotchkiss MG, Buckalew AR, Zorrilla LM, Cooper RL, Laws SC. Understanding the Effects of Atrazine on Steroidogenesis in Rat Granulosa and H295R Adrenal Cortical Carcinoma Cells. *Reprod Toxicol* (2011) 31(2):184–93. doi: 10.1016/j.reprotox.2010.11.005
23. Riffle BW, Klinefelter GR, Cooper RL, Winnik WM, Swank A, Jayaraman S, et al. Novel Molecular Events Associated With Altered Steroidogenesis Induced by Exposure to Atrazine in the Intact and Castrate Male Rat. *Reprod Toxicol* (2014) 47:59–69. doi: 10.1016/j.reprotox.2014.05.008
24. Eldridge JC, Fleenor-Heyser DG, Extrom PC, Wetzel LT, Breckenridge CB, Gillis JH, et al. Short-Term Effects of Chlorotriazines on Estrus in Female Sprague-Dawley and Fischer 344 Rats. *J Toxicol Environ Health* (1994) 43(2):155–67. doi: 10.1080/15287399409531912
25. Victor-Costa AB, Bandeira SM, Oliveira AG, Mahecha GA, Oliveira CA. Changes in Testicular Morphology and Steroidogenesis in Adult Rats Exposed to Atrazine. *Reprod Toxicol* (2010) 29(3):323–31. doi: 10.1016/j.reprotox.2009.12.006
26. Foradori CD, Zimmerman AD, Coder PS, Peachee VL, Handa RJ, Kimber I, et al. Lack of Immunotoxic Effects of Repeated Exposure to Atrazine

Associated With the Adaptation of Adrenal Gland Activation. *Regul Toxicol Pharmacol* (2017) 89:200–14. doi: 10.1016/j.yrtph.2017.07.017
27. van Vliet E, Melis M, van Ewijk W. The Influence of Dexamethasone Treatment on the Lymphoid and Stromal Composition of the Mouse Thymus: A Flowcytometric and Immunohistological Analysis. *Cell Immunol* (1986) 103(2):229–40. doi: 10.1016/0008-8749(86)90086-9
28. Blanchard RJ, Nikulina JN, Sakai RR, McKittrick C, McEwen B, Blanchard DC. Behavioral and Endocrine Change Following Chronic Predatory Stress. *Physiol Behav* (1998) 63(4):561–9. doi: 10.1016/s0031-9384(97)00508-8
29. Gamallo A, Villanua A, Trancho G, Fraile A. Stress Adaptation and Adrenal Activity in Isolated and Crowded Rats. *Physiol Behav* (1986) 36(2):217–21. doi: 10.1016/0031-9384(86)90006-5
30. Hu Y, Gursoy E, Cardounel A, Kalimi M. Biological Effects of Single and Repeated Swimming Stress in Male Rats: Beneficial Effects of Glucocorticoids. *Endocrine* (2000) 13(1):123–9. doi: 10.1385/ENDO:13:1:123
31. Aguilera G, Kiss A, Sunar-Akbasak B. Hyperreninemic Hypoaldosteronism After Chronic Stress in the Rat. *J Clin Invest* (1995) 96(3):1512–9. doi: 10.1172/JCI118189
32. Hattangady NG, Olala LO, Bollag WB, Rainey WE. Acute and Chronic Regulation of Aldosterone Production. *Mol Cell Endocrinol* (2012) 350 (2):151–62. doi: 10.1016/j.mce.2011.07.034
33. Krueger RJ, Orme-Johnson NR. Acute Adrenocorticotropic Hormone Stimulation of Adrenal Corticosteroidogenesis. Discovery of a Rapidly Induced Protein. *J Biol Chem* (1983) 258(16):10159–67. doi: 10.1016/S0021-9258(17)44619-9
34. Alberta JA, Epstein LF, Pon LA, Orme-Johnson NR. Mitochondrial Localization of a Phosphoprotein That Rapidly Accumulates in Adrenal Cortex Cells Exposed to Adrenocorticotropic Hormone or to Camp. *J Biol Chem* (1989) 264(4):2368–72. doi: 10.1016/S0021-9258(18)94186-4
35. Clark BJ, Wells J, King SR, Stocco DM. The Purification, Cloning, and Expression of a Novel Luteinizing Hormone-Induced Mitochondrial Protein in MA-10 Mouse Leydig Tumor Cells. Characterization of the Steroidogenic Acute Regulatory Protein (Star). *J Biol Chem* (1994) 269(45):28314–22. doi: 10.1016/S0021-9258(18)46930-X
36. Estabrook RW, Rainey WE. Twinkle, Twinkle Little StAR, How We Wonder What You are. *Proc Natl Acad Sci USA* (1996) 93(24):13552–4. doi: 10.1073/pnas.93.24.13552
37. Clark BJ, Stocco DM. Steroidogenic Acute Regulatory Protein: The StAR Still Shines Brightly. *Mol Cell Endocrinol* (1997) 134(1):1–8. doi: 10.1016/s0303-7207(97)00166-4
38. Cerny MA. Progress Towards Clinically Useful Aldosterone Synthase Inhibitors. *Curr Top Med Chem* (2013) 13(12):1385–401. doi: 10.2174/1568026611313120003
39. Mitani F, Miyamoto H, Mukai K, Ishimura Y. Effects of Long Term Stimulation of ACTH and Angiotensin II-Secretions on the Rat Adrenal Cortex. *Endocr Res* (1996) 22(4):421–31. doi: 10.1080/07435809609043728
40. Holland OB, Carr B. Modulation of Aldosterone Synthase Messenger Ribonucleic Acid Levels by Dietary Sodium and Potassium and by Adrenocorticotropin. *Endocrinology* (1993) 132(6):2666–73. doi: 10.1210/endo.132.6.8389287
41. Fuchs-Hammoser R, Schweiger M, Oelkers W. The Effect of Chronic Low-Dose Infusion of ACTH (1-24) on Renin, Renin-Substrate, Aldosterone and Other Corticosteroids in Sodium Replete and Deplete Man. *Acta Endocrinol (Copenh)* (1980) 95(2):198–206. doi: 10.1530/acta.0.0950198
42. Bird IM, Pasquarette MM, Rainey WE, Mason JI. Differential Control of 17 Alpha-Hydroxylase and 3 Beta-Hydroxysteroid Dehydrogenase Expression in Human Adrenocortical H295R Cells. *J Clin Endocrinol Metab* (1996) 81 (6):2171–8. doi: 10.1210/jcem.81.6.8964847
43. McMullin TS, Brzezicki JM, Cranmer BK, Tessari JD, Andersen ME. Pharmacokinetic Modeling of Disposition and Time-Course Studies With [14C]Atrazine. *J Toxicol Environ Health Part A* (2003) 66(10):941–64. doi: 10.1080/15287390306454
44. Campbell JLJr., Andersen ME, Hinderliter PM, Yi KD, Pastoor TP, Breckenridge CB, et al. Pbpk Model for Atrazine and Its Chlorotriazine Metabolites in Rat and Human. *Toxicol Sci* (2016) 150(2):441–53. doi: 10.1093/toxsci/kfw014
45. Lin J, Li HX, Xia J, Li XN, Jiang XQ, Zhu SY, et al. The Chemopreventive Potential of Lycopene Against Atrazine-Induced Cardiotoxicity: Modulation of Ionic Homeostasis. *Sci Rep* (2016) 6:24855. doi: 10.1038/srep24855
46. Gammon DW, Silva M, Aldous C, Sanborn JR, Carr WC, Pfeifer K, et al. *Atrazine Risk Characterization Document.* Sacramento, California: Medical Toxicology Branch, California Department Pesticide Regulation California Environment Protection Agency (2001).
47. EPA. *Iris Atrazine Casrn 1912-24-9 (01/01/91), Integrated Risk Information System.* UEP Agency, editor. Washington, DC: United State Environmental Protection Agency (1991).
48. EPA and Agency USEP. *Atrazine Label Amendment, Special Review Branch, Special Review and Reregistration Division, April 17, 1992.* Washington, DC United State Environmental Protection Agency (1992).
49. Brilla CG, Pick R, Tan LB, Janicki JS, Weber KT. Remodeling of the Rat Right and Left Ventricles in Experimental Hypertension. *Circ Res* (1990) 67 (6):1355–64. doi: 10.1161/01.res.67.6.1355
50. Young M, Fullerton M, Dilley R, Funder J. Mineralocorticoids, Hypertension, and Cardiac Fibrosis. *J Clin Invest* (1994) 93(6):2578–83. doi: 10.1172/JCI117269
51. Sun Y, Zhang J, Lu L, Chen SS, Quinn MT, Weber KT. Aldosterone-Induced Inflammation in the Rat Heart: Role of Oxidative Stress. *Am J Pathol* (2002) 161(5):1773–81. doi: 10.1016/S0002-9440(10)64454-9
52. Seccia TM, Caroccia B, Adler GK, Maiolino G, Cesari M, Rossi GP. Arterial Hypertension, Atrial Fibrillation, and Hyperaldosteronism: The Triple Trouble. *Hypertension* (2017) 69(4):545–50. doi: 10.1161/HYPERTENSIONAHA.116.08956
53. Bornstein SR, Ehrhart-Bornstein M, Scherbaum WA, Pfeiffer EF, Holst JJ. Effects of Splanchnic Nerve Stimulation on the Adrenal Cortex may be Mediated by Chromaffin Cells in a Paracrine Manner. *Endocrinology* (1990) 127(2):900–6. doi: 10.1210/endo-127-2-900
54. Foucart S, de Champlain J, Nadeau R. Modulation by Beta-Adrenoceptors and Angiotensin II Receptors of Splanchnic Nerve Evoked Catecholamine Release From the Adrenal Medulla. *Can J Physiol Pharmacol* (1991) 69(1):1–7. doi: 10.1139/y91-001
55. Shaw DM, Merien F, Braakhuis A, Dulson D. T-Cells and Their Cytokine Production: The Anti-Inflammatory and Immunosuppressive Effects of Strenuous Exercise. *Cytokine* (2018) 104:136–42. doi: 10.1016/j.cyto.2017.10.001
56. Meyer MR, Haas E, Barton M. Gender Differences of Cardiovascular Disease: New Perspectives for Estrogen Receptor Signaling. *Hypertension* (2006) 47 (6):1019–26. doi: 10.1161/01.HYP.0000223064.62762.0b
57. Caroccia B, Seccia TM, Campos AG, Gioco F, Kuppusamy M, Ceolotto G, et al. GPER-1 and Estrogen Receptor-Beta Ligands Modulate Aldosterone Synthesis. *Endocrinology* (2014) 155(11):4296–304. doi: 10.1210/en.2014-1416
58. Clark JT, Chakraborty-Chatterjee M, Hamblin M, Wyss JM, Fentie IH. Estrogen Depletion Differentially Affects Blood Pressure Depending on Age in Long-Evans Rats. *Endocrine* (2004) 25(2):173–86. doi: 10.1385/ENDO:25:2:173
59. Roesch DM, Tian Y, Zheng W, Shi M, Verbalis JG, Sandberg K. Estradiol Attenuates Angiotensin-Induced Aldosterone Secretion in Ovariectomized Rats. *Endocrinology* (2000) 141(12):4629–36. doi: 10.1210/endo.141.12.7822
60. Macova M, Armando I, Zhou J, Baiardi G, Tyurmin D, Larrayoz-Roldan IM, et al. Estrogen Reduces Aldosterone, Upregulates Adrenal Angiotensin II AT2 Receptors and Normalizes Adrenomedullary Fra-2 in Ovariectomized Rats. *Neuroendocrinology* (2008) 88(4):276–86. doi: 10.1159/000150977
61. Toering TJ, Gant CM, Visser FW, van der Graaf AM, Laverman GD, Danser AHJ, et al. Sex Differences in Renin-Angiotensin-Aldosterone System Affect Extracellular Volume in Healthy Subjects. *Am J Physiol Renal Physiol* (2018) 314(5):F873–F8. doi: 10.1152/ajprenal.00109.2017
62. Sealey JE, Laragh JH. The Renin–Angiotensin–Aldosterone System for Normal Regulation of Blood Pressure and Sodium and Potassium Homeostasis. In: JH Laragh, BM Brenner, editors. *Hypertension: Pathophysiology, Diagnosis, and Management.* New York, NY: Raven Press (1990). p. 1287.
63. Selye H. The General Adaptation Syndrome and the Diseases of Adaptation. *J Clin Endocrinol Metab* (1946) 6:117–230. doi: 10.1210/jcem-6-2-117
64. Selye H. Protection by a Steroid-Spirolactone Against Certain Types of Cardiac Necroses. *Proc Soc Exp Biol Med* (1960) 104:212–3. doi: 10.3181/00379727-104-25782
65. Monticone S, D'Ascenzo F, Moretti C, Williams TA, Veglio F, Gaita F, et al. Cardiovascular Events and Target Organ Damage in Primary Aldosteronism Compared With Essential Hypertension: A Systematic Review and Meta-Analysis. *Lancet Diabetes Endocrinol* (2018) 6(1):41–50. doi: 10.1016/S2213-8587(17)30319-4

66. Leopold JA, Dam A, Maron BA, Scribner AW, Liao R, Handy DE, et al. Aldosterone Impairs Vascular Reactivity by Decreasing Glucose-6-Phosphate Dehydrogenase Activity. *Nat Med* (2007) 13(2):189–97. doi: 10.1038/nm1545
67. Iwashima F, Yoshimoto T, Minami I, Sakurada M, Hirono Y, Hirata Y. Aldosterone Induces Superoxide Generation *Via* Rac1 Activation in Endothelial Cells. *Endocrinology* (2008) 149(3):1009–14. doi: 10.1210/en.2007-0864
68. Singh M, Sandhir R, Kiran R. Oxidative Stress Induced by Atrazine in Rat Erythrocytes: Mitigating Effect of Vitamin E. *Toxicol Mech Methods* (2010) 20 (3):119–26. doi: 10.3109/15376511003606253
69. Bhatti JS, Sidhu IP, Bhatti GK. Ameliorative Action of Melatonin on Oxidative Damage Induced by Atrazine Toxicity in Rat Erythrocytes. *Mol Cell Biochem* (2011) 353(1-2):139–49. doi: 10.1007/s11010-011-0780-y
70. Rogers JM, Ellis-Hutchings RG, Grey BE, Zucker RM, Norwood J Jr, Grace CE, et al. Elevated Blood Pressure in Offspring of Rats Exposed to Diverse Chemicals During Pregnancy. *Toxicol Sci* (2014) 137(2):436–46. doi: 10.1093/toxsci/kft248
71. Clark BJ, Pezzi V, Stocco DM, Rainey WE. The Steroidogenic Acute Regulatory Protein Is Induced by Angiotensin II and K+ in H295R Adrenocortical Cells. *Mol Cell Endocrinol* (1995) 115(2):215–19. doi: 10.1016/0303-7207(95)03683-0
72. Olala LO, Choudhary V, Johnson MH, Bollag WB. Angiotensin II-induced Protein Kinase D Activates the ATF/CREB Family of Transcription Factors and Promotes StAR mRNA Expression. *Endocrinology* (2014) 155(7):2524–33. doi: 10.1210/en.2013-1485
73. Nanba K, Chen A, Nishimoto K, Rainey WE. Role of Ca(2+)/calmodulin-dependent Protein Kinase Kinase in Adrenal Aldosterone Production. *Endocrinology* (2015) 156(5):1750–6. doi: 10.1210/en.2014-1782
74. Betancourt-Calle S, Calle RA, Isales CM, White S, Rasmussen H, Bollag WB. Differential Effects of Agonists of Aldosterone Secretion on Steroidogenic Acute Regulatory Phosphorylation. *Mol Cell Endocrinol* (2001) 173(1-2):87–94. doi: 10.1016/s0303-7207(00)00411-1
75. Yamazaki T, Kawasaki H, Takamasa A, Yoshitomi T, Kominami S. Ca2+ Signal Stimulates the Expression of Steroidogenic Acute Regulatory Protein and Steroidogenesis in Bovine Adrenal Fasciculata-Reticularis Cells. *Life Sci* (2006) 78(25):2923–30. doi: 10.1016/j.lfs.2005.11.019
76. Sanderson JT, Boerma J, Lansbergen GW, van den Berg M. Induction and Inhibition of Aromatase (CYP19) Activity by Various Classes of Pesticides in H295R Human Adrenocortical Carcinoma Cells. *Toxicol Appl Pharmacol* (2002) 182(1):44–54. doi: 10.1006/taap.2002.9420
77. Roberge M, Hakk H, Larsen G. Atrazine is a Competitive Inhibitor of Phosphodiesterase But Does Not Affect the Estrogen Receptor. *Toxicol Lett* (2004) 154(1-2):61–8. doi: 10.1016/j.toxlet.2004.07.005
78. Roberge MT, Hakk H, Larsen G. Cytosolic and Localized Inhibition of Phosphodiesterase by Atrazine in Swine Tissue Homogenates. *Food Chem Toxicol* (2006) 44(6):885–90. doi: 10.1016/j.fct.2005.11.014
79. Kucka M, Pogrmic-Majkic K, Fa S, Stojilkovic SS, Kovacevic R. Atrazine Acts as an Endocrine Disrupter by Inhibiting cAMP-specific Phosphodiesterase-4. *Toxicol Appl Pharmacol* (2012) 265(1):19–26. doi: 10.1016/j.taap.2012.09.019
80. Karmaus AL, Zacharewski TR. Atrazine-Mediated Disruption of Steroidogenesis in BLTK1 Murine Leydig Cells. *Toxicol Sci* (2015) 148 (2):544–54. doi: 10.1093/toxsci/kfv204
81. Tsai LC, Beavo JA. The Roles of Cyclic Nucleotide Phosphodiesterases (Pdes) in Steroidogenesis. *Curr Opin Pharmacol* (2011) 11(6):670–5. doi: 10.1016/j.coph.2011.09.003
82. Kitaoka K, Kawata S, Yoshida T, Kadoriku F, Kitamura M. Exposure to an Extremely-Low-Frequency Magnetic Field Stimulates Adrenal Steroidogenesis *Via* Inhibition of Phosphodiesterase Activity in a Mouse Adrenal Cell Line. *PloS One* (2016) 11(4):e0154167. doi: 10.1371/journal.pone.0154167
83. Szarek E, Stratakis CA. Phosphodiesterases and Adrenal Cushing in Mice and Humans. *Horm Metab Res* (2014) 46(12):863–8. doi: 10.1055/s-0034-1389916
84. Tao QH, Tang HX. Effect of Dye Compounds on the Adsorption of Atrazine by Natural Sediment. *Chemosphere* (2004) 56(1):31–8. doi: 10.1016/j.chemosphere.2004.02.029
85. Williams MM, Boydston RA, Peachey RE, Robinson D. Performance Consistency of Reduced Atrazine Use in Sweet Corn. *Field Crops Res* (2011) 121(1):96–104. doi: 10.1016/j.fcr.2010.11.020
86. Wu M, Quirindongo M, Sass J, Wetzler ACouncil NRD. (2010).
87. EPA. *Atrazine Monitoring Program Data and Results: United States Environmental Protection Agency* (2017). Available at: https://www.epa.gov/ingredients-used-pesticide-products/atrazine-monitoring-program-data-and-results.
88. Saito EAgency USEP. *Atrazine Registration Standard and Applied Experiment.* Washington D.C: EPA (1989).
89. Wiegand C, Krause E, Steinberg C, Pflugmacher S. Toxicokinetics of Atrazine in Embryos of the Zebrafish (Danio Rerio). *Ecotoxicol Environ Saf* (2001) 49 (3):199–205. doi: 10.1006/eesa.2001.2073
90. Chan YC, Chang SC, Hsuan SL, Chien MS, Lee WC, Kang JJ, et al. Cardiovascular Effects of Herbicides and Formulated Adjuvants on Isolated Rat Aorta and Heart. *Toxicol In Vitro* (2007) 21(4):595–603. doi: 10.1016/j.tiv.2006.12.007
91. Rajkovic V, Kovac R, Koledin I, Matavulj M. Atrazine-Induced Changes in the Myocardial Structure of Peripubertal Rats. *Toxicol Ind Health* (2014) 30 (3):250–8. doi: 10.1177/0748233712456058

Permissions

All chapters in this book were first published by Frontiers; hereby published with permission under the Creative Commons Attribution License or equivalent. Every chapter published in this book has been scrutinized by our experts. Their significance has been extensively debated. The topics covered herein carry significant findings which will fuel the growth of the discipline. They may even be implemented as practical applications or may be referred to as a beginning point for another development.

The contributors of this book come from diverse backgrounds, making this book a truly international effort. This book will bring forth new frontiers with its revolutionizing research information and detailed analysis of the nascent developments around the world.

We would like to thank all the contributing authors for lending their expertise to make the book truly unique. They have played a crucial role in the development of this book. Without their invaluable contributions this book wouldn't have been possible. They have made vital efforts to compile up to date information on the varied aspects of this subject to make this book a valuable addition to the collection of many professionals and students.

This book was conceptualized with the vision of imparting up-to-date information and advanced data in this field. To ensure the same, a matchless editorial board was set up. Every individual on the board went through rigorous rounds of assessment to prove their worth. After which they invested a large part of their time researching and compiling the most relevant data for our readers.

The editorial board has been involved in producing this book since its inception. They have spent rigorous hours researching and exploring the diverse topics which have resulted in the successful publishing of this book. They have passed on their knowledge of decades through this book. To expedite this challenging task, the publisher supported the team at every step. A small team of assistant editors was also appointed to further simplify the editing procedure and attain best results for the readers.

Apart from the editorial board, the designing team has also invested a significant amount of their time in understanding the subject and creating the most relevant covers. They scrutinized every image to scout for the most suitable representation of the subject and create an appropriate cover for the book.

The publishing team has been an ardent support to the editorial, designing and production team. Their endless efforts to recruit the best for this project, has resulted in the accomplishment of this book. They are a veteran in the field of academics and their pool of knowledge is as vast as their experience in printing. Their expertise and guidance has proved useful at every step. Their uncompromising quality standards have made this book an exceptional effort. Their encouragement from time to time has been an inspiration for everyone.

The publisher and the editorial board hope that this book will prove to be a valuable piece of knowledge for researchers, students, practitioners and scholars across the globe.

List of Contributors

Rebecca Dumbell, Olga Matveeva and Henrik Oster
Chronophysiology Group, Medical Department I, University of Lübeck, Lübeck, Germany

Nicolas C. Nicolaides, Evangelia Charmandari and George P. Chrousos
Division of Endocrinology, Metabolism and Diabetes, First Department of Pediatrics, National and Kapodistrian University of Athens Medical School, 'Aghia Sophia' Children's Hospital, Athens, Greece
Division of Endocrinology and Metabolism, Center of Clinical, Experimental Surgery and Translational Research, Biomedical Research Foundation of the Academy of Athens, Athens, Greece

Tomoshige Kino
Division of Experimental Genetics, Sidra Medical and Research Center, Doha, Qatar

Chiraz Ghaddhab and Johnny Deladoëy
Endocrinology Service and Research Center, Sainte-Justine University Hospital Center, Department of Pediatrics, Université de Montréal, Montreal, QC, Canada

Jean-Marc Vuissoz
Division of Pediatric Endocrinology, University Children's Hospital Basel (UKBB), University of Basel, Basel, Switzerland

Zachary J. Maben, Sundeep Malik, Liyi H. Jiang and Patricia M. Hinkle
Department of Pharmacology and Physiology, University of Rochester Medical Center, Rochester, NY, USA

Scott J. Moeller, Rachel Yehuda and Rita Z. Goldstein
Department of Psychiatry, Icahn School of Medicine at Mount Sinai, New York, NY, USA
Department of Neuroscience, Icahn School of Medicine at Mount Sinai, New York, USA

Lizette Couto, Vanessa Cohen, Yelena Lalazar and Eliza B. Geer
Department of Medicine, Icahn School of Medicine at Mount Sinai, New York, USA
Department of Neurosurgery, Icahn School of Medicine at Mount Sinai, New York, USA

Iouri Makotkine and Nia Williams
Department of Psychiatry, Icahn School of Medicine at Mount Sinai, New York, USA

Annabel S. Berthon, Eva Szarek and Constantine A. Stratakis
Section on Endocrinology and Genetics, Program on Developmental Endocrinology and Genetics and Pediatric Endocrinology Inter-Institute Training Program, Eunice Kennedy Shriver National Institute of Child Health and Human Development, National Institutes of Health, Bethesda, MD, USA

Djillali Annane
General Intensive Care Unit, Raymond Poincaré Hospital (AP-HP), Garches, France
Laboratory of Infection and Inflammation, U1173, University of Versailles Saint-Quentin-en-Yvelines University, INSERM, Garches, France

Nasha K. Nensey, Jonathan Bodager and Hershel Raff
Department of Medicine, Medical College of Wisconsin, Milwaukee, WI, USA
Endocrine Research Laboratory, Aurora St. Luke's Medical Center, Aurora Research Institute, Milwaukee, WI, USA

Ashley L. Gehrand
Endocrine Research Laboratory, Aurora St. Luke's Medical Center, Aurora Research Institute, Milwaukee, WI, USA

Jinwoo Lee
Department of Cell and Regenerative Biology, University of Wisconsin, Madison, WI, USA
Endocrinology and Reproductive Physiology Program, University of Wisconsin, Madison, WI, USA

Tiegang Tong, Yee Hoon Foong and Ibrahim Musaitif
Department of Cell and Regenerative Biology, University of Wisconsin, Madison, WI, USA

Haichuan Duan
Molecular and Cellular Pharmacology, University of Wisconsin, Madison, WI, USA

Colin Jefcoate
Department of Cell and Regenerative Biology, University of Wisconsin, Madison, WI, USA
Endocrinology and Reproductive Physiology Program, University of Wisconsin, Madison, WI, USA
Molecular and Cellular Pharmacology, University of Wisconsin, Madison, WI, USA
Molecular and Environmental Toxicology Center, University of Wisconsin, Madison, WI, USA

Takeshi Yamazaki
Graduate School of Integrated Arts and Sciences, Hiroshima University, Higashi-Hiroshima, Japan

Xavier Bertagna
Service des Maladies Endocriniennes et Métaboliques, Centre de Référence des Maladies Rares de la Surrénale, Faculté de Médecine Paris Descartes, Université Paris 5, Hôpital Cochin, Paris, France

Felicia Leccia, Isabelle Sahut-Barnola, Pierre Val, A-Marie Lefrançois-Martinez and Antoine Martinez
UMR6293, GReD, INSERM U1103, CNRS, Clermont Université, Clermont-Ferrand, France

Marie Batisse-Lignier
UMR6293, GReD, INSERM U1103, CNRS, Clermont Université, Clermont-Ferrand, France
Endocrinology, Diabetology and Metabolic Diseases Department, Centre Hospitalier Universitaire, School of Medicine, Clermont-Ferrand, France

Khalil Khoury
Department of Pediatrics, Faculty of Medicine, University of Sherbrooke, Sherbrooke, QC, Canada

Elie Barbar, Pierre Lavigne and Jean-Guy LeHoux
Department of Biochemistry, Faculty of Medicine, University of Sherbrooke, Sherbrooke, QC, Canada

Barbara J. Clark
Department of Biochemistry and Molecular Genetics, University of Louisville, Louisville, KY, USA

Agnès Desroches-Castan, Jean-Jacques Feige and Nadia Cherradi
Institut National de la Santé et de la Recherche Médicale, INSERM U1036, Grenoble, France
Commissariat à l'Energie Atomique et aux Energies Alternatives, Institut de Biosciences et Biotechnologies de Grenoble, Laboratoire Biologie du Cancer et de l'Infection, Grenoble, France
Université Grenoble Alpes, Unité Mixte de Recherche-S1036, Grenoble, France

Stefan R. Bornstein
Department of Internal Medicine III, Technische Universität Dresden, Dresden, Germany
Department of Endocrinology and Diabetes, King's College London, London, UK

Maria Candida Barisson Villares Fragoso, Ingrid Quevedo Wanichi, Isadora Pontes Cavalcante and Beatriz Marinho de Paula Mariani
Unidade de Suprarrenal, Disciplina de Endocrinologia e Metabologia, Laboratorio de Hormonios e Genetica Molecular LIM/42, Hospital das Clinicas, Faculdade de Medicina da Universidade de Sao Paulo, Sao Paulo, Brazil

John W. Funder
Hudson Institute of Medical Research and Monash University, Clayton, VIC, Australia

Aurélia E. Lewis
Department of Molecular Biology, University of Bergen, Bergen, Norway

Reidun Aesoy and Marit Bakke
Department of Biomedicine, University of Bergen, Bergen, Norway

Michel F. Rossier
Service of Clinical Chemistry and Toxicology, Hospital of Valais, Sion, Switzerland
Department of Human Protein Science, Faculty of Medicine, University of Geneva, Geneva, Switzerland

Cheryl L. Bell and Sandra A. Murray
Department of Cell Biology, University of Pittsburgh School of Medicine, Pittsburgh, PA, USA

Youssef Ainmelk and Annie Ouellet
Department of Obstetrics and Gynecology, Faculty of Medicine, University of Sherbrooke, Sherbrooke, QC, Canada

Antonio Marcondes Lerario, Isabella Finco and Christopher LaPensee
Department of Internal Medicine, Division of Metabolism, Endocrinology, and Diabetes, University of Michigan, Ann Arbor, MI, USA

Gary Douglas Hammer
Department of Internal Medicine, Division of Metabolism, Endocrinology, and Diabetes, University of Michigan, Ann Arbor, MI, USA
Endocrine Oncology Program, Comprehensive Cancer Center, University of Michigan, Ann Arbor, MI, USA
Center for Organogenesis, University of Michigan, Ann Arbor, MI, USA

Waldemar Kanczkowski and Mariko Sue
Department of Internal Medicine III, Technische Universität Dresden, Dresden, Germany

Gerard Ruiz-Babot, Irene Hadjidemetriou, Peter James King and Leonardo Guasti
Centre for Endocrinology, William Harvey Research Institute, Barts and the London School of Medicine and Dentistry, Queen Mary University of London, London, UK

Arthur D. Zimmerman, Laci Mackay, Robert J. Kemppainen, Melaney A. Jones, Casey C. Read, Dean Schwartz and Chad D. Foradori
Department of Anatomy, Physiology and Pharmacology, College of Veterinary Medicine, Auburn University, Auburn, AL, United States

Index

www.ingramcontent.com/pod-product-compliance
Lightning Source LLC
LaVergne TN
LVHW082156200926
848484LV00008B/2169